DRUG DELIVERY TO THE LUNG

T0203640

LUNG BIOLOGY IN HEALTH AND DISEASE

Executive Editor

Claude Lenfant
Director, National Heart, Lung and Blood Institute
National Institutes of Health
Bethesda, Maryland

1. Immunologic and Infectious Reactions in the Lung, *edited by C. H. Kirkpatrick and H. Y. Reynolds*
2. The Biochemical Basis of Pulmonary Function, *edited by R. G. Crystal*
3. Bioengineering Aspects of the Lung, *edited by J. B. West*
4. Metabolic Functions of the Lung, *edited by Y. S. Bakhle and J. R. Vane*
5. Respiratory Defense Mechanisms (in two parts), *edited by J. D. Brain, D. F. Proctor, and L. M. Reid*
6. Development of the Lung, *edited by W. A. Hodson*
7. Lung Water and Solute Exchange, *edited by N. C. Staub*
8. Extrapulmonary Manifestations of Respiratory Disease, *edited by E. D. Robin*
9. Chronic Obstructive Pulmonary Disease, *edited by T. L. Petty*
10. Pathogenesis and Therapy of Lung Cancer, *edited by C. C. Harris*
11. Genetic Determinants of Pulmonary Disease, *edited by S. D. Litwin*
12. The Lung in the Transition Between Health and Disease, *edited by P. T. Macklem and S. Permutt*
13. Evolution of Respiratory Processes: A Comparative Approach, *edited by S. C. Wood and C. Lenfant*
14. Pulmonary Vascular Diseases, *edited by K. M. Moser*
15. Physiology and Pharmacology of the Airways, *edited by J. A. Nadel*
16. Diagnostic Techniques in Pulmonary Disease (in two parts), *edited by M. A. Sackner*
17. Regulation of Breathing (in two parts), *edited by T. F. Hornbein*
18. Occupational Lung Diseases: Research Approaches and Methods, *edited by H. Weill and M. Turner-Warwick*
19. Immunopharmacology of the Lung, *edited by H. H. Newball*
20. Sarcoidosis and Other Granulomatous Diseases of the Lung, *edited by B. L. Fanburg*
21. Sleep and Breathing, *edited by N. A. Saunders and C. E. Sullivan*
22. *Pneumocystis carinii* Pneumonia: Pathogenesis, Diagnosis, and Treatment, *edited by L. S. Young*
23. Pulmonary Nuclear Medicine: Techniques in Diagnosis of Lung Disease, *edited by H. L. Atkins*
24. Acute Respiratory Failure, *edited by W. M. Zapol and K. J. Falke*
25. Gas Mixing and Distribution in the Lung, *edited by L. A. Engel and M. Paiva*

26. High-Frequency Ventilation in Intensive Care and During Surgery, *edited by G. Carlon and W. S. Howland*
27. Pulmonary Development: Transition from Intrauterine to Extrauterine Life, *edited by G. H. Nelson*
28. Chronic Obstructive Pulmonary Disease: Second Edition, *edited by T. L. Petty*
29. The Thorax (in two parts), *edited by C. Roussos and P. T. Macklem*
30. The Pleura in Health and Disease, *edited by J. Chrétien, J. Bignon, and A. Hirsch*
31. Drug Therapy for Asthma: Research and Clinical Practice, *edited by J. W. Jenne and S. Murphy*
32. Pulmonary Endothelium in Health and Disease, *edited by U. S. Ryan*
33. The Airways: Neural Control in Health and Disease, *edited by M. A. Kaliner and P. J. Barnes*
34. Pathophysiology and Treatment of Inhalation Injuries, *edited by J. Loke*
35. Respiratory Function of the Upper Airway, *edited by O. P. Mathew and G. Sant'Ambrogio*
36. Chronic Obstructive Pulmonary Disease: A Behavioral Perspective, *edited by A. J. McSweeny and I. Grant*
37. Biology of Lung Cancer: Diagnosis and Treatment, *edited by S. T. Rosen, J. L. Mulshine, F. Cuttitta, and P. G. Abrams*
38. Pulmonary Vascular Physiology and Pathophysiology, *edited by E. K. Weir and J. T. Reeves*
39. Comparative Pulmonary Physiology: Current Concepts, *edited by S. C. Wood*
40. Respiratory Physiology: An Analytical Approach, *edited by H. K. Chang and M. Paiva*
41. Lung Cell Biology, *edited by D. Massaro*
42. Heart–Lung Interactions in Health and Disease, *edited by S. M. Scharf and S. S. Cassidy*
43. Clinical Epidemiology of Chronic Obstructive Pulmonary Disease, *edited by M. J. Hensley and N. A. Saunders*
44. Surgical Pathology of Lung Neoplasms, *edited by A. M. Marchevsky*
45. The Lung in Rheumatic Diseases, *edited by G. W. Cannon and G. A. Zimmerman*
46. Diagnostic Imaging of the Lung, *edited by C. E. Putman*
47. Models of Lung Disease: Microscopy and Structural Methods, *edited by J. Gil*
48. Electron Microscopy of the Lung, *edited by D. E. Schraufnagel*
49. Asthma: Its Pathology and Treatment, *edited by M. A. Kaliner, P. J. Barnes, and C. G. A. Persson*
50. Acute Respiratory Failure: Second Edition, *edited by W. M. Zapol and F. Lemaire*
51. Lung Disease in the Tropics, *edited by O. P. Sharma*
52. Exercise: Pulmonary Physiology and Pathophysiology, *edited by B. J. Whipp and K. Wasserman*
53. Developmental Neurobiology of Breathing, *edited by G. G. Haddad and J. P. Farber*
54. Mediators of Pulmonary Inflammation, *edited by M. A. Bray and W. H. Anderson*
55. The Airway Epithelium, *edited by S. G. Farmer and D. Hay*

56. Physiological Adaptations in Vertebrates: Respiration, Circulation, and Metabolism, *edited by S. C. Wood, R. E. Weber, A. R. Hargens, and R. W. Millard*
57. The Bronchial Circulation, *edited by J. Butler*
58. Lung Cancer Differentiation: Implications for Diagnosis and Treatment, *edited by S. D. Bernal and P. J. Hesketh*
59. Pulmonary Complications of Systemic Disease, *edited by J. F. Murray*
60. Lung Vascular Injury: Molecular and Cellular Response, *edited by A. Johnson and T. J. Ferro*
61. Cytokines of the Lung, *edited by J. Kelley*
62. The Mast Cell in Health and Disease, *edited by M. A. Kaliner and D. D. Metcalfe*
63. Pulmonary Disease in the Elderly Patient, *edited by D. A. Mahler*
64. Cystic Fibrosis, *edited by P. B. Davis*
65. Signal Transduction in Lung Cells, *edited by J. S. Brody, D. M. Center, and V. A. Tkachuk*
66. Tuberculosis: A Comprehensive International Approach, *edited by L. B. Reichman and E. S. Hershfield*
67. Pharmacology of the Respiratory Tract: Experimental and Clinical Research, *edited by K. F. Chung and P. J. Barnes*
68. Prevention of Respiratory Diseases, *edited by A. Hirsch, M. Goldberg, J.-P. Martin, and R. Masse*
69. *Pneumocystis carinii* Pneumonia: Second Edition, *edited by P. D. Walzer*
70. Fluid and Solute Transport in the Airspaces of the Lungs, *edited by R. M. Effros and H. K. Chang*
71. Sleep and Breathing: Second Edition, *edited by N. A. Saunders and C. E. Sullivan*
72. Airway Secretion: Physiological Bases for the Control of Mucous Hypersecretion, *edited by T. Takishima and S. Shimura*
73. Sarcoidosis and Other Granulomatous Disorders, *edited by D. G. James*
74. Epidemiology of Lung Cancer, *edited by J. M. Samet*
75. Pulmonary Embolism, *edited by M. Morpurgo*
76. Sports and Exercise Medicine, *edited by S. C. Wood and R. C. Roach*
77. Endotoxin and the Lungs, *edited by K. L. Brigham*
78. The Mesothelial Cell and Mesothelioma, *edited by M.-C. Jaurand and J. Bignon*
79. Regulation of Breathing: Second Edition, *edited by J. A. Dempsey and A. I. Pack*
80. Pulmonary Fibrosis, *edited by S. Hin. Phan and R. S. Thrall*
81. Long-Term Oxygen Therapy: Scientific Basis and Clinical Application, *edited by W. J. O'Donohue, Jr.*
82. Ventral Brainstem Mechanisms and Control of Respiration and Blood Pressure, *edited by C. O. Trouth, R. M. Millis, H. F. Kiwull-Schöne, and M. E. Schläfke*
83. A History of Breathing Physiology, *edited by D. F. Proctor*
84. Surfactant Therapy for Lung Disease, *edited by B. Robertson and H. W. Taeusch*
85. The Thorax: Second Edition, Revised and Expanded (in three parts), *edited by C. Roussos*

86. Severe Asthma: Pathogenesis and Clinical Management, *edited by S. J. Szefler and D. Y. M. Leung*
87. *Mycobacterium avium*–Complex Infection: Progress in Research and Treatment, *edited by J. A. Korvick and C. A. Benson*
88. Alpha 1–Antitrypsin Deficiency: Biology • Pathogenesis • Clinical Manifestations • Therapy, *edited by R. G. Crystal*
89. Adhesion Molecules and the Lung, *edited by P. A. Ward and J. C. Fantone*
90. Respiratory Sensation, *edited by L. Adams and A. Guz*
91. Pulmonary Rehabilitation, *edited by A. P. Fishman*
92. Acute Respiratory Failure in Chronic Obstructive Pulmonary Disease, *edited by J.-P. Derenne, W. A. Whitelaw, and T. Similowski*
93. Environmental Impact on the Airways: From Injury to Repair, *edited by J. Chrétien and D. Dusser*
94. Inhalation Aerosols: Physical and Biological Basis for Therapy, *edited by A. J. Hickey*
95. Tissue Oxygen Deprivation: From Molecular to Integrated Function, *edited by G. G. Haddad and G. Lister*
96. The Genetics of Asthma, *edited by S. B. Liggett and D. A. Meyers*
97. Inhaled Glucocorticoids in Asthma: Mechanisms and Clinical Actions, *edited by R. P. Schleimer, W. W. Busse, and P. M. O'Byrne*
98. Nitric Oxide and the Lung, *edited by W. M. Zapol and K. D. Bloch*
99. Primary Pulmonary Hypertension, *edited by L. J. Rubin and S. Rich*
100. Lung Growth and Development, *edited by J. A. McDonald*
101. Parasitic Lung Diseases, *edited by A. A. F. Mahmoud*
102. Lung Macrophages and Dendritic Cells in Health and Disease, *edited by M. F. Lipscomb and S. W. Russell*
103. Pulmonary and Cardiac Imaging, *edited by C. Chiles and C. E. Putman*
104. Gene Therapy for Diseases of the Lung, *edited by K. L. Brigham*
105. Oxygen, Gene Expression, and Cellular Function, *edited by L. Biadasz Clerch and D. J. Massaro*
106. Beta$_2$-Agonists in Asthma Treatment, *edited by R. Pauwels and P. M. O'Byrne*
107. Inhalation Delivery of Therapeutic Peptides and Proteins, *edited by A. L. Adjei and P. K. Gupta*
108. Asthma in the Elderly, *edited by R. A. Barbee and J. W. Bloom*
109. Treatment of the Hospitalized Cystic Fibrosis Patient, *edited by D. M. Orenstein and R. C. Stern*
110. Asthma and Immunological Diseases in Pregnancy and Early Infancy, *edited by M. Schatz, R. S. Zeiger, and H. N. Claman*
111. Dyspnea, *edited by D. A. Mahler*
112. Proinflammatory and Antiinflammatory Peptides, *edited by S. I. Said*
113. Self-Management of Asthma, *edited by H. Kotses and A. Harver*
114. Eicosanoids, Aspirin, and Asthma, *edited by A. Szczeklik, R. J. Gryglewski, and J. R. Vane*
115. Fatal Asthma, *edited by A. L. Sheffer*
116. Pulmonary Edema, *edited by M. A. Matthay and D. H. Ingbar*
117. Inflammatory Mechanisms in Asthma, *edited by S. T. Holgate and W. W. Busse*
118. Physiological Basis of Ventilatory Support, *edited by J. J. Marini and A. S. Slutsky*

119. Human Immunodeficiency Virus and the Lung, *edited by M. J. Rosen and J. M. Beck*
120. Five-Lipoxygenase Products in Asthma, *edited by J. M. Drazen, S.-E. Dahlén, and T. H. Lee*
121. Complexity in Structure and Function of the Lung, *edited by M. P. Hlastala and H. T. Robertson*
122. Biology of Lung Cancer, *edited by M. A. Kane and P. A. Bunn, Jr.*
123. Rhinitis: Mechanisms and Management, *edited by R. M. Naclerio, S. R. Durham, and N. Mygind*
124. Lung Tumors: Fundamental Biology and Clinical Management, *edited by C. Brambilla and E. Brambilla*
125. Interleukin-5: From Molecule to Drug Target for Asthma, *edited by C. J. Sanderson*
126. Pediatric Asthma, *edited by S. Murphy and H. W. Kelly*
127. Viral Infections of the Respiratory Tract, *edited by R. Dolin and P. F. Wright*
128. Air Pollutants and the Respiratory Tract, *edited by D. L. Swift and W. M. Foster*
129. Gastroesophageal Reflux Disease and Airway Disease, *edited by M. R. Stein*
130. Exercise-Induced Asthma, *edited by E. R. McFadden, Jr.*
131. LAM and Other Diseases Characterized by Smooth Muscle Proliferation, *edited by J. Moss*
132. The Lung at Depth, *edited by C. E. G. Lundgren and J. N. Miller*
133. Regulation of Sleep and Circadian Rhythms, *edited by F. W. Turek and P. C. Zee*
134. Anticholinergic Agents in the Upper and Lower Airways, *edited by S. L. Spector*
135. Control of Breathing in Health and Disease, *edited by M. D. Altose and Y. Kawakami*
136. Immunotherapy in Asthma, *edited by J. Bousquet and H. Yssel*
137. Chronic Lung Disease in Early Infancy, *edited by R. D. Bland and J. J. Coalson*
138. Asthma's Impact on Society: The Social and Economic Burden, *edited by K. B. Weiss, A. S. Buist, and S. D. Sullivan*
139. New and Exploratory Therapeutic Agents for Asthma, *edited by M. Yeadon and Z. Diamant*
140. Multimodality Treatment of Lung Cancer, *edited by A. T. Skarin*
141. Cytokines in Pulmonary Disease: Infection and Inflammation, *edited by S. Nelson and T. R. Martin*
142. Diagnostic Pulmonary Pathology, *edited by P. T. Cagle*
143. Particle–Lung Interactions, *edited by P. Gehr and J. Heyder*
144. Tuberculosis: A Comprehensive International Approach, Second Edition, Revised and Expanded, *edited by L. B. Reichman and E. S. Hershfield*
145. Combination Therapy for Asthma and Chronic Obstructive Pulmonary Disease, *edited by R. J. Martin and M. Kraft*
146. Sleep Apnea: Implications in Cardiovascular and Cerebrovascular Disease, *edited by T. D. Bradley and J. S. Floras*
147. Sleep and Breathing in Children: A Developmental Approach, *edited by G. M. Loughlin, J. L. Carroll, and C. L. Marcus*

148. Pulmonary and Peripheral Gas Exchange in Health and Disease, *edited by J. Roca, R. Rodriguez-Roisen, and P. D. Wagner*
149. Lung Surfactants: Basic Science and Clinical Applications, *R. H. Notter*
150. Nosocomial Pneumonia, *edited by W. R. Jarvis*
151. Fetal Origins of Cardiovascular and Lung Disease, *edited by David J. P. Barker*
152. Long-Term Mechanical Ventilation, *edited by N. S. Hill*
153. Environmental Asthma, *edited by R. K. Bush*
154. Asthma and Respiratory Infections, *edited by D. P. Skoner*
155. Airway Remodeling, *edited by P. H. Howarth, J. W. Wilson, J. Bousquet, S. Rak, and R. A. Pauwels*
156. Genetic Models in Cardiorespiratory Biology, *edited by G. G. Haddad and T. Xu*
157. Respiratory-Circulatory Interactions in Health and Disease, *edited by S. M. Scharf, M. R. Pinsky, and S. Magder*
158. Ventilator Management Strategies for Critical Care, *edited by N. S. Hill and M. M. Levy*
159. Severe Asthma: Pathogenesis and Clinical Management, Second Edition, Revised and Expanded, *edited by S. J. Szefler and D. Y. M. Leung*
160. Gravity and the Lung: Lessons from Microgravity, *edited by G. K. Prisk, M. Paiva, and J. B. West*
161. High Altitude: An Exploration of Human Adaptation, *edited by T. F. Hornbein and R. B. Schoene*
162. Drug Delivery to the Lung, *edited by H. Bisgaard, C. O'Callaghan, and G. C. Smaldone*

ADDITIONAL VOLUMES IN PREPARATION

IgE and Anti-IgE in Asthma and Allergic Disease, *edited by R. B. Fick, Jr., and P. M. Jardieu*

Inhaled Steroids in Asthma: Optimizing Effects in the Airways, *edited by R. P. Schleimer, P. M. O'Byrne, S. J. Szefler, and R. Brattsand*

Clinical Management of Chronic Obstructive Pulmonary Disease, *edited by T. Similowski, W. A. Whitelaw, and J.-P. Derenne*

The opinions expressed in these volumes do not necessarily represent the views of the National Institutes of Health.

DRUG DELIVERY TO THE LUNG

Edited by

Hans Bisgaard

Copenhagen University Hospital, Rigshospitalet
Copenhagen, Denmark

Chris O'Callaghan

University of Leicester
Leicester, England

Gerald C. Smaldone

State University of New York
Stony Brook, New York

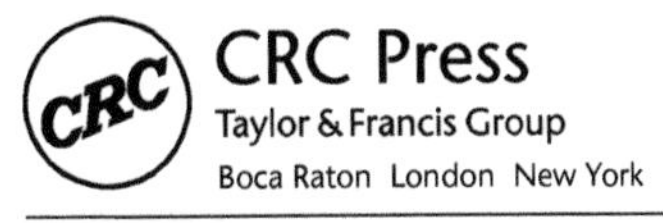

CRC Press is an imprint of the
Taylor & Francis Group, an **informa** business

CRC Press
Taylor & Francis Group
6000 Broken Sound Parkway NW, Suite 300
Boca Raton, FL 33487-2742

First issued in paperback 2019

© 2010 by Taylor & Francis Group, LLC
CRC Press is an imprint of Taylor & Francis Group, an Informa business

No claim to original U.S. Government works

ISBN-13: 978-0-8247-0541-1 (hbk)
ISBN-13: 978-0-367-39687-9 (pbk)

This book contains information obtained from authentic and highly regarded sources. While all reasonable efforts have been made to publish reliable data and information, neither the author[s] nor the publisher can accept any legal responsibility or liability for any errors or omissions that may be made. The publishers wish to make clear that any views or opinions expressed in this book by individual editors, authors or contributors are personal to them and do not necessarily reflect the views/opinions of the publishers. The information or guidance contained in this book is intended for use by medical, scientific or healthcare professionals and is provided strictly as a supplement to the medical or other professional's own judgement, their knowledge of the patient's medical history, relevant manufacturer's instructions and the appropriate best practice guidelines. Because of the rapid advances in medical science, any information or advice on dosages, procedures or diagnoses should be independently verified. The reader is strongly urged to consult the relevant national drug formulary and the drug companies' and device or material manufacturers' printed instructions, and their websites, before administering or utilizing any of the drugs, devices or materials mentioned in this book. This book does not indicate whether a particular treatment is appropriate or suitable for a particular individual. Ultimately it is the sole responsibility of the medical professional to make his or her own professional judgements, so as to advise and treat patients appropriately. The authors and publishers have also attempted to trace the copyright holders of all material reproduced in this publication and apologize to copyright holders if permission to publish in this form has not been obtained. If any copyright material has not been acknowledged please write and let us know so we may rectify in any future reprint.

Except as permitted under U.S. Copyright Law, no part of this book may be reprinted, reproduced, transmitted, or utilized in any form by any electronic, mechanical, or other means, now known or hereafter invented, including photocopying, microfilming, and recording, or in any information storage or retrieval system, without written permission from the publishers.

For permission to photocopy or use material electronically from this work, please access www.copyright.com (http://www.copyright.com/) or contact the Copyright Clearance Center, Inc. (CCC), 222 Rosewood Drive, Danvers, MA19023,978-750-8400. CCC is a not-for-profit organization that provides licenses and registration for a variety of users. For organizations that have been granted a photocopy license by the CCC, a separate system of payment has been arranged.

Trademark Notice: Product or corporate names may be trademarks or registered trademarks, and are used only for identification and explanation without intent to infringe.

A CIP record for this book is available from the British Library.

Library of Congress Cataloging-in-Publication Data available on application

Visit the Taylor & Francis Web
http://www.taylorandfrancis.com

and the CRC Press Web site at
http://www.crcpress.com

INTRODUCTION

As pointed out in the first chapter of this volume, inhalation therapy is not new! Granted, the drugs delivered to the lungs by this method, the propellants, and the methods themselves are undoubtedly new and constantly improving, but let's admit it: the basic principles were established a thousand years ago.

Asthma is certainly one of the diseases, if not the disease, that has benefited most from this therapeutic approach.

In the nineteenth century, one of the "Renaissance men" in the field of asthma therapy was Henry Hyde Salter, a Fellow of the Royal College of Physicians and a physician at Charing Cross Hospital. He was a strong advocate of inhalation therapy but, at least by today's standards, his remedies were horrifying. Indeed, one was tobacco!

That may be hard to believe, but just read the following: "For tobacco to cure asthma, as a depressant, it must produce collapse; as a sedative it merely produces that confusing and tranquilizing condition with which smokers are so familiar." And the story goes on, stating that even children may be cured with tobacco, but "in carefully measured quantities."

In his book *On Asthma: Its Pathology and Treatment*, Salter suggests many other remedies for the treatment of asthma.

The point of all this is that inhalation therapy has long been recognized as a treatment (not cure) of asthma. Of course, today we use pharmacological agents that are certainly more effective. Asthma is a disease that can be controlled, undoubtedly because of the inhalation administration of the many available drugs.

Since its beginning, the Lung Biology in Health and Disease series of monographs has recognized the importance of asthma and, at the same time, of finding better ways to administer medications for this disease and other conditions as well. This has led to the publication of many volumes on inhalation therapy, covering the methodology and the choice of medications as well.

Drug Delivery to the Lung is a different and timely addition to the series. As the editors point out in their preface, it is "aimed at clinicians, nurses, and respiratory therapists interested in the role of aerosol delivery for optimal management of lung disease." The beneficiaries of this interest will unquestionably be the patients.

I am grateful to the editors and the authors for this major contribution to the series. The series gains immeasurably from the opportunity to present this volume to its readership.

Claude Lenfant, M.D.
Bathesda, Maryland

PREFACE

Aerosolized delivery of drugs to the lungs has dramatically improved the treatment of a variety of respiratory diseases. For example, bronchodilator and anti-inflammatory aerosol medications are the cornerstone of asthma treatment; antibiotics, DNase, and hypertonic saline are established treatment options in cystic fibrosis; and nebulized adrenaline and steroids have been used to treat croup. There is great interest in using the lungs as a portal of entry for systemic drug therapy. Measles vaccination has been successfully administered via the inhaled route and the possibility of diabetics inhaling as opposed to injecting insulin is becoming a reality.

Aerosol drug delivery allows treatment to be targeted to the lower airways and total systemic exposure to be reduced. The device chosen has a major impact on aerosol delivery, and it should be considered an integral part of any prescription or drug approval. To date, this is rarely reflected in treatment guidelines for conditions such as asthma and cystic fibrosis, nor in day-to-day clinical practice or drug labeling. Inconsistent terminology, variations in study methodology and design, and the absence of guidelines have all led to confusion among practitioners.

Device development and documentation are driven by many different needs. For patients, important factors include device size, simplicity, irritants, taste and odors, and interactive features. Such factors impact on compliance, which is the main hindrance for effectiveness of aerosol treatment. The needs of the patient change significantly with age. On the other hand, clinicians require knowledge of the fraction of drug likely to reach the lungs when different delivery devices are used for patients of different ages. Finally, health regulators tend to emphasize only in vitro reproducibility. The choice of drug defines the need for accurate estimation of drug delivery; for example, less accurate dosing of β_2-agonists is acceptable due to their wide therapeutic index. Steroids and insulin, with narrower therapeutic indices, require more accurate drug delivery. Impact on the environment is an important concern, and risk of exposure of caregivers should be considered. Efficient devices may be a priority since they reduce the loss of drug, which improves safety of treatment as well as cost effectiveness. Such a multitude of needs determines the development, documentation, and, eventually, choice of device.

Aerosol treatment is maturing technically with recent advances in the understanding of lung dose and major innovations in device technology. If the important knowledge gained within this area is to have an impact on the management of our patients, it is mandatory that aerosol standards and principles be clearly communicated to the health professional. With this aim, a group of leading experts joined together to develop a milestone publication on the state-of-the-art knowledge in the area of aerosol treatment. This volume has compiled their very comprehensive knowledge into an easily readable text with an emphasis on clinical implications.

This book is intended for clinicians, nurses, and respiratory therapists interested in the role of aerosol delivery for optimal management of lung diseases. The content was inspired by a debate between the authors, with the editors serving as referees. This process was fertilized by a workshop in the spring of 1999, which defined the general principles and emphasized clinical relevance to the practitioner. The practical implications of the issues communicated have been strongly emphasized. Therefore, we hope this book will act as a bridge between basic aerosol science and good clinical practice in the treatment of lung diseases.

This meeting and the resulting book have been made possible through an educational grant from AstraZeneca. We wish to express our gratitude to the editor of this series, Dr. Claude Lenfant, for his interest and support.

Hans Bisgaard
Chris O'Callaghan
Gerald C. Smaldone

CONTRIBUTORS

Jacob Anhøj, M.D. Department of Pediatrics, Copenhagen University Hospital, Rigshospitalet, Copenhagen, Denmark

Hans Bisgaard, M.D., Ph.D. Professor of Pediatrics, Copenhagen University Hospital, Rigshospitalet, Copenhagen, Denmark

Lars Borgström, Ph.D. Senior Experimental Medicine Advisor, AstraZeneca R&D, Lund, and Uppsala University, Uppsala, Sweden

Andy Clark, Ph.D. Inhale Therapeutics Systems, San Carlos, California

John H. Dennis, Ph.D., M.Sc., B.Scl, M.B.I.O.H., Dip Occ Hyg. Senior Lecturer, Department of Environmental Science, University of Bradford, Bradford, West Yorkshire, England

Eric Derom, M.D., Ph.D. Professor, Department of Respiratory Diseases, Ghent University Hospital, Ghent, Belgium

Myrna B. Dolovich, P.Eng. Associate Clinical Professor, Department of Medicine, McMaster University, Hamilton, Ontario, Canada

Mark L. Everard, M.B., Ch.B., F.R.C.P.C.H., D.M. Department of Respiratory Medicine, Sheffield Children's Hospital, Sheffield, England

Joachim Heyder, Ph.D. Professor and Director, Institute for Inhalation Biology, GSF–National Research Center for Environment and Health, Munich, Germany

Alison A. Hislop, Ph.D. Reader, Developmental Vascular Biology, Institute of Child Health, University College, London, England

Michael E. Hyland, Ph.D. Professor of Health Psychology, University of Plymouth, Plymouth, England

Beth L. Laube, Ph.D. Associate Professor, Department of Pediatrics, Johns Hopkins University School of Medicine, Baltimore, Maryland

Peter N. LeSouef, M.D., M.R.C.P.(UK), F.R.A.C.P. Professor and Head, Department of Paediatrics, University of Western Australia, Perth, Australia

Ola Nerbrink, Lic. Eng., Ph.D. (MD) Associate Principal Scientist, AstraZeneca R&D, Lund, Sweden

Chris O'Callaghan, B.Med.Sci., B.M., B.S., F.R.C.P., F.R.C.P.C.H., Ph.D., D.M. Professor of Paediatrics, Department of Child Health, and Institute of Lung Health, University of Leicester, Leicester, England

Martyn R. Partridge, M.D., F.R.C.P. Chest Clinic, Whipps Cross University Hospital, London, England

Søren Pedersen, M.D., Ph.D. Professor, University of Southern Denmark, Odense, Denmark, and Adjunct Professor, McMaster University, Hamilton, Ontario, Canada

Cynthia S. Rand, Ph.D. Associate Professor, Department of Medicine, The Johns Hopkins School of Medicine, Baltimore, Maryland

Gerald C. Smaldone, M.D., Ph.D. Professor of Medicine, Physiology, and Biophysics, and Chief, Pulmonary/Critical Care Division, Department of Medicine, State University of New York, Stony Brook, New York

Janet Stocks, Ph.D. Professor of Respiratory Medicine, Portex Unit, Institute of Child Health, University College, London, England

Magnus U. Svartengren, M.D., Ph.D. Associate Professor, Department of Public Health Sciences, Karolinska Institutet, Stockholm, Sweden

Lars Thorsson, Ph.D. Experimental Medicine, AstraZeneca R&D, Lund, Sweden

Mika T. Vidgren, Ph.D. Professor, Department of Pharmaceutics, University of Kuopio, Kuopio, Finland

Johannes H. Wildhaber, M.D., Ph.D. Department of Respiratory Medicine, University Children's Hospital, Zurich, Switzerland

Ashley A. Woodcock, B.Sc., M.D., F.R.C.P. Professor of Respiratory Medicine, North West Lung Centre, Wythenshawe Hospital, Manchester, England

Paul Wright AstraZeneca R&D, Charnwood, Loughborough, England

Pieter Zanen, M.D., Ph.D. Department of Pulmonary Diseases, Heart Lung Centre Utrecht, Utrecht, The Netherlands

CONTENTS

1

The History of Inhaled Drug Therapy

CHRIS O'CALLAGHAN

University of Leicester
Leicester, England

OLA NERBRINK

AstraZeneca R&D
Lund, Sweden

MIKA T. VIDGREN

University of Kuopio
Kuopio, Finland

I. Introduction

The treatment of respiratory disorders such as bronchial asthma has varied greatly. Therapies have included hot and cold compresses or baths, concentrated showers to the back of the head, as well as dried fox lungs, owl blood in wine, and chicken soup (1). In this chapter we outline the history of inhaled medications in the treatment of respiratory disease.

II. Smokes and Vapors

Inhalation therapy was first described in Ayurvedic medicine more than 4000 years ago (2). The leaves of the *Atropa belladonna* plant, containing atropine, were smoked in diseases of the throat and chest (3). Often a paste consisting of *Datura* species was dried and fixed into a pipe. The length of the pipe controlled the strength of the inhalant. The Hindu physician Charaka advised the use of spices, gum resins, and fragrant wood that were ground into powder and made into a paste. The paste was then smeared over thin tubes or sticks and lighted. The smoke was inhaled to treat diseases of the throat and chest (3). A number of other ancient cultures recommended inhalation of a variety of substances for medicinal purposes. The ancient Greeks sent consumptive patients to the pine forests of Libya (3) to benefit from volatile gases released there. Ancient Egyptians inhaled vapors released when plants of *Hyosycamus muticus* were placed on hot bricks (4). Even Hippocrates supported the use of hot vapors for inhalation purposes (5).

More recently, in 1664, Bennet (3) employed inhalation therapy for the treatment of tuberculosis. In 1810, Laennec (3) used vapors released from a variety of sources including aromatic plants, balsams, and sulfur for the treatment of chest infections. In 1802, the Indian use of *Datura* was introduced into the United Kingdom (6). It was initially smoked in a pipe alone or in a mixture with tobacco. At the same time, *Datura stramonium* was substituted by *Datura ferox* for relief of the paroxysms of asthma. Later the *Datura*-tobacco mixture found its way to the cigarette (Fig. 1). Best known were Potter's asthma cigarettes, which contained shredded *D. stramonium* leaves (7). Since smoke is by definition a two-phase system where solid particles are mixed with a gas phase, cigarette smoke can be considered as a colloidal dry-powder aerosol system. The clinical effects of Potter's asthma cigarettes were studied by Elliot and Reid (8) in the randomized crossover study, which illustrated that smoking Potter's

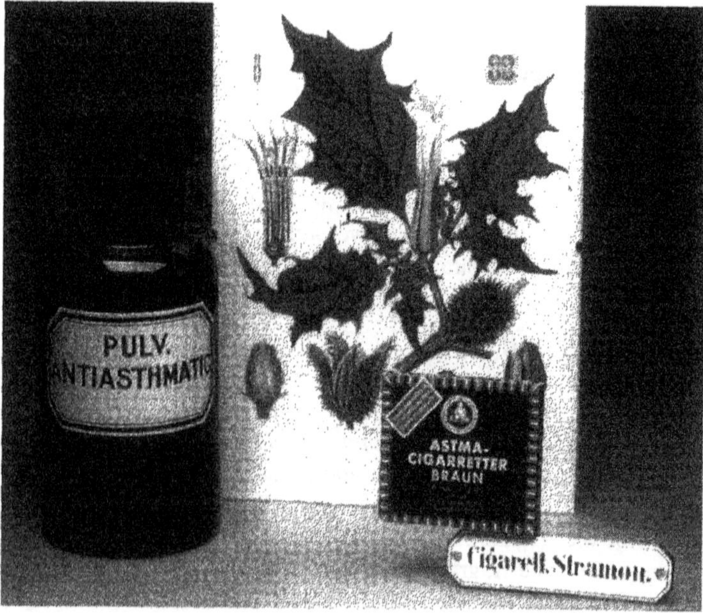

Figure 1 Asthma cigarettes containing shredded stramonium leaves.

asthma cigarettes caused a bronchodilator effect analogous to that seen with the inhalation of ipratropium by aerosol.

III. Inhalation of Droplets: The Early Nebulizers

Until the beginning of the nineteenth century, all inhalation therapy had relied on the use of vapors. In the late 1820s the inhalation of liquid droplets was developed and the use of nebulizers in inhalational therapy became established (3,9,10). In 1829, Schneider and Walz (10) constructed the first apparatus that could break liquid up into droplets. Later, Auphan constructed an "inhalatorium," where liquid in the form of mineral water was thrown against the walls of a room to form water droplets. In 1860 Sales-Girons presented a portable device (Fig. 2) constructed by Charrières. From this time an increasing number of devices were described and the inhalation of liquid droplets for inhalation therapy became more popular. The devices were often referred to as an apparatus for the "pulverization of liquids." Almost simultaneously, steam-driven devices such as the Seeger steam apparatus (11) were developed. Later on, compressed oxygen was also used to drive the atomization process. In 1872, the term *nebulizer* was defined in the Oxford dictionary.

There are many similarities between these early devices and modern nebulizers. Many of the devices had a detached "drug" container. Liquid was sucked

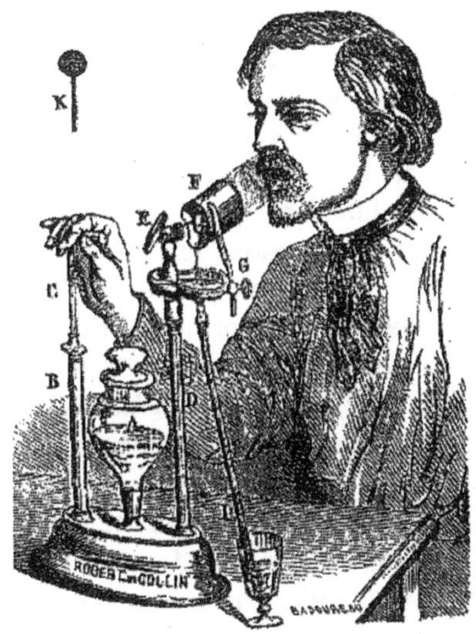

Figure 2 The Sales-Girons portable device from 1860. (From Ref. 12.)

to the atomization point by the negative pressure generated by steam or oxygen, under pressure, suddenly expanding at the exit nozzle. Baffle systems were not incorporated into the early nebulizer. Looking back, we would now define such early devices as atomizers. Today, nebulizers are regarded as atomizers that incorporate a baffle system to select out smaller particles for inhalation. This "modern" type of nebulizer appeared in the early twentieth century.

The inhalation of nebulized aerosols was advertised as beneficial for many ailments. The Sales-Girons device was advised for pharyngitis, laryngitis, bronchitis, pain, catarrh, asthma. tuberculosis, and sleeplessness (12). The liquids and substances inhaled varied widely and included mineral water containing sulfur, iodine, and chlorine; sedatives; antiseptics; and belladonna. In 1882, Yeo (3) prescribed the use of a mixture of creosote, carbolic acid, eucalyptus, or turpentine with equal parts of spirit and chloroform in his oronasal inhaler. The Yeo inhaler, which is poorly described, is probably more of a vaporizer than an early nebulizer. Earlier, in 1878, Lee (3) performed antiseptic experiments using a jet of steam containing a mixture of phenol and water. Iodoform, iodine, thymol, and terebene were also used (3).

Aerosols were advocated for other uses. In 1870, Sir Joseph Lister, professor of clinical surgery at Kings College, presented a method for the sterilization of the air during surgery (13). It consisted of a nebulizer apparatus called the Lister steam spray (Fig. 3). The nebulizer produced a steam containing carbolic acid by sucking the carbolic acid/water mixture, contained in a separate vessel, to the atomization point, with the aid of the expanding steam. The method was used to sterilize the air and to create an atmosphere where the surgical instruments could be kept without the danger of contamination. According to Pennington (13), the spray was also used when changing dressings. Less than 10 years after its introduction, it was questioned by von Bruns (14). Criticism of this method grew and Lister abandoned the technique in 1887. In his paper of 1890 (15), he commented, "I feel ashamed that I should have ever recommended it for the purpose of destroying the microbes of the air."

The question of whether aerosols, or "pulverised liquids," reached the lungs was debated intensively; that they did was not widely accepted until 1862, when Poggiale presented his report to the Paris Medical Academy (16). This triggered further investigations into the inhalation and deposition of aerosolized liquids in the airways. In 1872, Waldenbourg (17) conducted and presented several studies on the bronchial deposition of pulverized liquids. He concluded that approximately 25% of the dose was deposited in the mouth and larynx and approximately 30% passed beyond the larynx. Accordingly, he recognized that bronchial deposition depended on the physical characteristics of the patient, such as the position of the tongue in the mouth and the inspiratory volume, in addition to the patient's pathological conditions. As a conclusion, he even recommended gargling after the treatment. Heubner's (18) experi-

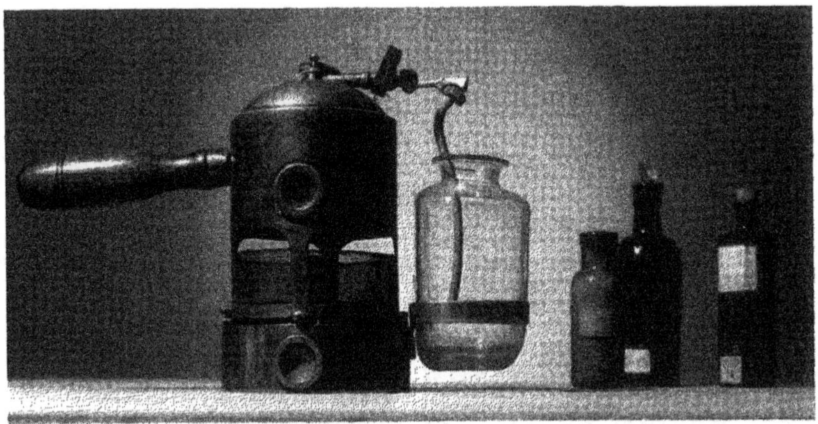

Figure 3 The Lister steam spray of 1870. (From Ref. 59.)

ments, reported in 1923, helped to convince others that aerosolized liquids reached the lungs.

Multiple large nebulizers with substantial output capabilities were used together as a collective inhalation chamber in the coal mines in South Africa and Germany in the 1930s (18). The nebulizer used was an 8- or 16-nozzle device placed in a cabinet in a corridor (Fig. 4). The corridor could be several hundred meters long and could contain a number of nebulizer cabinets (Fig. 5). The nebulizer was filled with what was considered to be a mucolytic and bronchodilating solution. At the end of the miners' shift, nebulization was commenced, and the miners walked slowly through the mist-containing corridor, inhaling the aerosol. A further example of collective inhalation was found in Germany (J. Heyder, personal communication). A large aerosol generator was located in a hallway of about 100 m long with piles of branches at the side. Salt solutions were allowed to drip onto the branches. Each time a falling drop struck a branch, smaller droplets were generated. Patients walked in the hallway inhaling the particles. This was considered a simple and efficient way to produce large volumes of therapeutic aerosols for inhalation.

The development and use of adrenaline in the treatment of asthma was a major advance. In 1900, Solis-Cohen (19) injected crude adrenal extract into patients with asthma and hay fever. Shortly afterwards, Bullowa and Kaplan (20) reported the successful use of adrenaline injection. This became established as a standard therapy for relief of severe attacks of asthma. By 1911 a nasal spray containing adrenaline was in use for asthma and as a decongestant for hay fever and rhinitis.

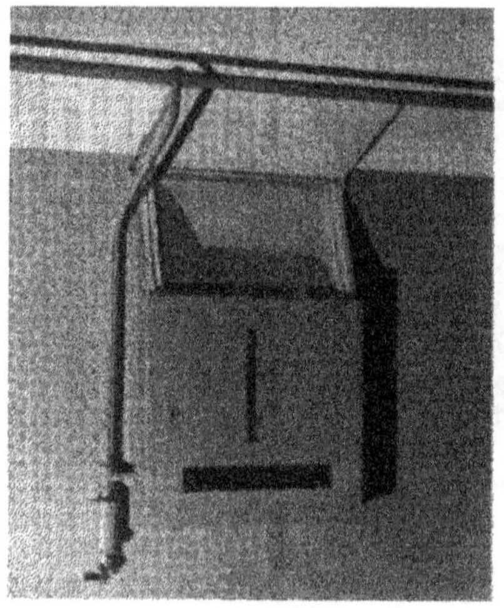
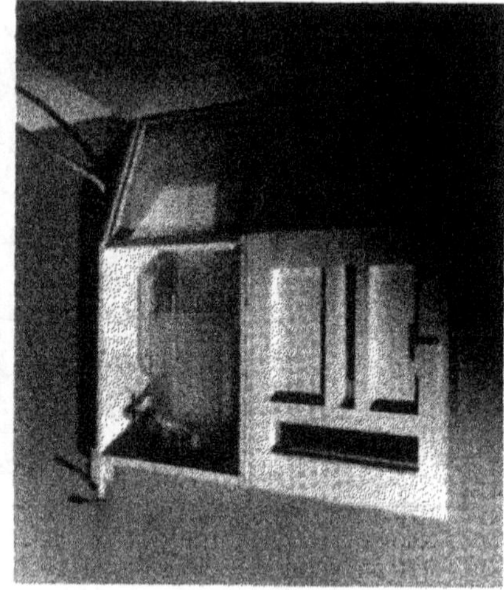

Figure 4 Collective inhalation device used in Germany and South Africa (1930). A 16-nozzle nebulizer is fitted in a wall-mounted cabinet. (From Ref. 18.)

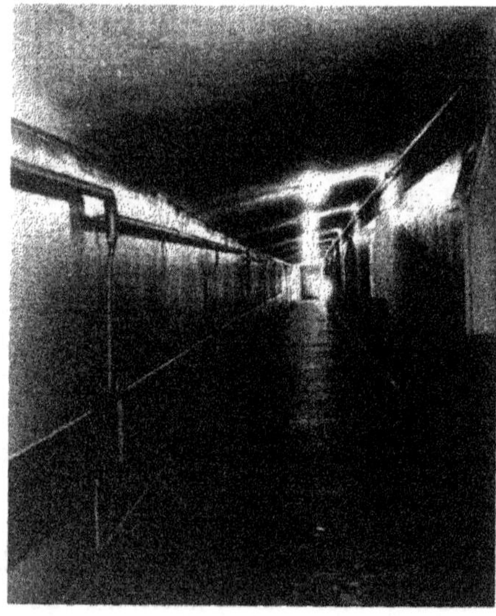

Figure 5 Collective inhalation device; the exposure corridor. (From Ref. 18.)

In 1911, Zeulzer (21) described the use of Glycerinan, a mixture of Epirenan, an adrenaline analogue, in water and glycerine. It was given via a Draeger nebulizer (constructed by Professor Spiess) to patients with chronic bronchitis, chronic laryngitis, croup-related pneumonia, interstitial pneumonia, and tuberculosis. The nebulizer used compressed air or compressed oxygen and was operated at 5 or 12 L/min. The first report of adrenaline being administered by an inhaler in the United Kingdom came from Guy's Hospital when it was used in the nebulized form in 1929 (22).

The Draeger or Hirth apparatus (22) and also a nebulizer called Apneu (23) became popular. Bulb nebulizers, where the patient operated the device by pressing a rubber bulb connected to the nebulizer to generate the gas flow, became popular (23). These nebulizers generated an aerosol with a wide droplet-size distribution and a large fraction of nonrespirable droplets. In the 1930s, glass-bulb nebulizers such as the DeVilbiss No. 40 and equivalent (Fig. 6) and the Vaponephrine nebulizers (Fig. 7) were popular. The Vaponephrine nebulizer was one of the first with a baffle close to the generation point. Not surprisingly, subsequent investigations showed that the DeVilbiss device produced larger droplets than the Vaponephrine device (24).

In 1946, electrical pumps providing a continuous flow of air were advocated. The Collison nebulizer (25), made of ebonite with a plate baffle to fil-

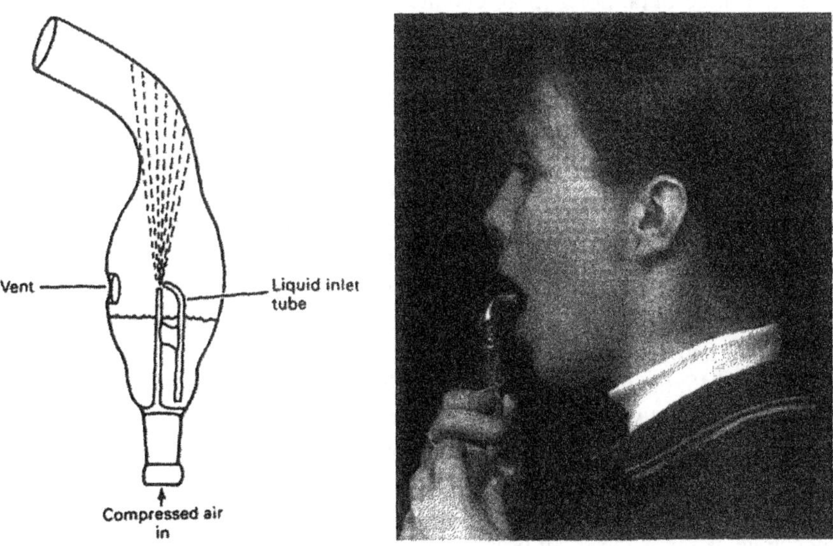

Figure 6 The Dyspne-Inhal. Laboratoire Du Dyspne-Inhal, Clermont-Ferrand, France, a copy of the DeVilbiss 40 nebulizer. (Courtesy of Kurt Nikander, AstraZeneca.)

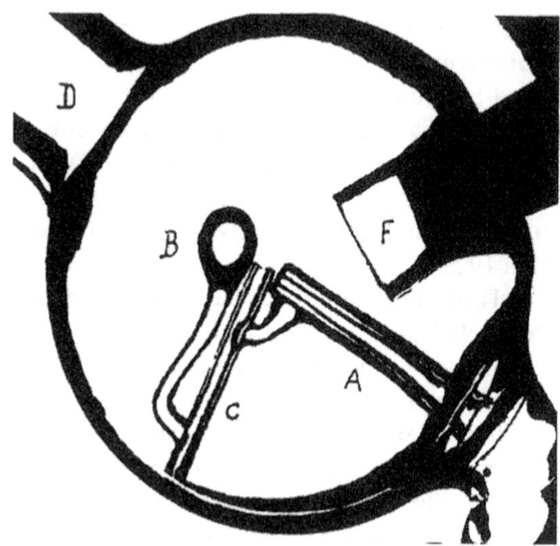

Figure 7 The Vaponephrine device with baffle (B). This was a blown-glass construction.

ter out large drug particles, became the most popular nebulizer in the United Kingdom. The Collison had one serious defect: the liquid was fed into the spray through three blind holes in an ebonite spray unit. Since most liquids used in nebulizers tended to form a deposit, these holes invariably became blocked and were difficult to clean. The glass spray-type of nebulizer had two serious defects. First, the sprays varied a good deal in their efficacy because they were "hand made." Second, the feed pipe of the spray was liable to become blocked after a period of use and attempts to clear it were often associated with breakage. In 1958, Wright (26), working in the pneumoconiosis research unit of the Medical Research Council, designed a nebulizer bearing his name, which was robust and easy to clean. It was entirely made of Perspex. In addition to being practically unbreakable and easy to clean, one of the criteria used as an indicator of good performance, was the ability of the nebulizer to produce droplets ranging in size between 1 and 6 μm in diameter at a given gas flow.

In 1945, the introduction of penicillin was followed swiftly by attempts to nebulize it directly to the lungs. A device know as the Deedon inhaler (Moore Medicinal Products Ltd., Aberdeen, Scotland) was a neat, hand-held inhaler made entirely from plastic and intended for the administration of penicillin or antispasmodics. It was suggested that the fine mist of penicillin was likely to penetrate as far as the small bronchi and bronchioles. Penicillin, in 30% glycerine, placed in the reservoir was administered in 6 to 7 min by squeezing the rubber bulb at each inspiration. The makers also advertised an electric pump, at a cost of £20, which was considered expensive by the *Lancet* (27). Other compounds, such as streptomycin, were also nebulized.

The next major advance in inhalational therapy for asthma was the introduction in 1951 of isoprenaline. In 1940, Konzett of Boehringer Ingelheim found that an analogue of adrenaline, its *N*-isopropyl derivative (28), helped to relieve the bronchospasm of asthma when inhaled. Knowledge of its development became available when the U.S. State Department investigated work carried out by German chemical manufacturers during the war. The drug, named isoprenaline, produced the bronchodilating effect of adrenaline, but was relatively free from troublesome pressor activity (29). The compound was introduced into clinical use in 1951.

The first ultrasonic nebulizer was introduced in the 1960s (11). It operated by vibrating a piezoelectric crystal inducing high-frequency waves, which caused droplets to break free from the surface of a liquid. Further developments of the nebulizer are dealt with in later chapters.

IV. The Pressurized Metered-Dose Inhaler

The most important development in antiasthma drug delivery was the advent of the metered-dose inhaler in 1956, which resulted in a huge increase in the use of antiasthma therapy. Sales of pressurized metered-dose inhalers now run at approximately 500 million per year. However, the introduction of this device was not without problems. This section of the chapter covers the early use of propellants in atomization, the origin of the metered-dose inhaler, and the epidemic of asthma deaths.

The power of propellants to atomize liquids was realized in the late nineteenth century. Helbing and Pertsch (30), from Lyon, France, described a patent for improving the preparation and application of coatings and insulating materials for medical purposes. Methyl and ethyl chlorides were mixed with certain "gummy or fatty materials." The heat of the hands surrounding the vessel in which the mixture was contained immediately caused the ethyl or methyl chloride inside the vessel to evaporate. Evaporation increased the internal pressure and the solution was ejected through the orifice in a fine jet or spray. On the surface of the target, the methyl or ethyl chloride in the ejected solution evaporated rapidly, leaving the residue as a uniform coat, layer, or varnish. Helbing and Pertsch felt that their invention would be particularly useful in forming a protective coating to a wound. At the turn of the century, Gebauer (31) found that partial vaporization of a propellant liquid prior to final atomization at the spray nozzle produced a finer spray; he went on to describe the first use of a twin-orifice expansion chamber. The discovery of freon propellants—such as 11, 12, 22, and 114 in the 1930s and 1940s—made liquefied gas generators a realistic option. The first commercial systems using propellants, introduced during the 1940s, were nonmetered devices designed for spraying insecticides.

The pressurized metered-dose inhaler (pMDI) for the delivery of anti-asthma drugs originated in the U.S. cosmetic industry. George Maison, the president of Riker Laboratories, and Irvin Porush, who worked in Riker's pharmaceutical development laboratory, are credited with the development of the first pMDI (32). Experiments were conducted to formulate pressurized aerosols of isoproterenol and epinephrine, which had been dissolved in alcohol, using the freon propellants 12 and 114.

In 1954, Philip Meshburg invented and patented a metering valve, intended for use by the perfumery industry, which allowed approximately 50 μL to be dispensed (33). The Meshberg valves were attached to plastic-coated glass vials that were used elsewhere as containers for the delivery of perfume aerosols. This initial MDI was connected to a 3-in. plastic mouthpiece, probably to decrease the impact of the inhaler's 50% ethyl alcohol solution on the oropharynx (Fig. 8). This mouthpiece was the forerunner of the modern extension tubes that are used to decrease the oropharyngeal deposition of drug. Initial clinical trials were carried out by Dr. Karr of the Veterans' Administration Hospital in Long Beach, California, in 1955 (32). The first published clinical trial showing successful treatment was by Friedman in 1956 (34). In March 1956, the Medihaler-Iso and Medihaler Epi were approved and launched.

At this very early stage, the possibility of using the lung to deliver systemic medication was considered possible. Other drug formulations intended for use in an MDI were also patented. These included both nicotine and insulin. Although insulin was shown in animal experiments to cause hypoglycemia, the effect was very variable and this initiative was not then pursued. It is of interest

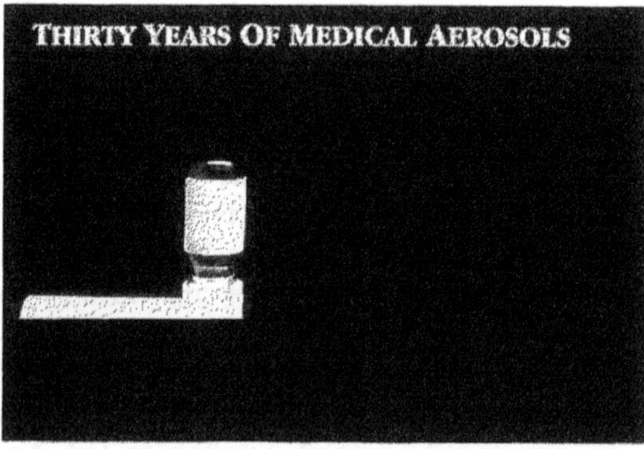

Figure 8 The original metered-dose inhaler with its 3-in. plastic mouthpiece. It was made of glass with a Meshburg metering valve attached. (Courtesy of 3M Pharmaceuticals.)

that inhaled insulin is now in phase 3 trials and may become a standard therapy for diabetic patients.

The next major development was by Dr. Charlie Thiel, a chemist at Riker (35). He used a surfactant, sorbitan trioleate (span 85), as a dispersing agent mixed with a suspension of micronized drug and propellant. The suspension aerosols appeared to deliver a respirable drug considerably more efficiently than the early alcohol solution formulations and allowed poorly soluble drugs to be aerosolized. In 1957, bronchodilator products were switched to suspensions. This switch resulted in many complaints because—although the suspensions appeared more effective—patients missed the taste of the alcohol, which they associated with a subsequent feeling of well-being!

Over the next years, the MDI was altered in a number of ways to improve the reproducibility of its output. It was noted very early on that if it stood upright for any length of time, it did not release a dose when fired for the first time. Significant drug was delivered only on the second shot. Therefore, a cup was introduced within the MDI, surrounding the valve, with an entrance at the top, so that the liquid formulation would not drain out when the valve sat upright. This markedly reduced loss of prime, although as we know that loss of prime with standing still occurs, as described in detail by Cyr and colleagues (36).

V. Asthma Deaths

The popularity of the MDI grew with advertisements for its use, which first appeared in the *British Medical Journal* in the early 1960s (Fig. 9). During the 1960s, in the United Kingdom and in a number of other countries, there was a sudden rise in the mortality of patients with asthma. From 1961, there was a steady and progressive rise in asthma mortality, which was most marked among patients aged 5 to 34. Reports of three deaths in which excessive use of a pMDI was considered to be a contributory factor were published in Australia in 1964, and a warning from the Autralian Minister of Health was given (37). In August 1965, Greenberg (38), a thoracic physician from Cambridge, sent a letter to the *Lancet* in which he recorded eight deaths associated with the use of the new MDI. In 1967, Greenberg and Pine (39) stated in the *British Medical Journal* their suspicion that patients with asthma were killing themselves with excessive use of MDIs. Richard Doll and Frank Spizer from Oxford and Peter Heaf and Leonard Strang from London (40) reported that there had been a 42% increase in the overall death rate between 1959 and 1964. The most seriously affected group were children between the ages of 5 and 14 years.

In June 1967, the Committee of Safety in Medicines (41) issued a warning about the need for care in prescribing and using aerosols, emphasizing their great

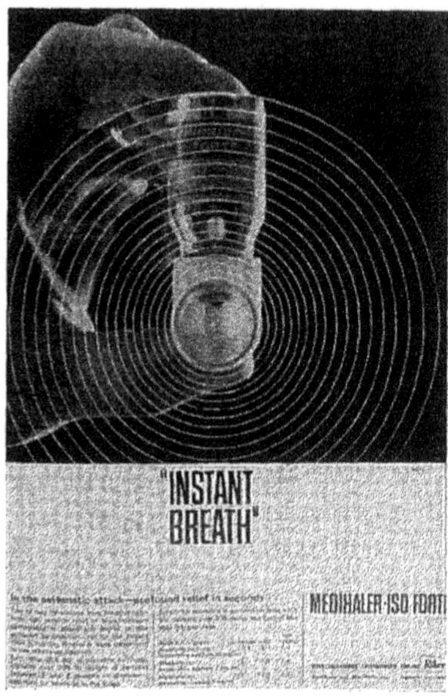

Figure 9 An early advertisment for pressurized metered dose inhalers appearing in the *British Medical Journal* in the early 1960s. (Courtesy of the *British Medical Journal.*)

value in treatment, but advising patients or parents to call their doctors if they failed to achieve the relief they usually experienced. From 1968 on, MDIs of antiasthma medications could be obtained in the United Kingdom only by prescription, having been available over the counter prior to this. In 1969, Bill Inman and Abe Edelstein (42), from the Committee on the Safety of Drugs, published a paper in the *Lancet* entitled "The Rise and Fall of Asthma Mortality in England and Wales in Relation to the Use of Pressurised Aerosols." In this paper, the true extent of the scale of asthma mortality was revealed.

When the changes in death rate were compared with estimates of prescriptions, it could be seen that the rise and fall in the death rates had followed the graph of sales of pressurized aerosols almost exactly (Fig. 10). In children 4 years of age and below, there had been no change in death rates. These patients had not been prescribed aerosols because they were not old enough to use them appropriately. Between the ages of 15 and 34, it was calculated that there had been more than 960 deaths, and in those over age 35, approximately 2300 in excess of those expected. Inman and Adelstein (42) proposed the subsequent fall in mortality might have been brought about either by a reduction in the number of patients using aerosols or by a reduction in the amount used. It was suggested that both

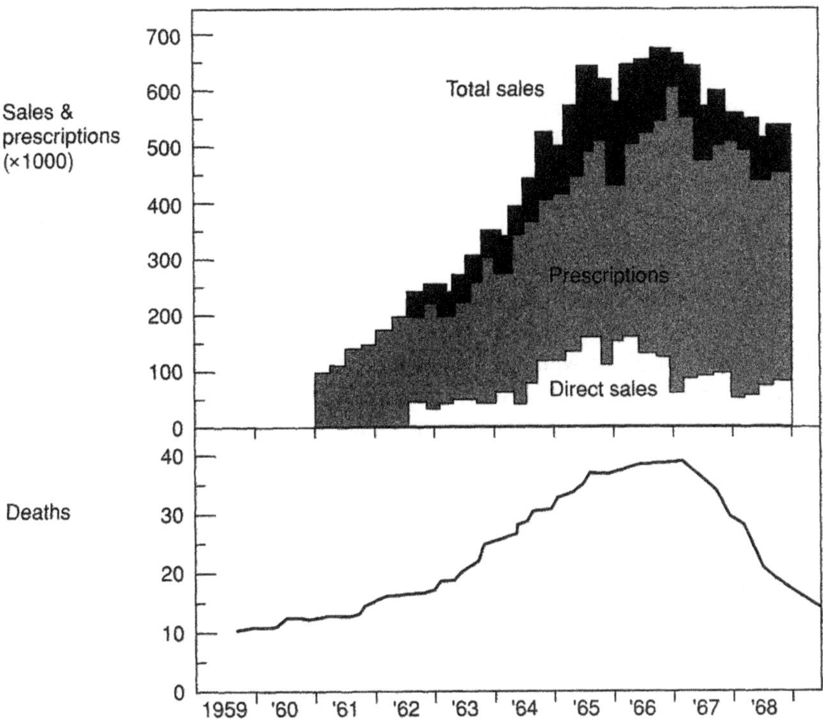

Figure 10 The rise and fall in death rates during the epidemic of asthma deaths was mirrored by the rise in sales of pressurized metered-dose aerosol inhalers. (From Ref. 42.)

doctors and patients may have been lulled into a false sense of security by effective bronchodilators. When medication failed to produce the expected relief, the patients may have continued to use the aerosol and thus to overdose. The doctor may have failed to recognize the resistance to treatment while the patient continued to deteriorate. The reason for the fall in the death rate may have been the greater understanding of the serious nature of an asthma attack and earlier admission to hospital with more effective treatment. It has been suggested that many lives would have been saved if steroids were started, or the dose already employed increased, whenever asthma deteriorated (43). Evidence that asthmatics actually overdosed themselves is circumstantial and is mainly derived from the accounts of those who witnessed the patients' excessive use of aerosols or who found such patients lying dead and clutching empty or partially empty canisters. Concentrations of isoprenaline or orciprenaline present in the body after death were not determined in these cases, and there were no characteristic postmortem changes attributable to the overdose.

However, the main toxicity of excess usage of an MDI was thought to be related to the fluorocarbon propellants. At a similar time as the asthma deaths were being investigated, there were reports from the United States that sudden deaths had occurred among individuals who were abusing aerosol propellants by filling plastic bags with them and then inhaling their contents (44). The mechanism of death was assumed to be cardiac arrhythmias, because autopsy failed to reveal any other cause. In the United Kingdom, the mechanism of death among asthmatics has never been clearly established.

It was shown that conscious dogs breathing moderate concentrations of fluorocarbon for 5 min would develop severe ventricular arrhythmia when challenged with intravenous bolus doses of adrenaline (45, 46). Dollery and colleagues (47), from the Hammersmith hospital, studied the toxicity of propellant gases in humans. The eight patients who volunteered for the study had severe asthma and took either one or two inhalations from their inhalers at intervals of 30 or 60 s. The arterial peak concentration of fluorocarbon occurred 10–20 s after the last inhalation. The fall in the concentration in arterial blood was rapid and declined to half in 18–38 s with fluorocarbon 11 and 12–24 s with fluorocarbon 12. The predicted peak myocardial levels were 10% or less than the predicted myocardial concentrations that sensitized the myocardium of dogs studied by Clark and Tinsten (46). To test extreme conditions, one volunteer took an inhalation from a pressurized aerosol placebo dispenser on every breath for 30, 60, and 120 s, breathing at a rate of 12 breaths per minute. The predicted peak myocardial concentration considerably exceeded the value that would sensitize the dog heart to circulating or injected adrenaline (48).

The results suggested that there should be a factor of safety of about 10 when the inhaler is used in the manner recommended by the manufacturers. As long as several normal breaths are taken before the inhaler is used again, the alveolar and thus the arterial and myocardial concentrations fall rapidly. Dollery (47) concluded that there was unlikely to be a hazard from the propellants if the inhaler was used as recommended, but there *could* be a hazard in conditions of excessive overdose. There are some concerns with regard to this interpretation, as in one of the dog experiments, one of the dogs tested was very much more sensitive than the others. In addition, we now know that in patients with severe asthma, the actual deposition of drug within the respiratory tract may vary greatly between patients. The effect of these factors and the use of isoprenaline, a nonselective $beta_2$ agonist, in patients during acute attacks of asthma (when they are likely to be hypoxic) can only be guessed.

The lesson that must not be forgotten is that any new treatment must be introduced gradually and under close supervision. The importance of pharmacovigilance and reporting cases of possible toxicity cannot be overemphasized.

VI. Dry-Powder Inhalers

The first inhalation system delivering solid drug particles was introduced in the late 1800s. This system, called the carbolic smoke ball, was patented by Frederick Augustus Roe in England in 1889 as a device to facilitate the distribution, inhalation, and application of medicated powders (49). The device consisted of a rubber ball containing fine powder charged with carbolic acid (phenol) (Fig. 11). Remedies such as glycyrrhiza and white hellebore (*Veratrum veride*) were commonly packed into the ball. The drug dose was released in puffs and inhaled via the mouth or nostrils. The carbolic smoke ball became a popular asthma and hay fever remedy (50). The product was marketed by offering a reward of £100 sterling to anyone contracting influenza after using the product three times daily for 2 weeks (Fig. 12). This resulted in several claims against the company (49) and the withdrawal of the offer.

Adrenocorticotropic hormone (ACTH) and cortisone became available in the 1940s (51). In 1949 Bordley and colleagues (52) reported the beneficial effect of intramuscular ACTH given to five asthmatic patients. Reeder and Mackey (53) reported that nebulized cortisone delivered directly to the lungs by inhalation in a patient with bacterial pneumonia caused remission of symptoms. Following this report, Gelfand (54) gave nebulized cortisone to five asthmatic patients. The drug was delivered via a DeVilbiss nebulizer on an hourly basis between 9 A.M. and 10 P.M. A total of 50 mg per day was given. In four of the five patients, a favorable response was observed. By the end of the seventh day, almost all signs of bronchospasm had disappeared. Relapses were observed in three of the four successfully treated cases 4 to 5 days after treatment had stopped. In 1955, Foulds (55), a registrar in ophthalmic surgery, and colleagues delivered hydrocortisone powder to 15 patients with bronchial asthma. The particle size of hydrocortisone powder was said to be less than 5 μm. Although the powder inhaler was not described, an estimated 7.5–15 mg was inhaled per day. After using hydrocortisone powder for 2 to 3 weeks, patients were given cartridges containing an inert powder for the same period. After this, some of them were changed back to hydrocortisone. In 11 patients, the treatment caused a definite improvement of the asthma with the number of isoprenoline inhalations dropping to half or less. When inert powder was substituted, the improvement persisted for up to 3 weeks. When the asthma had returned to its former severity, resumption of hydrocortisone again brought about relief. In contrast to these studies, a nebulized solution of hydrocortisone was found to be ineffective when trialed by Brockbank and colleagues in 1956 (56).

Although a number of patents for powder delivery devices for medicinal purposes were filed from the middle of the twentieth century, the first widely used powder inhaled was sodium cromoglycate.

In the mid-1950s, Khellin analogues were being investigated as potential

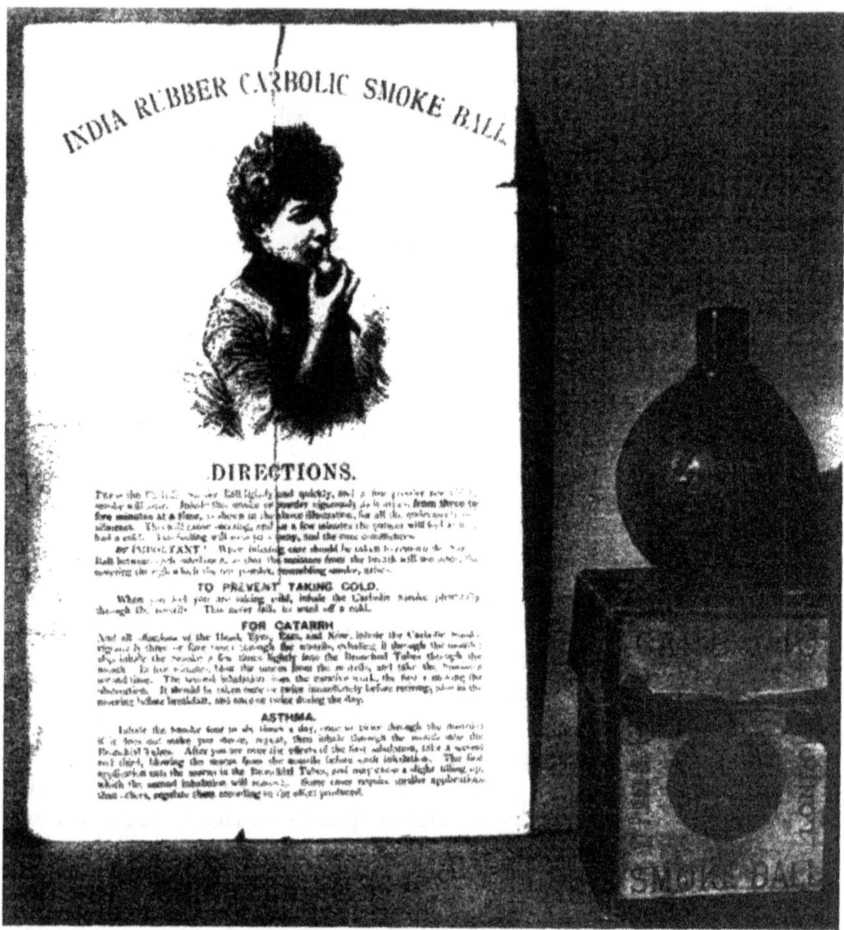

Figure 11 The India rubber carbolic smoke ball.

bronchodilators. Active compounds were examined in sensitized guinea pigs exposed to aerosols of egg white in order to induce a laboratory model of an asthma attack. Roger Altounyan, a physician who had severe asthma, tested compounds thought to have antiasthma properties on himself by inhaling a preparation of guinea pig hair, which he knew would induce an asthmatic attack. By 1958, he had found that several analogues of Khellin were protective. One in particular had no bronchodilating activity and afforded animals no protection against histamine; however, it protected Altounyan from the effects of guinea pig hair. The medication was effective only if inhaled, but as inhalation was found to

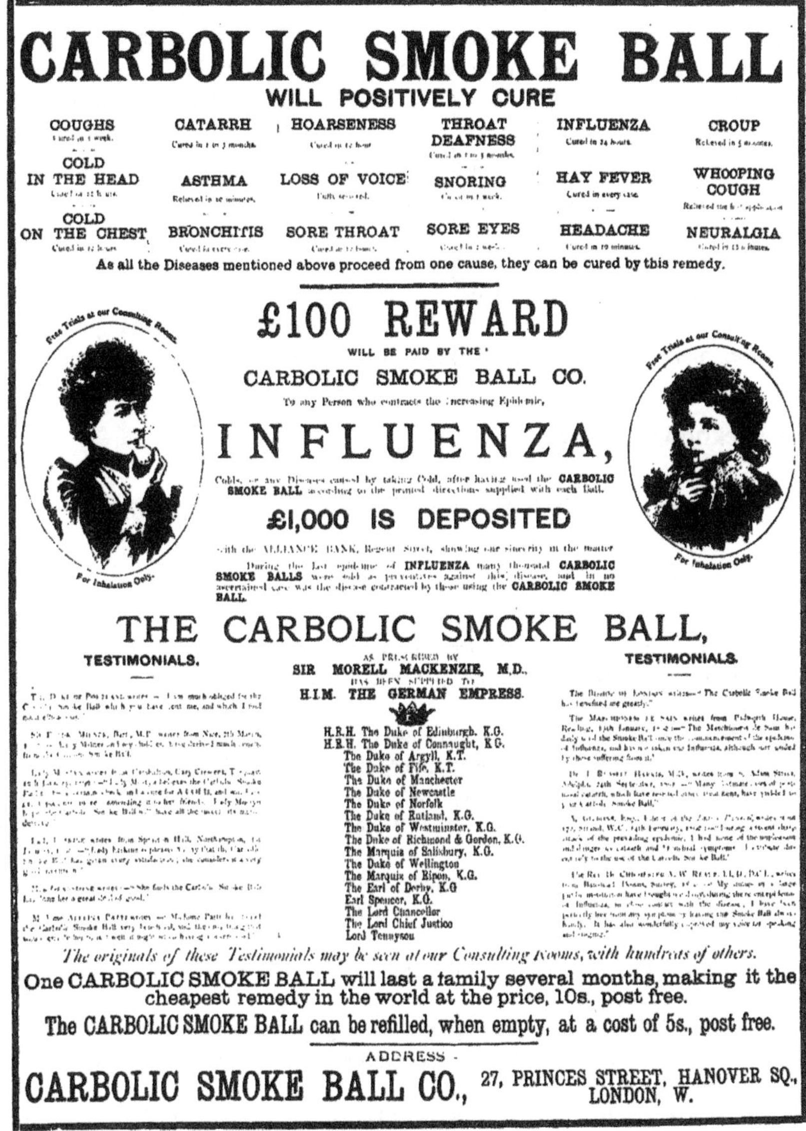

Figure 12 Advertising for the carbolic smoke ball. A reward of £100 was offered to those who genuinely caught influenza following use of the carbolic smoke ball.

irritate the lungs, the project was abandoned. However, in 1963, it was found that one of the compounds was contaminated with a highly active material. A series of bischromones were subsequently prepared for Altounyan to inhale. In 1965, he reported that sodium cromoglycate (57) was an ideal protective drug when inhaled. Altounyan and Howell, a company engineer, developed a special device that enabled the drug to be inhaled as a dry powder liberated from a pierced capsule. The results of the first clinical trial (58) were reported in 1967. Sodium cromoglycate, delivered in powder form from the Spinhaler, was marketed with great success.

The worldwide market for inhaled drug delivery is now approaching £5 billion each year. The drug delivery devices now used are described in detail in the remainder of this book. It will become obvious to the reader that while improvements have been made in aerosol drug delivery, further developments are still needed.

Acknowledgment

The 20th Century History of Medicine Department, The Wellcome Trust.

References

1. Larsson L. Incidence and Prevalence of Asthma—Relation to Differences in Utilisation of Asthma Drugs Between Two Neighbouring Swedish Provinces. Sweden: University of Umeå, 1995.
2. Gandevia B. Historical review of the use of parasympathicolytic agents in the treatment of respiratory disorders. Postgrad Med J 1975; 51:13–20.
3. Muthu DC. Pulmonary Tuberculosis: Its Etiology and Treatment—Record of Twenty-Two Years Observation and Work in Open-Air Sanatoria. London: Baillière, Tindall and Cox, 1922.
4. Brewis RAL. Classic Papers in Asthma. London: Science Press, 1990.
5. Miller WF. Aerosol therapy in acute and chronic respiratory disease. Arch Intern Med 1973; 131:148–155.
6. Sims J. Datura stramonium or thorn apple as a cure or relief of asthma. Edinburgh Med Surg J 1812; 8:364–367.
7. Grossman J. The evolution of inhaler technology. J Asthma 1994; 31(1):55–64.
8. Elliott HL., Reid JL. The clinical pharmacology of a herbal asthma cigarette. Br J Clin Pharmacol 1980; 10:487–490.
9. Hassal AH. The Inhalation Treatment of Diseases of the Organs of Respirations Including Consumption. London: Longmans, Green, 1885.
10. Moeller. Thérapeutique locales des maladies de l'appareil respiratoire par les inhalations médicamenteuses et les pratiques aérothérapiques. Paris: Baillière, 1882.
11. Muers MF. Overview of nebuliser treatment. Thorax 1997; 52:25–30.
12. Valet JS. To Breathe or Not to Breathe. Barcelona: Ancora SA, 1995.
13. Pennington TH. The lister steam spray in Aberdeen. Scott Med J 1988; 33:217–218.
14. von Bruns V. Fort mit dem Spray! Berl Klin Wochenschr 1880; 17:609–611.

15. Lister J. An address on the present position of antiseptic surgery. Br Med J 1890; 377–379.
16. Yernault JC. Inhalation therapy: an historical perspective. Eur Respir Rev 1994; 4:65–67.
17. Waldenbourg. Dic Locale Behandlung der Krankenheit der Athmungsorgane. Lehrbuch der Respiratorischen Therapie. Berlin: Reimer, 1872.
18. Dautrebande L. Microaerosols. New York: Academic Press, 1962.
19. Solis-Cohen S. J Am Assoc 1900; 34:1164
20. Bullowa GGM, Kaplan D. Med News 1903; 83:789
21. Zeulzer G. Die behandlung akuter Katarrhe der oberen Luftwege durch Inhalation von Nebennierenpräparaten. Berl Klin Wochenschr 1911; 285.
22. Camps PWL. A note on the inhalation treatment of asthma. Guy's Hosp Rep 1929; 79:496–498.
23. Graeser JB, Rowe AH. Inhalation of epinephrine for the relief of asthmatic symptoms. J Allergy 1935; 6:415–420.
24. Palmer F, Kingsbury SS. Particle size in nebulized aerosols. Am J Pharm 1952; 124:112–124.
25. Collison WE. Inhalation Therapy Technique. London: Heinemann Medical Books, 1937.
26. Wright BM. New inventions: a new nebuliser. Lancet 1958; 2:24–25.
27. Anonymous. Inhaler for penicillin: notes and news. Lancet 1946; 1:986.
28. Scheuing T. German Pat 1942; 723–728.
29. Siegemund OH, Grainger HR, Lands AM. J Pharmacol Exp Ther 1947; 90:254.
30. Helbinge H. Collodion mixture. 1999; U.S. Pat No 628,463.
31. Gebauer CL. Receptacles for containing and administering volatile liquids. U.S. Pat No 668,815.
32. Thiel CG. From Susie's question to CFC free: an inventor's perspective of 40 years of MDI development and regulation. Respir Tract Del 1996; 5:115–123.
33. Meshberg P. Aerosol containers and valves therefor. 1954 U.S. Pat No 457,189.
34. Friedman T. Medihaler for bronchial asthma: a new type of aerosol therapy. Postgrad Med 1956; 20:6:667–671.
35. Thiel CG. Dispensing device. 1957; U.S. Pat No 2,886,217.
36. Cyr TD, Graham SJ, Li KYR, Lovering EG. Low first spray drug contents in albuterol metered dose inhalers. Pharm Res 1991; 8:658–660.
37. McManis AG. Asthma deaths. Med J Aust 1964; 2:76.
38. Greenberg MJ. Isoprenaline in myocardial failure. Lancet 1965; 28:442.
39. Greenberg MJ, Pines A. Pressurised aerosols in asthma. Br Med J 1967; 1:563.
40. Doll R, Speizer F, Heaf P, Strong L. Increased deaths from asthma. Br Med J 1967; 1:756–759.
41. Aerosols in Asthma: Vaccines. Committee of Safety of Drugs Adverse Reaction Series, No 5. London: Wavel Press, June 1967.
42. Inman WHW, Adelstein AM. Rise and fall of asthma mortality in England and Wales in relation to the use of pressurised aerosols. Lancet 1969; 2:279–285.
43. Fraser PM, Speizer FE., Waters SDM, Doll R, Mann NM. The circumstances preceding death from asthma in young people in 1968–1969. Br J Dis Chest 1971; 65:71–84.
44. Bass M. Sudden sniffing death. JAMA 1970; 212:12:2075–2079.

45. Reinhardt CF, Azar A, Reinhardt CF, Smith PE, Mullin LS, Cardiac arrythmias and aerosol sniffing. Arch Environ Health 1971: 22:265–279.
46. Clark DG, Tinston DJ. Cardiac effects of isoproterenol, hypoxia, hypercapnia, and fluorocarbon propellants and their use in asthma inhalers. Ann Allergy 1972; 30:536–541.
47. Dollery CT, Williams FM, Draffan GH, Wise G, Sahyoun H, Patterson JW, Walker SR. Arterial blood levels of fluorocarbons in asthmatic patients following use of pressurised aerosols. Clin Pharmacol Ther 1973; 14:59–66.
48. Mullen LS, Azar A, Reinhardt CF, Smith PE, Fabryka EF. Halogenated hydrocarbon-induced cardiac arrhythmias associated with release of endogenous epinephrine. Am Industr Hygiene Assoc J 1972; 33:389–396.
49. Helfand WH. Historical images of the drug market. Pharm Hist 1995; 37(1):34–35.
50. Jackson WA. The carbolic smoke ball. Pharm Hist 1984; 14:9–10.
51. Kendal EC. Hormones of the adrenal cortex. Endocrinology 1942; 30:853–860.
52. Bordley JE, Carey RA, Harvey AM, Howard JE, Kattus AA, Newman EV, Winkenwerder WL. Preliminary observations on the effect of adrenocorticotrophic hormone (ACTH) in allergic disease. Bull Johns Hopkins Hosp 1949; 85:396–398.
53. Reeder WH, Mackay GS. Nebulised cortisone in bacterial pneumonia. Dis Chest 1950; 18:528–534.
54. Gelfand ML. Administration of cortisone by the aerosol method in the treatment of bronchial asthma. N Engl J Med 1951; 245:293–294.
55. Foulds WS, Greaves DP, Herxheimer H, Kingdom LG. Hydrocortisone in the treatment of allergic conjunctivitis, allergic rhinitis and bronchial asthma. Lancet 1955; 1:234–235.
56. Brockbank W, Brebner H, Pengelly CDR. Chronic asthma treatment with aerosol hydrocortisone. Lancet 1956; 2:807.
57. Fitzmaurice C, Lee DB. British Pat No 1969; 1144906.
58. Howell JBL, Altounyan REC. Lancet 1967; 2:539–542.
59. Courtesy of "A History of Medicine" by Morgan Samuel editions.

2

Basic Principles of Particle Behavior in the Human Respiratory Tract

JOACHIM HEYDER

GSF–National Research Center for Environment and Health
Munich, Germany

MAGNUS U. SVARTENGREN

Karolinska Institutet
Stockholm, Sweden

I. Introduction

If inspired particles were carried only convectively with the bulk of airflow, losses of these particles in the respiratory tract would be negligible. However, all inspired particles experience a nonzero chance of being lost. This is due to particle transport toward airway and airspace surfaces as a result of mechanical and electrical forces acting upon the particles. Upon contact with these surfaces, the particles are deposited. The human respiratory tract can therefore be considered as an "aerosol filter," removing particles from the inspired air. The effectiveness of this filter depends on

The physicochemical properties of the inspired particles
The breathing pattern and morphology of the subject inspiring the particles
The mode of breathing (nasal or oral)
The distribution of particles in the inspired air

The following pages discuss how the "filter characteristics" of the human respiratory tract or its regions are affected by these factors and what implications this has for an efficient aerosol therapy. This chapter also summarizes the development of the field over the last two decades:

Experimental determination of particle deposition in the human respiratory tract under laboratory conditions (summarized in Ref. 1).

Development of a semiempirical deposition model based on these experimental laboratory data (2).

Adaptation of the model to all available experimental deposition data and extension of the model to ultrafine particles by the International Commission on Radiological Protection (ICRP) (3).

Current applications of the ICRP model for predicting deposition of pharmaceutical particles.

Since pharmaceutical particles often look like spheres and these particles are usually administered per os, the behavior in the respiratory tract of *orally inspired spherical particles* is the focus of attention in this chapter.

II. Particle Transport onto Airway Surfaces

Because of the mechanical and electrical forces acting upon inspired particles, particle trajectories are different from airstream lines, so that particles are transported toward surfaces of the respiratory tract. However, whereas all inspired particles are exposed to mechanical forces, only charged particles are exposed to electrical forces. Since pharmaceutical particles are usually not heavily charged, particle transport in the human respiratory tract is governed by mechanical transport: diffusional, gravitational, and inertial (Fig.1). Since diffusional and gravitational transport are time-dependent transport phenomena, particles are simultaneously transported by both mechanisms. However, when particles cover more than about 30 $\mu m\ s^{-1}$ by diffusional transport, the contribution of gravitational transport becomes negligible. When they cover more than about 30 $\mu m\ s^{-1}$

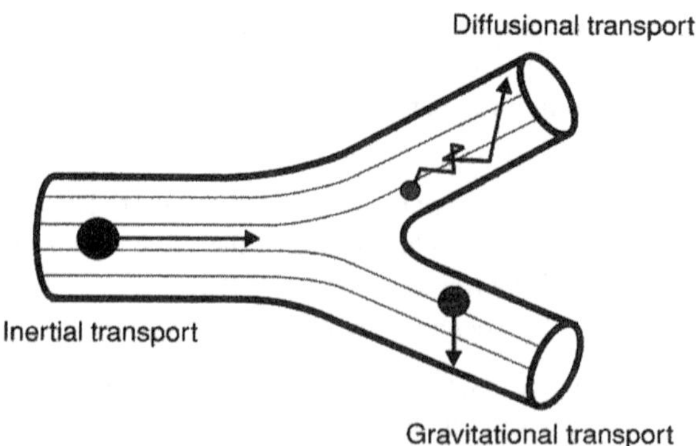

Figure 1 Illustration of particle transport onto airway surfaces.

by gravitational transport, the contribution of diffusional transport becomes negligible. On the other hand, inertial transport is a velocity-dependent transport phenomenon. It becomes effective for particle deposition only when particles cover more than 30 µm s^{-1} by this transport phenomenon.

A. Diffusional Particle Transport (Diffusion)

Aerosol particles of dimensions comparable with the mean free path of gas molecules (about 0.06 µm) recognize their gaseous surroundings as composed of individual molecules, and every collision of a particle with a gas molecule changes its kinetic energy and direction of motion; as a result, the particle moves at random through the gas (Brownian motion or diffusion). The random displacement a particle covers by this transport increases with time and with decreasing particle diameter. It is independent of the particle density.

In the respiratory tract, only ultrafine particles (particles smaller than 0.1 µm in diameter) are deposited solely due to diffusion, since those particles cover more than 30 µm s^{-1} by diffusional transport (Fig. 2). For all ultrafine particles of the same size, deposition is the same regardless of their density. Because of the time-dependence of diffusional particle transport, it is anticipated that diffusional deposition of ultrafine particles occurs mainly in lung regions of maximum residence time of the tidal air—i.e., in small airways and in the lung periphery.

B. Gravitational Particle Transport (Sedimentation)

Particles larger than 0.1 µm are less and less transported by diffusion but settle more and more under the action of gravity. The displacement of a particle by gravitational transport increases with time and with particle diameter and density. In the respiratory tract, spheres of 3 g cm^{-3} density larger than 0.5 µm, unit density spheres larger than 1 µm, and spheres of 0.1 g cm^{-3} density larger than 3 µm in diameter are no longer deposited due to diffusion but solely due to sedimentation, since those particles settle more than 30 µm s^{-1} (Fig. 2). Because of the time-dependence of gravitational particle transport, it is anticipated that gravitational deposition of particles occurs mainly in lung regions of maximum residence time of the tidal air—i.e., in small airways and in the lung periphery.

C. Inertial Particle Transport (Impaction)

In the branching network of airways, the inspired air is changing its velocity and direction of motion all the time while it is penetrating into the lungs. Particles carried with the air are therefore exposed to inertial forces all the time. For particles of sufficient mass, these forces result in an inertial displacement and thus in a particle transport toward airway surfaces. This displacement increases with particle

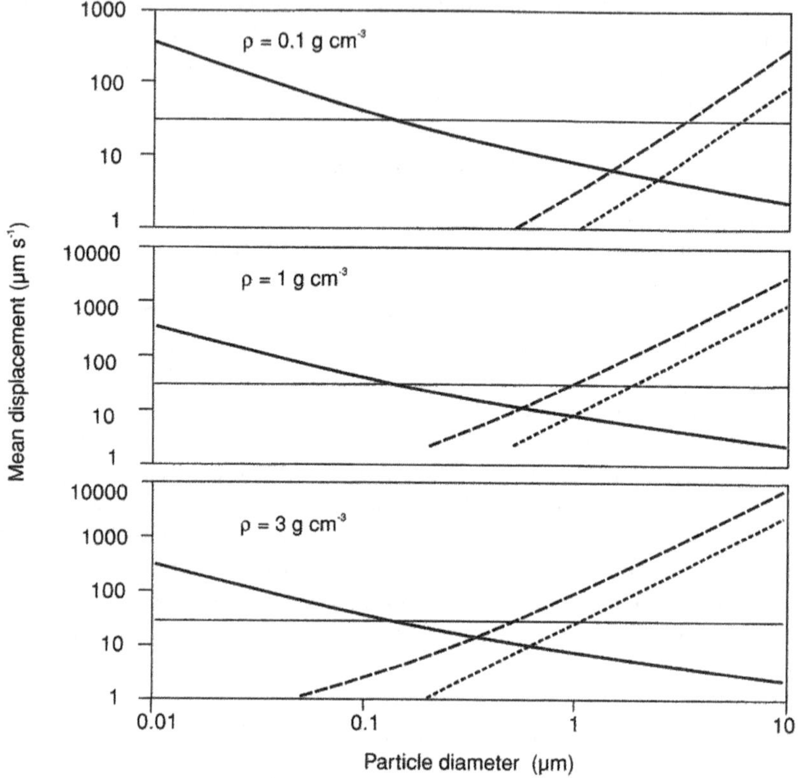

Figure 2 Mean displacement per second of particles of 0.1, 1 and 3 g cm^3 density undergoing diffusional, gravitational, and inertial transport (solid line: diffusional transport; dashed line: gravitational transport; dotted line: inertial transport).

velocity, diameter, and density. In the respiratory tract, inertial transport contributes to particle deposition for spheres of 3 g cm^{-3} density larger than 1 µm, unit density spheres larger than 2 µm, and spheres of 0.1 g cm^{-3} density larger than 6 µm in diameter, since these particles cover more than 30 µm s^{-1} by inertial transport (Fig. 2). Because of the velocity-dependence of inertial particle transport, it is anticipated that inertial deposition of particles in the respiratory tract occurs mainly in regions of maximum airflow velocity—i.e., in large airways.

D. Summary

In summary, particle transport onto airway surfaces depends on four parameters: particle diameter, particle density, particle velocity, and the time available for transport onto airway surfaces. Usually breathing cycle period and respiratory flow rate are used as substitutes for time and velocity; the dependence of the mean diffusional, gravitational, and inertial particle displacement on these four parameters can be summarized as follows:

	Particle size	Particle density	Breathing cycle period	Flow rate
Diffusional displacement	Decreases with size	Independent of density	Increases with time	Independent of flow rate
Gravitational displacement	Increases with size	Increases with density	Increases with time	Independent of flow rate
Inertial displacement	Increases with size	Increases with density	Independent of time	Increases with flow rate

III. Particle Deposition—Definitions and Fundamental Considerations

Deposition of ultrafine particles is due solely to diffusional transport. Deposition of larger particles is due to gravitational and/or inertial transport. It is therefore anticipated that the efficiency of the human respiratory tract to collect inspired particles decreases with particle size as long as deposition is governed by diffusion and increases with particle size when deposition is governed by sedimentation and/or impaction (Fig. 3). Deposition assumes a minimum when deposition due to diffusional transport is equal to that due to gravitational transport. For particles of 3 g cm^{-3} density, the lowest deposition is observed for 0.26-μm spheres; for unit-density particles, it occurs for 0.36-μm spheres. The shape of the fundamental filter characteristic of the respiratory tract schematically shown in Fig. 3 is typical for oral breathing of aerosols. The actual shape, however, is determined by particle density, breathing pattern, and gas volume in the lungs. It must therefore be emphasized that any statement about the filter characteristics of the respiratory tract is incomplete without mention of particle density, breathing pattern, and gas volume in the lungs for which it was obtained.

More time is available for transport toward airway surfaces for a particle inspired at the onset of a breath than for a particle inspired at the end of the breath. Therefore, even when indentical particles are inspired with the tidal air, the chance of being deposited will be different for each particle; thus the following definition is generally accepted:

> Definition: The fraction of inspired particles deposited in the respiratory tract, DF, is the *mean probability* that a particle inspired with the tidal air during steady-state breathing from functional residual capacity is deposited in the respiratory tract. DF is called *total deposition* throughout this chapter.

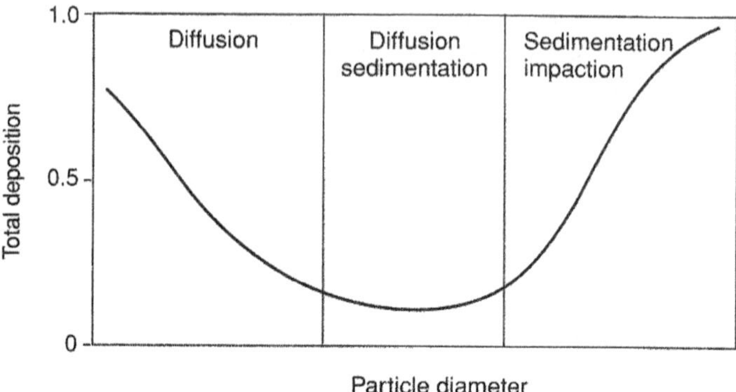

Figure 3 Schematic filter characteristic of the human respiratory tract for aerosol particles. Three domains can be recognized; the domain of deposition decreasing with particle size is solely due to diffusional particle transport, the domain of minimum deposition is due to simultaneous diffusional and gravitational particle transport, and the domain of deposition increasing with particle size due to gravitational and inertial particle transport.

Consequently, DF = 0.5 means that half the particles inspired per breath *are* deposited anywhere in the respiratory tract. Nevertheless, it is possible that all particles inspired at the onset of a breath are deposited but none of the particles inspired at the end of the breath.

The same considerations apply for particle deposition in regions of the respiratory tract:

> Definition: The fraction of inspired particles deposited in region X of the respiratory tract, DF_x, is the *mean probability* that a particle inspired with the tidal air during steady-state breathing from functional residual capacity is deposited in region X. DF_x are called *regional depositions* throughout this chapter.

Since each particle inspired with the tidal air can be deposited in only one region, the sum of all regional depositions equals total deposition.

As far as the behavior of aerosol particles is concerned, the respiratory tract can be partitioned into four regions:

Extrathoracic region: airways in head and neck
Upper bronchial region: trachea and bronchi (large ciliated thoracic airways)
Lower bronchial region: bronchioles (small ciliated thoracic airways)
Alveolar region: nonciliated thoracic airways and airspaces

Consequently, total deposition, DF, is the sum of extrathoracic deposition, DF_E, upper bronchial deposition, DF_{UB}, lower bronchial deposition, DF_{LB}, and alveolar deposition, DF_A:

$$DF = DF_E + DF_{UB} + DF_{LB} + DF_A$$

IV. Total Deposition

A. Experimental Methodology

According to the definition, total deposition is simply given by

$$DF = 1 - (\text{number of expired particles / number of inspired particles})$$

It must therefore be determined during steady-state breathing of well-defined monodisperse aerosols by counting the number of inspired and expired particles per breath. Since aerosol photometry is usually applied for monitoring particle number concentration, c, in inspired and expired tidal air and combined with pneumotachography for monitoring flow rate, Q, during breathing of the aerosol (Fig. 4), total deposition can be calculated by

$$DF = 1 - \left(\int_{t_e} c\,|Q|\,dt \Big/ \int_{t_i} c\,|Q|\,dt\right)$$

where t_i (t_e) is the time available for inspiration (expiration) of the tidal air.

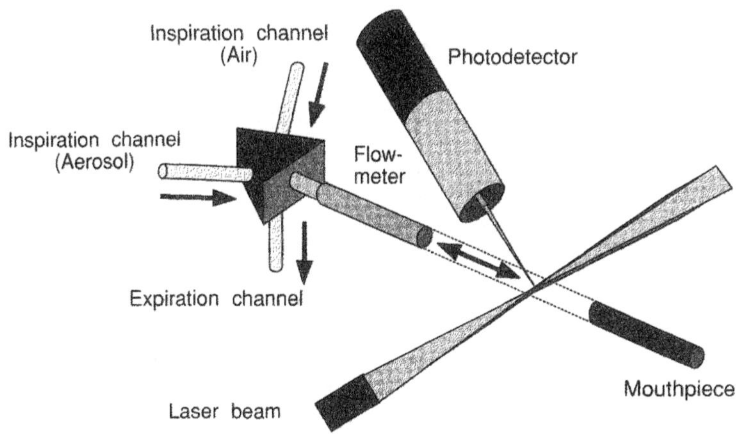

Figure 4 Scheme of the respiratory aerosol probe for determining total deposition of aerosol particles in the human respiratory tract.

Total deposition can also be determined by measuring the mean particle number concentration in samples taken from inspired and expired aerosols over periods of several breaths and taking into account particle losses due to the sampling procedure.

However, regardless of the technique used, the particle number concentration of the inspired aerosol must remain constant during the entire inspiration. In case the particle number concentration increases during inspiration, deposition will be different from that obtained for the case of a decreasing inspiratory particle number concentration. It must therefore be recognized that it is necessary to use only aerosols of uniform particle number concentration for the experimental determination of total deposition.

B. Effect of Particle Dynamics

The dependence of total deposition on particle dynamics is demonstrated in this chapter for monodisperse spherical particles of 0.9 and 3.2 g cm^{-3} density and diameters between 0.2 and 10 μm orally inspired with the tidal air from functional residual capacity by three subjects at patterns illustrated in Fig. 5 (1).

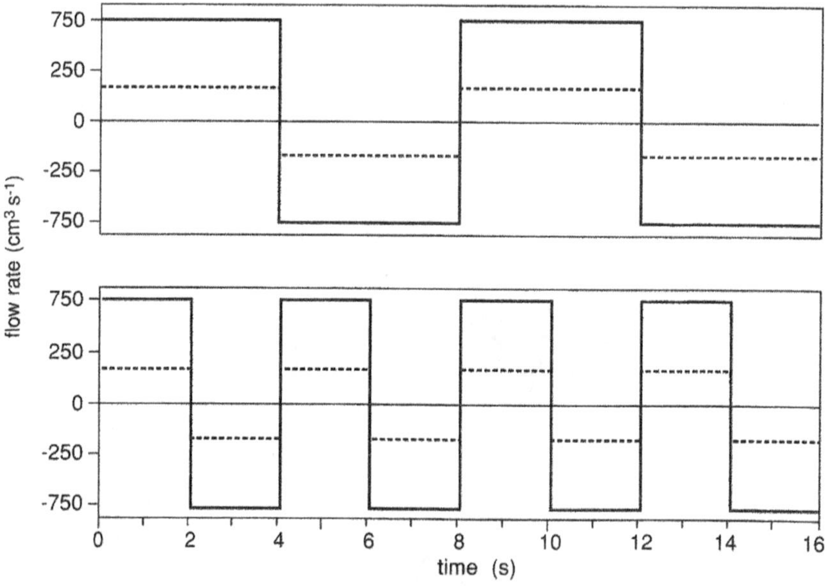

Figure 5 Breathing patterns used for studying total and regional particle deposition (lines: 4- and 8-s breathing-cycle periods and 750 cm^3 s^{-1} flow rate; dashed lines: 4- and 8-s breathing-cycle periods and 250 cm^3 s^{-1} flow rate).

For all particle sizes deposition increases with time (Fig. 6, top). At a flow rate of 250 $cm^3 s^{-1}$ deposition is governed by sedimentation but at 750 $cm^3 s^{-1}$ flow rate by impaction. Therefore, the time-dependency of deposition is less pronounced when the aerosols are respired at the high flow rate. When these data are plotted to illustrate the influence of flow rate on deposition (Fig. 6, bottom) it becomes obvious that inertial transport is not effective for deposition anywhere in the respiratory tract of orally inspired particles smaller than 2 μm in diameter.

In Fig. 7, top the effect of particle density on total deposition is demonstrated, and it can be seen that 2 μm particles of 3.2 g cm^{-3} density are deposited with the same efficiency than 4 μm particles of 0.9 g cm^{-3} density. This ambiguity can be eliminated by considering the aerodynamic size of the particles.

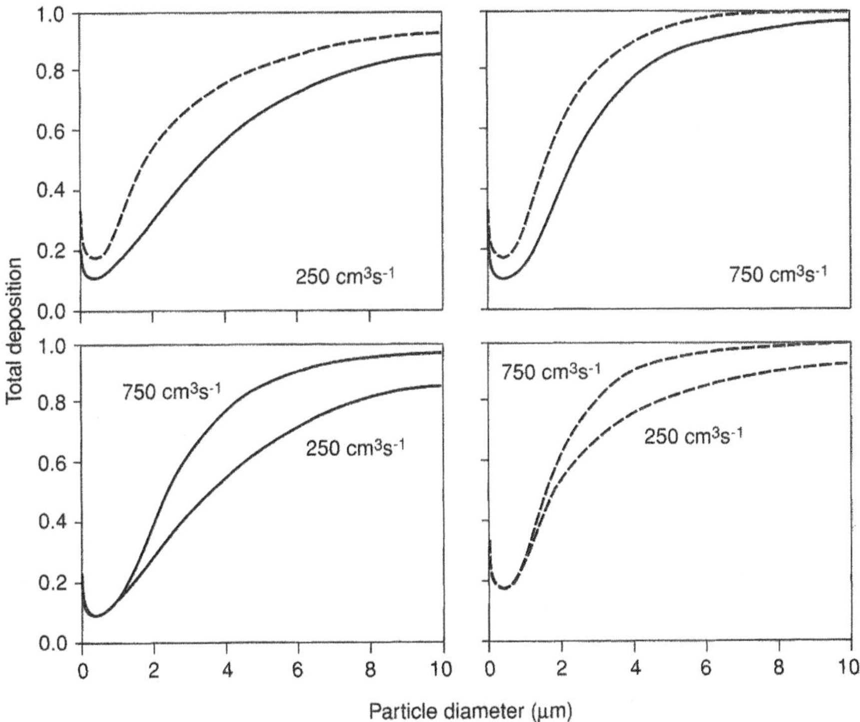

Figure 6 Oral tidal breathing of 0.9 g cm^{-3} density spheres with 4- and 8-s breathing-cycle periods and flow rates of 250 and 750 $cm^3 s^{-1}$ from functional residual capacity (lines: 4-s breathing cycle period, dashed lines: 8-s breathing-cycle period): upper graphs: effect of time on total deposition; lower graphs: effect of flow rate on total deposition.

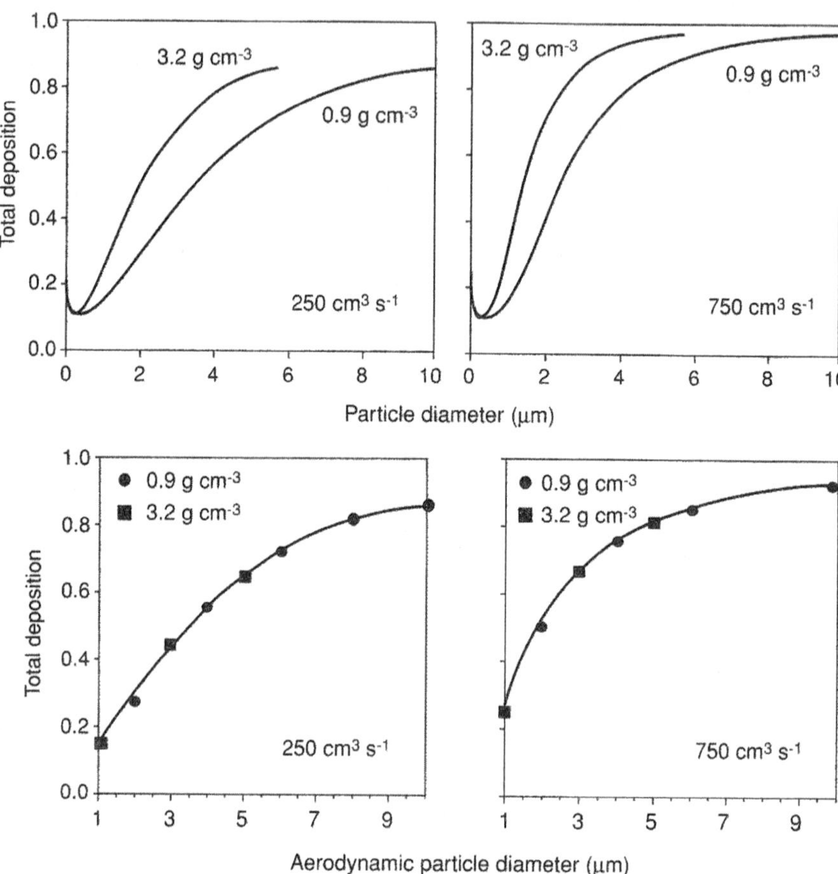

Figure 7 Oral tidal breathing of spheres of 0.9 and 3.2 g cm^{-3} density with 8-s breathing-cycle period and flow rates of 250 and 750 cm^3 s^{-1} from functional residual capacity: upper graphs: effect of particle density on total deposition; lower graphs: verification of the aerodynamic particle diameter concept for the human respiratory tract.

C. Concept of Aerodynamic Particle Diameter

Definition: The aerodynamic diameter of a particle is the diameter of a fictitious sphere of unit density which, under the action of gravity, settles with the same velocity as the particle in question.

From Fig. 7 (top) it is obvious that the transport properties of a small heavy sphere can be identical with that of a large light sphere. When both spheres are transported with the same velocity, they exhibit the same aerodynamic behavior and thus the same deposition. This velocity is determined by the geometrical size and the density of the particles. All particles of diameter, d, and density, ρ, behave aerodynamically in the same way as long as the value of the product (ρd^2) is the same. In this case, all these particles experience identical gravitational displacement. Since both gravitational and inertial transport are dependent on (ρd^2) they also experience identical inertial displacement.

In reality it is not entirely true, that particles characterized by identical (ρd^2) experience identical displacement due to the action of mechanical forces. The displacement is influenced by interactions between a particle and the gas molecules surrounding it. The so-called slip correction accounts for these interactions. If a particle is smaller than the mean free path of the gas molecules this correction is substantial. It decreases, however, for increasing particle size and becomes negligible far particles much larger than the mean free path of the gas molecules. In consequence, no correction has to be applied for estimating the transport of particles larger than 1 μm in diameter.

Considering a sphere of unit density, ρ_o, and diameter, d_{ae}, for which (ρ_o-d_{ae}^2) = (ρd^2), its transport properties are identical with those of all particles characterized by the same value of (ρd^2). Its diameter is called the aerodynamic diameter. The behavior of this fictitious sphere is representative of all particles collected with the same efficiency by the respiratory tract regardless of their density. Or, in other words, this sphere represents all these particles as far as their transport properties are concerned. However, it does not represent them as far as their physical properties are concerned (particle diameter, particle density, and consequently particle mass).

For each monodisperse aerosol with spheres of 0.9 and 3.2 g cm^{-3} density used to study deposition of the respiratory tract, the aerodynamic diameter can be calculated by

$$d_{ae} = d\,(\rho/\rho_0)^{0.5}$$

and total deposition can be plotted as a function of their aerodynamic diameter. For both flow rates, deposition is an unique function of the aerodynamic diameter (Fig. 7, bottom) and thus the concept of the aerodynamic diameter obviously applies to particle behavior in the human respiratory tract.

D. Limitations of the Concept of Aerodynamic Particle Diameter

This concept is confined to particles transported by gravitational sedimentation without interference of diffusion and, consequently, to particles larger than 1 μm in aerodynamic diameter. For smaller particles an aerodynamic diameter is not defined. Therefore, the abcissa in Fig. 7 (bottom) has to have a 1-μm origin.

Since both gravitational and inertial transport are dependent on (ρd^2), the aerodynamic diameter concept also applies in principle to inertial transport of particles larger than 1 μm in aerodynamic size. Inertial transport contributes to particle deposition in the human respiratory tract for particles larger than 2 μm in aerodynamic diameter. Therefore, particle deposition for spheres of different density is an unique function of the aerodynamic diameter.

Very often inertial deposition in impactors is used to characterize the aerodynamic behavior of aerosol particles. However, much larger inertial forces are applied for particle deposition in impactors than are available for particle deposition in the human respiratory tract. The particle size obtained by this technique is the "inertial diameter." This diameter is defined in the same way as the aerodynamic diameter but based on inertial rather than gravitational particle transport. When a particle is not only inertially but also gravitationally transported its inertial diameter is identical with its aerodynamic diameter.

Even ultrafine particles which are solely deposited in the lungs by diffusion can be classified with impactors. The inertial sizes of these ultrafine particles are however not suitable for estimating particle deposition in the respiratory tract. For instance, a 0.05-μm sphere of 3 g cm^{-3} density behaves in the lungs like a 0.05-μm particle. However, its inertial diameter is about 0.09 μm.

It must also be recognized that when only the aerodynamic diameter of a particle is known, its deposition efficiency in the respiratory tract can be estimated but it remains unknown what mass this particle delivers to the surfaces of the respiratory tract. This mass can be estimated only when either the density or the geometrical diameter of this particle is known. For instance, the mass of spheres that are 2 μm in aerodynamic size decreases by more than a factor of 5 when their density increases from 0.1 to 3 g cm^{-3} (Table 1). Although the particles are deposited with equal probability in the human respiratory tract, the mass they deliver to airway and airspace surfaces is far from being equal. For all spheres of equal aerodynamic size, the sphere with the lowest density carries the greatest mass into the lungs.

E. Intersubject Variability

Total deposition varies considerably among healthy individuals breathing monodisperse aerosols with identical pattern (Fig. 8). This huge variability is determined by the intersubject variability of airway and airspace morphometry.

Table 1 Mass (m) of Spheres of Equal Aerodynamic Diameter (d_{ae}) but Different Density (ρ)

d_{ae} (μm)	2.0	2.0	2.0
ρ (g cm^{-3})	0.1	1.0	3.0
d (μm)	6.3	2.0	1.2
m (pg)	13.1	4.2	2.4

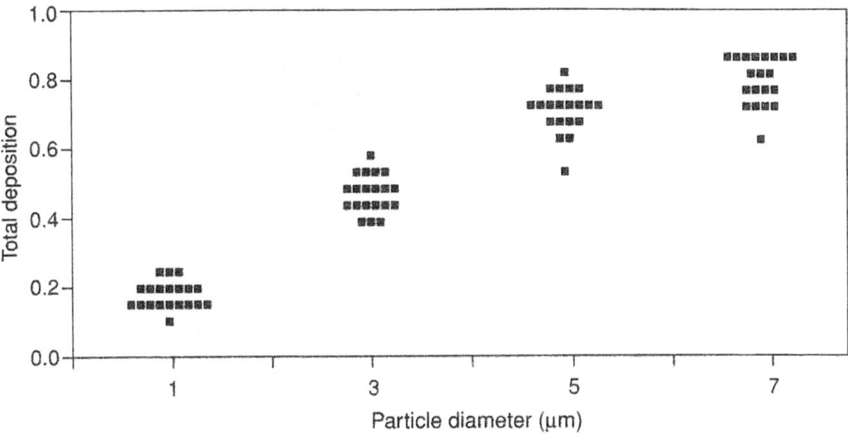

Figure 8 Total deposition of spheres 1, 3, 5, and 7 μm in diameter and 0.9 g cm^3 density in the respiratory tract of 20 healthy individuals breathing the aerosols orally with 4-s breathing-cycle period and flow rate of 400 $cm^3 s^{-1}$ from functional residual capacity.

Airway and airspace dimensions of these individuals estimated from deposition of 1-μm particles due to gravitational transport during end-inspiratory breath-holding are closely correlated with the total deposition of the individuals. The respiratory tract of individuals with wide airways collects particles less efficiently than that of individuals with narrow airways.

This huge intersubject variability of particle deposition has serious consequences for the therapeutic application of aerosols: monitoring the inspired mass of a drug is not sufficient; monitoring the deposited mass of the drug is necessary. A safe aerosol therapy with drugs of narrow therapeutic width requires therefore individual dosimetry.

V. Regional Deposition

A. Experimental Methodology

Determination of regional deposition is usually based on measurements of particle removal from the respiratory tract after short-term steady-state breathing of radiolabeled particles relatively insoluble in body fluids. First of all, total deposition can be partitioned into extrathoracic and thoracic components by external detection of the amount of radiotracer deposited in head and neck and in thorax immediately after particle administration with a number of scintillation detectors placed around head or thorax as schematically shown in Fig. 9. Thoracic deposition can then be

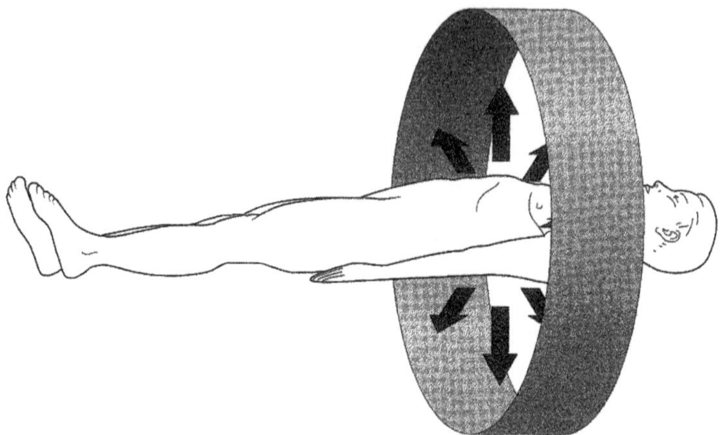

Figure 9 Scheme of the scintillation device for determining the amount of radiotracer deposited in head, neck, and thorax. The configuration of scintillation detectors and shielding allows detection of particle removal from the thorax regardless of the spatial distribution of particles within thorax and stomach.

partitioned into a bronchial and an alveolar component by external detection of the amount of radiotracer retained in the thorax over a couple of days after particle administration (Fig. 10). During this time the thoracic activity decreases in two distinct phases: a fast phase, complete within 40 h, due to mucociliary transport of particles to the glottis and subsequent swallowing of the particles, and a slow phase due to macrophage mediated particle removal from the thorax. The activity removed by mucociliary transport from the thorax is associated with particles deposited on surfaces of ciliated airways and that removed by macrophages with particles deposited on surfaces of nonciliated airways and airspaces. This radiotracer technique is confined to particles larger then 0.1 μm. Its sensitivity is not sufficient for studying regional deposition of ultrafine particles.

It has recently been recognized that a fraction of particles deposited on surfaces of ciliated thoracic airways is not removed from these airways within 40 h but retained for longer periods (4). This long-term retention phenomenon was observed for particles smaller than 6 μm in diameter. Although particle removal from thoracic airways is therefore overestimated by the radiotracer technique, it affects bronchial deposition by less than 10%.

B. Effect of Fluid Dynamics

When an aerosol enters the respiratory tract, its particles first experience inertial transport onto airway surfaces in the extrathoracic and upper bronchial region.

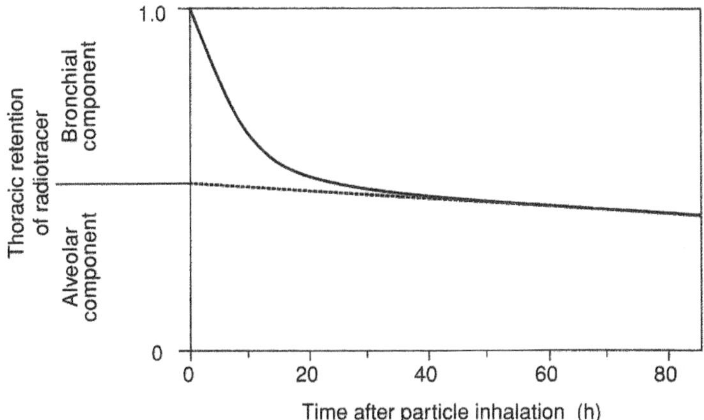

Figure 10 Temporal variation of thoracic retention.

As it penetrates further into the respiratory tract the efficacy of this transport diminishes and the efficacy of gravitational transport is enhanced. The upper respiratory tract can be considered as an impactor and the lower respiratory tract as an elutriator. This is due to the fluid dynamics of the respiratory tract.

An inspired aerosol flows through the upper respiratory tract at high velocity and remains in this region only for a short period, so that particle deposition is governed by inertial impaction. On the other hand, the long residence time of the aerosol in the lower respiratory tract is associated with low velocity, so that particle deposition is governed by diffusional and gravitational transport. Consequently, with increasing particle size and/or flow rate, the site of deposition is shifted from the lower to the upper respiratory tract. Because of the limitations of the radiotracer technique, this anticipation is, however, verified experimentally only for particles larger than 0.1 μm in diameter.

C. Effect of Particle Dynamics

To demonstrate the dependence of regional deposition on particle dynamics monodisperse radiolabeled spherical particles of 3.2 g cm^{-3} density and diameters between 0.3 and 10 μm were orally inspired with the tidal air from functional residual capacity by three subjects at the slow and fast patterns illustrated in Fig. 5 (1). Slow breathing is characterized by a breathing cycle period of 8 s and flow rate of 250 cm^3 s^{-1}; fast breathing by a 4-s cycle period and flow rate of 750 cm^3 s^{-1}. Total and regional depositions are presented in Fig. 11 as functions

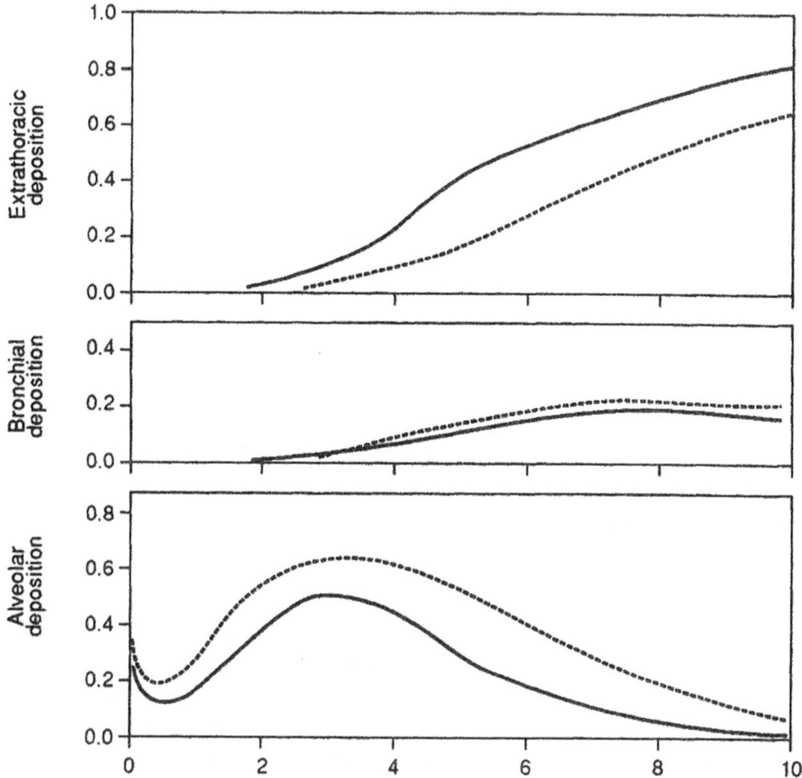

Figure 11 Experimentally determined deposition in extrathoracic, bronchial, and alveolar regions of the human respiratory tract for slow oral tidal breathing of unit-density spheres from functional residual capacity (lines: 8-s breathing-cycle period and flow rate of 250 $cm^3\ s^{-1}$) and fast oral breathing of unit-density spheres (dashed lines: 4-s breathing-cycle period and flow rate of 750 $cm^3\ s^{-1}$).

of the diameter of unit-density spheres which, for particles larger than 1 μm, is identical with the aerodynamic diameter.

Unit-density spheres smaller than about 2 μm in aerodynamic diameter are deposited in the alveolar region and deposition in other regions is undetectable (Fig. 11). Larger particles are already removed from the inspired air in extrathoracic as well as ciliated thoracic airways during inspiration with the result that alveolar deposition decreases with particle size in the range above 3 μm. Although alveolar deposition of 1- and 7-μm particles inspired at flow rate of 250

$cm^3\ s^{-1}$ is about the same, the behavior of these particles in the respiratory tract is entirely different. All inspired 1-μm particles penetrate to the alveolar region, where only a few of them are deposited. Although only a few of the inspired 7-μm particles penetrate to this region, all of them are deposited there. Above 8-μm bronchial deposition also decreases with particle size.

In the extrathoracic region, more particles are deposited during fast than during slow breathing (Fig. 11) and particle deposition is solely due to impaction in the larynx during inspiration. In the oral cavity, deposition is negligible, so that extrathoracic and larygeal deposition are identical.

In the bronchial region, particle deposition is less dependent on flow rate and breathing-cycle period (Fig. 11). It is due to impaction in upper thoracic airways and due to sedimentation in lower thoracic airways.

In the alveolar region, more particles are deposited during slow than during fast breathing (Fig. 11) and particle deposition is due to diffusion and/or sedimentation.

VI. Modeling of Particle Deposition

Experimentally determined regional deposition data have been used to obtain detailed insight into particle transport onto airway surfaces with a semiempirical deposition model, which considers extrathoracic, bronchial, and alveolar region of the respiratory tract as a series of aerosol filters (2). This model requires no assumptions with respect to either the geometric configuration of the respiratory tract, the particle dynamics in the respiratory tract, or the efficiency of each airway to collect inspired particles. However, it permits the conversion of regional deposition values into regional efficiencies, which can be used to estimate the contribution of particle transport mechanisms to regional deposition. In addition, this model can also be used to partition the bronchial region into an upper portion, in which deposition is mainly due to inertial particle transport, and a lower portion, in which particles are mainly collected by gravitational transport. Hence, it yields empirical analytical expressions for calculating deposition in extrathoracic airways, ciliated upper and lower bronchial airways, and the nonciliated portion of the lungs for oral breathing of aerosols with particles of a wide range of sizes and densities at a wide range of breathing patterns.

This model has been adopted by a Task Group of the International Commission on Radiological Protection (ICRP) to all available experimental total and regional deposition data and extended for calculating regional deposition of ultrafine particles (3). For oral breathing of unit-density spheres at rest, total and regional depositions calculated with the ICRP model are shown in Fig. 12.

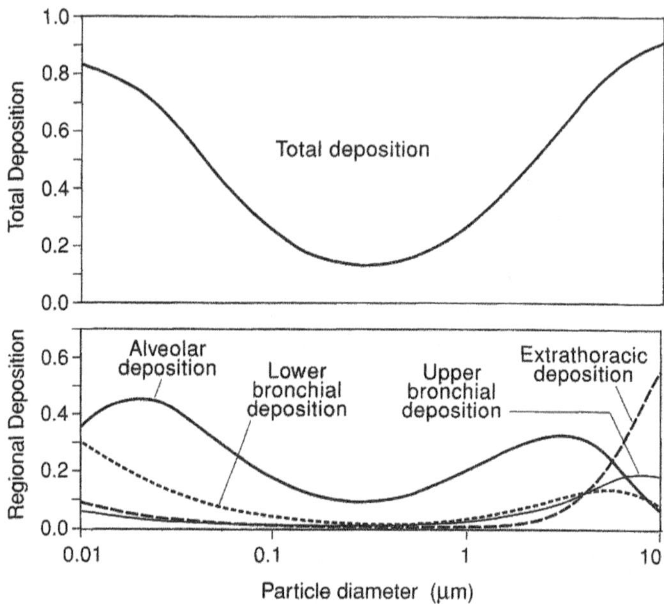

Figure 12 Total deposition and deposition in extrathoracic, upper and lower bronchial, and alveolar regions estimated with the ICRP semiempirical deposition model (3) for oral breathing of unit-density spheres at the reference resting pattern for an adult Caucasian male sitting awake (9): 15-s breathing-cycle period and flow rate of 300 $cm^3 s^{-1}$.

VII. Consequences for Aerosol Therapy of Particle Behavior in the Respiratory Tract

In aerosol therapy, particles are used to carry pharmaceuticals into the respiratory tract, where they become available upon deposition for the treatment of topical or systemic diseases. It must, however, be recognized that particle deposition in the human respiratory tract discussed so far is confined to particles with hydrophobic surfaces and fully entrained in the inspired air. However, in aerosol therapy, these ideal conditions are often not fulfilled. It must also be recognized that the deposited mass (dose) or the mass deposited per unit surface area (surface dose) rather than the number of deposited particles is of interest in aerosol therapy. Therefore, particles are suitable for therapy only if they deliver a sufficient dose of a pharmaceutical to the respiratory tract. These particles are usually larger than 1 μm in diameter.

A. Mass Deposition of Polydisperse Particles (Deposited Dose)

Usually, monodisperse aerosols are not available for aerosol therapy, but polydisperse aerosols are. For monodisperse aerosols, deposition is the same whether it is related to the number or the mass of inspired particles, but it is different for polydisperse particles. Regional mass depositions of polydisperse particles can be obtained by partitioning the polydisperse mass distribution (particle mass as a function of the geometric particle diameter) into monodisperse fractions, calculating regional depositions for each fraction and adding up these values for each region. For instance, if the mass of 1-μm particles in a polydisperse aerosol is 1 mg, and 20% of the 1-μm particles are deposited in the alveolar region, they contribute 0.2 mg to the mass deposited in this region. If the total mass inspired is 5 mg, the contribution of 1-μm particles to alveolar deposition is 4%. This procedure has to be performed for all monodisperse fractions and all regions. Alveolar mass deposition of 0.33 means that one-third of the inspired particle mass is deposited in this region.

For oral breathing at rest of unit-density spheres with log-normal mass distributions, regional mass depositions are illustrated in Fig. 13. Deposition for particles with a mass median diameter (MMD) of 1 μm occurs almost entirely by gravitational sedimentation on surfaces of small ciliated thoracic airways and on surfaces beyond these airways, and for particles with a MMD of 3 μm on surfaces throughout the respiratory tract but still mainly on surfaces comprising the alvolar region. When MMD increases alveolar deposition decreases, deposition in the lower bronchial region remains at a level observed for particles of 3-μm MMD, but deposition in extrathoracic airways increases considerably.

These data are confined to particles fully entrained in the inspired air. When particles are, however, inspired from propellant-based metered-dose or dry-powder inhalers, their velocity is much greater than that of the inspired air, and only a small mass fraction (nonballistic fraction) escapes inertial deposition in the oropharynx and enters the trachea. The mass fraction of particles deposited in the oropharynx (ballistic fraction) can be determined experimentally. It comprises more than 50% of the mass released from inhaler devices and therefore is much larger than that deposited in the larynx. It is usually assumed that the ballistic fraction is equal to the mass fraction collected in an induction port placed in front of a cascade impactor. Collection of particles in the impactor allows the estimation of the mass distribution of particles entering the respiratory tract. Finally, these distributions can be used to calculate regional mass depositions with a deposition model.

This approach for studying deposition in the human respiratory tract of ballistic and nonballistic mass fractions released from inhaler devices is thus based on

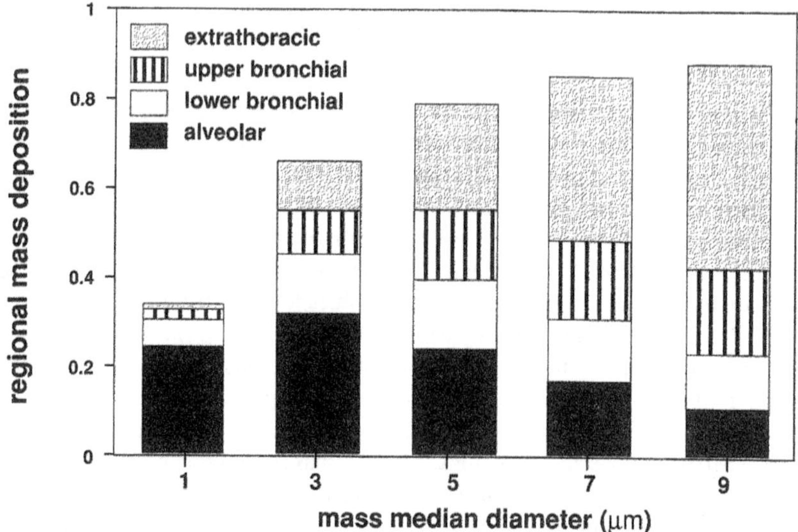

Figure 13 Regional mass depositions estimated with the ICRP semiempirical deposition model (3) for oral breathing of polydisperse aerosols with unit-density spheres at the reference resting pattern for an adult Caucasian male sitting awake (9) (5-s breathing-cycle period and flow rate of 300 cm^3 s^{-1}). The particle size distributions are log-normal mass distributions characterized by various mass median diameters and a geometric standard deviation of 2.

The experimental determination of extrathoracic (oropharyngeal) mass deposition.

The experimental determination of the mass distribution of the particles entering the respiratory tract.

The mathematical determination of regional mass depositions.

Using the ICRP deposition model, Pritchard et al. (6) were able to demonstrate that this approach is suitable to predict extrathoracic (oropharyngeal) and thoracic mass deposition of particles released from a dry powder inhaler obtained by the radiotracer technique (Fig. 14). The ballistic fraction comprised 50–70% of the particle mass but only about 12% were deposited in thoracic airways and airspaces of 19 patients.

B. Targeting Respiratory Tract Surfaces with Inspired Particles

Pharmaceutical particles are gravitationally and inertially transported onto airway and airspace surfaces. Extrathoracic and upper bronchial surfaces collect them by impaction and lower bronchial and peripheral airspace surfaces by sedi-

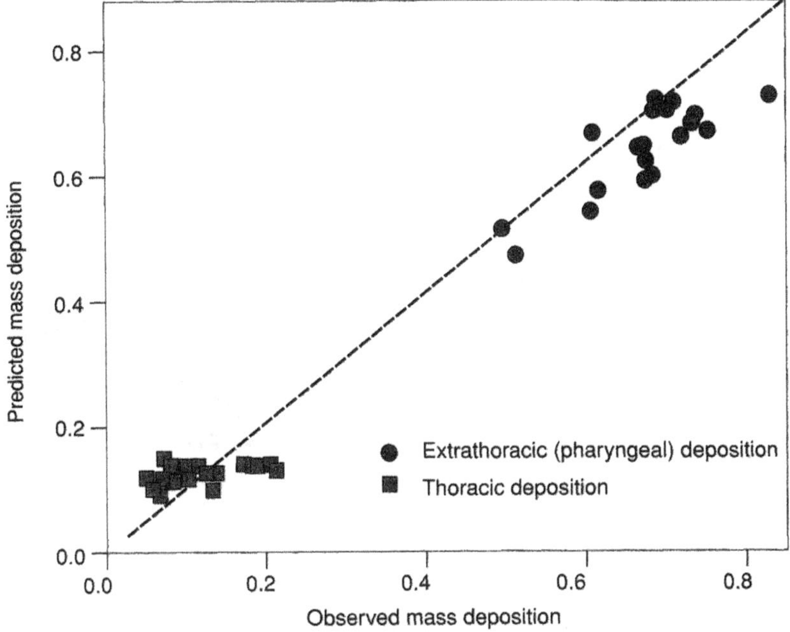

Figure 14 Predicted and observed extrathoracic and thoracic mass depositions of particles inspired by 19 patients from a dry-powder inhaler (6).

mentation. Targeting regions of the respiratory tract is therefore feasible. Optimum targeting can be obtained for the following conditions:

Targeting of extrathoracic airway surfaces can be achieved by inspiring at high flow rate particles much larger than 1 μm in aerodynamic size and suspended in tidal air of small volume.

Targeting of upper ciliated bronchial surfaces is not possible.

Targeting of lower ciliated bronchial surfaces can be achieved by inspiring as extremely low flow rate particles much larger than 1 μm in aerodynamic size and suspended in tidal air of large volume (5).

Targeting of peripheral airspace surfaces can be achieved by inspiring at low flow rate particles in the aerodynamic size range of about 1 μm and suspended in tidal air of large volume.

These conditions are specified in Fig. 15. More than 50% of the mass deposited in the entire respiratory tract can be specified in the extrathoracic, lower bronchial, and alveolar regions. Only targeting of the upper bronchial airways is not possible. However, when extrathoracic and upper bronchial regions are com-

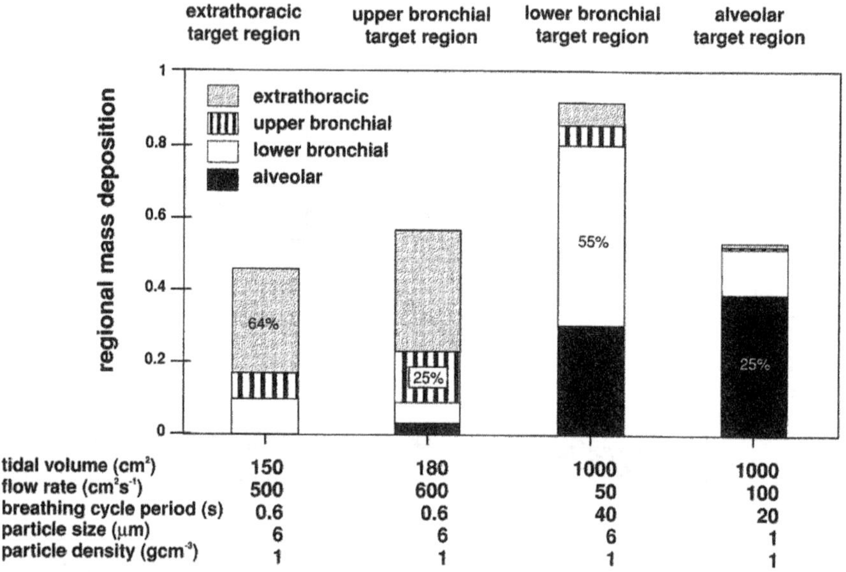

Figure 15 Targeting of extrathoracic, bronchial, and alveolar regions of the human respiratory tract with monodisperse aerosols inspired at specific breathing patterns. The estimation of regional mass deposition is based on the ICRP deposition model (3).

bined to an upper respiratory tract region and lower bronchial and alveolar regions to a lower respiratory tract region, targeting can considerably be improved and, even more important, targeting is independent of the particle size distribution. The inhalation of monodisperse particles and log-normally distributed polydisperse particles of identical mass median diameters result in a targeting efficiency of more than 90% for both the upper and lower respiratory tract regions (Fig. 16).

C. Hygroscopic Growth of Inspired Particles

In case of hydrophilic surfaces, particles absorb water vapor from the moist air in the respiratory tract. They grow therefore in size and diminish their density while they are penetrating with the convective air flow into the lungs. Consequently, when particles of identical size and density but different surface properties are inspired, the site of deposition is different. Particles with hydrophilic surfaces are deposited more proximal in the respiratory tract than those with hydrophobic surfaces.

Hygroscopic growth of monodisperse, solid 0.7-μm sodium chloride parti-

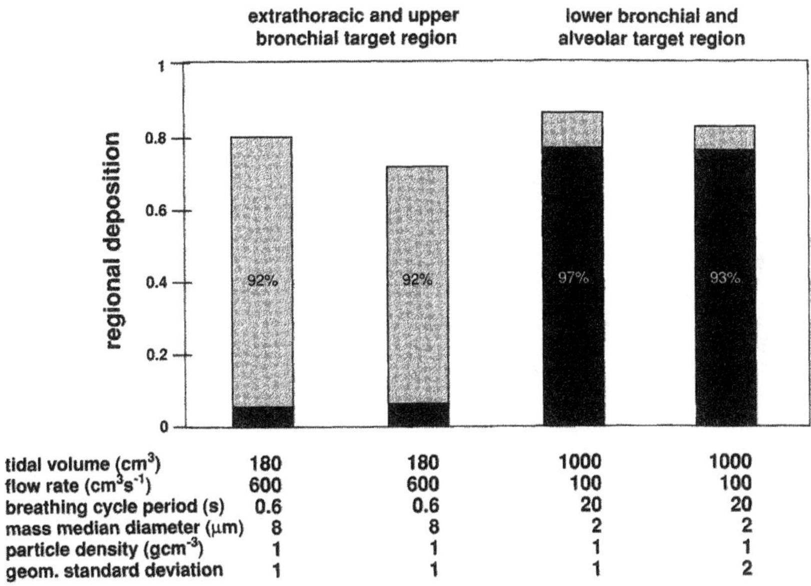

Figure 16 Targeting upper and lower respiratory tract regions of the human respiratory tract with mono- and polydisperse aerosols inspired at specific breathing patterns. The estimation of regional mass deposition is based on the ICRP deposition model (3).

cles in the human respiratory tract is demonstrated in Fig. 17. These particles were inspired within small aerosol boluses and carried to volumetric lung depths up to 800 cm^3 and recovered from these depths upon expiration. Their number concentration was so low that the photodetector of the respiratory aerosol probe (Fig. 4) received scattered light only from single particles so that the respiratory aerosol probe operated as a particle size spectrometer, and thus the particle size in inspired and expired air could be measured (7). When the 0.7-μm particles penetrated beyond 300 cm^3 lung depth, they were grown to 4-μm particles when expired. This was anticipated for water vapor exposure of the particles at 0.995 relative humidity, which is the maximum humidity generated by a saline solution. In lung depths smaller than 300 cm^3, the particles grew less in size, indicating that the relative humidity in these depths was less than 0.995.

The hygroscopic growth of pharmaceutical particles is usually less than that of sodium chloride particles. It is, however, not negligible, although it is often neglected in aerosol therapy. This was shown for a number of pharmaceutical aerosols. Particles were produced by nebulization of aqueous solutions of drugs, exposed to dry air and passed through a differential mobility analyzer for selec-

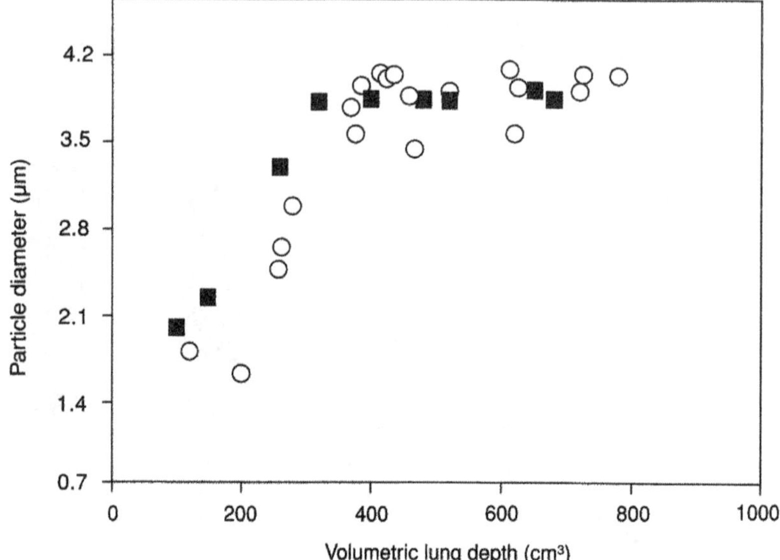

Figure 17 Hygroscopic growth of 0.7-µm sodium chloride particles in the respiratory tract of two volunteers as a function of the volumetric depth to which the particles are carried with the tidal air as aerosol boluses. The sizes of the grown particles were determined with the respiratory aerosol probe (Fig. 4) in the expired air.

tion of a monodisperse fraction in situ. The selected particles were then exposed to air of increasing relative humidity, and their size was analyzed with another differential mobility analyzer and a condensation particle counter. For instance, when the humidity was raised to 0.98, bricanyl particles increased their size by a factor of 2.44 (8).

References

1. Heyder J, Gebhart J, Rudolf G, Schiller CF, Stahlhofen W. Deposition of particles in the human respiratory tract in the size range 0.005–15 µm. J Aerosol Sci 1986; 17:811–825.
2. Rudolf G, Gebhart J, Heyder J, Scheuch G, Stahlhofen W. Mass deposition from inspired polydisperse aerosols. Ann Occup Hyg 1986; 32(suppl 1):919–938.
3. International Commission on Radiological Protection (ICRP). Human respiratory tract model for radiological protection. Ann ICRP 1994; 24:36–52.
4. Stahlhofen W, Scheuch G, Bailey MR. Investigation of retention of inhaled particles in the human bronchial tree. Radiat Prot Dosim 1995; 60:311–319.

5. Svartengren M, Svartengren K, Aghaie F, Philipson K, Camner P. Lung deposition and extremly slow inhalations of particles: limited effect of induced airway constriction. Exp Lung Res 1999; 25:353–366.
6. Pritchard JN, Layzell G, Miller JF. Correlation of cascade impactor data with measurements of lung deposition for pharmaceuticals aerosols. In: Drug Delivery to the Lungs VII. The Aerosol Society, 1996, 101–104.
7. Gebhart J, Heigwer G, Heyder J, Roth C, Stahlhofen W. The use of light scattering photometry in aerosol medicine. J Aerosol Med 1988; 1:89–112
8. Seemann S, Busch B, Ferron GA, Silberg A, Heyder J. Measurement of hygroscopicity of pharmaceutical aerosols in situ. J Aerosol Sci 1995; 26 (suppl 1):S527–538.
9. Cotes JE. Lung Function Assessment and Application in Medicine. Oxford, England: Blackwell Scientific Publications, 1979.

3

Structure and Function of the Respiratory System

Developmental Aspects and Their Relevance to Aerosol Therapy

JANET STOCKS and ALISON A. HISLOP

Institute of Child Health
University College
London, England

I. Introduction

The success of therapy using aerosolized medications depends on the ability to deliver sufficient drug to appropriate sites in the lung with minimal side effects. The recognized advantages of using aerosols compared with other forms of therapy include ease of administration, effectiveness with smaller doses than required for systemic administration, and rapidity of response to a drug in aerosol form. However, depositing aerosol in the lung involves not only generating sufficient quantities of suitable-sized particles or droplets but also ensuring that sufficient aerosol reaches the most appropriate region of the respiratory system. The efficacy of aerosol therapy is significantly related to the amount of drug deposited in the airways (1). This, in turn, depends on aspects of airway anatomy and physiology, which will alter with age and disease (2–4) and therefore need to be understood in considering both drug delivery and deposition.

As discussed below, airway size, structure, and branching pattern will all influence the delivery and deposition of aerosols. Airway caliber—which may be reduced due to bronchoconstriction, inflammation, edema, increased secretions, or simply age at both ends of the spectrum—is a major influence on site of deposition of aerosol in the lung. Considerations for delivering inhalant therapy to infants and children are similar to those for adults. However, in younger subjects, breathing pattern—with respect to higher respiratory rates, reduced tidal volumes, and the tendency to nose-breathe—is a prime influence in determining how much aerosol is inhaled into the lung.

Anatomic and physiological differences, together with the increased susceptibility of the very young and the elderly to respiratory problems, present a particular challenge in terms of developing efficient aerosol therapy for a variety of diseases throughout life. This challenge is one that is unlikely to be met without a firm understanding not only of the basic structure and function of the respiratory system but also of how these change with age. The purpose of this chapter is to provide such a background. In the space available, it is obviously both impossible and inappropriate to describe the anatomy and physiology of the respiratory system in detail, particularly when so many excellent reviews are already available (5–10). Instead, this chapter focuses specifically on those aspects of respiratory structure and function that are relevant to inhalation therapy, with particular emphasis on developmental changes.

II. Structural Organization of the Respiratory System

The respiratory system consists of the airways that carry the air to the alveoli, the gas-exchanging region of the lung, and the chest structures responsible for moving air in and out of the lungs—the respiratory pump. The lung is also supplied by blood vessels both to nourish the airways and for gas exchange. The respiratory system is divided into the upper and lower airways, the upper extending from the external nares to the larynx, the lower from the larynx to the respiratory bronchioli and alveoli. The lower airways exhibit a pattern of branching that maximizes efficient delivery of air to all parts of the lung as well as providing the maximal area for gas exchange (Fig. 1).

A. Functional Anatomy of the Respiratory Pump (Chest Wall)

The lungs are attached to the thoracic cage—which consists of the ribs, sternum, thoracic vertebrae, diaphragm, and intercostal muscles—by the visceral and parietal pleura. The two pleural membranes are sealed together by a film of pleural fluid that enables the lungs (which themselves contain no skeletal muscle) to be expanded and relaxed by movements of the chest wall. The balance between the inward recoil of the lung and the outward recoil of the chest wall determines the volume remaining in the lung at end expiration (functional residual capacity, or FRC) (Fig. 2).

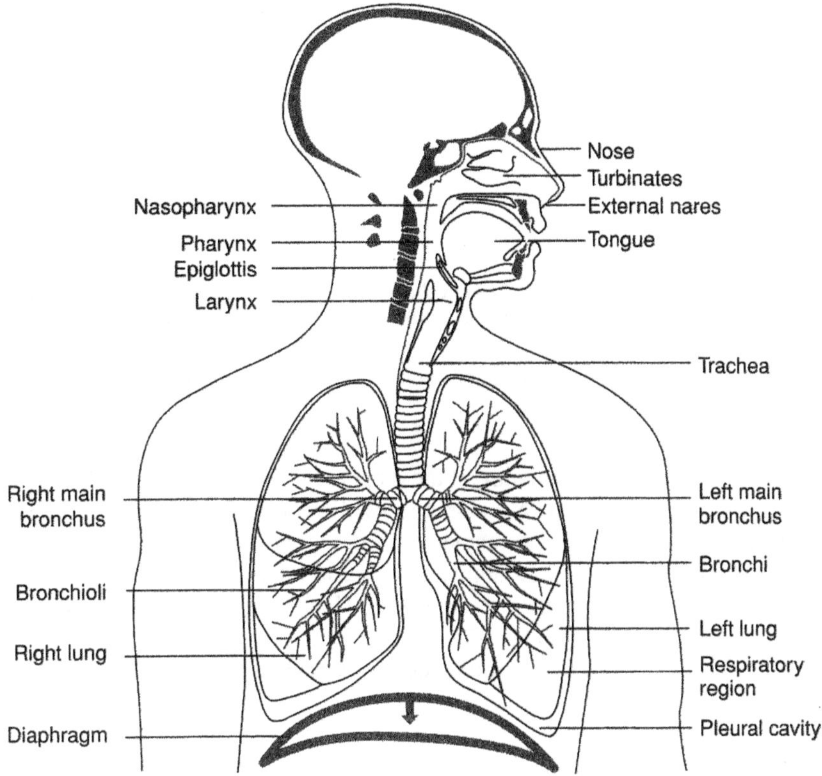

Figure 1 Gross structure of the respiratory system.

Diaphragm and Rib Cage

The diaphragm, which is innervated by the phrenic nerve, is the principal muscle of inspiration. Diaphragmatic activity is responsible for around 75% of the inhaled gas volume during quiet breathing, the remaining 25% being attributable to rib-cage movement. Contraction of the diaphragm leads to an increased depth of the thoracic cavity and an increase in abdominal pressure. The latter displaces the ribs outward and upward, thus enlarging the thoracic cage and lung and causing air to be drawn into the lungs by bulk flow. At end-inspiration, the respiratory muscles relax, allowing the lungs to recoil to FRC. During forced expiration, accessory muscles in the abdominal wall contract, thereby increasing abdominal pressure and forcing the diaphragm higher into the thorax.

Efficiency of breathing is reduced in the presence of hyperinflation (e.g.,

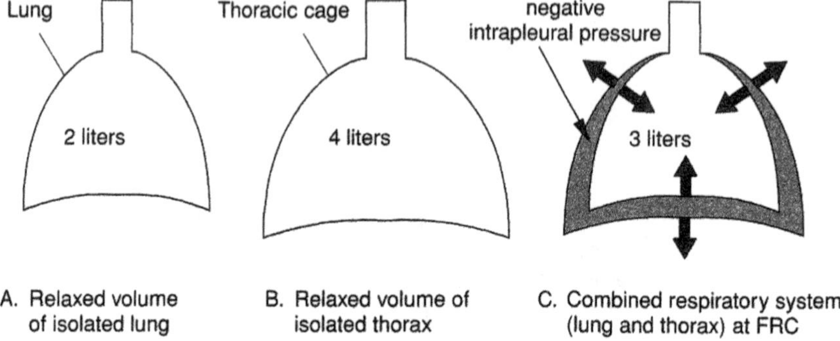

Figure 2 Relative relaxed volume of the isolated lungs, thorax, and intact respiratory system.

emphysema), due to the flattening of the diaphragm that occurs under these conditions. In adults, the downward-sloping ribs allow a significant increase in both the anteroposterior and lateral diameters of the thorax when the diaphragm descends. Infants have a limited ability to increase tidal or minute volume in response to increased ventilatory demands. This is largely because of their horizontally placed ribcage (11) (Fig. 3).

The adult rib-cage configuration develops gradually during the first 2 years

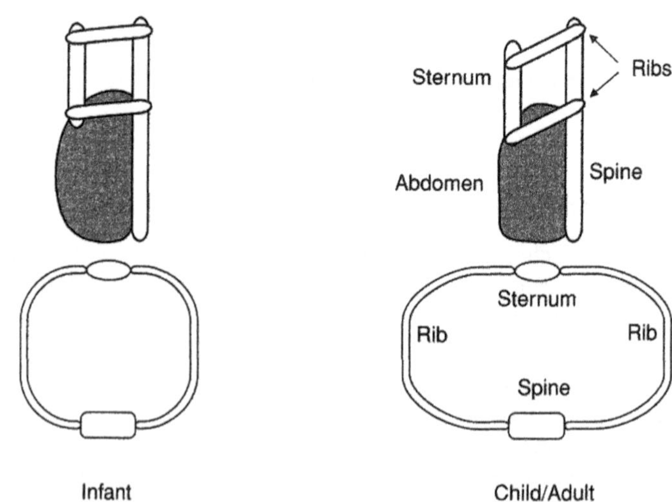

Figure 3 Changes in chest configuration from infancy to early adulthood. (Adapted from Ref. 11.)

of life. The external intercostal muscles play a vital role in stabilizing the rib cage. Although lung recoil is similar to that in adults, the outward recoil of the chest wall is low in infants and young children (12–14) (Fig. 4). Since FRC is determined by the balance of lung and chest wall recoil forces, this reduction in chest wall recoil will lead to a marked reduction in FRC unless it is maintained by other mechanisms (Fig. 5).

However, during the first months of life, infants partially compensate for this mechanical disadvantage by dynamically elevating their FRC. This is

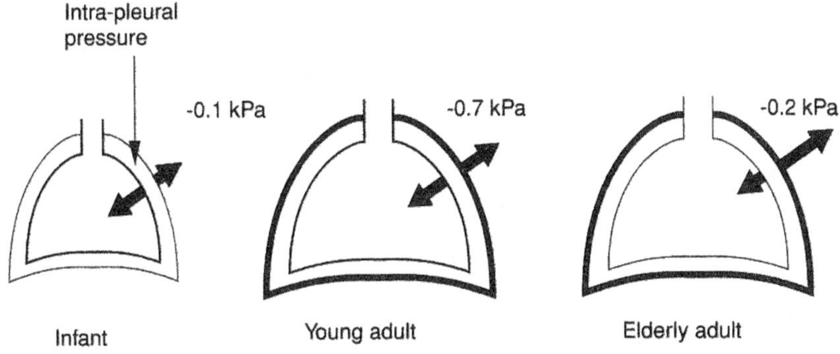

Figure 4 Determinants of transpulmonary pressure at functional residual capacity.

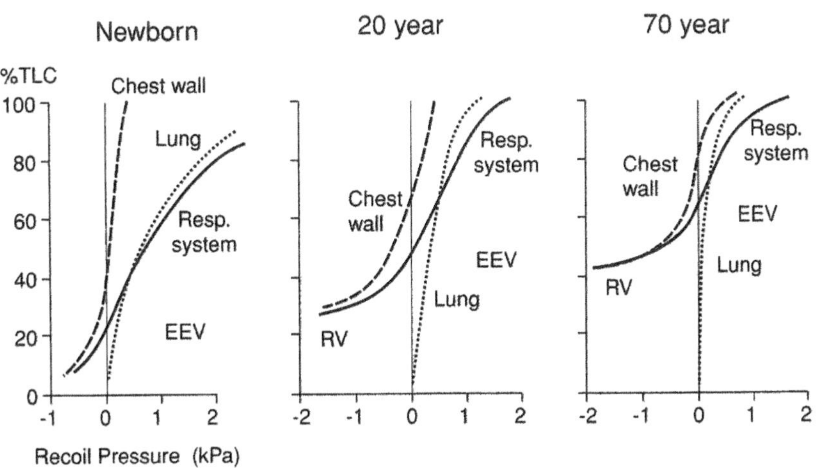

Figure 5 Shape of the pressure-volume curves of the chest wall, lung, and respiratory system. EEV=elastic equilibrium volume; RV=residual volume.

achieved by the combination of a short expiratory time (rapid respiratory rate) and modulation of expiratory flow by both laryngeal and postinspiratory diaphragmatic activity, which lengthens the expiratory time constant (15,16). End-expiratory volume is dynamically elevated until about 6 to 12 months of age, after which the passive characteristics of lung and chest wall appear to determine FRC, as in older subjects (17). While being an important physiological response to the anatomic immaturity of the chest wall, such modifications of breathing patterns, which are highly dependent on sleep state, may at times have an unpredictable influence on aerosolized drug delivery.

Maturational Changes in Chest Wall Compliance

The reduced chest wall compliance in early life may also have a marked effect on airway patency in infants, since, by supplying less distending pressure to the intrathoracic airways, there will be an increased tendency to airway closure during tidal breathing (18) (Fig. 6). Airway closure during tidal breathing (i.e., above FRC) is one of the main causes of hypoxemia in the very young as well as the elderly and will have a marked effect on the distribution of ventilation and inhaled aerosols (Sec. III.D) The highly compliant chest wall in young infants also increases the tendency to chest wall recession, particularly in the presence of lung disease and following premature delivery. This, in turn, increases the work of breathing, since much of the inspiratory effort is wasted in distorting the chest wall and may lead to respiratory failure in the presence of severe respiratory disease. Such chest wall distortion will also cause marked regional differences in transpulmonary pressure, which will affect distribution of inspired particles (Sec. III.B).

Ossification of the rib cage, sternum, and vertebrae begins in utero and continues until about age 25, while calcification of the costal cartilage can con-

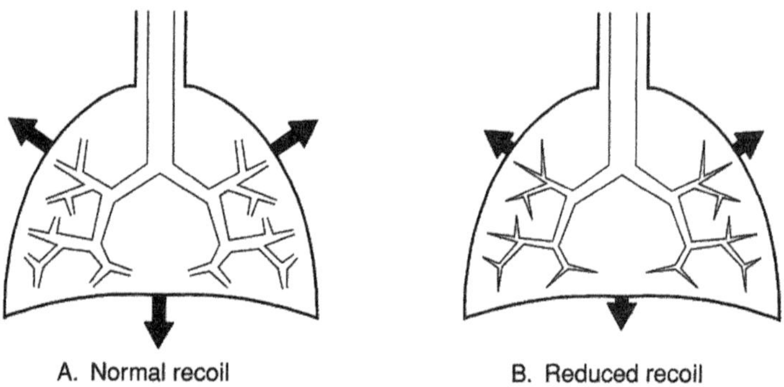

Figure 6 Effect of distending pressure on airway caliber.

tinue into old age. There is a progressive decrease in chest wall compliance with aging, due both to this increased calcification and narrowing of the intervertebral disk spaces. This results in lower force-generating capabilities, as reflected by the age-related decline in forced volumes and flows (19). Compliance is also reduced when the mobility of the chest wall is impaired (e.g., ankylosing spondylitis) and by obesity. This, together with decreased respiratory muscle strength in elderly patients, may have an adverse influence on their ability to generate high enough peak inspiratory flows (PIF) to actuate certain types of aerosol devices effectively (Sec. III.B, under "Peak Inspiratory Flow").

B. Normal Airway Anatomy

Air may enter the respiratory passages via the nose or mouth (Fig. 1), although—as a result of anatomical differences—babies rarely breathe through their mouths until at least 3–6 months of age (20,21). The route of inhalation during aerosol therapy is therefore difficult to standardize until children are old enough to use a mouthpiece, which is usually around 3 years of age.

The Nose

The function of the nose is to warm, humidify, and filter the air and to provide olfaction. Regrettably for those requiring aerosol therapy, it also acts as a very efficient barrier, with lung deposition being approximately halved during nose versus mouth breathing (22) (Sec. III.A, "Inhalation Route—The Influence of Nose Breathing"). The nasal vestibule, which is located immediately posterior to the external nasal opening, is lined with stratified squamous epithelium and numerous hairs that filter out large particulate matter. This vestibule funnels air towards the nasal valve. This part of the airway accounts for approximately 50% of the total resistance to respiratory airflow between the nostril and the alveoli, the relative contribution appearing to remain similar throughout life (23–25) (Sec. III.A, "Inhalation Route—The Influence of Nose Breathing," and Sec. II.B, under "Partitioning of Resistance").

The pattern of airflow changes from laminar before and at the nasal valve to that of a more turbulent nature posteriorly. The latter encourages impaction of large inhaled particles. The lateral nasal wall has turbinates or conchae that increase the nasal mucosal surfaces. When the mucous membrane is inflamed or irritated by head colds or allergic reactions, it swells and the entire nasal cavity may become blocked, again severely limiting aerosol delivery to the lower airways in nose-breathing subjects (26). It has been argued that the relatively large upper airway in infants (27) together with absence of nasal hair in the preadolescent, may make nasal breathing less of a problem for aerosol delivery in young children than might be expected. However, the upper airway appears to be a more efficient aerodynamic filter in infants than in older subjects (28).

The entire nasal cavity is lined by pseudostratified squamous epithelium with a cover of a thin layer of mucus providing immune and mechanical protection. Cilia beat in the mucus about 1000 times per minute and surface material is moved along at a rate of 3–25 mm/min. This transport is unidirectional and moves mucus and any trapped inhaled particles back toward the nasopharynx, where it is periodically swallowed. Drug delivery to the lung is therefore likely to be markedly reduced in the presence of excess mucous secretion. Further details of the anatomy and physiology of the nasal cavity can be found in published reviews (24,29,30).

The Pharynx and Larynx

Having passed through the nose or mouth, air and any inhaled particles it contains enters the pharynx, a funnel-shaped tube that starts at the internal nares (nasal passages) and extends to the level of the cricoid cartilage (the laryngeal cartilage lying immediately above the trachea) (Fig. 1). Its wall is composed of skeletal muscles and lined with mucous membrane. The pharynx is again a major site of impaction, particularly in the presence of high flows and large particle size. Age-related anatomic changes in the shape of the throat influence patterns of aerosol deposition (31). A recent study demonstrated that the deposition pattern of aerosolized rhDNase in patients with cystic fibrosis (CF) is strongly influenced by developmental changes in respiratory physiology and the clinical status of the patient. In children with CF, as much as 48% of the deposited aerosol was found in the pharynx. With increasing age and tidal volume, there was a decrease in upper airway deposition and more particles reached the lungs. Similarly, enhanced pulmonary deposition was found in patients with more severe airway disease (32). Deposition of particles in the upper airway is reduced if the subject inhales against an external resistance due to changes in the shape of the oropharyngeal aperture. Some drug delivery devices have been designed to take this into account in order to increase lung deposition (33).

The lowest portion of the pharynx (laryngopharynx) divides into the larynx, through which air passes on its way to the trachea and lungs, and the esophagus. The larynx, or voice box, is composed of pieces of cartilage and is lined with mucous membrane. The small larynx of young children is particularly susceptible to spasm when inflamed and may become partially or totally obstructed causing severe respiratory distress and inspiratory stridor (croup). As mentioned previously (Sec. II.A, under "Diaphragm and Rib Cage"), the larynx also plays a major role in modulating patterns of breathing, especially in young infants, which may, in turn, influence drug delivery to the lung.

The Trachea

The trachea is a cylindrical tube, 10–12 cm long, about half of which is extrathoracic and half intrathoracic. The trachea is lined with ciliated epithelium, which assists in filtering and warming inspired air. Its wall is composed of 16–20 incomplete (C-shaped) rings of cartilage joined together by fibrous and muscular tissue that provide rigidity to the trachea and prevent collapse when airway pressure becomes negative during inspiration. During coughing, the elastic, muscular posterior wall moves forward and narrows the trachea to a U-shaped slit. Coughing should therefore be avoided, if at all possible, during aerosol delivery. At the level of the fifth thoracic vertebra the trachea divides into the two primary bronchi. There is an internal cartilaginous ridge at the point of bifurcation, called the carina. This is lined with mucous membrane and is an extremely sensitive area, closely associated with the cough reflex (34).

The right bronchus is a shorter, wider tube than the left and the angle of branching from the trachea is only 20–30°. Consequently any foreign bodies that enter the trachea are more likely to be inhaled into the right main bronchus. This may also influence the distribution of aerosol delivery to the lungs. The trachea is funnel-shaped at birth, with the upper end wider than the lower, but it becomes cylindrical with increasing age. Tracheal growth is fastest during the first few years of life (35), but the ratio of cartilage to muscle appears to remain constant throughout childhood.

Intrapulmonary Airways

For air to reach the alveolar surface, it must pass through a series of branching airways that become progressively more numerous and smaller in diameter. The first divisions within the lung give rise to lobar and segmental main branches. This pattern of division varies and is probably genetically determined (36). The branching pattern resembles that of a tree, with large branches giving rise to successively smaller branches. Occasionally these are true dichotomous branches, but the subdivisions are more commonly of unequal diameter and length. The number of branches between the hilum and periphery varies between 8 in some segments of the upper lobe to 24 in the longest segments of the lower lobes. It is thus difficult to describe the lung in terms of a simple model, though many have tried (37–40). Whichever model is used, it appears that the diameters of the conducting airways are well designed to ensure optimal conditions for airflow.

The average number and dimensions of airways in the different orders are given in Fig. 7. This branching pattern is the most efficient way of producing a large surface area within a small volume. The decrease in airway caliber (from 1.8 cm to 0.6 mm) together with a relatively small increase in cross-sectional area (from 2.5 to 180 cm^2) between the trachea and terminal bronchioles provides optimal conditions for bulk flow of air through the conducting airways. Dichotomous branching continues in the terminal airways that comprise the respiratory zone and acini, but there is very little subsequent reduction in diameter of the respiratory bronchioles and alveolar ducts with each new generation (0.6

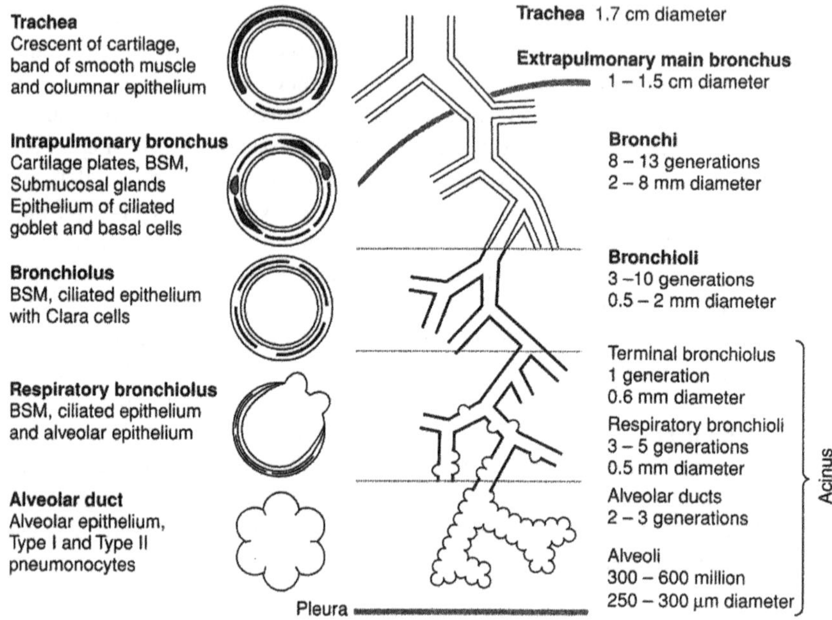

Figure 7 Number and dimensions of airways in the adult lung and the structure of the airway wall.

to 0.3 mm). Consequently, total cross-sectional area of the airways virtually doubles with each generation beyond generation 16 [rising from 180 to 10,000 cm^2 (100 m^2)]. The cross-sectional alveolar surface area in adults approaches 150 m^2, considerably larger than that of a tennis court! The way in which airway dimensions change between the trachea and the peripheral airways has a marked influence on the partitioning of airway resistance, ventilation, velocity distribution of airflow, and both the distribution and deposition of inhaled particles (Sec. II.B, under "Partitioning of Resistance", and III.D, "Distribution of Ventilation").

The airways are known as bronchi while they contain cartilage in the wall; thereafter they are called bronchioles or bronchioli, which in the adult are usually less than 1 mm in diameter. There are approximately 8–13 divisions from the trachea to the smallest bronchi, depending upon the length of the main pathway, with a further 3–10 divisions of bronchioli before the terminal bronchiolus. The bronchioli have an internal diameter of 0.3–1 mm, the total number in the two lungs being about 25,000. The cartilage provides essential support to the extrathoracic airways, preventing deformation against the negative airway pressure that develops during inspiratory efforts. The anatomic structure of the large airways generally prevents any significant reduction in airway patency due to bronchospasm or abnormalities of the mucosa and renders the caliber of the intrathoracic bronchi less dependent on changes in lung volume than that of smaller peripheral airways.

The diameter of the bronchioli reaches a peak in the fourth decade and declines thereafter. Declining small airway diameter may contribute to the decrement in expiratory flow with ageing. However, since peripheral airways contribute marginally to total resistance of the airways in adults (Sec. II.B, under "Partitioning of Resistance") age has no significant effect on airway resistance when adjusted for lung volume (41).

Partitioning of Resistance

The extent to which different types of airways contribute to total airway resistance has a major impact on manifestation of airway disease at different ages. It also influences the methods used to assess the nature, severity, and response to therapy of such disease, and the design of devices that aim to deliver drugs directly into the lungs. During normal, quiet respiration, the largest component of airways resistance resides in the upper airways, with nasal resistance contributing approximately 50% total resistance during nose breathing. During mouth breathing, the trachea represents the site of the smallest airway cross-sectional area and highest resistance and, together with the glottis and larynx, is responsible for almost 70% of total airway resistance. Within the lung itself, resistance is mainly in the larger airways, those with diameters of 3–8 mm, contributing up to 20% during mouth breathing. Although the small airways are themselves tiny, the dichotomously branching pattern of the bronchial tree results in an increasingly large number of airways in peripheral generations (Sec. II.B). This results in very low resistance of each generation of small airways, so that in total they contribute only about 10% of total airway resistance. Consequently, most of the small airways can be damaged or obstructed before any symptoms occur and before conventional lung function tests, in particular measures of airway resistance, show any functional loss. This is why the small airways are sometimes labeled "the silent zone of the lung" (42). Newer methods of aerosol-derived airway morphometry should make it easier to distinguish small airway and alveolar dimensions (43).

Structure of the Airway Wall

Since so much aerosol therapy is directed toward reducing airway inflammation and/or minimizing bronchoconstriction, some knowledge of airway wall structure is essential for those prescribing and administering such treatment (44). The left and right main bronchi have the same wall configuration as the trachea. Within the lung, the horseshoe-shaped cartilage gives way to irregular plates of cartilage; these reduce in number and size as the airways decrease in diameter. In addition, within the wall, there are bundles of smooth muscle cells and submucosal glands. Bronchioli have a wall of connective tissue and smooth muscle. The walls of bronchi and bronchioli are supplied with oxygenated blood by the bronchial circulation. The terminal bronchiolus is the last subdivision of the bronchial tree in which the lumen is surrounded by a continuous layer of cuboidal epithelium and a subepithelium (Fig. 7).

The portion of the lung distal to one terminal bronchiolus is called an acinus. Beyond each terminal bronchiolus there are two to five generations of respiratory airways, which have part of their wall lined by cuboidal cells and part by flattened alveolar cells. A typical acinus contains about 14 of these respiratory bronchioli, each of which has shallow alveoli in its wall. Beyond these are alveolar ducts (approximately 100 per acinus) lined by alveolar epithelium. These have a diameter ranging from 0.6 to 2 mm and an increasing number of alveoli opening from their walls. Between the alveoli is a thin spiral of collagen and elastin that acts as a scaffold but is also able to lengthen like a spring. In the adult lung there are between 300 and 600 million alveoli, each measuring about 250–300 μm when expanded (45). As a result of the enormous increase in surface area, bulk flow of air decreases rapidly within the respiratory zone until movement of air within alveoli is entirely by diffusion.

Surface Epithelium

The airways condition the inspired air before it reaches the gas-exchange region by warming and humidifying the air and removing pollutants. While this partly depends upon the branching pattern, the cells lining the airways also play an important part. In the trachea and the major airways, the epithelium is pseudostratified and columnar; that is, all cells rest on a basement membrane but not all reach the airway lumen. Further into the lungs the epithelium is columnar, and by the terminal bronchioli, the cells are cuboidal in shape. In the human, four major cell types make up the surface epithelium (46).

Ciliated cells are present throughout the airways as far as the respiratory bronchioli. The surface of the ciliated cell is covered by cilia, about 200 per cell, which beat synchronously with those on adjacent cells, the stroke being generally in a cranial direction (47). The cilia move the overlying mucous layer only with their tips, which have hooklets that probably help grasp the mucous layer. Genetically determined defects in this arrangement may lead to dyskinetic or immotile cilia and impairment of mucociliary transport. In the human trachea there are between 6 and 7 thousand mucus-secreting *goblet cells* per square millimeter (48). Their density decreases toward the periphery, with few found in the bronchioli. In the adult between 30 and 40% of the total cells in the larger airways are mucous cells. The number of mucous cells increases in chronic bronchitis and in smokers. The *basal cells* are thought to be the major stem cell from which ciliated and mucous cells drive. They may also strengthen the adhesion of the overlying columnar cells to the basement membrane. In the adult, surface epithelium is replaced slowly, with less than 1% of the cells undergoing division (49).

In addition, there are *Clara cells*, which are restricted to the terminal bronchioli, where they make up 20% of the cell population; they are the principal stem cells of the small airways. They may produce a bronchiolar surfactant and have oxidase activity as well as being involved in fluid absorption.

The alveolar epithelium is made up of *type I cells* or *pneumonocytes,* which cover most of the alveolar surface. These prevent fluid loss and form the thin gas-exchange barrier. *Type II cells* are cuboidal and are twice as numerous as the type I cell but cover only about 7% of the surface area. They are metabolically active and responsible for both epithelial cell renewal and synthesizing surfactant, a phospholipid that reduces surface tension forces in the lung (50). Airway epithelium is differentiated by 12 weeks' gestation, whereas alveolar epithelium differentiates from 23 weeks of gestation (51).

The Submucosal Glands

The submucosal glands are continuous with the epithelium and are found from the trachea to the end of the small bronchi. A narrow ciliated tract is continuous with a collecting duct that leads into mucous and serous tubules. The submucosal glands are the major source of tracheobronchial mucus and increase in chronic bronchitis and asthma. Glands appear early in gestation; during childhood, the gland area is relatively large in comparison with that in the adult (52). This may have implications for relative hypersecretion in small airways during early life (53). Any airway obstruction as the result of excess secretions or mucus will obviously have a deleterious effect on aerosol delivery to the more distal airways.

Bronchial Smooth Muscle

Bronchial smooth muscle is found in the gaps between the cartilage plates in the trachea and extrapulmonary bronchi, whereas in the intrapulmonary airways, muscle entirely circles the lumen internal to the cartilage. This is in two spirals such that, with contraction, the airways shorten and constrict. Muscle first appears at 6–8 weeks of gestation and has been found in all the airways to the adult level by 26 weeks of gestation (54). The muscle in the airway wall in humans is structurally mature at birth and has been since the third trimester. At this time human lung buds demonstrate spontaneous contractions and also respond to carbachol, acetylcholine, and isoproterenol (55).

Measurements of bronchial smooth muscle in fetal life and infancy show that there is an increase up to 1 year of age. There is a particularly rapid increase in the relative amount of bronchiolar smooth muscle immediately after birth (54), which is probably related to the change to air breathing. There is excessive bronchial smooth muscle in babies who have been artificially ventilated, those with bronchopulmonary dysplasia, and in children with asthma (54,56,57), which increases reactivity and may affect aerosol delivery due to the resultant diminution of airway caliber. Relative changes in bronchial reactivity through life remain controversial (Sec. III.C, under "Maturational Changes in Airway Responsiveness"). In animal studies, maximal airway narrowing during bronchoconstriction has been shown to be greater in immature than mature rabbits and may result in increased ventilation inhomogeneity in early life (58,59). However, while changes in airway resistance are reflected by morphometrically assessed changes in airway caliber during methacholine challenge (58), the mechanisms underlying this association have yet to be elucidated (60) (Sec. III.C, under "Maturational Changes in Airway Responsiveness").

Bronchial Arteries and Veins

The bronchial arteries originate from the aorta or intercostal arteries, and there are commonly two to each lung entering at the hilum. They divide to form a subepithelial plexus and an adventitial plexus on either side of the bronchial smooth muscle layer. The blood flow to these arteries is about 1% of the cardiac output, but it covers a large surface area. True pulmonary veins drain the trachea and upper bronchi and return blood to the right atrium, while the veins in the more peripheral airways drain via the pulmonary veins to the left atrium. The bronchial supply appears at the end of the first trimester and extends down the airway wall as the bronchial smooth muscle, cartilage, and glands differentiate. There are also bronchial blood vessels in the adventitia of large pulmonary arteries and veins.

The primary function of the bronchial circulation is to supply oxygen and nourishment to the lung, but by maintaining the fluid balance it also facilitates efficient mucociliary clearance. It also responds to inhaled noxious substances by vasodilatation (61). Sympathetic and parasympathetic nerves control the bronchial vasculature. Stimulation of the α receptors causes vasoconstriction, while stimulation of the β receptors results in vasodilatation. Changes in temperature of the inspired airflow will influence blood flow. However, neuromodulators given by aerosol do not have a great effect on blood flow (62). The bronchial circulation is important for the uptake of drugs from aerosols in that any drug passing through the epithelium will diffuse into the bronchial vessels. It will then move downstream to the periphery of the lung or will return to the heart via the bronchial veins and thus into the systemic system. This will lead to modification of effect on peripheral smooth muscle. The bronchial circulation may therefore be of assistance in delivering drugs to other areas in the lung and elsewhere in the body but could also decrease delivery to the more peripheral airways. A vasodilator administered at the same time as aerosol therapy will increase absorbency of a drug that could be exploited therapeutically (63).

Interstitium

The framework of the lung is made up of bundles of elastic and collagen fibers, which extend from the larger airways to the alveoli and pleura. During development, collagen appears first in the primitive airways and blood vessels, while immature elastin appears in what will become the mouths of the alveoli. Both types of fiber increase in number after birth, with elastin contributing approximately 12% of dry lung weight by about 6 months. The proportion of collagen continues to increase throughout childhood. Though collagen and elastin are relatively indistensible, they can move with respect to each other, thereby facilitating lung expansion. They also make a major contribution to the elastic recoil of the lung (approximately equal to that of surface tension forces), thereby providing an essential traction to maintain airway patency and influencing the pattern of ventilation distribution throughout the lungs (Secs. III.C. and III.D).

Innervation and Receptors

Within the lung there are nerve bundles running alongside airways and blood vessels as far as the acinar region; within the alveolar region, individual fibers are found. Nerve plexuses supply the submucosal glands, bronchial smooth muscle, and epithelium. The lungs are innervated by afferent sensory nerves and efferent motor nerves. Sensory nerves respond through a central nervous system–mediator reflex arc. Irritant or rapidly adapting receptors within the epithelium and between smooth muscle cells respond to chemical or particulate irritants. Afferent C-fibers are also located in the epithelium and between smooth muscle cells and are activated by chemical and mechanical stimuli. Both lead to reflex bronchoconstriction via efferent cholinergic motor nerves. Slowly adapting sensory receptors in the smooth muscle of central airways respond to airway stretch and maintain respiratory drive.

The efferent nerves to the airways are autonomic excitatory cholinergic nerves and inhibitory nonadrenergic, noncholinergic (NANC) nerves. Cholinergic nerves release acetylcholine into the bronchial smooth muscle and submucosal glands to cause bronchoconstriction and an increase in the production of mucus. NANC nerves provide inhibitory bronchodilation via vasoactive intestinal peptide (VIP), and recent evidence suggests that neural nitric oxide may also be involved. There are no functional adrenergic nerves to the bronchial smooth muscle, but they do help regulate mucus production and bronchial and pulmonary blood flow. Bronchoconstriction can, however, be inhibited by circulating epinephrine acting via β receptors. In addition, the airway epithelium produces a relaxing factor, which may be nitric oxide (64). Further discussion on the pharmacology of airways and receptors is beyond the scope of this chapter but has been the subject of several excellent reviews (65–69).

In humans, the nerves appear early in development alongside bronchial smooth muscle; at birth, the infant has as many nerves as the adult. In vitro studies show a similar level of responsiveness of tracheal muscle between 36 days of gestation and birth but a decrease in response to acetylcholine after 4 weeks of age. A greater number of neuropeptides causing bronchodilation has been reported in the newborn than in children over 3 years of age (70). We have little information on the development of receptors, although functional studies by Tepper (71) suggest that they are present in the first year of life. Indeed, despite the minimal bronchodilator response in young infants, there is clear evidence that β_2-adrenoreceptors are present and functional in the airways from birth. During infancy, nebulized salbutamol reduces the response to inhaled histamine or nebulised water (72–75). Current data suggest that the number of β_2-receptors may remain relatively consistent through life. However, the level of sensitivity appears to peak in early adult life, with a progressive increase throughout the early childhood years and a decline in responsiveness with increasing age in patients over 40 years of age (76) (Sec. III.C, under "Maturational Changes in Airway Responsiveness").

C. Factors Influencing Airway Structure and Function

Anything that influences the size and elasticity of the lungs or airway caliber may affect the efficacy of aerosol therapy in any particular individual. There is increasing recognition that the level of airway function may be established during fetal development and the first year of life, with little subsequent remodeling (77–79). Adverse events during fetal life and infancy may therefore have long-term and irreversible effects throughout life and have a significant effect on aerosol delivery and deposition (2,4,80). Since airway structure and function in the adult are dependent on normal growth and development of the lung during early life, an appreciation of the sequence and timing of the major developmental changes is an important prerequisite to understanding respiratory disease and its treatment. Several recent articles have described pre- and postnatal lung growth in detail (51,81,82).

Early Lung Development

The lung appears as a diverticulum of the foregut at 4 weeks of gestation. As a result of dichotomous branching of this bud within the surrounding mesenchyme, all airways to the level of the terminal bronchiolus are present by 16 weeks of gestation (83) (Fig. 8). Further division leads to the development of the respiratory airways, nearly all of which are present by birth. Airway wall structure is mature by 26 weeks of gestation (54,84), and by this stage type II cells in the respiratory region are capable of producing surfactant. Although gas exchange is feasible earlier, as witnessed by the survival of some extremely premature infants from about 23 weeks gestation onward, true alveoli first appear at

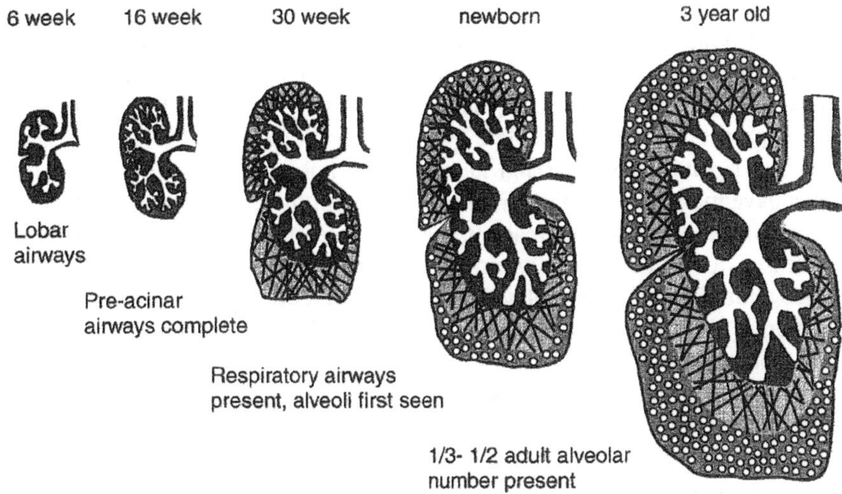

Figure 8 The main features of lung development.

around 30 weeks of gestation. By term, approximately one-third to one-half the adult number are present (85,86). The blood/gas barrier is the same thickness as in the adult. The alveolar stage is followed by an additional and final stage in lung development—that of microvascular maturation (87). In the human lung, rapid alveolar multiplication occurs during the last few weeks of intrauterine life and the first few months of postnatal life. A large proportion of the human lung looks mature by 6 months of age in that many parenchymal septa no longer exhibit the double capillary network needed for the formation of new interalveolar walls. This does not, however, mean that alveolar formation is terminated A slower phase probably continues up to at least 2 years of age. In the adult lung, there is collateral ventilation between alveoli via the pores of Kohn. These are not present at birth or for the first year of life; they then gradually increase in number. This will influence the distribution of inhaled particles, especially in the presence of airway obstruction. Lung volume is closely related to the weight and length of the infant (85,88,89), but there is more controversy about the relationship between airway and lung or body size (2–4), as discussed below (Sec. II.C, under "Dysanaptic Growth").

Postnatal Lung Growth

While most of our knowledge about prenatal lung growth comes from structural studies, information about postnatal growth has been largely derived from lung function studies. In the first 2 years after birth, alveoli multiply with their accompanying arteries and veins. The time point of completion of alveolar formation remains the subject of debate. Studies have suggested varying times between 2 and 20 years of age, but it seems likely that most human alveolar development is virtually complete by 18 months of age (90,91). The final adult number depends upon size and lung volume, but from early in development boys have more alveoli than girls for their height (45,91). After multiplication is complete, the alveoli increase in diameter and surface area as lung volume increases. Alveoli are 50–100 μm at birth, increasing to 300 μm in the adult. Once multiplication is complete, airways and alveoli appear to grow in a proportionate (i.e., isotropic manner) at least until puberty (Sec. II.C, under "Dysanaptic Growth").

In healthy individuals, most parameters of respiratory function remain remarkably constant when related to either surface area or body size, reflecting the fact that respiration is closely attuned to the metabolic requirements of the body (Table 1). However the underlying factors determining these parameters may vary considerably according to age (2,4,89). Indeed, the rapid somatic growth that occurs during the first year of life is accompanied by major developmental changes in respiratory physiology that may influence both the pattern of respiratory disease (92,93) and that of aerosol delivery.

Lung volume increases approximately 10-fold between 1 month and 7 years (Table 1), but it then slows down until the age of 18 years (Fig. 9). The associated increase in elastic recoil pressure combined with a progressive decrease in closing volume will affect patterns of aerosol distribution and may

Table 1 "Typical" Values of Lung Function in Healthy Individuals[a]

	Preterm	Newborn	1 Year	7 Year	Adult
Body weight (kg)	1	3	10	25	70
Crown–heel length (cm)	35	50	75	120	175
Respiratory rate (min^{-1})	60	45	30	20	15
Tidal volume (mL)	7	21	70	180	500
Anatomic dead space (mL)	3	6	20	50	150
Maximal flow at FRC ($mL{\cdot}s^{-1}$)	80	150	300	—	—
Functional residual capacity (mL)	25	85	250	750	2100
Lung compliance ($mL{\cdot}kPa^{-1}$)	15	50	150	500	2000
Airway resistance ($kPa{\cdot}L^{-1}{\cdot}s$)	8	4	1.5	0.4	0.2
Specific compliance (kPa^{-1})	0.6	0.6	0.6	0.7	0.8
Specific conductance ($s^{-1}{\cdot}kPa^{-1}$)	5.0	2.9	2.7	2.7	2.3

[a]For approximate conversion from SI to traditional units (kPa to cmH_2O), divide lung compliance, specific compliance, and specific conductance by 10 and multiply airway resistance by 10 (1 kPa= 10.2 cmH_2O).

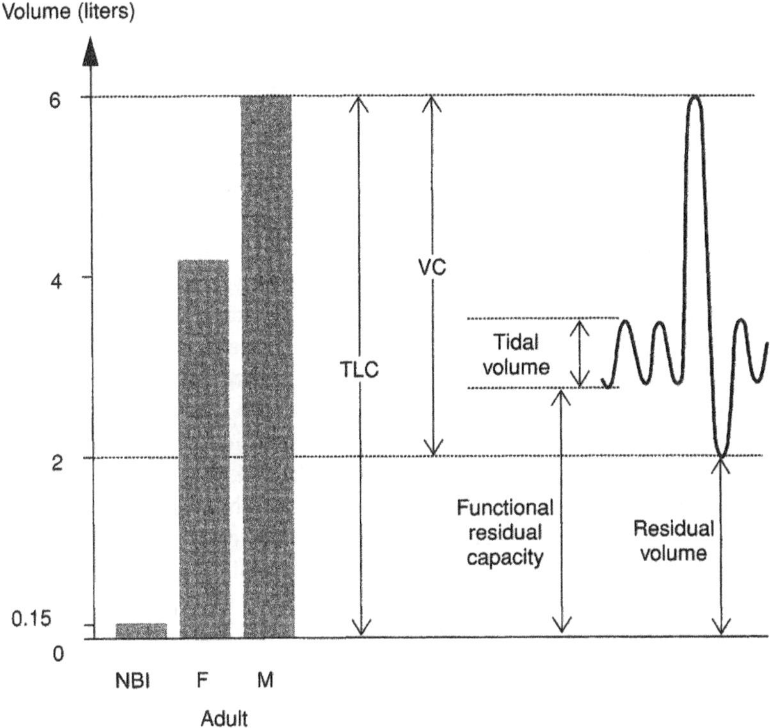

Figure 9 Growth and divisions of lung volumes.

explain the increased mixing efficiency in children during growth (18,93,94). Lung growth is rapid as children enter puberty and continues until the completion of skeletal growth in girls and for 2 to 3 years beyond that in boys (95). Forced expiratory volume in 1 s (FEV_1) and forced vital capacity (FVC) increase up to about 20 years of age in females and 27 years of age in males. These then diminish with advancing age, this decline being greater in males than females and more rapid in patients with increased airway reactivity (41). The factors determining residual volume (RV) change with age. In young adults, it is reached when the respiratory muscles cannot compress the lung any further; whereas in children and older adults, it reflects the patency of small airways and the duration of expiratory effort. RV increases by approximately 50% between 20 and 70 years of age due to air trapping and loss of lung recoil (Fig. 5). During this same period, vital capacity (VC) decreases to about 75% of the best values achieved within an individual.

Postnatal Airway Growth

In a study of fetal and infant lungs, a linear and continuous increase in airway size, which was not interrupted by birth, was observed (54). Between birth and adulthood, airways increase in diameter and length symmetrically throughout the lung two- to threefold in total (54,96). While Horsfield reported that the peripheral airways were large relative to the proximal airways (38), Hogg et al. (97) suggested that the peripheral airways may contribute more to total airway resistance in the first 5 years of life than in older subjects, though this has never been confirmed. Functional studies suggest that airway caliber is relatively large compared to lung volume at birth and is enhanced in females (92,98–100). Thus, while airway resistance is much higher in infants than adults due to the small absolute size of the airways, specific airway conductance (the reciprocal of resistance, corrected for lung volume) is similar in a nose-breathing infant and in a mouth-breathing adult (101) (see Sec. III. A, "Inhalation Route—The Influence of Nose Breathing"). As mentioned previously, the lack of outward chest wall recoil has a marked influence on the caliber of the peripheral airways during early life and predisposes their closure during tidal breathing (2) (Sec. II, A). This not only impairs gas exchange but, together with the small absolute size of the airways, renders the infant and young child particularly susceptible to airway obstruction and contributes to the high prevalence of wheezing during the first year of life (92,93,102).

Longitudinal estimates of lung and airway growth demonstrate a high degree of tracking within individuals, with increase in age and lung volume; in other words, an individual's airway function tends to remain in the same relative position within a population throughout life (3,103–106).

Dysanaptic Growth

The concept of dysanapsis [i.e., disproportionate growth of the airways and lung parenchyma (Fig. 10)] is potentially relevant to aerosol therapy. The relationship of airway to lung volume may play a major role in determining the pattern of deposition of inhaled particles in the bronchial tree (107). Many authors have concluded that airways and lung parenchyma develop disproportionately in size at least during the first few years of life (105,108–113) because the conducting airways are complete in number at birth and increase only in size, whereas alveoli increase both in size and in number (85, 91, 96). After about 2 years of age, parenchymal growth is mainly due to alveolar enlargement. It is therefore likely that airways and airspaces grow isotropically (i.e., in proportion to each other) thereafter throughout childhood (3). A recent longitudinal study suggested that airways and airspaces continue to grow isotropically in boys during adolescence, whereas in girls, airway growth lags behind that of the parenchyma at this stage (114).

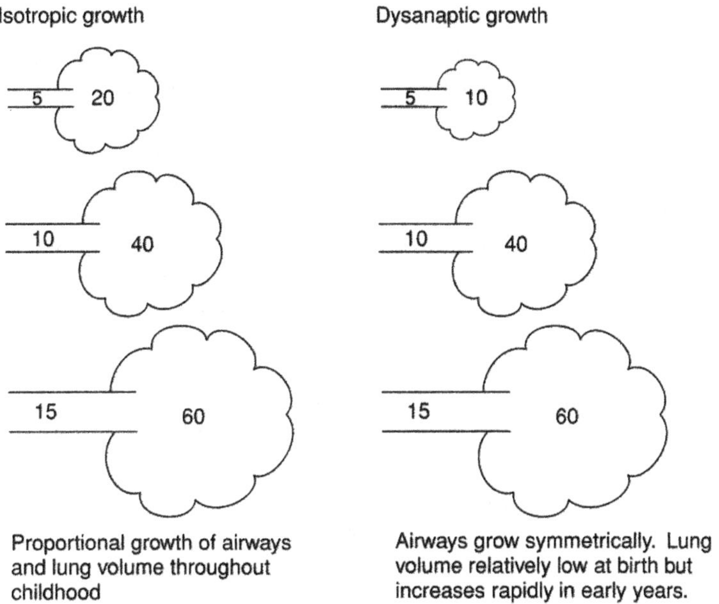

Figure 10 Diagrammatic representation of isotropic and dysanaptic growth of the lungs and airways.

Effect of Gender

Gender-and age-related differences in airway function and their implications have been discussed previously (3,4). Although lung volume and alveolar number are greater in boys than girls (115–117), airway function is diminished in boys compared with girls during both infancy and childhood (118–123). Girls have larger expiratory flows than boys (99,118,124), and the narrower peripheral airways of boys seem to predispose them to wheeze (77,113,122,125,126). The relatively lower airflow in boys prepubertally may also result in gender differences in aerosol delivery and distribution.

During growth, vital capacity increases more slowly in girls than boys, as indicated by the rise in RV/TLC during growth among girls. Thus, although girls have wider and/or shorter airways in childhood than boys, by adulthood boys have larger airways relative to lung size than girls. This enhanced airway growth in adolescent males (3,121) may partly explain the more marked clinical improvement in males with respiratory disease as they become adults (114,127,128). Tracheal size does not differ between sexes during early life (129), but adult males have larger tracheas than do females (109,110).

Effect of Ethnic Group

Marked ethnic differences in infant mortality and respiratory morbidity have been reported (130). Prematurely delivered Afro-Caribbean infants are less likely to develop the respiratory distress syndrome (RDS) than white infants of similar gestational age (131), which suggests that the respiratory system is either more mature or that airway function is enhanced in black preterm infants (132). Some of these differences may be attributed to differences in nasal anatomy, since the lower total airway resistance found in Afro-Caribbean infants when compared with Caucasian infants of similar age and weight (101) was accounted for by their lower nasal resistance (23). Such differences would be expected to influence both breathing patterns and the distribution of inhaled aerosols.

In adults and older children, lung volume and forced expiratory flows are lower in black than white subjects, based on values predicted from standing height (133,134). These discrepancies have been largely attributed to ethnic differences in trunk–leg ratio, since no such discrepancies are observed when respiratory function is related to sitting height.

Aging

Changes in respiratory function associated with aging have recently been reviewed (19). Physiological aging of the lung is associated with:

Dilatation of alveoli, enlargement of airspaces, and a decrease in surface area for gas exchange.
Reduction in lung elastic recoil to support peripheral airways, which contributes to an increased residual volume and FRC (Figs. 5 and 6).
Diminished chest wall compliance.
Decreased respiratory muscle strength.
Diminished expiratory flows suggestive of small airway disease.
Increased inhomogeneity of ventilation/perfusion ($\dot{V}/\dot{Q}$) distribution due to premature closing of dependent airways (see Sec. III.D, under "Determinants of Regional Ventilation").
Decreased carbon monoxide transfer, reflecting the loss of surface area.

D. Adverse Developmental Influences on Airway Caliber

In addition to the natural influences of factors such as growth, gender, and aging that affect all individuals, there are numerous additional factors that may affect lung and airway function. Adverse influences during infancy and early childhood may operate by:

Diminishing airway or alveolar growth and hence maximal lung and airway size attained.

Increasing airway responsiveness to allergens, viruses, and air pollutants in later childhood or adult life.

Impairing development of collagen and elastin in the lung parenchyma, with secondary effects on airway function or by some combination of all three of the listed factors.

The age-related decline in respiratory function commencing in mid-adult life may be more rapid or reach a critical threshold at an earlier age in those in whom maximal fetal and early childhood growth potential has not been achieved (77,135–137).

Early Influences

Recent epidemiological evidence has shown a relationship between adult airway function and birth weight (77,138). During early intrauterine life, adverse factors will influence airway growth (135,139,140), while factors having their effect in later weeks of gestation and infancy will affect alveolar development (141). Abnormalities in airway branching cannot be corrected once the period of airway multiplication is complete. Thus airflow is likely to be abnormal in these subjects throughout life. Infants with congenital diaphragmatic hernia, renal agenesis and dysplasia, and thoracic dystrophy all have reduced airways and subsequently fewer alveoli (142,143). Both pre- and postnatal experimental studies have shown that nutrition, gas tensions, hypoxia, or hyperoxia, amniocentesis, drugs, and nicotine all affect alveolar growth and airway responsiveness (144,142).

Pre- and Postnatal Therapy

The use of glucocorticoids to accelerate lung maturation or prevent inflammation may affect lung growth, especially since lung morphogenesis is regulated by glucocorticoid-affecting growth factors (145,146). To date, human functional studies have not demonstrated differences in lung function between babies who have been treated with betamethasone and those who have not (147). However, it must be remembered that the tools currently available for assessing lung volumes and airway caliber in infants (89) are not able to detect a reduction in alveolar number if this has been compensated for by increased alveolar size. Experimental structural studies in animals (144,148,149) have shown that the administration of glucocorticoids prevents normal alveolar development (87,150) and reduces the multiplication of bronchial smooth muscle cells in culture (151).

Inhaled terbutaline does not seem to affect epithelial appearance (152) but β-agonists do appear to inhibit proliferation of smooth muscle cells (153). Long-term use of bronchodilators may therefore lead to abnormally small amounts of muscle in the airway walls, which, in turn, could lead to changes in airway growth and responsiveness Such factors must be taken into account in prescribing corticosteroids during fetal and early postnatal life and warrant long-term follow-up studies of subsequent lung growth.

Influence of Exposure to Tobacco Smoke and Nicotine

Exposure to tobacco smoke, whether pre- or postnatally, has a detrimental effect on lung health and respiratory function throughout life (154). The age-related decline in airway function is accelerated in those who smoke, and the prevalence of respiratory illness greatly increased (155–160). The potential effects of smoking during pregnancy on lung and airway development may include structural alterations (161) as well as interference with the control of respiration (162,163) and the developing immune system (164). Animal studies have shown that maternal exposure to cigarette smoke or nicotine results in offspring with small lungs and decreased airspaces (144), reduced elastin production (165), and increased collagen around the airways (166). These findings fit with results from functional studies in human infants shortly after birth, which have shown changes in the pattern of breathing and diminished airflow in those whose mothers smoked during pregnancy (100,167,168). Recent measurements in preterm infants have shown that these changes are evident at least 7 weeks before an infant is due to be born (124). Such changes in airway function may be sufficient to alter both the need for and response to aerosol therapy.

Neonatal Lung Disease and Subsequent Airway Function

Premature delivery has little effect on overall alveolar multiplication or airway growth (54,85,169), although there is some evidence of increased bronchial reactivity in later childhood among those born very preterm (170–172). Artificial ventilation leads to long-term abnormalities of alveolar growth and architecture and also influences airway wall structure (54,56,173), these changes being worse in infants who develop bronchopulmonary dysplasia (BPD) after ventilatory assistance (174–176). Wheezing occurs more frequently in adolescents and young adults who had BPD in infancy than in age-matched controls of similar or normal birth weight (177). Follow-up studies have suggested relatively mild long-term sequelae in survivors (178), although an increased prevalence of symptoms and/or reduced airway function is still present in adults (179). With the increased survival of severely affected infants and more sophisticated methods of assessment, recent studies have demonstrated a greater prevalence of abnormalities. Abnormal central and peripheral airway function has been detected in survivors with chronic respiratory symptoms, while there is evidence of unequal ventilation (see Sec. III.D) even in those without symptoms (135,180,181).

Asthma and Cystic Fibrosis

Two of the commonest diseases for which aerosol therapy is prescribed during childhood are asthma and cystic fibrosis. Asthma might be expected to interfere with normal development of the lungs and airways. However, despite intensive investigation, this remains a very controversial area (182). Although reduced expiratory flows have been documented prior to bronchodilator therapy, several longitudinal studies have suggested that anti-inflammatory treatment improves airway caliber to within the normal range (183–185). Airways of symptomatic teenagers with asthma seem to grow in parallel with those of their asymptomatic peers, albeit with airway size remaining smaller. Asthmatic adults who have had symptoms since childhood have lower flows for any given lung size, and airway closure occurs at a greater lung volume when they enter adulthood. These differences may reflect irreversible processes such as smaller airway geometry, reduced alveolar attachments, or reduced lung elastic recoil (186).

In cystic fibrosis (CF), the structural abnormalities appear to result from the repeated injury of infections that initially affect the small airways, causing serious impairment of growth of the intraacinar structures (187–189). Further damage is caused by the collapse of nonventilated lung parenchyma and abscesses, and airways become obstructed by mucus (190–192). In view of the thick mucous secretions and inflamed airways, specialized devices may need to be developed to optimize drug delivery to the lung of patients with CF, especially during infancy and childhood (193–197).

III. Developmental Changes in Respiratory Function That Will Influence Aerosol Therapy

Having discussed relevant aspects of lung and airway structure that may influence the efficacy of aerosol therapy, it is important that we consider the potential impact of differences in respiratory function between individuals as a result of age, maturity, or clinical status. Particular problems may be encountered in delivering drugs to the respiratory tract of young children as a result of anatomic and physiological variations due to age (198). The most relevant aspects of respiratory physiology with respect to aerosol therapy include the

Route of inhalation
Pattern of breathing
Airway caliber and responsiveness
Distribution of ventilation

A. Inhalation Route—The Influence of Nose Breathing

Nasal filtration has been shown to reduce pulmonary deposition of inhaled aerosol by up to 50% of that observed during mouth breathing (22). This presents a particular problem in infants who are preferential nose breathers (20) and children who are too young to use a mouthpiece Thus, while lung deposition of jet-nebulized medications varies from 8 to 17% in adults (199–202), as little as 1% may be deposited in the lungs of wheezy infants (203).

Patient-related factors in nebulised drug delivery to children have been reviewed recently (204,205). During childhood, nasal deposition appears to increase with age. This may reflect the influence of changes in tidal volume and flows (Sec. III.B, "Pattern of Breathing") as much as any structural changes with growth, since nasal deposition increases with increasing flow and particle size (206). Although most young children nose breathe at rest, the mode of breathing during nebulization is unclear, making estimations of drug delivered at this age particularly difficult. Every attempt must therefore be made to train young children to breathe through a mouthpiece at the earliest opportunity—a task facilitated by the recent development of novel devices (207). This is particularly important, since use of a face mask and absorption through the nasal mucosa may lead to unwanted local as well as systemic side effects (208). It should also be remembered that nasal resistance, which contributes approximately 50% total airway resistance (Sec. II.B, under "Age-Related Changes in Aerosol Deposition"), will be included when measuring resistance in infants. This may mask changes in lower airway resistance with disease or therapeutic interventions, especially if there has been a recent upper respiratory infection.

B. Pattern of Breathing

As a result of its direct influence on the efficacy of aerosol therapy, the effect of changes in breathing pattern has been intensively investigated (205,209,210). During larger breaths, aerosol is likely to penetrate further into the lung, increasing peripheral deposition. Conversely, with the higher flows associated with deep or fast breathing, turbulence is more likely to occur with increasing inertial deposition in the upper airway and major bronchi.

Minute Ventilation

Both tidal volume and respiratory rate vary enormously according to age and clinical status, with resting minute ventilation being approximately 6 L/min in an adult compared with less than 1 L/min in an infant (Table 1). The rapid respiratory rates (ranging from 20–90 breaths per minute) (211) and lower tidal volumes (20–100 mL—i.e., approximately 7–10 mL/kg) (212–214) found in infants translate into reduced drug delivery when compared with older, larger subjects. High respiratory rates usually result in increased deposition in the more proximal airways; a reduction in breathing rate can therefore result in improved lung deposition in children (215).

During inspiration, gas enters the lung by the process of bulk flow, in which molecules travel together by convection generally to the level of the alveolar ducts, after which gas movement occurs only by diffusion. Shallow, rapid breathing should be avoided during inhalation therapy, since the smaller the tidal volume, the greater the proportion that will he wasted in the dead space. Dead space varies with age and body size but is relatively large in infants due to the increased size of their heads in relation to their bodies (27). Normal elderly subjects breathe with identical minute ventilation to that of younger adults at rest, but with a smaller tidal volume and higher respiratory frequency and hence an increased ratio of dead space to tidal volume (19). This decreased alveolar ventilation will, in turn, influence patterns of aerosol deposition.

Peak Inspiratory Flow

The success of most inhaled therapy is dependent on the subject producing an adequate inspiratory flow. During childhood, peak inspiratory flows (PIF) range from less than 0.05 to over 40 L/min, depending on age, maturity, and clinical status (197). PIF is reduced in children and in the presence of severe asthma. However, even during acute exacerbations, most subjects over the age of 6 can generate an adequate PIF (i.e., > 30 L/min) to actuate most of the commonly used devices, particularly if a pattern of deep, forceful breathing is encouraged (216). In considering topical bronchodilator or anti-inflammatory treatment with a powder inhaler for older subjects, determination of PIF may be relevant, since lung deposition of such drugs is flow-dependent with many currently available devices, and the very elderly may not be able to achieve the recommended minimal inspiratory flows (217). In infants and young children, inability to coordinate breathing patterns with actuation, together with a lower PIF, usually requires the use of specialized delivery devices (204,218). The dead space of such devices, including the spacer, needs to be considered carefully, since the combination of a small tidal volume and large spacer dead space will markedly reduce the amount of drug inhaled with each breath (205,209,210,219,220).

While nebulizer output is usually diluted as a result of air entrainment in children and adults, infants may inhale pure nebulizer as a result of their low PIF (221) (Fig. 11). The quantity of aerosol that can be inspired, including that deposited in the nose and upper airways, appears to be similar in children and adults once inspired flow exceeds nebulizer flow, and minute ventilation is high enough to ensure that the entire nebulizer output is inhaled. The former appears to be the case in most young children after 6 months of age (Sec. III.B, "Age-Related Changes in Aerosol Deposition"). However, the smaller minute ventilation means that younger infants will not inspire all the nebulizer output (221), unless a breath synchronized device and prolonged administration time are used (220).

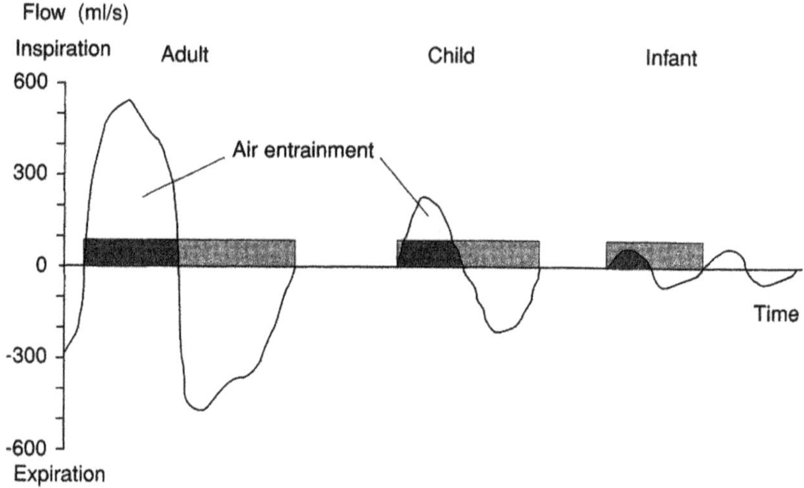

Figure 11 Diagrammatic representation of air entrainment. (Adapted from Ref. 221.)

Pattern of Airflow

Changes in airway caliber, will alter the pattern and speed of gas through the airways, and hence influence the distribution and deposition of inhaled particles. As mentioned in Sec. II.B, under "Intrapulmonary Airways," and II.B, under "Partitioning of Resistance," airways are of small diameter in the periphery of the lung, but there are so many of them that the total cross-sectional area is large. Hence air moves relatively slowly in a streamlined or laminar manner. By contrast, central airways are much larger, but—since there are fewer of them—total cross-sectional area is smaller. For any given flow, velocity is much higher in such airways, which may result in turbulence, gas molecules then traveling transversely across the airway as well as longitudinally. Under these conditions, frictional resistance is markedly increased.

In the trachea, flow is partly turbulent during quiet breathing, but it becomes progressively more turbulent with increasing minute ventilation. By contrast, in the bronchi, the gas stream only becomes turbulent at flows of around 5 L/s, whereas in the bronchioles it remains nearly laminar at all levels of ventilation except at bifurcations, where there are local eddies that dissipate energy. These flow profiles may differ in early life, with relatively low flows through the narrow trachea in infants favoring more laminar flow through the upper airways than found in older subjects. This, together with the diminished traction in the presence of a high chest wall compliance (Sec. II.A, under "Maturational Changes in Chest Wall Compliance"), could alter the relative partitioning of resistance throughout the respiratory tree (Sec. II.B, under "Partitioning of Resistance"), with the peripheral airways contributing relatively more than in older subjects (93). This despite the fact that, anatomically, the airways at birth appear to be a miniature of those found in the adult (Figs. 7 and 8) and to grow symmetrically thereafter. The complex relationships between the structure and function of the respiratory system (4) must be borne in mind when attempting to predict patterns of aerosol distribution from simple anatomical models.

Duty Cycle

The amount of aerosol inhaled depends not only on minute or alveolar ventilation but also on the duty cycle—i.e., the ratio of inspiratory (t_I) to total respiratory cycle time (t_{tot}) (221) (Fig. 12). Since most of the aerosolized output is delivered during inspiration, any reduction in duty cycle, as may occur in the presence of obstructive airways disease, will lead to a reduction in the inhaled mass of the drug. Duty cycle is remarkably constant in healthy infants and young children at around 0.42 (213,222), but in the presence of airway disease, it may be significantly lower. During crying, duty cycle may be so low that virtually no drug will be inhaled. Every effort must therefore be made to ensure that infants and young children are calm before any attempt to administer aerosolized treatment is made (28) (Fig. 13). In older children and adults, duty cycle tends to range from 0.32 to 0.50 in health, but again may be considerably lower in the presence of disease (K. Nikander, personal communication).

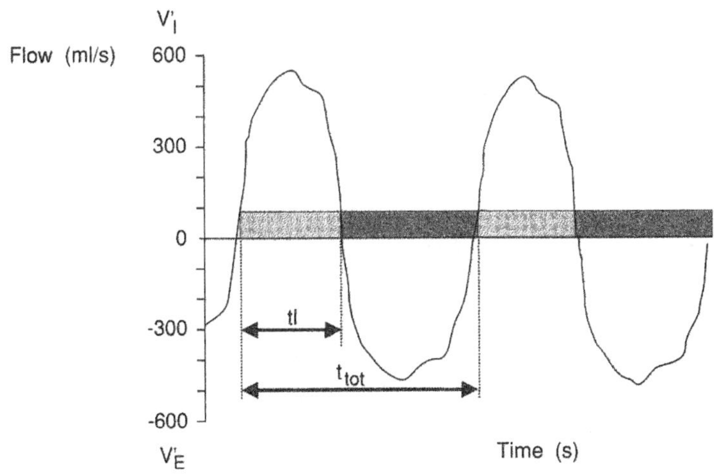

Figure 12 Importance of duty cycle on efficacy of aerosol therapy.

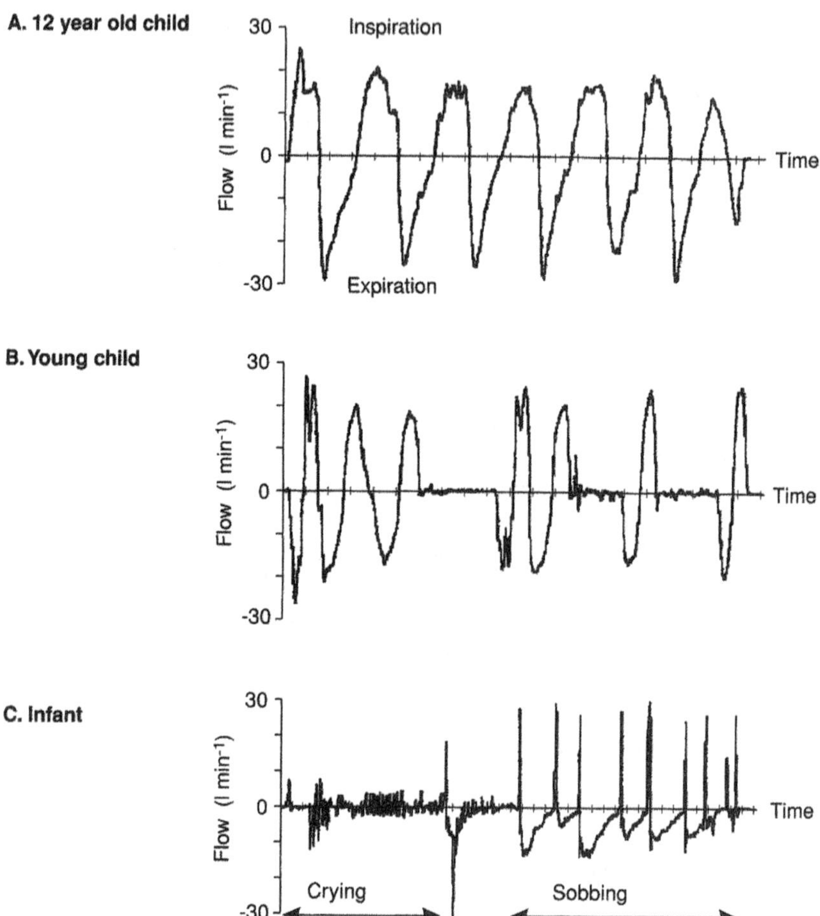

Figure 13 Range of typical breathing patterns in infants and children. (Adapted from Ref. 222.)

Age-Related Changes in Aerosol Deposition

Several models have been proposed to calculate deposition of particles within the respiratory tract of children, but these remain highly controversial because of the assumptions about the breathing pattern and structure of the upper and lower respiratory tract that have been made (223,224). Drug delivery to the very young child is enhanced by the fact that infants with PIFs below 100 mL/s (6 L/min—generally those less than 6 months of age) will inhale pure aerosol from a nebulizer, whereas air which does not contain aerosol will be entrained in older subjects, resulting in some dilution of the delivered dose (Fig. 11) (221,225).

Since airway resistance is inversely related to the fourth power of airway radius, any degree of airway narrowing due to bronchospasm, inflammation, secretions, or simply small body size may result in a considerable increase in resistance, which will encourage central airways deposition. It has therefore been suggested that optimal particle size for inhaled therapy in children may be smaller than in adults and smaller still for children with bronchoconstriction. However, if smaller droplets are produced, more may be exhaled. Furthermore, it may be impractical to nebulize some medications in small enough particles to produce a therapeutic effect. There have been relatively few deposition studies of nebulized aerosols in children, but those published have generally reported increased lung deposition with age (22,226,227). Using radiolabeled budesonide, Wildhaber et al. showed that mean lung deposition was significantly correlated with age, peak inspired flow, and height when dry-powder inhalers were used (227). Nevertheless, lung deposition was generally satisfactory even in the younger children in this study, since all those over 6 years of age could produce a PIF greater than the required 45 L/min. Indeed, while there may be relatively poor drug deposition in infant lungs during aerosol therapy due to low minute ventilation and nasal breathing, this is at least partially compensated for by the small body size and lack of air entrainment. Consequently, the final weight-corrected dose reaching the lungs may in fact be similar in infants and adults (221) (Fig. 14).

It is of course not just the weight-corrected dose of inhaled aerosol that is relevant but also the regional distribution and the ratio of peripheral to centrally deposited particles (Sec. III.D). Prediction of the effect of age on patterns of aerosol distribution is difficult. In young children, the smaller airways will favor central deposition by impaction, but the lower flows will tend to decrease impaction in central airways. Decreased residence time (faster respiratory rate) will tend to decrease peripheral deposition by reducing diffusion and sedimentation. Lower inspired flows in the very young may reduce absolute levels of nasal deposition, but smaller noses are more effective filters. Severity of lung disease will also affect efficacy of aerosol deposition and distribution by changing both airway caliber and the relative partitioning of resistance (Sec. II.B).

C. Factors Influencing Airway Caliber and Responsiveness

The flow-resistive properties of the airways are of major relevance to aerosol therapy in that they directly influence the pattern of distribution and deposition of inhaled particles within the lungs. Airway resistance increases, and hence aerosol delivery will be reduced, if the airways become partially blocked or narrowed by factors such as bronchospasm, inflammation, or secretions. Small changes in airway caliber can have dramatic effects on airway resistance. In a healthy adult, airway resistance is approximately 0.2 kPa/L/s (2 cmH_2O/L/s)

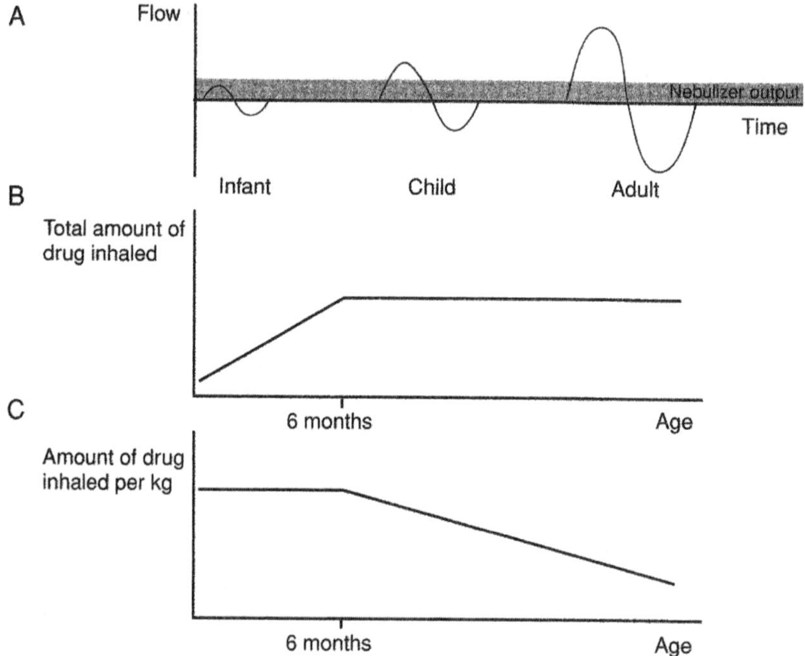

Figure 14 Hypothetical effect of age on amount of aerosol that can be inhaled.

during mouth breathing; whereas in a newborn infant, it is some twenty times higher (Table 1). However, the airways are relatively large in the very young in relation to lung volume, with specific conductance (a measure of airway caliber corrected for lung volume) in a nose-breathing infant being similar to that in a healthy adult during mouth breathing (23). Airway caliber and the maximum speed at which air can flow through the airways is the result of a delicate balance between forces generated by the airway smooth muscle and a number of opposing factors (228) and may be affected by numerous physical, chemical, and neural factors (Fig. 15).

Changes in Lung Volume and Elastic Recoil Pressure

Resistance falls during inspiration and rises during expiration due to changes in intrathoracic pressure surrounding the airways. Although the larger airways are well supported by cartilage, the cross-sectional area of the smaller airways depends heavily upon the elastic properties of the lung parenchyma. Destruction of elastic tissue and loss of recoil due to aging or emphysema results in reduced

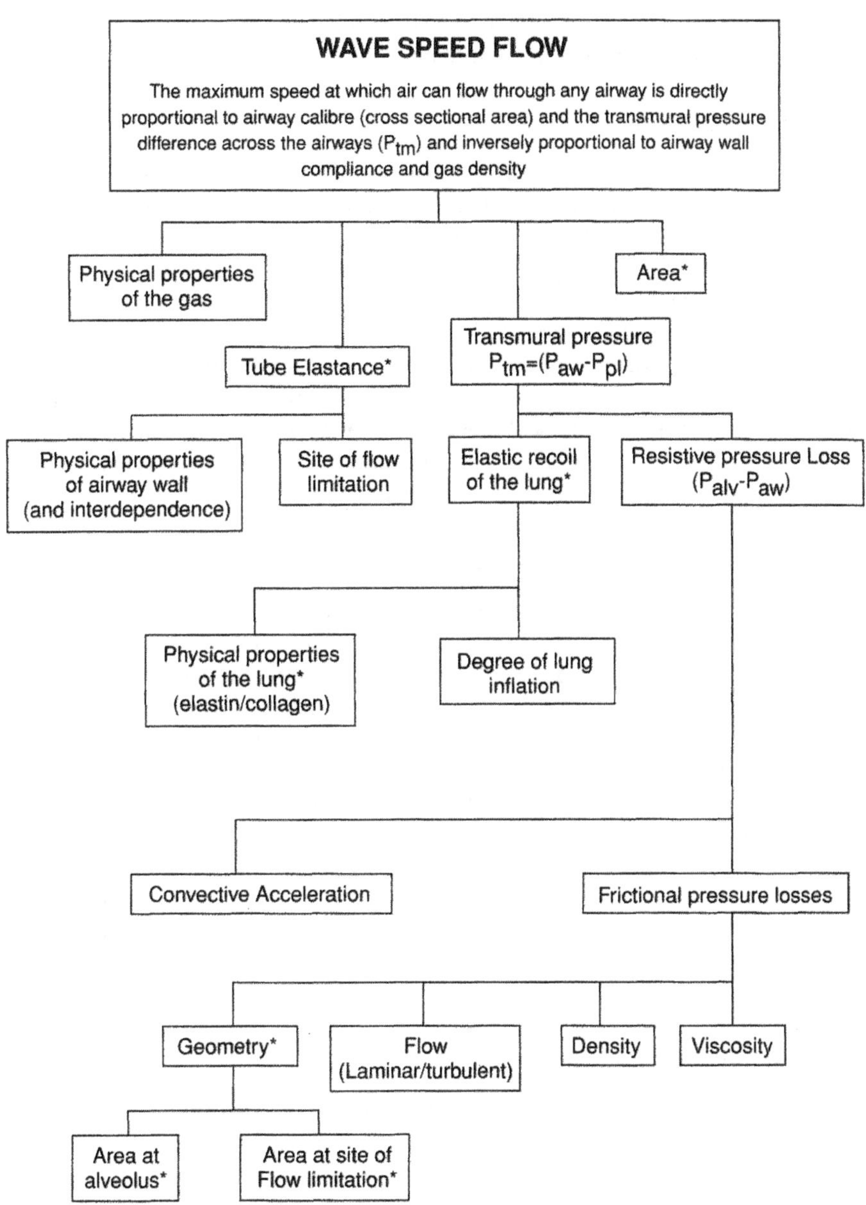

* Factors that change with growth. P_{pl}: pleural pressure; P_{tm}: transmural pressure (intra-airway pressure-pleural pressure); P_{alv}:alveolar pressure; P_{aw}: intra-airway pressure. Modified from Wohl (4)

Figure 15 Factors influencing airway caliber and the wave speed of airflow.

traction to the airway walls and decreased peripheral airway caliber, especially during expiration, when airway closure may occur (Fig. 6).

Smooth Muscle Tone

As discussed previously (Sec. II.B), bronchial smooth muscle tone is under autonomic control. Cold air and stimulation of receptors by irritants such as cigarette smoke, dust particles, and sulfur dioxide can also cause increased tone and hence bronchoconstriction (229). Bronchomotor tone is also modulated by vagal stretch reflexes and varies inversely with lung volume. Paradoxically, the rise in bronchomotor tone and/or increase in FRC during an attack of asthma may partially reverse the reduction in airway caliber that occurs in this condition, making assessment of response to therapy complex. Similarly, bronchodilators have been shown to cause paradoxical reductions in airflow and desaturation in some infants with history of wheeze, a phenomenon that has been attributed at least partially to changes in airway wall compliance (230–232).

Lung Volume—Airway Interdependence

The way in which airway dimensions change with lung volume is of great importance for the manifestation, assessment, and treatment of airway disease, but it is a poorly understood area. The effect of smooth muscle contraction on lung–airway interdependence is even less well understood. Recent measurements in dogs using high-resolution computed tomography have suggested that, contrary to previous hypotheses, relaxed bronchi do not expand isotropically with the lungs. Rather, they are highly compliant at low lung volumes close to FRC but very noncompliant at high lung volumes. By contrast, in the presence of even moderate bronchoconstriction, such airways become much stiffer, so that it may be impossible to achieve maximal airway caliber even when very high airway pressures are applied (233). These findings are in keeping with the observation that inability to dilate airways during lung inflation appears to be a primary defect in asthma (234).

Maximal Airway Responsiveness In Vivo

Previous observations have suggested that, in contrast to asthmatic subjects, healthy individuals usually exhibit an airway response plateau effect during bronchial challenge (235). However, this concept has recently been challenged, since it has been shown that when airways constrict in vitro, they do not exhibit a plateau effect but continue to constrict to increasing concentrations of agonist until complete airway closure occurs (236). The same authors found that while airway responses reached a plateau when a standard aerosol challenge was used in vivo, airways could easily be narrowed to complete closure at normal agonist concentrations where methacholine was delivered directly to the airway luminal surface. Since neither the elastic recoil of the lung nor limitations of smooth muscle shortening can be responsible for these observations, the apparent plateauing of the dose-response curves in vivo is probably attributable to difficulties in delivering high concentrations of agonists by the aerosol route. These findings are of considerable relevance in attempting to optimize drug delivery to the lungs in individuals with airway obstruction, whether it is due to bronchospasm or other causes.

Maturational Changes in Airway Responsiveness

Reviews of the etiology and control of bronchial hyperresponsiveness in children have been published recently (237). In infants, heightened responsiveness may result not only from anatomically small airways or increased smooth muscle tone but also from relatively thicker airway walls, decreased chest wall recoil, increased airway wall compliance (225,231,238), or excess secretions. Together with the difficulties in estimating the dose of agonist that will actually be delivered to the lung in infants and young children (Sec. III.B, under "Age-Related Changes in Aerosol Deposition"), such factors currently make it virtually impossible to determine relative changes in bronchial reactivity during the first few years of life (225).

While airway reactivity is clearly present from early life (71), the response to bronchodilators is less clear. Failure of infants and young children to respond to inhaled bronchodilators may be partially attributed to difficulties in delivering adequate amounts of aerosolized drugs in this age group (Sec. III.B, under "Age Related Changes in Aerosol Deposition"), but this is unlikely to be the only explanation. It may also be due to differences in the underlying pathology, with airway narrowing and wheezing in younger children being more due to congenitally small airways (77) (Sec. II.D), airway wall edema, and/or secretions than to smooth muscle shortening. Whereas increased airway responsiveness is evident in asthmatic adults and older wheezy children, this is not routinely the case in wheezy infants (239,240). The degree of bronchodilator response appears to be age-related, being minimal or absent below 18 months of age (72,73,241–243) but well established by 8 years of age (244,245). Several recent studies have suggested that reactivity appears to rise between 2 and 9 years of age and then to decrease somewhat (246,247). Bronchial reactivity is more prevalent in boys than girls prepubertally, and children who are not atopic are most likely to outgrow such hyperreactivity as they enter adolescence (248).

Functional Effect of Changes in Airway Caliber and Resistance

The functional consequences of alterations in bronchial tone depend on the site at which the change occurs. Bronchoconstriction of the large airways is more commonly the result of neural stimulation and mainly causes changes in airway resistance. By contrast, bronchoconstriction of the smaller airway, which is usually due to humoral factors such as histamine, prostaglandins, or changes in P_{CO_2}, primarily influences lung volumes and the distribution of ventilation. The determinants of airway resistance and maximal expiratory flow remain controversial (249,250) (see Fig. 15). A recent investigation of the relationship between structure and function of the airways found that airway obstruction correlated well with lung elastic recoil and airway conductance but not with airway collapsibility or the amount of airway cartilage present (251). When airway narrowing does occur, it does not affect all airways equally. Regions where the airways are most affected incur the greatest reduction in ventilation. In this way a high airway resistance often causes very uneven distribution of inspired air, which may, in turn, decrease the efficacy of aerosol therapy (Sec. III.D).

Assessment of Airway Disease and Response to Therapy

Tests of pulmonary function provide objective, quantifiable measurements that are used for various purposes (232). The fact that forced expiratory maneuvers are relatively independent of the resistance of the upper airways and hence more sensitive to changes in intrathoracic caliber has made these measurements a popular means of assessing airway disease and response to aerosol therapy.

Airway elastic properties and cross-sectional area interact to determine maximum flow through the airways (249,253) (Fig. 15). Generally, flows measured during forced expiration reflect the functional anatomy of more central airways at high lung volumes and more peripheral airways at lower lung volumes (254). However, the interdependent airway-emptying behavior tends to mask airway nonhomogeneities. This potentially diminishes the usefulness of such measurements for assessing disease severity or response to therapy unless particular care is taken to inspect the shape of the resultant flow-volume curves (255) and to relate changes in ventilatory capacity to absolute lung volume (TLC) rather than FVC (256–258).

D. Distribution of Ventilation

The efficiency of inhalation therapy depends not only on the weight corrected dose of aerosol that is delivered to the lung but also on the pattern of aerosol distribution and deposition throughout the respiratory system. This, in turn, is critically influenced by the way in which ventilation is distributed (259–261). By using inert radiolabeled gases, it has been shown that the first gas to be inhaled during slow inspiration goes to the upper parts of the lung, whereas during midinspiration, air is distributed throughout the regions. By contrast, toward end-inspiration, a larger proportion goes to the lower regions until, at near total lung capacity, the apex is almost fully inflated and the last air to be inhaled goes mainly to the bases. During expiration, the emptying of different lung regions occurs in a reverse order from inspiration, with the bases tending to empty before the apices, hence "first in is last out" (262).

In the presence of regional ventilation inequalities, the precise distance and distribution of the inhaled particles depends on numerous factors including breathing pattern, the lung volume at which the inhalation is made (259), and the degree of the inequalities. Lobar and segmental atelectasis may be considered an extreme form of ventilation maldistribution, where alveolar ventilation is zero. However, less obvious regional differences in ventilation will still have a marked influence on aerosol distribution and deposition. New methods of investigating regional deposition may help to clarify the way in which inhaled particles are distributed and retained within the airways. This, in turn, may help to optimize the therapeutic effects of aerosolized medications in the future (263–265).

Determinants of Regional Ventilation

The determinants of regional ventilation can best be understood by considering the simplified equation of motion (7,8), which states that pressure applied during a breathing cycle is that required to overcome the combined elastic and resistive forces of the lungs and airways—i.e.,

$$\Delta Ppl = \Delta V/C + \Delta V' \times R$$

where: ΔPpl = the tidal change in pleural pressure (the driving pressure)
ΔV = the local tidal volume change
C = the local static inspiratory compliance
$\Delta V'$ = local inspiratory flow
R = the local airway resistance

When flow and/or resistance are small compared with $\Delta V/C$ (as is the case in normal lungs), ΔV is proportional to $\Delta Ppl \times$ compliance. Since the *change* in pleural pressure during a breathing cycle is reasonably uniform over most of the lung surface, regional changes in volume vary directly with local compliance, which in health depends primarily on the shape of pressure-volume curve of the lung (Fig. 16).

In the normal erect adult, both ventilation and perfusion are preferentially distributed to the lower zones as a result of gravity. This normal gravitational distribution of ventilation is determined by the weight of the lungs, which in adults creates a vertical pressure gradient of approximately 0.8 kPa (8 cmH_2O) from top to bottom of the lung. The more negative pleural pressure surrounding the upper zones means that they are more distended than the lower ones, and regional alveolar *volume* is therefore greater. However, this greater background distending pressure also means that they lie on the flatter (stiffer) upper portion of the sigmoid pressure/volume curve of the lung (Fig. 16a). Since local com-

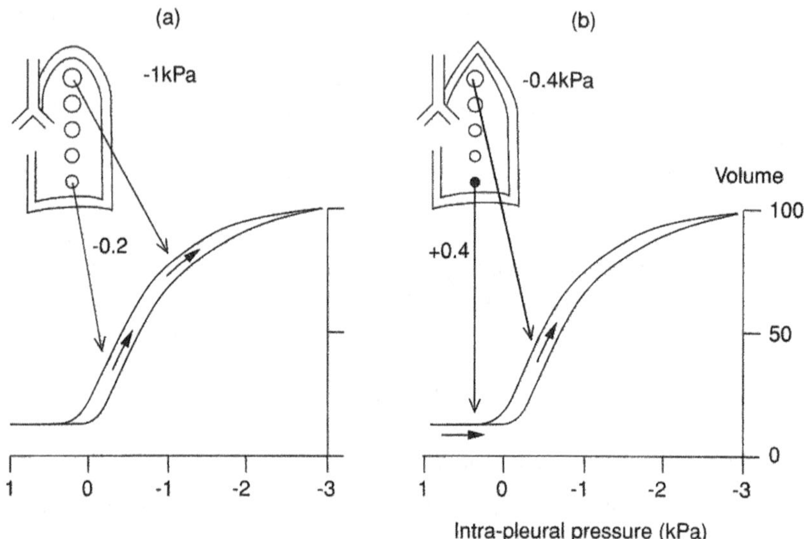

Figure 16 Effect of gravity on regional differences in ventilation (a) at functional residual capacity and (b) at residual volume.

pliance is lower, there is a decreased *change* in volume for any given change in pleural pressure. Lung units in the upper zones therefore resist expansion more than those in the lower zones that lie on the steeper central portion of the pressure-volume curve (7).

Thus, alveoli in the apices of the lung are well inflated but poorly ventilated, whereas those toward the base are poorly inflated but better ventilated. In normal subjects in the erect posture, the ratio of alveolar ventilation to volume in the upper parts of the lung is approximately 60% of that at the lung bases. In the lateral (decubitus) posture, the inferior (dependent) lobe has better ventilation than that which is superior; whereas in the supine position, the ventilation per unit of lung volume is relatively uniform. These gravitational differences disappear at total lung capacity, when all alveoli are fully expanded.

The preferential distribution of ventilation to dependent parts of the lungs is not observed in either the young or the elderly due to the reduced recoil pressure from the chest wall and lung respectively (Sec. II. A, under "Maturational Changes in Chest Wall Compliance"). In both these age groups, the upper portions of the lung lie on the central steep portion of the pressure/volume curve and therefore tend to be better expanded *and* ventilated than dependent areas (Fig. 16b). Indeed, the low distending pressure in dependent parts of the lungs predisposes to airway closure, inhomogeneity of gas exchange, and development of patchy atelectasis in infants and preschool children (266,267). This may have a significant effect on aerosol distribution in infants. Similar changes may occur in the elderly due to loss of lung recoil (19).

Influence of Airway Disease

In health, these regional inequalities cause minimal interference with intrapulmonary gas exchange because of concurrent regional distribution of pulmonary blood flow (7,268). However, in the presence of disease, regional differences in alveolar ventilation will cause considerable disturbances in gas exchange. In diseased lungs, the distribution of ventilation will be compromised by units with high local resistance or low compliance (increased stiffness). The sequence of filling during inspiration is determined by the relative time constants of the various acini or lung units. The time constant is a measure of the filling/emptying time and is the product of local compliance and resistance. Lung units with a short time constant (in other words, alveoli that have a low compliance and/or are served by airways with a low resistance) tend to fill quickly and hence early in the inspiration. By contrast, those which are served by relatively narrow airways (high resistance and hence a long time constant) tend to fill later on in inspiration, thereby causing temporal inequalities in ventilation distribution (Fig. 17). Furthermore, regions with a short time constant will tend to receive proportionally

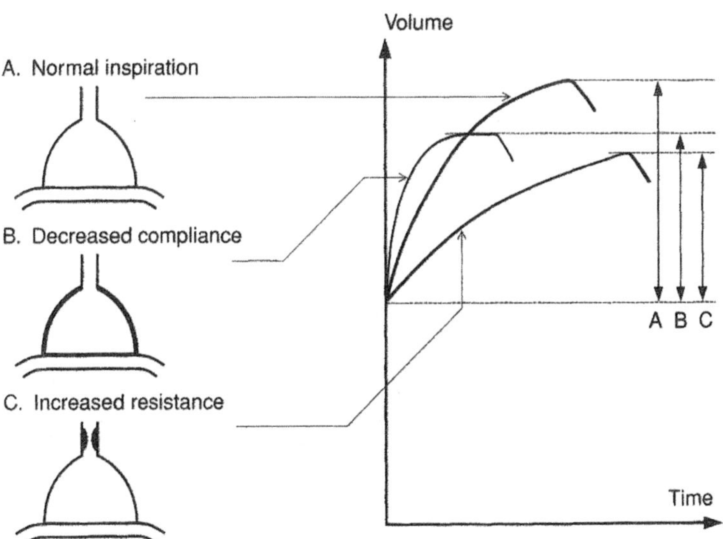

Figure 17 Temporal effects of differences in compliance and airway resistance on ventilation of lung units.

more of the common deadspace than those with a long time constant, whether the latter is due to increased resistance (narrow airways) or high compliance (e.g., emphysematous loss of elastic recoil) (7,250).

Whether or not there are also spatial inequalities, i.e., in the proportion of ventilation (and hence aerosol) that is delivered to different regions will depend both on the duration of inspiration and the extent to which there are local difference in compliance as well as resistance. If compliance is equally distributed and inspiration is prolonged, then, for a given change in pleural pressure, all alveoli will eventually achieve the same expansion ratio. However, if inspiration is brief, lung units having a high resistance will expand less than the low-resistance units (Fig. 18). In the presence of airway disease and a rapid respiratory rate, there may be insufficient time for the inhaled aerosol to reach the most relevant areas of the lung, in terms of treatment effects, before exhalation commences.

Where there are coexistent differences in local compliance due to either normal gravitational effects (Fig. 16) or disease, the situation becomes even more complex. Under these circumstances, some units may fill and empty slowly due to the high resistance of the airways supplying them; yet, provided inspiratory time is long enough, they may receive a large proportion of the ventilation due to a local loss of elastic recoil (high compliance), whereas others may fill

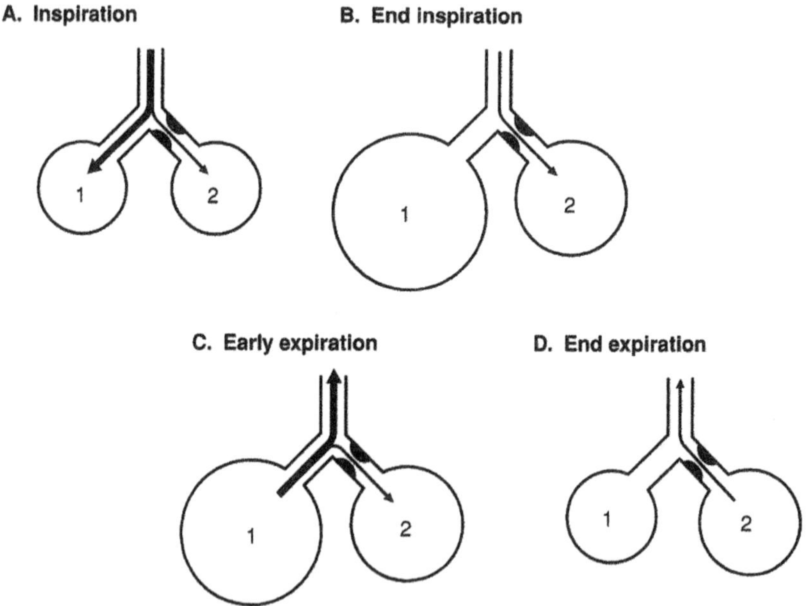

Figure 18 Effects of uneven time constants in the lung on ventilation distribution.

rapidly but receive very little ventilation due to a combination of stiff units supplied by normal airways. The resultant mix of spatial and temporal inequalities in ventilation distribution makes prediction of the pattern of aerosol distribution in the presence of disease extremely complex. In addition, this pattern may vary within individuals on a daily or even hourly basis according to clinical status and response to therapy.

When two compartments have different time constants due to differences in resistance or compliance, gas can be flowing out of one at the same time as it is flowing into the other. This "pendelluft" phenomenon reduces effective tidal volume results in frequency dependence of dynamic compliance and resistance measurements, and again makes prediction of aerosol distribution in the presence of disease highly complex (269) (Fig. 18).

Distribution of Inhaled Aerosols

In the healthy lung, the distribution of inhaled aerosol is largely due to convective mixing and nonreversal of the axial streaming. However, nonuniform distribution of ventilation due to regional differences in pulmonary resistance and compliance may become an increasingly important factor affecting aerosol distribution in the presence of lung disease (270–273). Enhanced pulmonary deposition of aerosolized rhDNAase occurs in CF patients with more severe airway disease (32). There is more central deposition in adults with bronchoconstriction than in those with normal lung function, and there may be marked regional differences in peripheral lung deposition This pattern may be due to functional narrowing of the large airways during expiration at flow-limiting segments. In the presence of chronic obstructive airway disease, dynamic airway compression at these flow-limited segments may reduce peripheral and enhance central deposition of inhaled particles (273–274). As the lungs shift from a single, well-ventilated system towards a multicompartment system with both healthy and obstructed lung regions, aerosol recovery (which is the ratio of exhaled to inhaled particles) decreases. Increased residence time in slow regions and sites of airway obstruction with ventilatory inhomogeneities may enhance regional deposition in poorly ventilated areas if aerosol is conveyed to smaller airway dimensions than would occur with more uniform ventilation patterns (224,270,272). Again, this makes it very difficult to predict pattern of aerosol distribution or optimal dosage in the presence of severe disease.

IV. Conclusions and Future Directions

During recent years, there have been considerable technological advances in aerosol therapy and increasingly sophisticated methods of assessing how such aerosols are distributed and deposited throughout the lung. However, in order to optimize aerosol therapy, it is essential to consider the influence of the structure and function of the respiratory system and the effect that normal growth and development, aging and disease will have on airway caliber and patterns of airflow. The major physiological factors influencing aerosol delivery include the route of inhalation, pattern of breathing, airway caliber and responsiveness, and the distribution of ventilation. Anatomic and physiological differences in the very young and the elderly present particular challenges in delivering sufficient aerosol to appropriate parts of the lung according to the age and clinical status of the individual. Developmental changes in airway structure and function that will influence aerosol deposition are summarized in Table 2.

The complexity of the relationship between structure and function of the airways means that mathematical models based simply on gross airway anatomy—without taking into account the influence of the chest wall, lung parenchyma, airway compliance and pattern of airflow—are unlikely to provide accurate prediction of aerosol deposition in vivo. Similarly, the results of studies using animal models must be interpreted with caution, since aerosol deposition is critically dependent on branching pattern, and that of the dog or rat does not necessarily reflect that of the human. The search for a relevant animal model in which to investigate both short- and long-term effects of various interventions on the developing lung is therefore critical. It is also very difficult to extrapolate results from adults to infants and young children, particularly since the latter have such high chest wall compliance, lower flows, and the tendency to nose breathe.

Table 2 Summary of Developmental Changes in Airway Structure and Function That May Affect Aerosol Therapy

- Body size is a major determinant of lung and airway size, and hence function.
- Airway resistance is very high in infants and young children but decreases with growth.
- Lung growth is most rapid during late fetal life and the first year postnatally. Adverse influences during this period may have long-term effects on airway caliber. Thus, if airway function is diminished during infancy, it is likely to remain so throughout life.
- Infants are preferential nose-breathers.
- Airway function is enhanced in girls as compared with boys throughout childhood; this relative advantage is reversed after puberty.
- Dysanaptic (disproportionate) growth probably occurs during infancy and early childhood, with lung parenchyma and volumes increasing faster than airway caliber. Thereafter lung and airway growth is likely to be more isotropic, at least until puberty, when growth may once again become dysanaptic in females.
- Distribution of ventilation is likely to be more uneven in the very young and the elderly due to the diminished elastic recoil from the chest wall and lung tissue respectively.
- Aging is associated with a gradual decline in airway function.

In the past, knowledge about in vivo airway caliber has been severely limited by the rather blunt tools available for assessment of lung function. However, the introduction of exciting new techniques based on aerosol-derived morphometry, using high-resolution computed tomography, promises to provide far more accurate information about aerosol distribution and deposition in the near future. Nevertheless, caution will again need to be exercised in trying to extrapolate the results of these studies to young children, in whom such investigations may be less feasible. Future challenges include the need to develop more sensitive, noninvasive tests for longitudinal and cross-sectional studies. These would enable more precise measurements of normal lung growth and development to be made, thereby improving our ability to evaluate the effects of disease and individual response to therapy in patients of all ages. Longitudinal measurements of lung growth and development are essential if we are to identify any potentially adverse side effects from delivering various agents directly into the lung during critical phases of growth and development or to assess any sparing effects of early interventions on subsequent airway remodeling in "at risk" subjects (63,186).

For many drugs, the optimum site of action remains unknown, and the dose of many therapeutic agents may be less pertinent than their delivery profile down the tracheobronchial tree. Whereas it is likely that steroid therapy for asthma is best delivered to the larger airways, antibiotics for cystic fibrosis may need to be delivered to the more distal airways and alveoli. However, further improvements in aerosol and nebulizer technologies may be required before anti-inflammatory agents can be effectively delivered to the periphery of the lung.

In conclusion, if the potential of recent technological advances in improved aerosol delivery devices is to be fully realized, it is important that we focus on how to get the aerosol to the right site according to the age, maturity, and disease status of the individual. This can be achieved only if both drug delivery and assessment of effectiveness are based on a firm knowledge of the underlying structure and function of the respiratory system in the individual concerned.

Acknowledgments

We should like to thank Jillian Ridgwell for secretarial assistance as well as David Smithson and Dr. Susan Hall for their help with the illustrations. Janet Stocks is supported by SIMS Portex plc and Alison Hislop by the British Heart Foundation.

References

1. Pauwels R, Newman S, Borgström L. Airway deposition and airway effects of antiasthma drugs delivered from metered-dose inhalers. Eur Respir J 1997; 10:2127–2138.

2. Stocks J. Developmental physiology and methodology. Am J Respir Crit Care Med 1995; 151:S15–S17.
3. Martin TR, Feldman HA, Fredberg JJ, Castile RG, Mead J, Wohl MEB. Relationship between maximal expiratory flows and lung volumes in growing humans. J Appl Physiol 1988; 65:822–828.
4. Wohl MEB. Developmental physiology of the respiratory system. In: Chernick V, Boat TF, Kendig EL, editors. Kendig's Disorders of the Respiratory Tract in Children, 6th ed. Philadelphia: Saunders, 1998:19–27.
5. O'Brodovich HM, Haddad GG. The functional basis of respiratory pathology and disease. In: Chernick V, Boat TF, Kendig EL, eds. Kendig's Disorders of the Respiratory Tract in Children, 6th ed. Philadelphia: Saunders, 1998:27–73.
6. Brewis RAL, White FE. Anatomy of the thorax. In: Brewis RAL, Corrin B, Geddes DM, Gibson GJ, eds. Respiratory Medicine, 2d ed. London: Saunders, 1995:22–53.
7. West JB. Respiratory Physiology—The Essentials, 5th ed. Baltimore: Williams & Wilkins, 1995.
8. Cotes JE. Lung Function. In: Leathart GL, ed. Lung Function: Assessment and Applications in Medicine. Oxford: Blackwell, 1993.
9. Taylor AE, Rehder K, Hyatt RE, Parker JC. Anatomy and function of the lung. In: Taylor AE, Rehder K, Hyatt RE, Parker JC, eds. Clinical Respiratory Physiology. Philadelphia: Saunders, 1989:3–24.
10. Sauleda J, Gea J, Orozco-Levi M, Corominas J, Minguella J, Aguar C, et al. Structure and function relationship of the respiratory muscles. Eur Respir J 1998; 11:906–911.
11. Openshaw P, Edwards S, Helms P. Changes in rib cage geometry during childhood. Thorax 1984; 39:624–627.
12. Agostoni E. Volume-pressure relationships of the thorax and lung in the newborn. J Appl Physiol 1959; 14:909–913.
13. Helms P, Beardsmore CS, Stocks J. Absolute intraesophageal pressure at functional residual capacity in infancy. J Appl Physiol 1981; 51:270–275.
14. Papastamelos C, Panitch HB, England SE, Allen JL. Developmental changes in chest wall compliance in infancy and early childhood. J Appl Physiol 1995; 78:179–184.
15. Kosch PC, Stark AR. Dynamic maintenance of end-expiratory lung volume in full-term infants. J Appl Physiol 1984; 57:1126–1133.
16. Rabbette PS, Stocks J. Influence of volume dependency and timing of airway occlusions on the Hering-Breuer reflex in infants. J Appl Physiol 1998; 85:2033–2039.
17. Colin AA, Wohl MEB, Mead J, Ratjen FA, Glass G, Stark AR. Transition from dynamically maintained to relaxed end-expiratory volume in human infants. J Appl Physiol 1989; 67:2107–2111.
18. Mansell A, Bryan C, Levison H. Airway closure in children. J Appl Physiol 1972; 33:711–714.
19. Janssens JP, Pache JC, Nicod LP. Physiological changes in respiratory function associated with ageing. Eur Respir J 1999; 13:197–205.

20. Rodenstein DON, Perlmutter N, Stanescu DC. Infants are not obligatory nasal breathers. Am Rev Respir Dis 1985; 131:343–347.
21. deAlmeida VL, Alvaro RA, Haider Z, Rehan V, Nowaczyk B, Cates D, et al. The effect of nasal occlusion on the initiation of oral breathing in preterm infants. Pediatr Pulmonol 1994; 18:374–378.
22. Chua HL, Collis GG, Newbury AM, Chan K, Bower GD, Sly PD. The influence of age on aerosol deposition in children with cystic fibrosis. Eur Respir J 1994; 7:2185–2191.
23. Stocks J, Godfrey S. Nasal resistance during infancy. Respir Physiol 1978; 34:233–246.
24. Hey EN, Price JF. Nasal conductance and effective airway diameter. J Physiol 1982; 330:429–437.
25. Lorino AM, Lofaso F, Abi-Nader F, Drogou I, Dahan E, Zerah F, et al. Nasal airflow resistance measurement: forced oscillation technique versus posterior rhinomanometry. Eur Respir J 1998; 11:720–725.
26. Widdicombe JG. Nasal pathophysiology. Respir Med 1990; 84(suppl A):3–10.
27. Numa AH, Newth CJL. Anatomic dead space in infants and children. J Appl Physiol 1996; 80:1485–1489.
28. Mallol J, Rattray S, Walker G, Cook D, Robertson CF. Aerosol deposition in infants with cystic fibrosis. Pediatr Pulmonol 1996; 21:276–281.
29. Eiser N. The hitch-hikers guide to nasal airway patency. Respir Med 1990; 84:179–183.
30. Baroody FM. Anatomy and physiology. In: Naclerio RM, Durham SR, Mygind N, eds. Rhinitis: Mechanisms and Management. New York: Marcel Dekker, 1999:1–22.
31. Berg E. In vitro properties of pressurised metered dose inhalers with and without spacer devices. J Aerosol Med 1995; 8:S3–S11.
32. Diot P, Palmer LB, Smaldone A, DeCelie-Germana J, Grimson R, Smaldone GC. RhDNase 1 aerosol deposition and related factors in cystic fibrosis. Am J Respir Crit Care Med 1997; 156:1662–1668.
33. Svartengren K, Lindestad PA, Svartengren M, Bylin G, Philipson K, Camner P. Deposition of inhaled particles in the mouth and throat of asthmatic subjects. Eur Respir J 1994; 7:1467–1473.
34. Chang AB. Cough, cough receptors, and asthma in children. Pediatr Pulmonol 1999; 28:59–70.
35. Wailoo MP, Emery JL. Normal growth and development of the trachea. Thorax 1982; 37:584–587.
36. Shannon JM, Deterding RR. Epithelial-mesenchymal interactions in lung development. In: McDonald JA, ed. Lung Growth and Development. New York: Marcel Dekker, 1997:81–118.
37. Horsfield K. Diameters, generations, and orders of branches in the bronchial tree. J Appl Physiol 1990; 68:457–461.
38. Horsfield K, Gordon WI, Kemp W, Phillips S. Growth of the bronchial tree in man. Thorax 1987; 42:383–388.
39. Weibel ER. Functional morphology of the growing lung. Respiration 1970; 27:27–35.

40. Weibel ER. Lung morphometry and models in respiratory physiology. In: Chang HK, Paiva M, eds. Respiratory Physiology: An Analytical Approach. New York: Marcel Dekker, 1989:1–56.
41. Crapo RO The aging lung. In: Mahler DA, ed. Pulmonary Disease in the Elderly Patient, 63rd ed. New York: Marcel Dekker, 1993:1–21.
42. Macklem PT. The physiology of small airways. Am J Respir Crit Care Med 1998; 157:S181–S183.
43. Brand P, Kohlhaufl M, Meyer T, Selzer T, Heyder J, Haussinger K. Aerosol-derived airway morphometry and aerosol bolus dispersion in patients with lung fibrosis and lung emphysema. Chest 1999; 116:543–548.
44. Forrest JB, Lee RMKW. The bronchial wall: Integrated form and function. In: Crystal RG, West JB, eds. The Lung: Scientific Foundations. New York: Raven Press, 1991:729–739.
45. Angus GE, Thurlbeck WM. Number of alveoli in the human lung. J Appl Physiol 1972; 32:483–485.
46. Jeffery PK. Microscopic structure of normal lung. In: Brewis RAL, Corrin B, Geddes DM, Gibson GJ, eds. Respiratory Medicine London: Saunders, 1995:54–72.
47. Sleigh MA. The nature and action of respiratory tract cilia. In: Brain JD, Proctor DF, Reid L, eds. Respiratory Defense Mechanisms. New York: Marcel Dekker, 1977:247–267.
48. Ellefsen P, Tos M. Goblet cells in the human trachea: quantitative studies of a pathological biopsy material. Arch Otolaryngol 1972; 95:547–555.
49. Evans MJ, Plopper CG. The role of basal cells in adhesion of columnar epithelium to airway basement membrane. Am Rev Respir Dis 1988; 138:481.
50. Crapo JD, Barry BE, Cehr P, Bachofen M, Weibel ER. Cell characteristics of the normal lung. Am Rev Respir Dis 1982; 125:740–745.
51. Jeffrey PK, Hislop AA. Embryology and growth. In: Brewis RAL, Corrin B, Geddes DM, Gibson GJ, eds. Respiratory Medicine. London: Saunders, 1995:3–21.
52. Matsuba K, Thurlbeck WM. A morphometric study of bronchial and bronchiolar walls in children. Am Rev Respir Dis 1972; 105:908–913.
53. Wong YC, Beardsmore CS, Meek JH, Stocks J, Silverman M Bronchial hypersecretion in preterm neonates. Arch Dis Child 1982; 57:117–122.
54. Hislop AA, Haworth SG. Airway size and structure in the normal fetal and infant lung and the effect of premature delivery and artificial ventilation. Am Rev Respir Dis 1989; 140:1717–1726.
55. McCray PB. Spontaneous contractility of human fetal airway smooth muscle. Am J Respir Cell Mol Biol 1993; 8:573–580.
56. Margraf LR, Tomashefski JFJ, Bruce MC, Dahms BB Morphometric analysis of the lung in bronchopulmonary dysplasia. Am Rev Respir Dis 1991; 143:391–400.
57. James AL, Pare PD, Hogg JC. The mechanics of airway narrowing in asthma. Am Rev Respir Dis 1989; 139:242–246.
58. Tepper RS, Wiggs B, Gunst SJ, Pare PD. Lower shear modulus of the lung for immature than mature rabbits. Am J Respir Crit Care Med 1999; 159:A406.
59. Shen X, Bhargava V, Wodicka GR, Doerschuk CM, Gunst SJ, Tepper RS. Greater

airway narrowing in immature than in mature rabbits during methacholine challenge. J Appl Physiol 1996; 81:2637–2643.
60. Ramchandani RP, Shen X, Gunst SJ, Tepper RS. Comparison of inner wall areas of non-constricted airways from immature and mature rabbits. Am J Respir Crit Care Med 1999; 159:A406.
61. Baile EM. The anatomy and physiology of the bronchial circulation. J Aerosol Med 1996; 9:1–6.
62. Widdicombe JG. Comparison between the vascular beds of upper and lower airways. Eur Respir J 1990; 3:564–571.
63. Wanner A. Clinical perspectives: Role of the airway circulation in drug therapy. J Aerosol Med 1996; 9:19–23.
64. Vanhoutte PM. Epithelium derived relaxation factor: myth or reality? Thorax 1988; 43:665–668.
65. Barnes PJ. Pharmacology of airway smooth muscle. Am J Respir Crit Care Med 1998; 158:S123–S132.
66. Barnes PJ. Neural mechanisms in asthma: new developments Ped Pulmonol 1997; 16:82–83.
67. Adcock IM, Stevens DA, Barnes PJ. Interactions of glucocorticoids and β_2-agonists. Eur Respir J 1996; 9:160–168.
68. Altiere RJ, Thompson DC. Physiology and pharmacology of the airways. In: Hickey AJ, editor. Inhalational Aerosols: Physical and Biological Basis for Therapy. Marcel Dekker, 1996:85–137.
69. Barnes PJ. Beta-adrenergic receptors and their regulation. Am J Respir Crit Care Med 1995; 152:838–860.
70. Hislop AA, Wharton J, Allen KM, Polak J, Haworth SG. Immunohistochemical localisation of peptide-containing nerves in the airways of normal young children. Am J Respir Cell Mol Biol 1990; 3:191–198.
71. Tepper RS. Airway reactivity in infants: a positive response to methacholine and metaproterenol. J Appl Physiol 1987; 62:1155–1159.
72. Prendiville A, Green S, Silverman M. Bronchial responsiveness to histamine in wheezy infants. Thorax 1987; 42:92–99.
73. O'Callaghan C, Milner AD, Swarbrick A. Nebulised salbutamol does have a protective effect on airways in children under 1 year old. Arch Dis Child 1988; 63:479–483.
74. O'Callaghan C, Milner AD, Webb MSC, Swarbrick A. Nebulised water as a bronchoconstricting challenge in infancy. Arch Dis Child 1991; 66:948–951.
75. Henderson AJ, Young S, Stick SM, Landau LI, Le Souëf PN. Effect of salbutamol on histamine induced bronchoconstriction in healthy infants. Thorax 1993; 48;317–323.
76. Ullah MI, Newman GB, Saunders KB. Influence of age on response to ipratropium and salbutamol in asthma. Thorax 1981; 36:523–529.
77. Dezateux CA, Stocks J. Lung development and early origins of childhood respiratory illness. Br Med Bull 1997; 53:40–57.
78. Shaheen SO, Barker DJP, Shiell AW, Crocker FJ, Wield GA, Holgate ST. The relationship between pneumonia in early childhood, and impaired lung function in late adult life. Am J Respir Crit Care Med 1994; 149:616–619.

79. Martinez FD, Wright AL, Taussig LM, Holberg CJ, Halonen M, Morgan WJ, et al. Asthma and wheezing in the first six years of life. N Engl J Med 1995; 332:133–138.
80. Chan KN, Noble-Jamieson CM, Elliman A, Bryan EM, Silverman M. Lung function in children of low birth weight. Arch Dis Child 1989; 64: 1284–1293.
81. Burri PH. Structural aspects of prenatal and postnatal development and growth of the lung. In: McDonald JA, ed. Lung Growth and Development. New York: Marcel Dekker, 1997:1–35.
82. Merkus PJFM, ten Ilave-Opbroek AAW, Quanjer PH. Human lung growth: a review. Pediatr Pulmonol 1996; 21:383–397.
83. Bucher U, Reid L. Development of the intrasegmental bronchial tree: the pattern of the branching and development of cartilage at various stages of intra-uterine life. Thorax 1961; 16:207–218.
84. Bucher U, Reid L. Development of the mucus-secreting elements in human lung. Thorax 1961; 16:219–225.
85. Hislop A, Wigglesworth JS, Desai R. Alveolar development in the human fetus and infant. Early Hum Dev 1986; 13:1–11.
86. Langston C, Kida C, Reed M, Thurlbeck WM. Human lung growth in late gestation and in the neonate. Am Rev Respir Dis 1984; 129:607–613.
87. Burri PH. Lung development and pulmonary angiogenesis. In: Gaultier C, Bourbon JR, Post M, eds. Lung Development. New York: Oxford University Press, 1999:122–151.
88. Stocks J, Quanjer PH. Reference values for residual volume, functional residual capacity and total lung capacity. ATS Workshop on Lung Volume Measurements. Official statement of the European Respiratory Society. Eur Respir J 1995; 492–506.
89. Stocks J, Sly PD, Tepper RS, Morgan WJ. Infant Respiratory Function Testing. New York: Wiley, 1996.
90. Zeltner TB, Caduff JH, Gehr P, Pfenninger J, Burri PH. The postnatal development and growth of the human lung: I. Morphometry Respir Physiol 1986; 67:247–267.
91. Thurlbeck WM. Postnatal human lung growth. Thorax 1982; 37:564–571.
92. Stocks J. Respiratory physiology during early life. Monaldi Arch Chest Dis 1999; 54:358–364.
93. Helms PJ. Lung growth: implications for the development of disease. Thorax 1994; 49:440–441.
94. Cooper DM, Mellins RB, Mansell AL. Changes in distribution of ventilation with lung growth. J Appl Physiol 1981; 51:699–705.
95. Borsboom GJJM, Van Pelt W, Quanjer PH. Interindividual variation in pubertal growth patterns of ventilatory function, standing height, and weight. Am J Respir Crit Care Med 1996; 153:1182–1186.
96. Hislop A, Muir DCF, Jacobsen M, Simon G, Reid L. Postnatal growth and function of the pre-acinar airways. Thorax 1972; 27:265–274.
97. Hogg JC, Williams J, Richardson JB, Macklem PT, Thurlbeck WM. Age as a factor in the distribution of lower airway conductance and in the pathological anatomy of obstructive lung disease. N Engl J Med 1970; 282:1283–1287.

98. Tepper RS, Reister T. Forced expiratory flows and lung volumes in normal infants. Pediatr Pulmonol 1993; 15:357–361.
99. Stocks J, Henschen M, Hoo A-F, Costeloe K, Dezateux CA. The influence of ethnicity and gender on airway function in preterm infants. Am J Respir Crit Care Med 1997; 156:1855–1862.
100. Jones M, Castile R, Davis S, Kisling J, Filbrun D, Flucke R, et al. Forced expiratory flows and volumes in infants. Am J Respir Crit Care Med 2000; 161:353–359.
101. Stocks J, Godfrey S. Specific airway conductance in relation to postconceptional age during infancy. J Appl Physiol 1977; 43:144–154.
102. Dezateux C, Stocks J, Dundas I, Fletcher ME. Impaired airway function and wheezing in infancy: the influence of maternal smoking and a genetic predisposition to asthma. Am J Respir Crit Care Med 1999; 159:403–410.
103. Hibbert ME, Hudson IL, Lanigan A, Landau LI, Phelan PD. Tracking of lung function in healthy children and adolescents. Pediatr Pulmonol 1990; 8:172–177.
104. Strope GL, Helms RW. A longitudinal study of spirometry in young black and white children. Am Rev Respir Dis 1984; 130:1100–1107.
105. Sherrill D, Holberg CJ, Lebowitz MD. Differential rates of lung growth as measured longitudinally by pulmonary function in children and adolescents. Pediatr Pulmonol 1990; 8:145–154.
106. Dockery DW, Berkey CS, Ware JH, Speizer FE, Ferris BG Jr. Distribution of forced vital capacity and forced expiratory volume in one second in children 6 to 11 years of age Am Rev Respir Dis 1983; 128:405–412.
107. Becklake MR, Toyota B, Stewart M, Hanson R, Hanley J. Lung structure as a risk factor in adverse pulmonary responses to asbestos exposure Am Rev Respir Dis 1983; 128:385–388.
108. Sherrill DL, Camilla A, Lebowitz MD. On the temporal relationships between lung function and somatic growth. Am Rev Respir Dis 1989; 134:956–961.
109. Mead J. Dysanapsis in normal lungs assessed by the relationship between maximal flow, static recoil and vital capacity. Am Rev Respir Dis 1980; 121:339–342.
110. Martin TR, Castile RG, Fredberg JJ, Wohl B, Mead J. Airway size is related to sex but not lung size in normal adults. J Appl Physiol 1987; 63:2042–2047.
111. Lanteri CJ, Sly PD. Changes in respiratory mechanics with age. J Appl Physiol 1993; 74:369–378.
112. Sly PD, Willet K. Developmental physiology. In Silverman M, ed. Childhood Asthma and Other Wheezing Disorders. London: Chapman & Hall, 1995:55–66.
113. Green M, Mead J. Turner JM. Variability of maximum expiratory flow-volume curves. J Appl Physiol 1974; 37:67–74.
114. Merkus PJFM, Borsboom GJJM, Van Pelt W, Schrader PC, Van Houwelingen HC, Kerrebijn KF, et al. Growth of airways and air spaces in teenagers is related to sex but not to symptoms. J Appl Physiol 1993; 75:2045–2053.
115. Thurlbeck WM. Postnatal growth and development of the lung. Am Rev Respir Dis 1975; 3:803–844.
116. Mansell AL, Bryan AC, Levison H. Relationship of lung recoil to lung volume and maximum expiratory flow in normal children. J Appl Physiol 1977; 42:817–823.

117. Zapletal A, Paul T, Samanek A. Pulmonary elasticity in children and adolescents. J Appl Physiol 1976; 40:953–961.
118. Tepper RS, Morgan WJ, Cota K, Wright A, Taussig LM, The Group Health Medical Associates' Pediatricians Physiologic growth and development of the lung during the first year of life. Am Rev Respir Dis 1986; 134:513–519.
119. Rona RJ, Chinn S. Lung function, respiratory illness, and passive smoking in British primary school children. Thorax 1993; 48:21–25.
120. Hanrahan JP, Tager IB, Castile RG, Segal MR, Weiss ST, Speizer FE. Pulmonary function measures in healthy infants: variability and size correction. Am Rev Respir Dis 1990; 141:1127–1135.
121. Hibbert M, Lannigan A, Raven J, Landau L, Phelan P. Gender differences in lung growth. Pediatr Pulmonol 1995; 19:129–134.
122. Taussig LM, Cota K, Kaltenborn W. Different mechanical properties of the lung in boys and girls. Am Rev Respir Dis 1981; 123:640–643.
123. Pagtakhan RD, Bjelland JC, Landau LI, Loughlin G, Kaltenborn W, Seeley G, et al. Sex differences in growth patterns of the airways and lung parenchyma in children. J Appl Physiol 1984; 56:1204–1210.
124. Hoo A-F, Henschen M, Dezateux C, Costeloe K, Stocks J. Respiratory function among preterm infants whose mothers smoked during pregnancy. Am J Respir Crit Care Med 1998; 158:700–705.
125. Martinez FD, Morgan WJ, Wright AL, Holberg C, Taussig LM, The Group Health Medical Associates. Initial airway function is a risk factor for recurrent wheezing respiratory illnesses during the first three years of life. Am Rev Respir Dis 1991; 143:312–316.
126. Gold DR, Wypij D, Wang X, Speizer FE, Pugh M, Ware JH, et al. Gender and race-specific effects of asthma and wheeze on level and growth of lung function in children in six U.S. cities. Am J Respir Crit Care Med 1994; 149:1198–1208.
127. Gerritsen JGH, Koeter GH, Postma DS, Schouten JP, Knol K. Prognosis of asthma from childhood to adulthood. Am Rev Respir Dis 1989; 140:1325–1330.
128. Schwartz J, Gold D, Dockery DW, Weiss ST, Speizer FE. Predictors of asthma and persistent wheeze in a national sample of children in the United States: association with social class, perinatal events and race. Am Rev Respir Dis 1990; 142:555–562.
129. Griscom NT, Wohl MEB, Fenton T. Dimensions of the trachea to age 6 years related to height. Pediatr.Pulmonol 1989; 6:186–190.
130. Greenberg DN, Yoder BA, Clark RH, Butzin CA, Null DM. Effect of maternal race on outcome of preterm infants in the military. Pediatrics 1993; 91:572–577.
131. North AF, MacDonald HM. Why are neonatal mortality rates lower in small black infants than in white infants of similar birth weight? J Pediatr 1977; 90:809–810.
132. Stocks J, Gappa M, Rabbette PS, Hoo A-F, Mukhtar Z, Costeloe KL. A comparison of function in Afro-Caribbean and Caucasian infants. Eur Respir J 1994; 7:11–16.
133. Pool JB, Greenough A. Ethnic variation in respiratory function in young children. Respir Med 1989; 83:123–125.
134. American Thoracic Society. Lung function testing: selection of reference values and interpretative strategies. Am Rev Respir Dis 1991; 144:1202–1218.

135. Wohl MEB. Pulmonary sequelae of insults to the lung in early life. Pediatr Pulmonol 1995; 19:90–95.
136. Samet JM, Tager IB, Speizer FE. The relationship between respiratory illness in childhood and chronic air-flow obstruction in adulthood. Am Rev Respir Dis 1983; 127:508–523.
137. Weiss ST, Tager IB, Munoz A, Speizer FE. The relationship of respiratory infections in early childhood to the occurrence of increased levels of bronchial responsiveness and atopy. Am Rev Respir Dis 1985; 131:573–578.
138. Shaheen SO, Barker DJP. Early lung growth and chronic airflow obstruction. Thorax 1994; 49:533–536.
139. Thibeault DW, Sigalet DL. Congenital diaphragmatic hernia from the womb to childhood. Curr Probl Pediatr 1998; 28:1–25.
140. Ijsselstijn H, Tibboel D, Hop WJC, Molenaar JC, de Jongste JC. Long-term pulmonary sequelae in children with congenital diaphragmatic hernia. Am J Respir Crit Care Med 1997; 155:174–180.
141. Harding R. Fetal breathing: relation to postnatal breathing and lung development. In: Hanson MA, Spencer JAD, Rodeck CH, Walters D, eds. Fetus and Neonate: Physiology and Clinical Applications. Vol 2. Breathing. Cambridge, UK: Cambridge University Press, 1994:63–84.
142. Hislop AA. Developmental anatomy and cell biology. In: Silverman M, ed. Childhood asthma and other wheezing disorders. London: Chapman and Hall Medical, 1995:35–54.
143. Burri PH, Hislop AA. Structural considerations. Eur Respir J 1998; 12:59s–65s.
144. Massaro GD, Massaro D. Formation of pulmonary alveoli and gas exchange surface area quantitation and regulation. Annu Rev Physiol 1996; 58:73–92.
145. Jaskoll T, Choy HA, Melnick M. The glucocorticoid-glucocorticoid receptor signal transduction pathway, transforming growth factor-β, and embryonic mouse lung development in vivo. Pediatr Res 1996; 39:749–759.
146. Melnick M, Choy HA, Jaskoll T. Glucocorticoids, tumor necrosis factor-α, and epidermal growth factor regulation of pulmonary morphogenesis: a multivariate in vitro analysis of their related actions. Dev Dyn 1996; 205:365–378.
147. Wong YC, Beardsmore CS, Silverman M. Antenatal dexamethasone and subsequent lung growth. Arch Dis Child 1982; 57:536–538.
148. Pinkerton KE, Willet KE, Peake JL, Sly PD, Jobe AH, Ikegami M. Prenatal glucocorticoid and T_4 effects on lung morphology in preterm lambs. Am J Respir Crit Care Med 1995; 156:624–630.
149. Johnson JWC, Mitzner W, Beck JC, London WT, Sly DL, Lee PA, et al. Long-term effects of betamethasone on fetal development. Am J Obstet Gynecol 1981; 141:1053–1061.
150. Tschanz SA, Damke BM, Burri PH. Influence of postnatally administered glucocorticoids on rat lung growth. Biol Neonate 1995; 68:229–245.
151. Stewart AG, Fernandes D, Tomlinson PR. The effect of glucocorticoids on proliferation of human cultured airway smooth muscle. Br J Pharm 1995; 116:3219–3226.
152. Laitinen LA, Laitinen A, Haahtela T. A comparative study of the effects of an in-

haled corticosteroid, budesonide, and a β_2-agonist, terbutaline, on airway inflammation in newly diagnosed asthma: a randomized, double-blind, parallel group controlled trial. J Allergy Clin Immunol 1992; 90:32–42.

153. Tomlinson PR, Wilson JW, Stewart AG. Salbutamol inhibits the proliferation of human airway smooth muscle cells grown in culture: relationship to elevated cAMP levels. Biochem Pharmacol. 1995; 49:1809–1819.
154. Upton MN, Watt GCM, Davey-Smith G, McConnachie A, Hart CL. Permanent effects of maternal smoking on offspring's lung function. Lancet 1998; 352:453.
155. Althuis MD, Sexton M, Prybylski D. Cigarette smoking and asthma symptom severity among adult asthmatics. J Asthma 1999; 36:257–264.
156. Burr ML, Anderson HR, Austin JB, Harkins LS, Kaur B, Strachan DP, et al. Respiratory symptoms and home enviroment in children: a national survey. Thorax 1999; 54:27–32.
157. Cook DG, Strachan DP. Summary of effects of parental smoking on the respiratory health of children and implications for research. Thorax 1999; 54: 357–366.
158. Li JS, Peat JK, Xuan W, Berry G. Meta-analysis on the association between environmental tobacco smoke (ETS) exposure and the prevalence of lower respiratory tract infection in early childhood. Pediatr Pulmonol 1999; 27:5–13.
159. Bodner CH, Ross S, Little J, Douglas JG, Legge JS, Friend JAR, et al. Risk factors for adult onset wheeze. Am J Respir Crit Care Med 1998; 157:35–42.
160. Di Stefano A, Capelli A, Lusuardi M, Balbo P, Vecchio C, Maestrelli P, et al. Severity of airflow limitation is associated with severity of airway inflammation in smokers. Am J Respir Crit Care Med 1998; 158:1277–1285.
161. Collins MH, Moessinger AC, Kleinerman J. Fetal lung hypoplasia associated with maternal smoking: a morphometric analysis. Pediatr Res 1985; 19:408–412.
162. Milerad J, Larsson H, Lin J, Sundel HW. Nicotine attenuates the ventilatory response to hypoxia in the developing lamb. Pediatr Res 1995; 37:652–660.
163. Lewis KW, Bosque EM. Deficient hypoxia awakening response in infants of smoking mothers; possible relationship to sudden infant death syndrome. J Pediatr 1995; 127:691–699.
164. Taylor B, Wadsworth J. Maternal smoking during pregnancy and lower respiratory tract illness in early life. Arch Dis Child 1987; 62:786–791.
165. Maritz GS, Woolward K. Effect of maternal nicotine exposure on neonatal lung elastic tissue and possible consequences. S Afr Med J 1992, 81:517–519.
166. Sekhon HS, Jia Y, Raab R, Kuryatov A, Pankow JF, Whitsett JA, et al. Prenatal nicotine increases pulmonary $\alpha 7$ nicotine receptor expression and alters fetal lung development in monkeys. J Clin Invest 1999; 103:637–647.
167. Young S, Le Souëf PN, Geelhoed GC, Stick SM, Turner KJ, Landau LI. The influence of a family history of asthma and parental smoking on airway responsiveness in early infancy. N Engl J Med 1991; 324:1168–1173.
168. Tager IB, Hanrahan JP, Tosteson TD, Castile RG, Brown RW, Weiss ST, et al. Lung function, pre- and post-natal smoke exposure, and wheezing in the first year of life. Am Rev Respir Dis 1993; 147:811–817.
169. Merth IT, de Winter JP, Borsboom GJJM, Quanjer PH. Pulmonary function during

the first year of life in healthy infants born prematurely. Eur Respir J 1995; 8:1141–1147.
170. Pelkonen AS, Hakulinen AL, Turpeinen M. Bronchial lability and responsiveness in school children born very preterm. Am J Respir Crit Care Med 1997; 156:1178–1184.
171. von Mutius E, Nicolai T, Martinez FD. Prematurity as a risk factor for asthma in preadolescent children. J Pediatr 1993; 123:223–229.
172. Nikolajev K, Heinonen K, Koskela H, Korppi M, Lansimies E, Jokela V. Determinants of bronchial responsiveness at school age in prematurely born children. Pediatr Pulmonol. 1999; 28:408–413.
173. Hislop A, Wigglesworth JS, Desai R, Abet V. The effects of preterm delivery and mechanical ventilation on human lung growth. Early Hum Dev 1987; 15:147–164.
174. Hislop AA. Bronchopulmonary dysplasia: pre- and postnatal influences and outcome. Pediatr Pulmonol 1997; 23:71–75.
175. Pierce MR, Bancalari E. The role of inflammation in the pathogenesis of bronchopulmonary dysplasia. Pediatr Pulmonol 1995; 19:371–378.
176. Abman SH, Groothius JR. Pathophysiology and treatment of bronchopulmonary dysplasia; current issues. Pediatr Clin North Am 1994; 41:277–315.
177. Northway WHJ, Moss RB, Carlisle KB, Parker BR, Popp RL, Pitlick PT, et al. Late pulmonary sequelae of bronchopulmonary dysplasia. N Engl J Med 1990; 323:1793–1799.
178. Lamarre A, Linsao L, Reilly BJ, Swyer PR, Levinson H. Residual pulmonary abnormalities in survivors of idiopathic respiratory distress syndrome. Am Rev Respir Dis 1973; 108:56–61.
179. Northway WH, Moss RB, Carlisle KB, Parker BR, Popp RL, Pitlock PT, et al. Late pulmonary sequelae of bronchopulmonary dysplasia. N Engl J Med 1990; 323:1793–1799.
180. Bader D, Ramos AD, Lew CD, Platzker ACG, Stabile MW, Keens TG. Childhood sequelae of infant lung disease: exercise and pulmonary function abnormalities after bronchopulmonary dysplasia. J Pediatr 1987; 110:693–699.
181. Cano A, Payo F. Lung function and airway responsiveness in children and adolescents after hyaline membrane disease: a matched cohort study. Eur Respir J 1997; 10:880–885.
182. Buist AS, Vollmer WM. Prospective investigations in asthma: what have we learned from longitudinal studies about lung growth and senescence in asthma? Chest 1987; 91:119s–126s.
183. Redline S, Tager IB, Segal MR, Gold D, Speizer FE, Weiss ST. The relationship between longitudinal change in pulmonary function and nonspecific airway responsiveness in children and young adults. Am Rev Respir Dis 1989; 140:179–184.
184. Merkus PJFM, Van Essen-Zandvliet EEM, Kerrebijn KF, Quanjer PH. Large lungs after childhood asthma: a case control study. Am Rev Respir Dis 1993; 148:1484–1489.
185. Sherrill D, Sears MR, Lebowitz MD, Holdaway MD, Hewitt CJ, Flannery EM, et al. The effects of airway hyperresponsiveness, wheezing, and atopy on longitudinal pulmonary function in children: a 6-year follow-up study. Pediatr Pulmonol 1992; 13:78–85.

186. Elias JA. Airway remodeling in asthma: unanswered questions. Am J Respir Crit Care Med 2000; 161:S168–S171.
187. Armstrong DS, Grimwood K, Carlin JB, Carzino R, Gutièrrez JP, Hull J, et al. Lower airway inflammation in infants and young children with cystic fibrosis. Am J Respir Crit Care Med 1997; 156:1197–1204.
188. Durieu I, Peyrol S, Gindre D, Bellon G, Durand V, Pacheco Y. Subepithelial fibrosis and degradation of the bronchial extracellular matrix in cystic fibrosis. Am J Respir Crit Care Med 1998; 158:580–588.
189. Wagener JS, Kahn TZ, Copenhaver SC, Accurso FJ. Early inflammation and the development of pulmonary disease in cystic fibrosis. Pediatr Pulmonol 1997; 16:267–268.
190. Bronsveld I, Bijman J, Mekus F, Ballmann M, Veeze HJ, Tummler B. Clinical presentation of exclusive cystic fibrosis lung disease. Thorax 1999; 54:278–281.
191. Hiatt PW, Grace SC, Kozinetz CA, Raboudi SH, Treece DG, Taber LH, et al. Effects of viral lower respiratory tract infection on lung function in infants with cystic fibrosis. Pediatrics 1999; 103:619–626.
192. Campbell PW, Saiman L. Use of aerosolized antibiotics in patients with cystic fibrosis. Chest 1999; 116:775–788.
193. Devadason SG, Everard ML, Linto JM, Le Souëf PN. Comparison of drug delivery from conventional versus "Venturi" nebulizers. Eur Respir J 1997; 10:2479–2483.
194. Wilson D, Burniston M, Moya E, Parkin A, Smye S, Robinson P, et al. Improvement of nebulised antibiotic delivery in cystic fibrosis. Arch Dis Child 1999; 80:348–352.
195. Conway SP. Evidence for using nebulised antibiotics in cystic fibrosis. Arch Dis Child 1999; 80:307–309.
196. Bisgaard H. A metal aerosol holding chamber devised for young children with asthma. Eur Respir J 1995; 8:856–860.
197. Coates AL, Ho SL. Drug administration by jet nebulization. Pediatr Pulmonol 1998; 26:412–423.
198. O'Callaghan C. How to get drugs into the respiratory tract. Arch Dis Child 1993; 68:441–443.
199. Lewis R. Nebulisers for lung aerosol therapy. Lancet 1983; 2:849.
200. Thomas SHL, O'Doherty MJ, Graham A, Page CJ, Nunan TO. Pulmonary deposition of nebulised amiloride in cystic fibrosis: comparison of two nebulisers. Thorax 1991; 46:717–721.
201. Ilovite JS, Gorvoy J, Smaldone GC. Quantitative deposition of aerosolized gentamicin in cystic fibrosis. Am Rev Respir Dis 1987; 136:1445–1449.
202. Clay MM, Pavia D, Clarke S. Effect of aerosol particle size on bronchodilation with nebulised terbutaline in asthmatic subjects. Thorax 1986; 41:364–368.
203. Salmon B, Wilson NM, Silverman M. How much aerosol reaches the lungs of wheezy infants and toddlers? Arch Dis Child 1990; 65:401–403.
204. Barry PW, O'Callaghan C. Nebuliser therapy in childhood. Thorax 1997; 52:S78–S88.
205. Bisgaard H. Patient-related factors in nebulized drug delivery to children. Eur Respir Rev 1997; 7:376–377.

206. Becquemin MH, Swift DL, Bouchikhi A, Roy M, Teillac A. Particle deposition and resistance in the nose of adults and children. Eur Respir J 1991; 4:694–702.
207. Bisgaard H. Towards improved aerosol devices for the young child. Pediatr Pulmonol 1999; 18:78.
208. Dubus JC, Marguet C, Le Roux P, Brouard J, Heraud MC, Fayon M, et al. Local side effects of inhaled corticosteriods in infantile asthma. Eur Respir J 1999; 14:(Suppl 30):280s.
209. Agertoft L, Pedersen S. Importance of the inhalation device on the effect of budesonide. Arch Dis Child 1993; 69:130–133.
210. Pedersen S, Hansen O, Fuglsang G. Influence of inspiratory flow rate upon the effect of a Turbuhaler. Arch Dis Child 1990; 65:308–310.
211. Gagliardi L, Rusconi F. Respiratory rate and body mass in the first three years of life. Arch Dis Child 1997; 76:151–154.
212. Rabbette PS, Fletcher ME, Dezateux CA, Soriano-Brucher H, Stocks J. The Hering-Breuer reflex and respiratory system compliance in the first year of life: a longitudinal study. J Appl Physiol 1994; 76:650–656.
213. Stick S. Measurements During Tidal Breathing. In: Stocks J, Sly PD, Tepper RS, Morgan WJ, eds. Infant Respiratory Function Testing. New York: Wiley, 1996:117–138.
214. American Thoracic Society/European Respiratory Society. Respiratory mechanics in infants: physiologic evaluation in health and disease. Am Rev Respir Dis 1993; 147:474–496.
215. Dolovich M. Aerosol delivery to children: what to use, how to choose. Pediatr Pulmonol 1999; 18:79–82.
216. Crompton GK. Inhalational flows in adult patients populations, including those with acute asthma. J Aerosol Med 1997; 10:S23–S29
217. Borgström L, Bondesson E, Moren F, Trofast E, Newman S. Lung deposition of budesonide inhaled via Turbuhaler: a comparison with terbutaline sulphate in normal subjects. Eur Respir J 1994; 7:69–73.
218. Chernick V, Boat TF, Kendig EL. Kendig's Disorders of the Respiratory Tract in Children, 6th ed. Philadelphia: Saunders, 1998.
219. Pedersen S. Delivery options for inhaled therapy in children over the age of 6 years. J Aerosol Med 1997; 10:S41–S44.
220. Nikander K, Bisgaard H. Impact of constant and breath-synchronized nebulization on inhaled mass of nebulized budesonide in infants and children. Pediatr Pulmonol 1999; 28:187–193.
221. Collis GG, Cole CH, Le Souëf PN. Dilution of nebulised aerosols by air entrainment in children. Lancet 1990; 336:341–343.
222. Nikander K. Adaptive aerosol delivery: the principles. Eur Resp Rev 1997; 7:385–387.
223. Thomas RG. Regional human lung dose following inhalation of radioactive particles at ages one month to adulthood. Ann Occup Hyg 1988; 32:1025–1033.
224. Xu GB, Yu CP. Effects of age on deposition of inhaled aerosol in the human lung. Aerosol Sci Technol 1986; 5:349–357.
225. Le Souëf PN. Validity of methods used to test airway responsiveness in children. Lancet 1992; 339:1282–1284.

226. Alderson PO, Secker-Walker RH, Strominger DB, Markham J, Hill RL. Pulmonary deposition of aerosols in children with cystic fibrosis. J Pediatr 1974; 84:479–484.
227. Wildhaber JH, Devadason SG, Wilson JM, Roller C, Lagana T, Borgström L, et al. Lung deposition of budesonide from turbuhaler in asthmatic children. Eur J Pediatr 1998; 157:1017–1022.
228. Brusasco V, Crimi E, Pellegrino R. Airway hyperresponsiveness in asthma: not just a matter of airway inflammation. Thorax 1998; 53:992–998.
229. Widdicombe JG. Neurophysiology of the cough reflex. Eur Respir J 1995; 8:1193–1202.
230. O'Callaghan C, Milner AD, Swarbrick A. Paradoxical deterioration in lung function after nebulised salbutamol in wheezy infants. Lancet 1986; 2:1424–1425.
231. Croteau JR, Cook CD. Volume-pressure and length-tension measurements in human tracheal and bronchial segments. J Appl Physiol 1961; 16:170–172.
232. Prendiville A, Green S, Silverman M. Paradoxical response to nebulised salbutamol in wheezy infants, assessed by partial expiratory flow-volume curves. Thorax 1987; 42:86–91.
233. Brown RH, Mitzner W. Effect of lung inflation and airway muscle tone on airway diameter in vivo. J Appl Physiol 1996; 80:1581–1588.
234. Brusasco V, Crimi E, Barisione G, Spanevello A, Rodarte JR, Pellegrino R. Airway responsiveness to methacholine: effects of deep inhalations and airway inflammation. J Appl Physiol 1999; 87:567–573.
235. Woolcock AJ, Salome CM, Yan K. The shape of the dose-response curve to histamine in asthmatic and normal subjects. Am Rev Respir Dis 1984; 130:71–75.
236. Brown RH, Mitzner W. The myth of maximal airway responsiveness in vivo. J Appl Physiol 1998; 85:2012–2017.
237. Spahn JD, Szefler SJ. The etiology and control of bronchial hyperresponsiveness in children. Curr Opin Pediatr 1996; 8:591–596.
238. Frey U, Jackson AC, Silverman M. Differences in airway wall compliance as a possible mechanism for wheezing disorders in infants. Eur Respir J 1998; 12:136–142.
239. Stick SM, Arnott J, Turner DJ, Young S, Landau LI, Le Souëf PN. Bronchial responsiveness and lung function in recurrently wheezy infants. Am Rev Respir Dis 1991; 144:1012–1015.
240. Hopp RJ, Bewtra AK, Nair MN. Methacholine inhalation challenge studies in a selected pediatric population. Am Rev Respir Dis 1986; 134:994–998.
241. Silverman M. Bronchodilators for wheezy infants? Arch Dis Child 1984; 59:84–87.
242. Lenney W, Milner AD. At what age do bronchodilator drugs work? Arch Dis Child 1978; 53:532–535.
243. Soto ME, Sly PD, Uren E, Taussig LM, Landau LI. Bronchodilator response during acute viral bronchiolitis in infancy. Pediatr Pulmonol 1985; 1:85–90.
244. Robertson CF, Smith F, Beck R, Levison H. Response to frequent low doses of nebulised salbutamol in acute asthma. J Pediatr 1985; 106:672–674.
245. Greenough A, Loftus BG, Pool J, Price JF. Response to bronchodilators assessed by lung mechanics. Arch Dis Child 1986; 61:1020–1023.

246. Turner DJ, Landau LI, Le Souëf PN. The effect of age on bronchodilator responsiveness. Pediatr Pulmonol 1993; 15:98–104.
247. Mochizuki H, Shigeta M, Kato M, Maeda S, Shimizu T, Mirokawa A. Age-related changes in bronchial hyperreactivity to methacholine in asthmatic children. Am J Respir Crit Care Med 1995; 152:906–910.
248. Burrows B, Sears MR, Flannery EM, Herbison GP, Holdaway MD, Silva PA. Relation of the course of bronchial hyperresponsiveness from age 9 to age 15 to allergy. Am J Respir Crit Care Med 1995; 152:1302–1308.
249. Castile RG. Pulmonary function testing in children. In: Chernick V, Boat TF, Kendig EL, eds. Kendig's Disorders of the Respiratory Tract in Children, 6th ed. Philadelphia: Saunders, 1998:196–214.
250. Castile RG, Hyatt RE, Rodarte JR. Determinants of maximal expiratory flow and density dependence in normal humans. J Appl Physiol 1980; 49:897–904.
251. Tiddens HAWM, Bogaard JM, de Jongste JC, Hop WCJ, Coxson HO, Paré PD. Physiological and morphological determinants of maximal expiratory flow in chronic obstructive lung disease. Eur Respir J 1996; 9:1785–1794.
252. Hughes JMB, Pride NB. Lung Function Tests: Physiological Principles and Clinical Applications. London: Saunders, 1999.
253. Dawson SV, Elliott EA. Wave-speed limitation on expiratory flow—a unifying concept. J Appl Physiol Respir Environ Exerc Physiol 1977; 43:498–515.
254. McNamara JJ, Castile RG, Glass GM, Fredberg JJ. Heterogeneous lung emptying during forced expiration. J Appl Physiol 1987; 63:1648–1657.
255. McNamara J, Castile R, Ludwig M. Interdependent regional emptying during forced expiration. J Appl Physiol 1994; 76:356–360.
256. Cotes JE. Lung function throughout life: determinants and reference values. In: Leathart GL, ed. Lung Function: Assessment and Applications in Medicine. Oxford: Blackwell, 1993.
257. Quanjer PH, Tammeling GJ, Cotes JE, Pedersen OF, Peslin R, Yernault J-C. Lung volumes and forced ventilatory flows. Eur Respir J 1993; 6:5–40.
258. Taylor AE, Rehder K, Hyatt RE, Parker JC. Clinical pulmonary function tests. In: Wonsiewicz M, ed. Clinical Respiratory Physiology. Philadelphia: Saunders, 1989:147–168.
259. Bennett WD, Scheuch G, Zeman KL, Brown JS, Kim C, Heyder J, et al. Regional deposition and retention of particles in shallow, inhaled boluses: effect of lung volume. J Appl Physiol 1999; 86:168–173.
260. Wagner EM, Bleecker ER, Permutt S, Liu MC. Direct assessment of small airways reactivity in human subjects. Am J Respir Crit Care Med 1998; 157:447–452.
261. Wagner PD, Hedenstierna G, Rodriguez-Roisin R. Gas exchange, expiratory flow obstruction and the clinical spectrum of asthma. Eur Respir J 1996; 9:1278–1282.
262. Bhuyan U, Peters AM, Gordon I, Davies H, Helms P. Effects of posture on the distribution of pulmonary ventilation and perfusion in children and adults. Thorax 1989; 44:480–484.
263. Drummond GB. Computed tomography and pulmonary measurements Br J Anaesth 1998; 80:665–671.
264. Coren ME, Ng V, Rubens M, Rosenthal M, Bush A. The value of ultrafast

computed tomography in the investigation of pediatric chest disease. Pediatr Pulmonol 1998; 26:389–395.

265. Okazawa M, Müller N, McNamara AE, Child S, Verburgt L, Pare PD. Human airway narrowing measured using high resolution computed tomography. Am J Respir Crit Care Med 1996; 154:1557–1562.
266. Davies H, Kitchman R, Gordon I, Helms P. Regional ventilation in infancy: Reversal of adult pattern. N Engl J Med 1985; 313:1626–1628.
267. Davies H, Helms P, Gordon I. Effect of posture on regional ventilation in children. Pediatr Pulmonol 1992; 12:227–232.
268. Lauzon A-M, Prisk GK, Elliott AR, Verbanck S, Paiva M, West JB. Paradoxical helium and sulfur hexafluoride single-breath washouts in short-term vs. sustained microgravity. J Appl Physiol 1997; 82:859–865.
269. Sala H, Veriter C, Rodenstein D, Alzaibar C, Liistro G. Can "pendelluft" explain supramaximal flows (SF) during interrupted forced expirations? Eur Respir J 1999; 14.
270. Brown JS, Gerrity TR, Bennett WD. Effect of ventilation distribution on aerosol bolus dispersion and recovery. J Appl Physiol 1998; 85:2112–2117.
271. Rosenthal FS, Blanchard JD, Anderson PJ. Aerosol bolus dispersion and convective mixing in human and dog lungs and physical models. J Appl Physiol 1992; 73:862–873.
272. Rosenthal FS. The effect of nonuniform ventilation on the dispersion of inspired aerosol bolus: a modelling study. J Aerosol Med 1993; 6:177–197.
273. Smaldone GC, Messina MS. Enhancement of particle deposition by flow-limiting segments in humans. J Appl Physiol 1985; 59:509–514.
274. Smaldone GC, Messina MS. Flow limitation, cough, and patterns of aerosol deposition in humans. J Appl Physiol 1985; 59:515–520.

4

In Vitro Testing of Pharmaceutical Aerosols and Predicting Lung Deposition from In Vitro Measurements

ANDY CLARK

Inhale Therapeutics Systems
San Carlos, California

LARS BORGSTRÖM

AstraZeneca R&D
Lund
Uppsala University
Uppsala, Sweden

I. Introduction

The relationship between a pharmaceutical aerosol product's physical performance and its clinical safety and efficacy are of primary importance to product developers, regulators, and prescribing physicians alike. Being able to predict lung deposition, and the resulting safety and efficacy of a product, from physical characteristics measured on the laboratory bench has therefore been one of the "holy grails" of pharmaceutical aerosol science. With the advent of better laboratory sizing techniques and more accurate in vivo lung deposition methodologies, the grail is nearer than ever to being found. However, as one would expect from the diverse array of aerosol generation systems used in the delivery of inhaled medications, the correlations, such as they are, between laboratory and clinic are complex and to a large extent product- or at least modality-specific.

Beyond their potential value in predicting lung deposition, in vitro laboratory tests are a major component of the quality-control and product-release process for pharmaceutical aerosol products. In this context they are not required to have any in vivo predictive power. Demonstrating that different batches of product possess the same physical characteristics is all that is needed. However, understanding a test's relevance to clinical performance is important.

When considering the performance of an inhalation aerosol, the important in vivo parameters are the total dose that reaches the patient (a measure of the total drug exposure to the body and hence safety) and the deposition pattern of the inhaled dose in the airways (a measure of the drug distributed between the pharmacologically active and nonactive sites hence a measure of safety and efficacy). In principle the former of these can be measured in vitro using simple filter techniques. However, because of the effects that breathing patterns and peak flows can have on aerosol generation, this simple measure does not always return a valid in vivo prediction. Obtaining realistic estimates of delivered dose can be far more complex than would initially be expected. The second parameter, deposition and distribution of the inhaled aerosol within the airways, can by definition be determined only in vivo. In vitro laboratory tests must therefore use a surrogate measurement. Deposition patterns in the human airways are controlled by three major factors: airway geometry, the aerodynamic particle size distribution of the inhaled aerosol and the inhalation flow rate at which it is inhaled. The first of these is strictly a patient characteristic and, although of major importance, is not related to the aerosol generation system. However, the latter two can both be characteristics of a delivery device/formulation. The particle size because the device is generating the aerosol that is being inhaled. The inspiratory profile because a devices resistance characteristics can and does influence inspiratory flows. Of these two factors, it is the aerodynamic particle size that is the "surrogate" for deposition. However, a devices effect on inhalation profiles and the interaction of the dynamics of the aerosol with the airways must always be taken into account when carrying out laboratory tests. For this reason a variety of approaches are used to determine delivered dose and aerosol size distributions. The popular techniques and methods are discussed below. Suffice to say here that different modalities often require very different instrumental approaches if useful "predictive" data are to be obtained.

Assuming that a reliable aerodynamic size distribution has been determined in vitro, the theoretically correct way to proceed in order to compute lung deposition is to carry out a mathematical convolution of the aerosol size distribution with the functions describing deposition in the various compartments of the airways. In principle this can be done using deterministic type approaches to lung deposition modeling (1) or by using empirical correlations that approximate deposition in the various lung compartments (2). For a stable nonhygroscopic aerosol that is traveling at the same velocity as the inspired airstream under normal tidal breathing conditions, this type of calculation usually result in reasonable estimates of the average deposition in the airways. For example, we will see later that this approach appears to work reasonably well for nebulized aerosols delivered under normal tidal breathing conditions provided the droplet size is measured in an appropriate manner (3). However, in general, these calculations are tedious and, because of the highly dynamic nature of some aerosols, such as pressurized metered-dose inhaler (pMDI), and the "artificial" breathing patterns used when inhaling most medical aerosols, this approach rarely results in correct predictions without considerable data manipulation being performed. A further complication is that the nature of dynamic aerosols results in sizing data that are very often dependent upon the particular apparatus used to measure them. In most cases, therefore, deposition estimates are made from correlations relating the fraction of the inhaled aerosol in the particular size range, with the potential to penetrate and deposit in the lungs, to actual deposition values determined by scintigraphy or pharmacokinetics. This aerosol fraction is usually referred to as the fine particle fraction (FPF) or fine particle dose (FPD) and is discussed in more detail below. FPF and FPD are, however, at best, only measures of aerosol quality that correlate with deposition and no single size fracion, no matter how carefully chosen, can ever truly represent the complex convolution of deposition probabilities with an aerodynamic size distribution. In the search for the holy grail, we should not necessarily look for as close a numerical prediction as possible but instead look for a technique that gives the lowest variability in "predicted" lung deposition. Provided a good correlation can be demonstrated, the actual lung deposition could be easily calculated.

The following sections detail existing in vitro/in vivo correlations for the major aerosol modalities and, where appropriate, comparisons are made with lung model predictions. Measures of particle diameter, particle size statistics, and aerosol test methods are also discussed. Aerosol test methodologies are included in the discussion because, as described above, sizing results are highly dependent upon the method and apparatus used. The correlations that have been developed and any predictions that can be made from them are therefore specific to the use of particular experimental methods, and it is important that the applicability of the different instruments/methods be understood.

II. Aerosol Characterization Techniques

A. Aerosol Size

There are many ways to describe the "size" of an aerosol particle. For example it may be described by its longest dimension or by a sphere of equivalent volume. It may be described by its light scattering properties or by the way it behaves in an airstream. In a very real sense there is no such thing as the "correct" size or diameter of an aerosol particle. There are as many "correct" diameters as there are ways of measuring it, and it is up to the researcher to measure a size parameter relevant to the particular application under investigation. From a deposition perspective, it is the inertial behavior of the particle in an airstream that defines how and where it will deposit (Chap. 2). This characteristic diameter is known as the aerodynamic diameter and is the characteristic diameter that is normally measured for inhalation aerosol products. It is defined as the diameter of a sphere of unit density which has the same settling velocity in air as the aerosol particle being measured. Mathematically this is

$$d_{ae} = d_p\sqrt{\rho_p}$$

Where d_{ae} is the aerodynamic diameter, ρ_p is the particle density, and d_p is its physical diameter. For a sphere, d_p is the sphere's diameter; for an irregular particle, d_p will depend on particle shape. By definition, a water droplet with density of 1 g/cm^3 will have the same aerodynamic and physical diameter. It is the aerodynamic size distribution which is measured as the in vitro surrogate for inhalation aerosols.

The Log-Normal Distribution Function

Aerosols generally consist of particles or droplets with a range of sizes. It is advantageous to describe these size distributions by distribution functions. Many functions are in use (4); however, it is the log-normal distribution that is generally used to describe inhalation aerosols. Mathematically, this is described by the function

$$df = \frac{1}{\sqrt{2\pi}\ln\sigma_g}\exp\left\{\frac{\left(\ln d_p - \ln\bar{d}\right)^2}{2\left(\ln\sigma_g\right)^2}\right\}d\ln d_p$$

where σ_g is the geometric standard deviation (GSD) and represents the width of the distribution, d_p is particle diameter, and $\bar{d}$ is the median diameter (50% of the particles are larger than the median and 50% are smaller). The distribution can be expressed in particle number terms, in which case the median diameter is the count median, or particle mass, in which case it is the mass median diameter. In drug delivery, it is the mass of drug at a particular deposition site (or, more correctly, the concentration of drug at a particular site) that is important. It is therefore the mass median aerodynamic diameter (MMAD) and the associated GSD that are usually used to describe pharmaceutical aerosol size distributions. Figure 1 illustrates mass and count distributions for a log-normally distributed aerosol with a GSD of 2. The conversion between the count and mass distribution was performed using the Hatch Coate equations (5). The equation for conversion from MMAD to count median diameter (CMAD) is shown in the figure insert. Also shown are the FPFs for 3 and 5 μm (see below). It should be noted that when the distribution is expressed as a count distribution, the aerosol "appears" to be much finer. This is a ploy that is sometimes used when trying to make an aerosol distribution appear to be of a much higher quality than it really is. Statements such as "the number of particle less than 5 μm" should always be regarded as indicating a poor-quality aerosol.

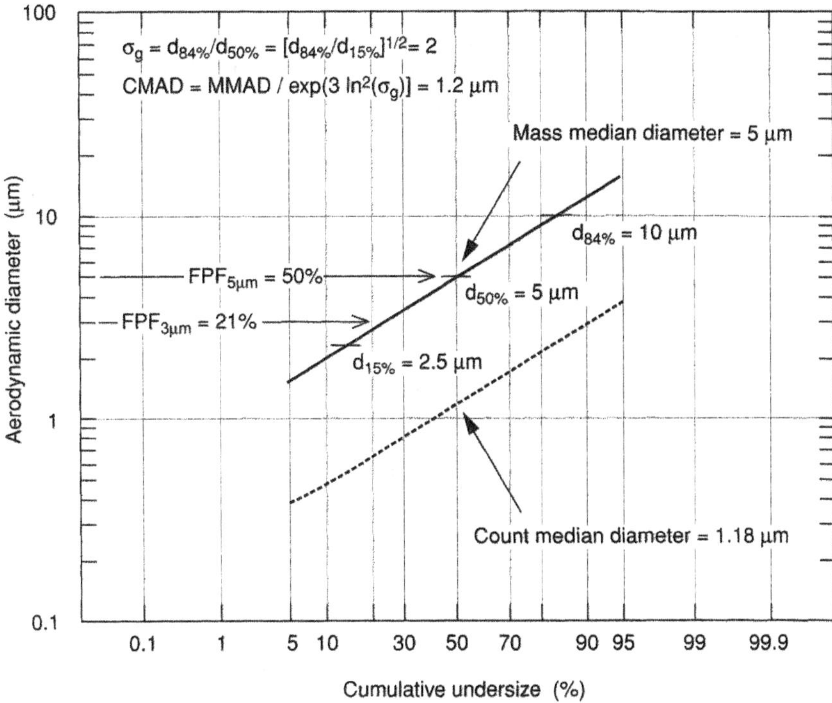

Figure 1 Example of log-normal aerosol size distribution illustrating MMAD, CMAD, GSD, and FPF values for an aerosol with mass median aerodynamic diameter of 5 μm and a geometric standard deviation of 2.

Fine Particle Fraction and Fine Particle Dose

As discussed above and elucidated below, because of the highly dynamic nature of inhalation aerosols, it is often erroneous to try and calculate deposition from in vitro size distributions and mathematical lung models. For this reason, and to simplify data interpretation, FPF or FPD is often used to describe the quality of an inhalation aerosol. FPF refers to that fraction of an aerosol that is in a size range with the potential to penetrate and deposit in the airways. FPD refers to the mass of drug in the potential deposition size range. The particular size ranges chosen can vary greatly and are usually defined more as a matter of experimental convenience than as an exact representation of that fraction of the aerosol that would deposit in the lung. For example, a value corresponding to a particular cut-off diameter for the cascade impactor being used to measure the size distribution may be chosen ($FPF_{4.7\mu m}$ for stage 3 of the Andersen impactor) or a diameter corresponding to a particular channel on a diffraction analyzer ($FPF_{5\mu m}$ for channel 22 on a Malvern Mastersizer) may be used. Although somewhat arbitrary, the diameter ranges are loosely based on the 1- to 5-μm aerodynamic size range believed to be capable of the greatest penetration into the intermediate and peripheral lung. However, FPFs may vary in range from as small as 0.5–3 μm to as large as 1–10 μm, depending upon what purpose it is being used for and by whom it is being defined. Although, in general, these FPFs and FPDs do not represent lung deposition per se; (in fact, they are usually overestimates of lung deposition (see below)). They do serve as a relative measure of aerosol quality and they are often used as the independent variable in in vitro/in vivo deposition correlations.

In Vitro Aerosol Characterization Techniques

Inertial Impaction

As described above and elsewhere in this text, it is the inertial behavior and the aerodynamic properties of an inhalation aerosol which dictate its deposition profile within the airways. It should therefore not be too surprising that an inertial separation method should constitute the "gold standard" for in vitro characterization of inhalation aerosols. Although there are a variety of ways of embodying inertial separation into a sizing instrument, it is the jet and impaction plate, and the cascade or multistage versions of it, that have proven to be the most effective. In this technique the airflow carrying the aerosol is directed by a jet, or nozzle, at an impaction plate. The airflow is forced to make a sharp turn as it impinges on the plate and the particles with the highest inertia, which cannot make the turn, impact out. "Finer" particles with less momentum follow the flow lines more easily and pass the plate without impacting. By carefully controlling the flow rate, or air velocity, impinging on the plate and geometry of the collection plate itself, a fairly precise aerodynamically size-selective instrument can be produced. When a size distribution is required, a "cascade" of jets and impaction plates are employed. Each successive stage is designed to increase the velocity of the airstream emanating from the jet(s) so that particles with successively less and less mass, or smaller and smaller aerodynamic diameters, are impacted out. In practice, because of the limitations of stage geometry, the capture efficiency of an impactor stage varies with particle diameter and usually exhibits a sigmoid nature. Impactor stages are therefore defined by their d_{50} or "cutoff" diameters—that is, the aerodynamic diameter for which the probability of capture is 50%. In most cases, over a reasonable range of operational flow rates, the d_{50} varies in a manner consistent with a dimensionless number known as the Stokes number.

$$St = \frac{4\rho_p C_c d_p^2 Q}{9\pi\eta D_n^3}$$

where ρ_p is particle density, C_c is Cunningham's slip correction factor, d_p is particle diameter, Q is volumetric flow rate, η is air viscosity, and D_n is the nozzle diameter. This leads to the conclusion that the d_{50} for an impactor stage generally scales as $Q^{1/2}$ (i.e., d^2Q = const) (6,7).

One of the main problems with cascade impaction is carryover of the particles to lower or "finer" stages than their aerodynamic diameter would suggest. This can occur either because of reentrainment into the airstream or simply because particles bounce of the collection plates (4). A detailed description of the methods used to minimize these phenomena can be found elsewhere. Suffice to say here that a variety of impactor designs have evolved to combat these issues and to facilitate assay of impacted drug. Figure 2 presents schematics of the three most popular instruments used in pharmaceutical aerosol testing (6). The Andersen cascade impactor, originally developed for environmental monitoring, and the Multi-Stage Liquid Impinger, originally developed for airborne bacterial sampling, have enjoyed the highest popularity with regulators and pharmaceutical scientists. More recently the Marple-Miller impactor was developed with the intention of minimizing the labor involved in impactor analysis. Calibrations have been developed for these instruments that allow them to be operated across a reasonably wide range of flows. (Tables 1 and 2) (6, 8, 9).

As can be seen, the cutoff diameters generally follow the $Q^{1/2}$ relation, as would be expected from the Stokes relationship described above. The ability to operate an impactor over a wide range of flow rates is particularly important in testing dry powders inhalers (see below).

After inertial separation of the particles within these instruments, it is necessary to quantify the amount of drug in each of the size fractions in order to derive an aerosol size distribution. This is usually performed by chemical assay for drug substance and may entail a variety of analytical techniques. However, it is important that drug substance be assayed, because most pharmaceutical aerosols contain excipients and the distribution of the drug and excipients will not necessarily be uniform and in equal proportion across the entire size distribution.

One last obstacle remains before cascade impactors can be effectively used for the analysis of pharmaceutical aerosols; that is, how to introduce the aerosol into the instruments. From a practical perspective, most aerosol products deliver their aerosols in the horizontal plane and cascade impactors have generally been designed to operate in the vertical plane. An inlet bend or manifold is therefore required. Additionally, as described below, the dynamic nature of some aerosols requires that the inlet mimic the oropharyngeal cavity. For these reasons a variety of inlet bends or "throats" have been developed. Figure 3 presents seven popular inlet configurations (10). They range from oropharyngeal casts to simple right-angle bends. Traditionally, despite their limited representation of the oral cavity, the twin impinger inlet and USP-2 inlet have been used the most. Although, with the advent of advanced imaging techniques such

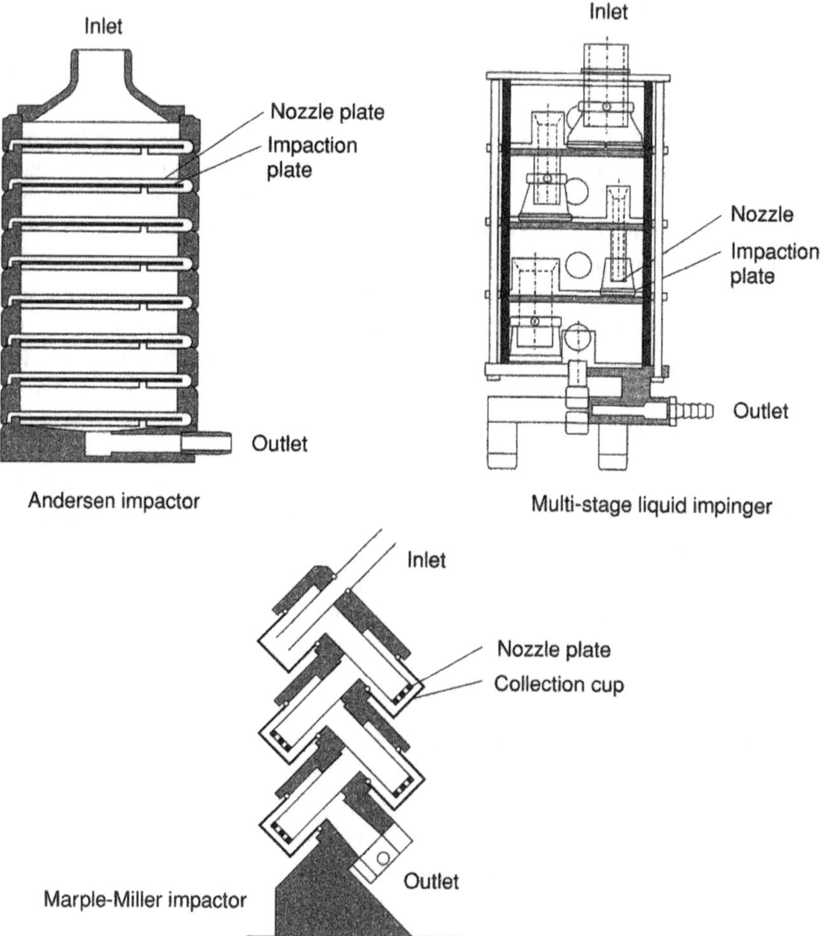

Figure 2 Cross-sectional views of the Andersen sampler Mark II impactor, the Multi-Stage Liquid impinger, and the Marple-Miller impactor. (From Ref. 6.)

as magnetic resonance, spiral computed tomography and stereo lithography, replica oropharyngeal casts are becoming more popular. A consortium of pharmaceutical companies in Europe is currently developing, if possible, a range of standard anatomic casts, beginning with adults.

Light-Scattering Techniques

As described above, inertial cascade impaction is the gold standard for characterization of pharmaceutical aerosols. However, it is not the only method avail-

Table 1 Nominal Cutoff Diameters of the MLI in the Flow Range 30–100 L/Min

Stage	Cutoff Diameter (µm) at Flow Rate Q (L/min)
Stage 1	$ECD_{50\%,Q} = 13.0(Q/60)^{-1/2}$
Stage 2	$ECD_{50\%,Q} = 6.8\ (Q/60)^{-1/2}$
Stage 3	$ECD_{50\%,Q} = 3.1\ (Q/60)^{-1/2}$
Stage 4	$ECD_{50\%,Q} = 1.7\ (Q/60)^{-1/2}$

ECD = Effective cut-off diameter.
Source: Ref. 9.

Table 2 Nominal Cutoff Diameters for the Mark II Eight-Stage Andersen Impactor at Flow Rates of 28.3 and 60 L/Min

	Operational Flow Rate 28 L/min		Operational Flow Rate 60 L/min
Stage	dae_{50} Theory	dae_{50} Actual	dae_{50} Actual
0	9.0	8.6	5.6
1	5.8	5.9	4.3
2	4.7	4.6	3.4
3	3.3	3.1	2.0
4	2.1	2.0	1.1
5	1.1	0.9	0.5
6	0.7	0.5	0.3
7	0.4	0.2	0.1

Source: Ref. 6.

able, and a number of other characterization techniques are being used. The two most popular are the laser diffraction technique and the single particle aerodynamic sizer.

Diffraction Analyzers

Diffraction instruments were initially developed to size liquid droplet fuel aerosols (11). They have therefore found a natural application in the characterization of the liquid droplet aerosols produced by nebulizers. In the diffraction analyzer, the aerosol droplets are illuminated with a monochromatic, spatially expanded laser beam. The resulting far-field diffraction pattern produced by the droplets is a function of their size distribution and is generally described by a set of first-and second-order Bessel functions. Large droplets scatter light at small angles; small droplets scatter light at high angles. With the aid of mathematical techniques, the diffraction pattern can be analyzed and inverted to pro-

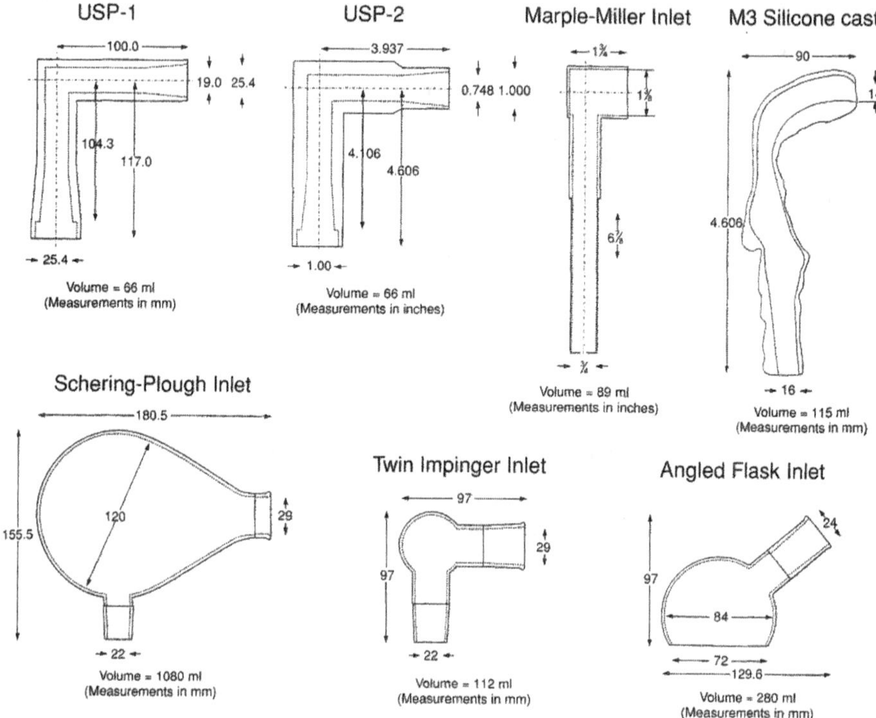

Figure 3 Dimensions and volumes of seven popular inlet "throats" used with cascade impactors for the analysis of pharmaceutical aerosols. The USP-1, USP-2, and twin impinger inlet are the most popular. (From Ref. 10.)

duced the size distribution of the illuminated droplets. The technique's advantages are that it is extremely quick, requires no chemical assays, and can measure droplet diameters immediately as droplets exit a nebulizer mouthpiece (3). A typical experimental configuration is shown in Fig. 4. In general, for aqueous solutions, the physical diameter measured is equivalent to aerodynamic diameter, since the density of nebulized droplets is close to unity. However, the technique does have its disadvantages, it suffers from lack of resolution for aerosols of the order of 1 μm and the inversion routines can produce erroneous results if the refractive index of the droplets is not known. Also, diffraction analysis cannot be applied to suspension nebulizer formulations, since it measures droplet size and cannot determine which droplets contain drug particles. The use of the technique in developing predictive deposition correlation for nebulized aerosols is described below (3).

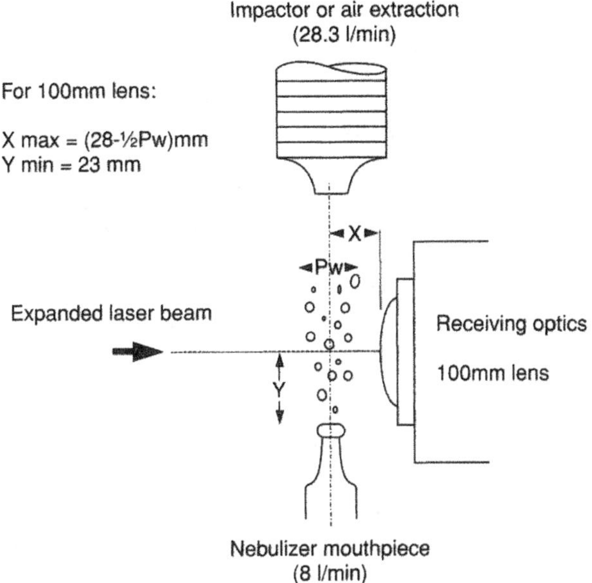

Figure 4 Experimental configuration of laser diffraction analyzer used to measure droplet distributions produced by aqueous nebulizers. Droplet collection may be by impactor, as shown, or by simple filtration. (From Ref. 3.)

Single-Particle Counters

A number of single-particle counting instruments have also been used for pharmaceutical aerosol characterization. The most popular of these are the so-called time-of-flight instruments (12, 13). These devices measure the deceleration of aerosol particles as they are injected into a laser sensing zone. Since they measure aerodynamic behavior, they do give a direct measure of aerodynamic size. However, while they are valuable research instruments with undoubted application to the study of pharmaceutical aerosols, they have not been used extensively because of severe experimental limitations. Like all light-scattering instruments, they do not measure the size distribution of the drug but rather the combined distribution of the drug and excipients. Also, they are limited in terms of the aerosol concentration they can operate with, and usually considerable aerosol dilution is required. This introduces experimental sampling problems and the possibility of large sampling errors. They also primarily determine aerodynamic number distributions, and as described above, it is really the mass distribution that is required when working with pharmaceutical aerosols. In the single-particle analyzer, mass distribution is always a calculated quantity. In general, then, these instruments have been used, but great care should be taken in interpreting the data they produce.

The second class of single-particle counting instruments that have been used with pharmaceutical aerosols are the phase Doppler analyzers (PDA)(14). PDAs use two intersecting laser beams to generate a set of interference fringes. As the droplets, or particles, traverse the interference zone, the Doppler signal generated by passage through the light and dark interference bands gives information about both the size and velocity of the droplets. The main limitations of this approach are that the sensing zone is small, it requires spherical droplets if "accurate" sizing data are required, and, off course, the instrument determines a number distribution as its primary distribution function. As with the time-of-flight instruments, weight distribution is a calculated quantity. The small interference zone means that measurements can be made at specific positions in a spray plume, thus affording spatial resolution that is not available with other techniques. However, while this is advantageous if spray structure is being investigated, a technique for averaging over an entire spray plume has to be developed if the overall size distribution of the spray is required. Dunbar et al. (15) have used the PDA to investigate pMDI spray structure. Finlay et al. (16) have successfully developed and applied an averaging technique and used it in conjunction with a deposition model to estimate lung doses from commercial nebulizer devices.

III. In Vivo Characterization Techniques

It might at first seem that correlations between in vitro data and the clinical efficacy of an inhaled pharmaceutical compound would be far more useful than correlations with deposition. However, because clinical measures of efficacy are generally much less precise than lung deposition measurements and since different molecules have different sites of action within the airways, this approach has not enjoyed much favor. Correlations based on lung deposition have a much broader application, are generally molecule-independent, and better describe device or delivery system performance. There are two classical ways of measuring lung deposition, scintigraphy, and pharmacokinetics.

A. Scintigraphy

In gamma scintigraphy, the formulation is labeled with a gamma ray–emitting isotope, and the fate of the inhaled drug, together with that retained in the delivery device, is followed by an external gamma camera (17). The labeling process varies from ad hoc mixing, resulting in a "loose" association of label and drug, to more sophisticated molecular labeling if a suitable atomic species is present. However, molecular labeling has been used only once as means of following a drug moiety, and direct mixing, using a variety of techniques, is the really the mainstay of the scintigraphy technique. The general process employed in aerosol scintigraphy is outlined in Fig. 5. The imaging technique normally used for pharmaceutical aerosols is planar scintigraphy (17). That is quantification of the deposited dose is performed from 2D images of the thorax and head. Although 3D imaging, by the way of single particle emission computed tomography, has been used and has advantages in terms of spatial resolution, it requires more sophisticated cameras, more complex data handling, longer acquisition times, and a higher level of radioactivity.

Two main difficulties exist with scinitgraphy. The first is labeling of the formulation and ensuring that the label follows the active drug sufficiently well to act as a valid marker for its aerodynamic behavior. The second is interpretation of the activity images in terms of anatomy and lung structure. The labeling techniques generally result in a label that associates with the aerosol in a way that mimics the size distribution of the drug and, as described above, it is rare that the molecule itself is labeled. Validation of the labeling process is performed using cascade impaction. Drug-specific assays are compared to radioactivity for

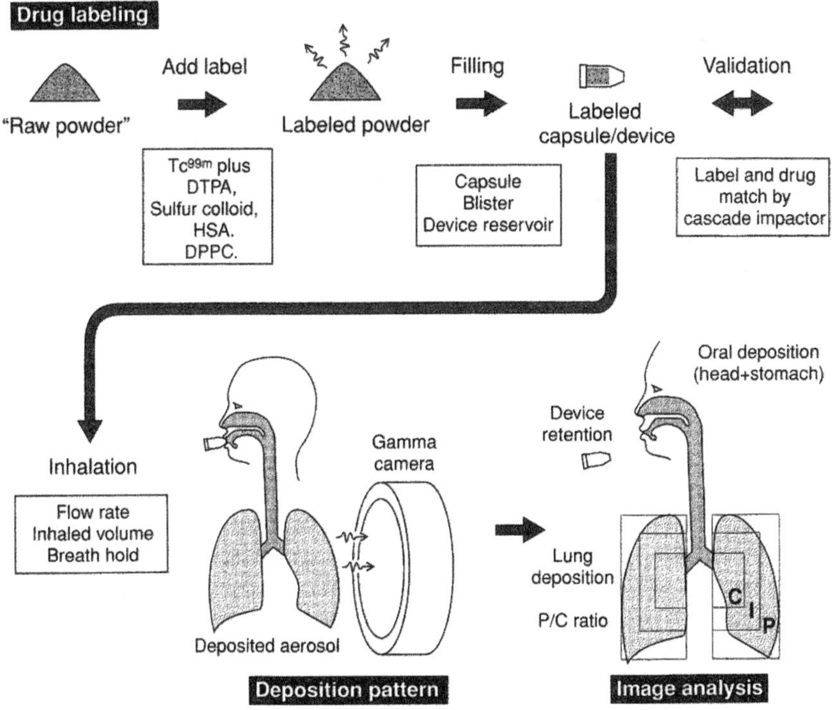

Figure 5 Schematic illustration of the application of gamma scintigraphy to the estimation of airway deposition profiles.

each stage fraction. The standard way of analyzing lung images is to use so called "regions of interest." These are defined arbitrarily and range from standard box matrices placed over the right and left lung images (19) to sophisticated routines that outline the lung and divide the image into central and peripheral zones by equal division of radius vectors or by area (20). The problem in all cases, however, is being able to interpret the "regions of interest" in terms of anatomic structures—i.e., conducting airways versus peripheral alveolar sacs. Some work has been done to calibrate peripheral-to-central (P/C) ratios (21,22) in terms of 24-h clearance measurements, but the relationships are fairly broad and certainly cannot be used on a individual basis. [Such 24-h clearance measurements are used to define deposition in the nonciliated region of the airways. Since the majority of insoluble particles deposited in the conducting ciliated airways are cleared by the mucociliary ladder and swallowed within 24 h, activity remaining after 24 h therefore represents alveolar, or at least nonciliated, airways (23) deposition.] Because of this lack of anatomic resolution, most of the in vivo/in vitro correlations that have been developed for pharmaceutical aerosols focus on whole-lung deposition rather than deposition patterns within the lungs. Gamma scintigraphy,however, does have an advantage over other techniques of assessing deposition profiles in that a "mass balance" (more correctly an activity balance) can be performed easily. The distribution of drug (label) throughout the delivery device, the body, including the distribution within the lung, and the exhaled air can be quantified individually. It is also noninvasive. For these reasons the technique has become the mainstay of in vivo drug deposition investigations. The major criticism of the technique is that the labeling process invariably results in manipulation of the product being tested and hence a product can never be tested in its original "unadulterated" form. In practice this concern can usually be mitigated by the demonstration of correspondence of the original and labeled aerosol size distributions.

B. Pharmacokinetics

The pharmacokinetic estimation of whole-lung deposition is based on the fact that, for some drug molecules, either because of their intrinsic properties or because their oral absorption can be blocked, drug appearing in the systemic circulation (24) or urine (25) represents drug initially deposited in the lung. This approach requires that the molecule not be metabolized in lung and that either oral absorption be intrinsically negligible or can be blocked by ingestion of an absorbing agent such as charcoal. Figure 6a and b summarize the steps involved in determining whole-lung deposition using the charcoal-block method. For molecules with negligible oral absorption, the ingestion of charcoal is obviously not necessary. Borgström (24) and others have used this technique effectively for terbutaline, budesonide, formoterol,

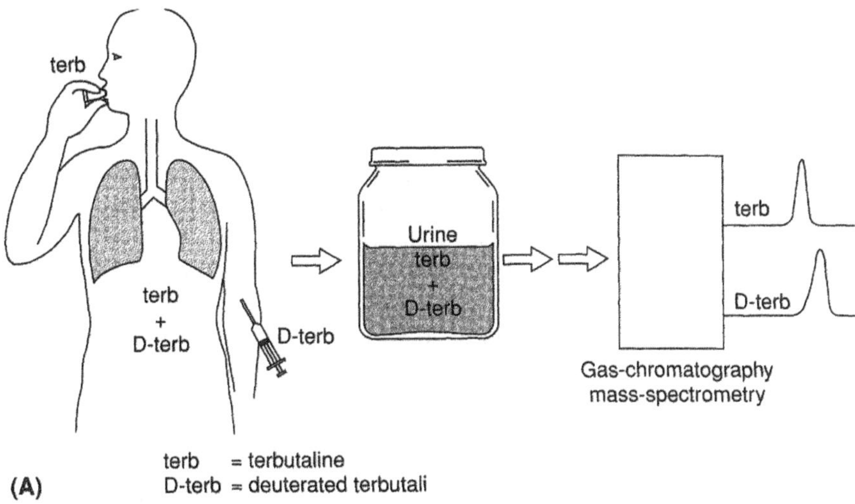

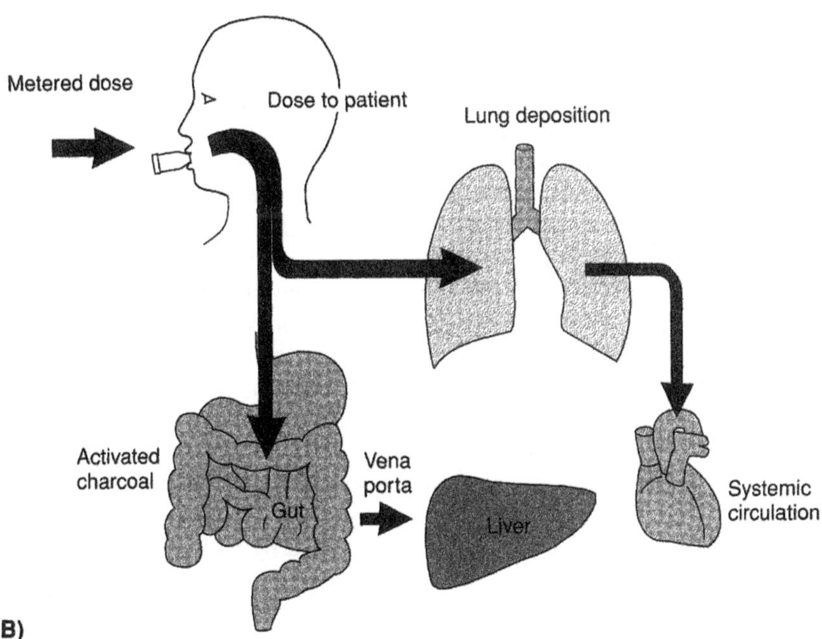

Figure 6 Schematic illustration of the application of pharmacokinetics and the charcoal block method to the estimation of lung deposition. (A) Use of urine collection. (B) Use of plasma collection. (From Ref. 24.)

salbutamol, sodium cromoglycate, nedocromil sodium, and ipratrpium bromide. Biddiscombe (26) has recently applied it to salbutamol. The main limitation of the technique is that it determines only the total amount of drug absorbed from the lung, and no information on regional distribution can be obtained. However, delivered dose, device retention, and the amount of drug exhaled can be quantified simultaneously by chemical assay techniques and the fraction of the nominal or inhaled dose deposited in the lung can be calculated. Borgstrom et al. (27) have shown that pharmacokinetically determined lung deposition is in agreement with that determined scintigraphically, both in terms of the mean fraction deposited and in terms of intersubject variability. A number of studies investigating the correlation between charcoal-block determinations of lung deposition and in vitro data have now been reported (see below).

IV. In Vitro Characterization: Issues and Limitations

A. Nebulizers

The production of aqueous droplets by pneumatic shear forces probably represents the oldest method of therapeutic aerosol generation. In more recent times, high-frequency ultrasonic transducers, low-frequency ultrasonic meshes, and mechanical extrusion have also been used. All of these systems generate liquid droplet streams that are entrained in humid airflows. In the pneumatic devices, the droplet distribution produced at the atomizer is usually very coarse (~ 50–80 μm) and baffles are needed to condition the aerosol and ensure that only "fine" droplets are inhaled by the patient. The recirculation caused by this baffling process can represent in excess of 95% of the atomizer flow. The air being pumped through the nebulizer therefore emerges moist and in quasiequilibrium with the vapor pressure of the droplets. Indeed, the major component of the temperature drop seen in the solution reservoir of a nebulizer during nebulization is caused by evaporation from these recirculated droplets. The other forms of nebulization also generally result in a humidified airstream in quasiequilibrium with the droplets. The term *quasiequilibrium* is used to describe the relationship between the droplets and the transporting airstream because they are not in true equilibrium and are unstable to evaporation/growth. The curvature of a droplet surface causes an excess vapor pressure, described by the Kelvin equation (4), which is proportional to the exponent of the inverse of the droplet diameter. The Kelvin effect means that a droplet size distribution can never be truly stable under uniform relative humidity conditions.

However, a further and much more important stability issue is that any entrained ambient air that enters the sizing instrument can be considerably drier than the humidified droplet-laden airstream emanating from the nebulizer. This can result in rapid droplet evaporation. The problem that these instabilities induce from a characterization perspective is that it is difficult to characterize an aqueous aerosol in a reproducible manner and in a way that is relevant to its deposition kinetics. Evaporation or growth can also take place in the airways after inhalation, and thus it is also questionable as to what diameter is actually "seen" during passage through the airways. This latter issue has led to a number of complex deposition models that incorporate, and try to account for, hygroscopic growth effects (29). The pragmatic approach of measuring the distribution in a reproducible way and correlating either MMAD or FPF has also been used (3).

There are only two experimental strategies that have the potential to yield reliable "predictive" results for nebulized aerosols. The first is to measure the droplets in their fully hydrated state. This can be done either immediately as they exit the mouthpiece, using a real-time sizing instrument, or by reducing the evaporation kinetics sufficiently to allow measurement downstream with an off-line technique such as inertial cascade impaction. The second is to completely dry the aerosol, size the dry particles, and then calculate back to obtain the original size distribution. Measuring the aerosol at intermediate hydration states between these two extremes is obviously problematic because the hydration state would have to be measured in order to correct the size distribution back to the original "inhaled" size.

The latter approach—completely drying the aerosol—while valid, is difficult to perform experimentally (29). The low solids content of pharmaceutical nebulizer solutions results in dry aerosols that are too fine for reliable enough measurements to be made to allow back calculation with any accuracy. For example a typical nebulizer droplet distribution with a mass median diameter of 3 μm generated from a 0.1% drug solution would result in a dry particle distribution with a mass median diameter of ~0.1 μm. Obtaining size distribution data with any reasonable resolution at this size is very problematic. A further issue is that the solids content of the original droplets must be known in order to perform the calculation, and this can vary considerably during the course of nebulization. This technique has therefore not been used extensively.

The former approach, attempting to measure the droplets in their fully hydrated state, has enjoyed more widespread use. Experimentally, this has been accomplished in a number of ways. The use of low-flow impactors that entrain minimal quantities of ambient air and hence maintain the quasiequilibrium humidity exiting the nebulizer is one approach (30). Adding humidified dilution air, rather than ambient air, to a high-volume cascade impactor is another. Cooling the impactor to the same temperature as the nebulizer cloud (reservoir) has also been shown to be an effective way of providing sufficient stabilization for aerosol measurement purposes (31). However, a technique that has been used extensively in conjunction with a large number of deposition studies is laser diffraction (3). As described above, this technique measures the physical diameter of aqueous droplets by deconvolution of a laser-derived diffraction pattern. It has the advantage that it can be used to measure the droplet distribution immediately as the aerosol exits the nebulizer mouthpiece, and the physical diameter it measures is equivalent to aerodynamic diameter for aqueous solutions with a density close to 1 g/cm^3. However, the diffraction technique is limited in that it can be applied only to nebulized solutions. Where suspension are to be measured and droplet occupancy is an issue, inertial impaction and chemical assay appears to be the only viable option.

B. Pressurized Metered-Dose Inhalers

The aerosol cloud delivered from a pMDI consists of a collection of evaporating droplets moving at high speeds (32). At the spray orifice, the droplets can be as large as 30–40 μm, and they can be moving at velocities of 30–60 m/s. As the plume moves away from the spray orifice and into the respiratory tract, the droplets evaporate and the cloud slows down. This highly dynamic behavior is at the heart of the problem of developing techniques to characterize pMDI clouds in a way that allows prediction of their in vivo performance. The difficulty stems from the fact that the aerodynamic size surrogate that can be used for nebulizer clouds and passive dry-powder aerosols no longer adequately describes the variables that control deposition. The probability of inertial impaction is controlled by an aerosol particles stopping distance ψ,

$$\Psi = \frac{\rho d^2 \upsilon}{18\eta}$$

where ρ is the particle density, υ is the particle velocity, d is the particle's aerodynamic diameter, and η is the viscosity of air. Here, ψ is literally the distance it takes an aerosol particle to stop when it is injected into still air at velocity υ. (Note: ψ is a special dimensional case of the nondimensional Stokes number described above in the context of inertial impactors.) As can be seen, the probability of impaction is dependent upon particle velocity as well as aerodynamic diameter. Thus, for pMDI clouds, with their high-velocity plumes, it is imperative that velocity be taken into account. The stopping distance of a unit-density 3-μm particle in the mouth when inhaled at 30 L/min is approximately 0.030 mm. The stopping distance of the same particle moving at a typical pMDI cloud velocity of 20 m/s in the mouth is 4 cm. It is for this reason that instruments such as single-particle counters or diffraction analyzers, which measure only droplet or particle size, are of little use in developing in vitro/in vivo correlations for pMDIs.

From an experimental perspective two basic approaches are possible. The first is to characterize the droplet/particle distribution and the velocity distribution separately and then compute some measure proportional to ψ. The second is to take a more empirical approach and use an apparatus that resembles the mouth and oropharynx. This latter approach is by far the most popular. However, its adoption has led to a wide selection of inlet manifolds or "throats" being used as entry ports for cascade impactors (Fig. 3), and since different throats can result in different values for FPFs and FPDs this has made it difficult to develop true global correlations that are useful for the prediction of deposition.

Cascade impaction has also been the method of choice for pMDI aerosols because they are generally multicomponent systems and drug assays are required if the drug size distributions are to be obtained. It is of course where the drug deposits and hence the drug size distribution that is of importance.

Spacers and Holding Chambers

A spacer puts distance, or "space," between a pMDI's actuator and a patient's pharynx so as to allow the initial velocity of the aerosol cloud to decay and the large propellant droplets to evaporate. A holding chamber, in addition, facilitates aerosol actuation into a chamber from which the patient can inhale without the need for coordination.

In order to assess the "efficacy" of a spacer at performing its task in vitro, it is necessary to take the aerosol cloud's velocity and droplet kinetics into account. Spacer testing is therefore carried out with similar test configurations to those used for standard pMDIs. Outside of the need for an inlet throat, a further and more subtle issue is whether flow through the spacer and sizing apparatus should be initiated before or after aerosol actuation. In that spacers still require a fairly high degree of coordination when used by a patient, and the intention is to actuate the aerosol during inspiration, it would appear that flow initiation prior to actuation is the most appropriate.

The possible pMDI exception to the use of model inlet throats is the characterization of the clouds produced by valved holding chambers. Holding chambers are designed to hold the aerosol cloud so that the initial velocity completely decays and the droplets evaporate prior to the patient's inhalation. From this perspective the aerosol inhaled from a holding chamber is "stable" and will travel at the same velocity as the airstream when it is inhaled. There is therefore no need for model inlets because, in principle at least, the standard deposition factors apply, and it is only aerodynamic particle size that is important. Thus, simple measurement of aerodynamic size distribution should correlate with deposition and lung model predictions. However, in reality, a lot of the work carried out with spacers and chambers in the in vitro setting is aimed at comparing efficiencies between the valved chambers, spacers, and standard pMDIs. As a result, oropharyngeal models are still popular. One of the golden rules of pharmaceutical aerosol science is that, wherever possible, the same methodology should be used if attempts are being made to compare the quality of different aerosols. Since valved holding chambers are designed to be used by the patient in a delay mode, fired, and then inhaled, aerosol testing should be performed by actuation and followed by flow initiation rather than with a continuous flow through the sizing apparatus/chamber.

C. Dry-Powder Inhalers

Dry-powder aerosol delivery offers yet another set of challenges from an in vitro/in vivo correlation perspective. There are two main types of dry-powder inhaler; those that are "passive" and rely on the patient's inspiratory effort to generate the aerosol and those that are "active" and use some form of internal power source. Examples of the former would be the Turbuhaler, Accuhaler/Diskus, and the like. Examples of the latter are the Dura Spiros and the Inhale pulmonary delivery system. Characterizing the aerosol clouds generated by these devices in a manner useful for deposition predictions can require different experimental approaches.

For the passive devices it is the patient's inspiratory effort that supplies the energy to disperse the powder and to draw the aerosol from the device (33). The aerosol particles are therefore moving at the same velocity as the airstream when they pass into the airways and, at least in principle, there is no need to consider the dynamics of the aerosol cloud when carrying out an in vitro characterization experiment. However, passive DPIs vary greatly in their resistance to airflow and as a result there are considerable differences in the flow rates at which different inhalers are used. Since the efficiency of powder dispersion and hence the particle size of the delivered aerosol is usually dependent upon effort and flow rate, the problem from an in vitro characterization perspective becomes "What is the appropriate flow rate to test at and what is the size fraction that should be used to define FPF or FPD?" The flow rate at which to test a device can be determined empirically by simply asking a group of patients to inhale through a device and recording their flow profiles, or by using one of the published relationships between device resistance and peak inspiratory flow. Figure 7 presents a typical flow/resistance correlation for healthy volunteers (54). The definition of the FPF size range, however, is a little more subtle. As described elsewhere in this book, the capture efficiency of the oropharynx and upper airways is a function of flow rate. The stopping distance parameter ψ, described above, would suggest that it is d^2Q that is the important parameter (where Q is the inhalation flow rate, which in this case is proportional to the air and particle velocity). Hence, it has been suggested that the size fraction considered to be "fine" should decrease as the square root of the inhalation flow rate or, since inertial impactors generally operate under the d^2Q law (see above), that the fraction below a particular stage be used to define FPF regardless of the flow rate at which a test is carried out. A further proposal is the use of the oral deposition function developed by Stahlhofen et al. to define FPF (14). The idea behind this approach is that it is oropharyngeal filtering which prevents most of the inhaled aerosol particles from reaching the

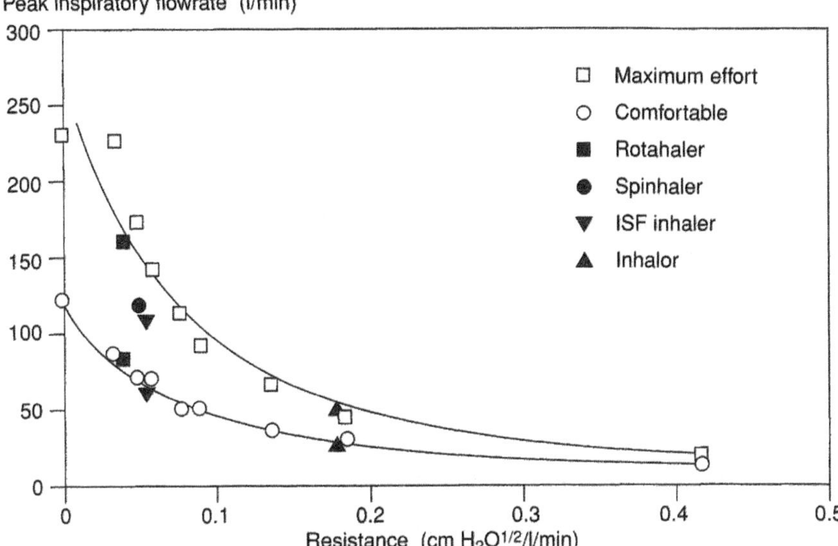

Figure 7 Peak inspiratory flow rate versus device resistance for patient-driven dry-powder inhalers illustrating "comfortable" and "maximum effort" curves for healthy volunteers. (From Ref. 34.) The United States Pharmacopiea specifies that DPIs should be tested at a device pressure drop of 4 kPa.

lung and hence it is how oropharyngeal deposition varies with flow rate that should define FPF. While this function generally follows the d^2Q law, the exponents are slightly modified to compensate for changes of oropharyngeal geometry with inhalation flow rate. The Stahlhofen equation (2) states that

$$\eta_{oral} = 1 - \left[1.5x10^{-5} \left(d_{ae}^2 Q^{\frac{2}{3}} V^{-\frac{1}{4}} \right)^{1.4} + 1 \right]^{-1}$$

where η_{oral} represent the probability of capture in the oropharyngeal region of the airways and V is the inspired volume. This function leads to FPF_{oral} being based on the d_{50}, or cut-off diameter, for the oropharynx, where the d_{50} is defined as

$$d_{oral} = (57.74/Q^{0.3})_{V=4\ \text{liters}}\ \mu m$$

In some cases, however, the fraction below a fixed size—for example, $FPF_{5\mu m}$—regardless of the test flow rate has been used to compare DPI performance; hence the effect of flow rate on particle behavior has not been accounted for correctly.

In nearly all cases, cascade impactors with inlet throats are used for the analysis of DPI clouds. In most instances this is because DPI clouds contain excipients as well as drug particles, and chemical drug-specific assays are required in order to measure the drug size distribution. Although inlet bends are not strictly necessary, because the aerosol particles are moving at the same speed as the "inhaled" air, they are usually used as a matter of experimental convenience.

For active devices the situation can be similar to the passive case in terms of the device resistance dictating the inhaled flow rate and hence the flow rate at which the device should be tested. However, just like the pMDI, if the device generates an aerosol that has a velocity relative to the inspired airstream, some form of stopping distance measurement, such as an oropharyngeal cast or inlet bend, is mandatory.

V. Predicting Lung Deposition

A. In Vitro/In Vivo Deposition Correlations for Nebulizers

Outside of the droplet sizing difficulties described above for nebulizer clouds, some further problems arise when trying to make droplet size/deposition correlations for use in predicting lung deposition from an inhaled dose. These are related to the interpretation of gamma camera images and fall into two categories. Experimental problems associated with accurately quantifying the deposited dose as a fraction of the inhaled dose and the use of different data reduction techniques by different investigators. The common practice is to express the lung dose as a fraction of that placed in the nebulizer or as a fraction of that deposited in the body and not as a fraction of the inhaled dose. This is mainly because of the experimental difficulty of splitting and separately quantifying the inhaled and exhaled aerosol. The former of these two practices is not useful in developing general droplet size deposition correlations because nebulizer efficiencies vary greatly from one device to another. The latter is more useful, but it is limited because it cannot be directly related to the dose inhaled by the patient, since—for nebulized aerosols used in a normal tidal breathing mode—a large fraction of the inhaled aerosol is exhaled, and this exhaled fraction is, as would be expected, also a function of droplet size. For these reasons the literature data that can be correlated must be presented as lung or peripheral dose expressed as a fraction, or percentage, of that deposited in the body, and the dose deposited as a fraction of that inhaled must be inferred by calculation from lung deposition models. This approach seems reasonably reliable, since, as will be seen below, deposition models appear to give reasonable predictions for nebulized aerosols.

This approach has been taken by Clark et al. (3), and the correlation plots are shown in Figs. 8 and 9. Fig. 8 presents a compilation of the available data relat-

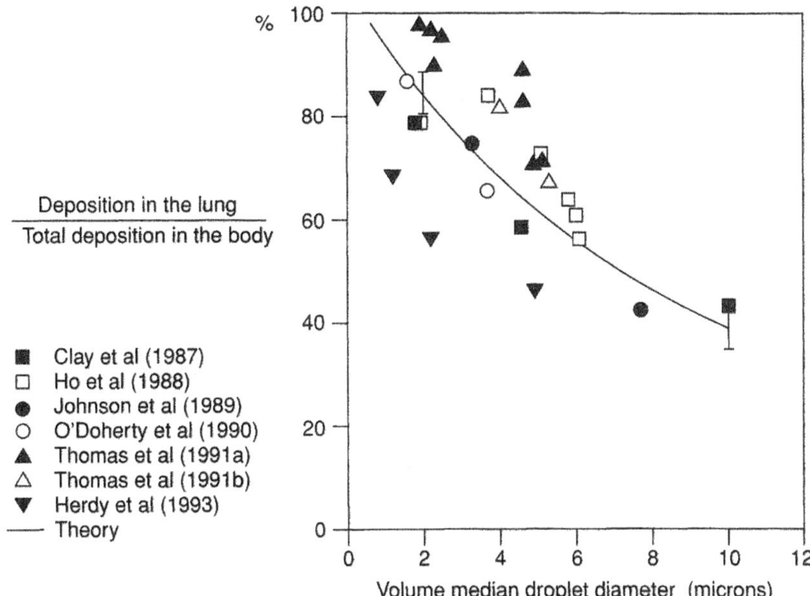

Figure 8 Correlation between the volume median diameter of a nebulized aerosol, measured by laser diffraction, and thoracic deposition expressed as percent of total body deposition. The 95% confidence intervals represent the variability between volunteer groups and not true intersubject variability. (From Ref. 3.)

ing volume median droplet diameter, as measured by laser diffraction, to whole-lung deposition. For the reasons described above, lung dose is expressed as a percentage of the total dose deposited in the body rather than a fraction of the inhaled dose. It can be seen that an excellent correlation exists, although there is a fairly large spread in the data. However, this variability is perhaps no more than would be expected from studies involving different groups of volunteers and from the application of the laser sizing methodology at different laboratories. (Unfortunately there are no data enabling one to distinguish between these two causes of variability.) Figure 9 presents a similar compilation for peripheral deposition as a function of droplet size. Peripheral deposition is expressed as a percentage of the dose deposited in the body and was determined by the 24-h clearance technique using human serum albumin. Again there is a good correlation between droplet size and deposition. In this case there is apparently less variability, but this may simply be due to fewer data on which to base the correlation. In both figures the deposition curves predicted by an empirical model have been overlaid on the data. It can be seen that there is generally good agreement between the

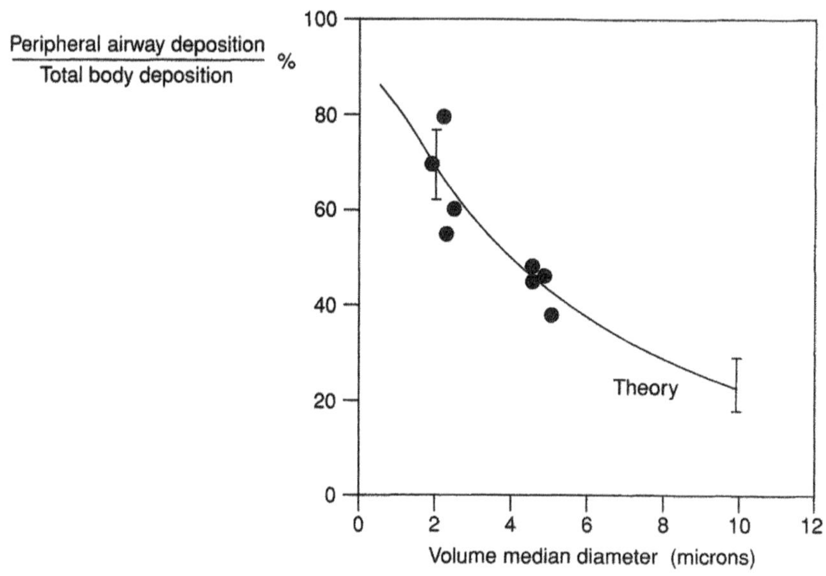

Figure 9 Peripheral deposition (defined by 24-h clearance measurements) for nebulized aerosols as a function of volume median diameter measured by laser diffraction analyzer. Peripheral deposition is expressed as a percent of total body deposition. (From Ref. 3.)

model (2) and experimental data. This confirms the validity of the size measurement technique and gives confidence in the application of the model to the calculation of deposited dose as a function of that inhaled.

The data presented above are derived using light-scattering techniques. However, it was also stated earlier that either low-volume impactors, humidification of entrained air, or possibly cooling the impactor results in sufficient quenching of the evaporation kinetics to be able to obtain droplet sizes by cascade impaction. The predicted deposition profiles presented above should thus be applicable to impactor-derived MMADs if they are determined appropriately. Indeed, Price et al. (35) have shown excellent agreement between LUDEP (23) (a deposition program developed by the NRPB, Chilton, UK) and lung deposition estimated by gamma camera for three studies carried out by Newman's group. The impactor technique also has an advantage over the light-scattering approach with respect to nebulizer suspensions such as budesonide. As discussed above, light-scattering measures the droplet distribution and cascade impaction coupled to drug assay can measure the distribution of the drug within the droplet distribution.

B. Model Predictions for Nebulizers

Figure 10 presents model calculations for normal airways when nebulized aerosols with a GSD of 2.2 and a median droplet diameter in the range 0.5–10 μm are "inhaled." The model does not make allowances for droplet size changes due to hygroscopic growth and does not represent diseased lungs (see below). The important features of the deposition predictions are that the total deposition in the body decreases as the median droplet size decreases, due to a higher proportion of the aerosol being exhaled. At the same time, the fraction of the aerosol deposited in the oropharynx and central airways shows a concomitant decrease. The net result of these effects is that peripheral deposition peaks at approximately 3 μm. However, over the 1- to 6-μm range, peripheral deposition varies by less than 20%, ranging between 30 and 38% of the inhaled dose. This means that the dose deposited in the peripheral lung remains almost constant over the size range 1–6 and that the only reason to use a "fine" nebulized aerosols in a reasonably

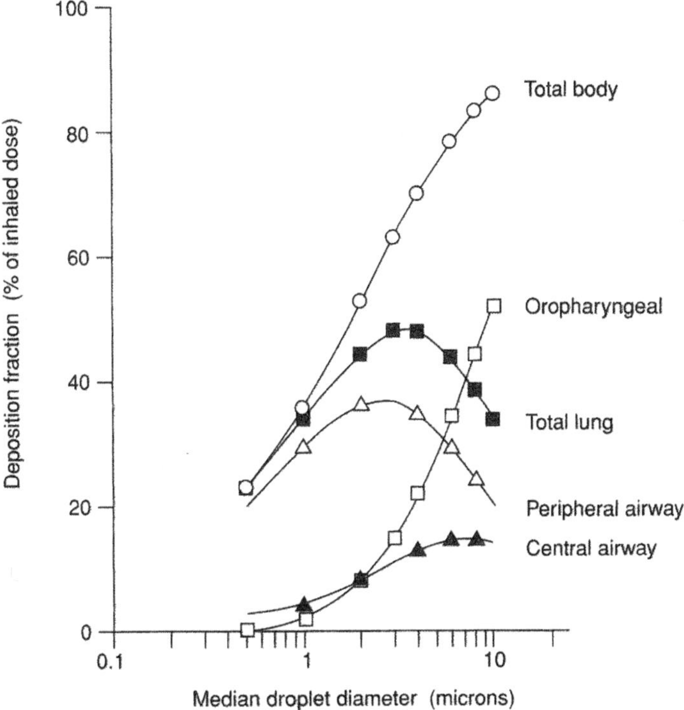

Figure 10 Deposition predictions of the Rudolf algebraic model for aqueous aerosols delivered from a nebulizer under normal tidal breathing conditions. (From Ref. 3.)

healthy airway is to avoid oral and conducting airway deposition, not to enhance the dose deposited in the lung periphery. However, for diseased lungs, the situation may be different.

C. Effects of Hygroscopic Growth

The data presented in Figs. 8 and 9 obviously take into account any changes in droplet size during passage of the aerosol through respiratory tract, since they summarize in vivo deposition studies. However, the modeling curves in the figures do not. It is thus instructive to ask what effect allowing for hygroscopic factors would have on the calculated deposition. A number of models incorporating growth kinetics have been developed. However, most assume infinite sink conditions, i.e., that the growth or evaporation of droplets does not affect ambient airway conditions. More recently, however, two-way coupled heat and mass transfer models have been developed (28). These models suggest that the isotonic nature of current nebulizer products would result in only small deviations from the simple deposition models. The two-way models generally predict a slightly higher lung deposition than would be expected for a given droplet size, but the predictions are within the scatter in Fig. 8. Finlay et al. (28) did show excellent agreement with two published studies for their model.

D. In Vitro/In Vivo Correlations for pMDIs and DPIs

Numerous attempts have been made to correlate lung deposition data for pMDIs and DPIs with in vitro FPF measurements. The most comprehensive reports are those presented by Newman et al. (36) and Olsson et al. (37). Newman et al. compared gamma camera data with FPFs determined with either a standard or high-precision MLI equipped with a glass bulb inlet or a standard USP inlet for 11 clinical studies. Olsson et al. used the charcoal-block pharmacokinetic method applied to studies involving salbutamol to determine whole-lung deposition as a function of FPFs determined by an Andersen impactor equipped with either a glass bulb inlet or an oropharyngeal model. The oropharyngeal model was based on a design developed by Swift. These studies involved a mixture of pMDIs, with and without spacers, and DPIs. Figure 11 presents a compilation of the data from both groups in terms of $FPF_{5.0\mu m}$ versus whole-lung deposition. It will be seen that there is a general correlation between $FPF_{5.0\mu m}$ and lung deposition, higher FPFs giving higher whole-lung deposition. However, $FPF_{5.0\mu m}$ overestimates lung deposition by a factor of approximately 1.7 and variability is high. The data indicate that a 20% $FPF_{5.0\mu m}$ could result in lung deposition as low as 8% or as high as 20%, depending upon the particular product under investigation. The correlation using standard inlets is therefore not very powerful as a predictive tool.

The two groups both implemented experimental improvements designed

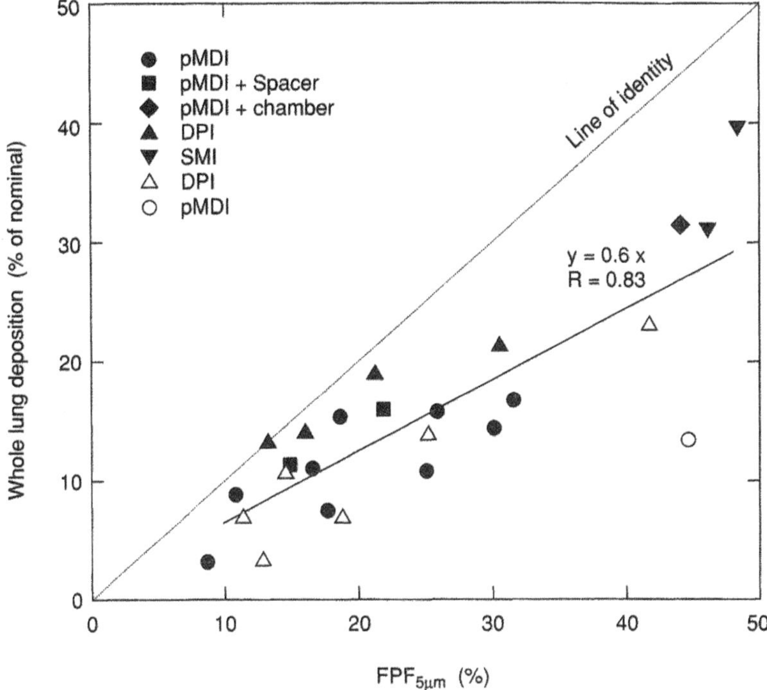

Figure 11 A compilation of $FPF_{5.0\mu m}$ versus whole lung deposition for the work of Newman et al. (36) (filled symbols) and Olsson et al. (37) (open symbols). Newman measured deposition by gamma camera. Olsson used the Charcoal block pharmacokinetics technique. Both groups used the twin impinger glass inlet (see Fig. 3).

to enhance the agreement between FPF and lung deposition. Newman redefined the FPF as $FPF_{5.0\mu m}$ (equivalent to the drug deposited on stage 4 and filter of the MLI). Olsson utilized an orophayngeal model in an attempt to more realistically represent the orophryngeal airspace. Figure 12 present Newman's $FPF_{3.1\mu m}$ correlation. Figure 13 presents the oropharyngeal model $FPF_{5.0\mu m}$ correlation of Olsson. It can be seen that Newman's approach improves the agreement and results in a slope of approximately 1, but fails to improve variability. Olsson's method on the other hand reduces variability, but it continues to "overestimate" lung deposition by a factor of 1.7. From the deposition data presented in earlier chapters this overestimate of lung deposition when using $FPF_{5.0\mu m}$ would seem quite logical in that none of the deposition models predict complete deposition of this size fraction. It would also be expected that an oropharyngeal model would bring pMDI data more in line with DPI data and reduce scatter since it deals more correctly

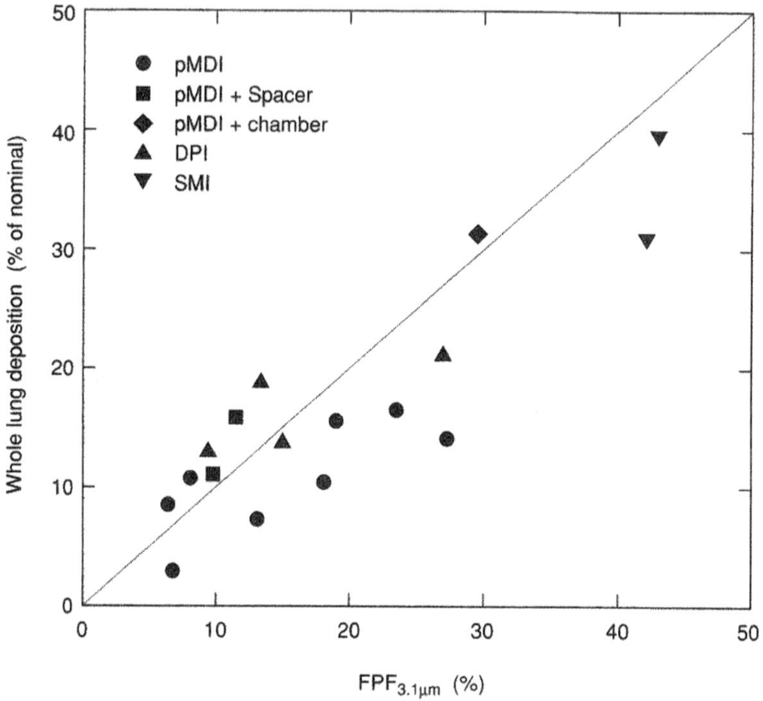

Figure 12 Correlation of $FPF_{3.1\mu m}$ versus whole lung deposition from Newman et al. (36). Note the data clusters close to the line of identity, but variability is still high.

with the dynamic plume. From Newman's data, $FPF_{3.1\mu m}$ appears to predict deposition more accurately—i.e., the linear fit gives a gradient close to the line of identity. However, this is probably because it underestimates the size range over which particles have some finite probability of deposition. Again, no single size fraction can really represent the complex convolution of a size distribution with the deposition probability equations that describe aerosol behavior in the human respiratory tract. As was stated above, a method that shows lower variability, not necessarily one that predicts the race more accurately, will take us closer to finding the holy grail.

E. Modeling Predictions for pMDIs and DPIs

A number of attempts have been made to use lung deposition models and in vitro size distributions to predict deposition profiles for both DPIs and pMDIs. These studies have always been performed in hind sight and are limited in extent because of the expense of performing lung deposition studies in human volunteers.

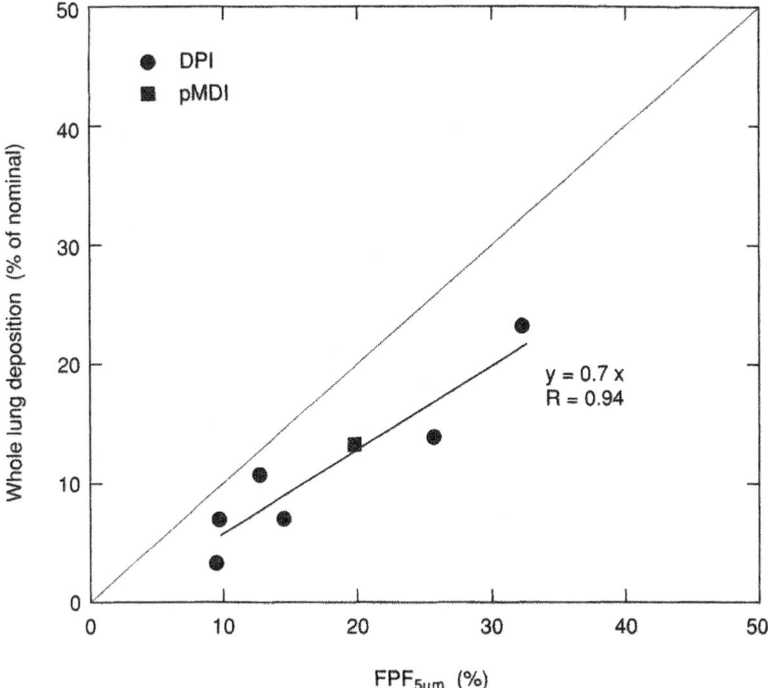

Figure 13 Correlation of $FPF_{5.0\mu m}$ when using an anatomic cast as the inlet "throat" versus whole-lung deposition from Olsson et al. (37). Note, that scatter has been reduced due to the more "correct" in vitro representation of the pMDI data point; however, as would be expected, the DPI points have been affected only marginally. The in vitro data continues to overestimate of lung deposition.

A lot of the studies have also been carried out using numerous and varied in vitro sizing techniques and this makes data evaluation doubly difficult. It was noted above how aerosol size distributions can be instrument- and technique-dependent. It should also be apparent that the mathematical calculation techniques used for DPIs and MDIs have to be different in order to take the different aerosol cloud dynamics into account.

Theil (39) recently proposed a method for dealing with pMDI "prediction" calculations. As described above, the main issue with pMDIs is the ballistic nature of the aerosol plumes they produce. Theil's approach is simply to remove the ballistic component, that fraction retained on the inlet "throat" of the impactor, from the deposition calculations by assuming it will all deposit in the mouth. Using only the data from the stages of the impactor and a proprietary fitting routine, he fits a log-normal distribution to the data and calculates a MMAD and GSD. The deposition prediction is then performed by applying a deposition model to the log-normal distribution to calculate the deposition pattern. Theil chose an empirical algebraic model, suitably modified to include a breath-holding pause after inhalation. Having determined the split between head and lungs for the nonballistic aerosol, the ballistic or "throat" fraction is then added to the calculated oral deposition to complete the calculation. Table 3 summarizes Thiel's calculations for five clinical studies comparing gamma camera deposition measurements with deposition model calculations. It can be seen that there really is a remarkable agreement between the model's "predictions" and the experimentally determined deposition. Typical differences between prediction and reality are less than 5%. This is all the more remarkable when one considers the huge intergroup variability highlighted in the nebulizer correlations shown above and the large individual variability seen in most deposition studies.

Clark et al. (40) developed what is a mathematically similar approach to Theil's, which was applied to both DPIs and pMDIs plus spacer and chambers. (Clark et al. deliberately avoided using data from pMDIs alone because of the difficulties associated with the ballistic nature of the plume.) The basis of the technique is the assumption that lung deposition is simply the inhaled dose minus that deposited in mouth and oropharynx. This approach does not require the application of a lung deposition model and is justified for most DPIs and pMDI since the fractions exhaled after a typical 5- to 10-s breath-hold are always close to zero. As an oral deposition function, Clark et al. chose to use the function proposed by Stahlhofen et al. and Rudolf et al., which is then numerically integrated with the size distribution derived from cascade impactor data to calculate oral deposition. Subtracting oral deposition from the inhaled dose allows calculation of the lung dose. Clark used gamma camera data from seven clinical studies, four DPI and three pMDI, to evaluate the approach. On analysis, it was seen that

Table 3 Comparison of Theoretical and Actual Deposition for Thiel's Model

	% Lung deposition	
Aerosol	Measured	Theoretical Prediction
Albuterol	35.1	33.8
Terbutaline DPI	32.4	31.6
Nacystelyn MDI with spacer	49.5	53.2
Albuterol DPTI	41.6	39.9
Steroid –50, breathing pattern A	50.9	49.7
Steroid –50, breathing pattern B	39.6	36.21

Source: Ref. 39.

calculated deposition is higher than actual deposition, suggesting that the oral deposition function, originally developed for application to environmental exposure situations, underestimates oral deposition from pharmaceutical aerosols. The approach generally overestimates lung deposition by a factor of 1.7. It should also be noted that this conclusion is not model specific and that convolution with other oropharyngeal functions, such as those proposed by Phalen or Yu, was also shown to result in a similar underestimation.

A further data set generated using LUDEP has been developed by Pritchard and colleagues (35,41,42). In series of three reports, they used a combination of LUDEP, and the Theil approach to ballistic fractions, to compare modeling predictions and deposition from the clinical work reported by Biddiscombe. Deposition was estimated using the charcoal block pharmacokinetic technique for four pMDI and three DPI formulations containing salbutamol. It was concluded that there is generally good agreement between theory and practice. However, the LUDEP model does not make allowances for a breath hold pause and always dramatically overestimates the exhaled fraction. There also appears to be a systematic underestimate of oral deposition in the data set. While these two generally compensate for each other and lead to the correct calculated lung deposition it does appear to be a case of two wrongs making a right. If lung deposition is assumed to be inhaled dose minus oral deposition the combined approach of ballistic component plus LUDEP underestimates oral deposition and overestimates whole-lung deposition, again suggesting that oral deposition for pharmaceutical aerosols is higher than predicted by the functions used by the environmental aerosol community.

Figure 14 presents a compilation of the data sets discussed above. In the case of the data generated by Clark and Pritchard, the data have been plotted as 100% minus oral deposition versus lung deposition. In the case of Theil, since his model included a breath-hold, the calculated lung deposition is reported against actual lung deposition. It can be seen that Clark's approach overestimates lung deposition by a factor of 1.7, Pritchard's approach, suitably modified to account for the exhaled fraction, overestimates it by 1.3 and Theil's approach appears to predict lung deposition correctly. It is interesting to speculate as to why Theil's approach appears to be so successful when Clark's and Pritchard's calculations show an overestimate of lung deposition. This is particularly perplexing as all three model's are based in the same empirical deposition equation's developed by Stahlhofen and Rudolf. It is even more fascinating since, because of the high oral deposition of the > 10 μm fraction and the low exhaled fractions, the three techniques appear to be mathematically equivalent. Unfortunately, direct comparison between the data sets is not possible because different clinical data were used by each group. It would appear that more work is needed before this issue will be resolved. However, these problems do highlight the fact that great care must be taken when attempting to predict deposition using in vitro sizing coupled to lung modeling.

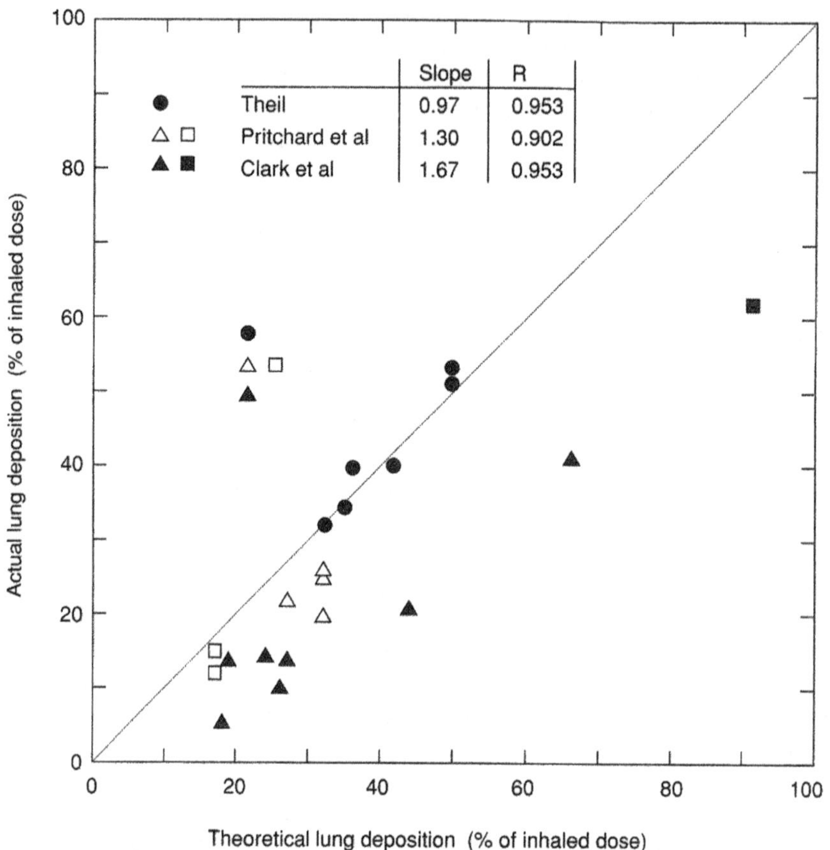

Figure 14 A comparison of model predictions and in vivo deposition for DPIs, pMDIs, and pMDIs plus spacers as developed by Clark et al. (40), Pritchard et al. (42), and Theil (59). Data generated by Pritchard have been plotted as inhaled dose minus oral deposition, so as to make it comparable to that of Clark et al. Theil's data have been plotted directly, since a breath-holding pause was incorporated in his calculations.

F. In Vitro Versus In Vivo Variability

The data reported in the sections above may, if viewed in a favorable light, lead to the conclusion that there are reasonable correlations between in vitro sizing data and mean lung deposition determined in vivo. (The predictive power of these correlations is discussed in more detail below.) However, one of the other factors that determines the suitability of an inhalation product for use with a particular drug is variability of deposition. As one would perhaps expect a priori, in vitro and in vivo variability can be very different. In vitro variability is made up of intrinsic product variability (differences in particle size distribution and delivered dose from shot to shot) and variability in the experimental methods. In vivo variability consists of product variability, variability caused by the way the product is used (for example, coordination with a pMDI or inhaled flow rate with a DPI) and anatomic differences between volunteers or patients. Borgström (43) investigated the relationship between in vitro and in vivo variability for a pMDI and a DPI, Turbuhaler, both of which delivered terbutaline. In addition the variability of lung dose determined by the charcoal block and gamma scintigraphic methods was compared. Table 4 summarizes the data. It can be seen that the in vitro and in vivo variability is reversed for the two products. The pMDI being the most reproducible in vitro and the DPI being the most reproducible in vivo. This is perhaps not too surprising, since pMDIs require a good deal of coordination in order to ensure correct delivery whereas DPIs only require the patient to inhale through them to ensure delivery. These data strongly suggest, for Turbuhaler at least, that the variability in aerosol quality that is caused by variations in the flow rate at which patients inhaled is far smaller than variability caused by incorrect coordination for the pMDI. These data illustrate that interpretation of in vitro dose uniformity data in terms of clinical variability is far from straightforward.

G. The Effect of Lung Disease

With some minor exceptions, the data presented above were obtained in healthy volunteers and patients with mild to moderate asthma. In part the heterogeneity of the volunteer groups may have contributed to the variance and spread of the data in the correlation plots. Theoretical calculations presented in the figures where derived from an empirical model based on mean deposition data in healthy volunteers. It is thus instructive to consider how airways disease would affect deposition. A detailed discussion is beyond the scope of this chapter. However, in general, airways disease affects the caliber of the airways and

Table 4 Comparison of In Vitro and In Vivo variability (CV%) for Terbutaline pMDI and Terbutaline DPI (Turbuhaler)

	Turbuhaler	pMDI
In vitro $FPF_{5.0\mu m}$ ($n = 100$)	18.2	6.4
Intrasubject variation ($n = 4$)	32.9	64.7
Intersubject variation ($n = 12$)	28.4	61.8

Source: Ref. 43.

would therefore be expected to affect regional deposition within the lung but not necessarily the total dose entering and depositing in the lung. This appears generally to be the case, with constricted airways causing higher central deposition. Indeed, Melchor et al. (44) have shown that, for DPI and pMDI products, regional distribution, not total lung deposition, is altered in disease. However, the situation with nebulized aerosols may be a little more complex, because the lack of a breath-hold pause during nebulizer therapy means that the total dose deposited in the lung may be dependent upon airway caliber. That is, the fraction of the dose lost to exhalation may be reduced due to higher lung deposition at airway constriction sites.

VI. Summary

The purpose of this chapter has been to review the literature and data that are available in relation to predicting lung deposition from in vitro measurements of pharmaceutical aerosols. In vitro test methods where described and discussed in the context of the dynamic behavior of inhalation aerosols, the issue being that an understanding of the behavior of the aerosol, coupled to and an understanding of the principles of operation of the sizing instruments, leads to a more detailed appreciation of the value and limitations of the correlations between in vitro and in vivo data.

Over the past few decades different sizing strategies have evolved for the different modalities and the relationships between in vitro tests and lung deposition have been studied more in terms of correlations than modeling predictions. Recently, as more clinical data has become available, attempts have been made to use lung deposition models to more accurately predict in vivo deposition. However, because of the complex interplay of aerosol generation and patient use, predictions of deposition from mere aerosol sizing data are and probably always will be limited. The work of Borgstrom et al. (39) on in vitro versus in vivo variability is an excellent example of this issue. The differences in the way a device is "used" in vitro by the researcher and in vivo by the patient are critical in determining how useful or useless an in vitro/in vivo correlation can be. Despite these problems, correlations have been developed. Generally FPFs or FPDs are used as a measure of aerosol quality and in a very general sense, although extra care must be taken when comparing different delivery systems, larger FPFs usually mean higher lung deposition. However, the correlations, such as they are, being based on particular sizing techniques are far from the point of being able to give accurate lung deposition predictions. For example the 95% confidence intervals for $FPF_{5.0\mu m}$ for the DPIs and pMDIs (Figs. 11 and 13) are extremely broad: 3 to 1 in terms of predicted lung dose. However, it should also be remembered that these data have typically been obtained using simple inlet bends and in some cases have been generated without due consideration for in vivo test conditions. As in vitro tests are carried out under more and more in vivo–like conditions—i.e., anatomic throats and appropriate test flow rates—variability would be expected to improve and predictive power to increase.

If the potentially more "precise" modeling techniques are applied to size distributions, rather than the simple FPF values, the picture becomes better. However, scatter between studies is still high and predictive power is still limited. Currently it would appear that mean deposition from nebulizers is amenable to the application of modeling techniques, whereas there is still some confusion over the application of deposition models to DPI and pMDI clouds. Three groups applying essentially the same techniques obtained different degrees of agreement between modeling and reality. It would appear that accounting for breathing patterns of individuals brings modeling calculations more in line. However, even though this may make the modelers happier, it does not improve the predictive power of the technique in the normal clinical situation were breathing is not controlled or measured.

The in vivo data presented above are also limited to studies involving healthy volunteers and as such say little about the relationship between in vitro characteristics and deposition profiles in diseased airways. However, it does appear that in general total deposition is similar, but profiles within the lung are changed in disease. Correlations between in vitro data and deposition in children and infants have also not been discussed. Because of the different airway structure in young children and the different breathing profiles, deposition patterns and the relationships between laboratory and clinic are likely to be different.

References

1. Clark AR, Egan MJ. Modelling the deposition of inhaled powdered drug aerosols. J Aerosol Sci. 1994:25, 1:175–186.
2. Rudolf G, Kobrich R, Stahlhofen W. Modelling and algebraic formulation of regional aerosol deposition in man. J Aerosol Sci. 1990; 21 (suppl 2):403–406.
3. Clark AR. The use of laser diffraction for the evaluation of the aerosol clouds generated by medical nebulizers. Int J Pharm 1995; 115:69–78.
4. Hinds WC. Aerosol Technology; Properties, Behavior, and Measurement of Airborne Particles. New York: Wiley, 1982.
5. Hatch T, Choate SP. Statistical Description of Size Properties of Non-Uniform Particle Substances. Franklin Institute, 1929: 207, 369.
6. Marple V, Olson BA, Miller NC. The role of inertial particle collectors in evaluating pharmaceutical aerosol delivery systems. J Aerosol Med 1998; 11(1):S139–S153.
7. Rao AK, Whitby KT. Non-ideal collection characteristics of single stage and cascade impactors. Am Ind Hyg Assoc J 1977; 38(4):174–179.

8. Nichols SC, Brown DR, Smurthwaite M. New concept for variable flow rate Andersen cascade impactor and calibration data. J Aerosol Med 1998; 11(1):S133–S138.
9. Asking L, Olsson B. Calibration of the multistage liquid impinger at different flows. Pittsburgh, PA: AAAR, 1995;185.
10. Dolovich M, Rhem R. Impact of oropharyngeal deposition on inhaled dose. J Aerosol Med 1998; 11(1): S112–SS115.
11. Felton PG, Hamidi AA, Aigai AK. Measurement of drop-size distribution in dense sprays by laser diffraction. Proceedings, ICLAS-85. Third International Conference on Liquid Atomization and Spray Systems (The Institute of Energy, London, 1985), IVA/4/1.
12. Mitchell JP, Nagel MW. Time-of-flight aerodynamic particle size analyzers: their use and limitations for the evaluation of medical aerosols. J Aerosol Med 1999: 12(4):217–240.
13. Mitchell JP, Nagel MW, Archer AD. Size analysis of a pressurized metered dose inhaler–delivered suspension formulation by API aerosizer particle size analyzer. J Aerosol Med 1999; 12(4): 255–264.
14. Clifford RH, Ishi I, Montaser A. Dual beam light-scattering interferometry for simultaneous measurements of droplet-size and velocity distributions of aerosols from commonly used nebulizers. Chemistry 1990; 62:309–394.
15. Dunhar C. An experimental investigation of the spray issued from a pMDI using laser diagnostic techniques. J Aerosol Med. 1997; 10 (4) 351–358.
16. Finlay W, Stapleton K, Zuberbuhaler P. Variations in predicted regional lung deposition of salbutamol sulphate between 19 nebulizer types. J Aerosol Med 1998; 11 (2):65–80.
17. Snell NJC, Ganderton D. Assessing lung deposition of inhaled medications. Respir Med 1999; 93:123–133.
18. Perring S, Summers QA, Fleming JS, Nassim MA, Holgate ST. A new method of quantification of pulmonary regional distribution of aerosols using combined CT and SPECT and its application to nedocromil sodium administered by metered dose inhaler. Br J Radiol 1994; 67:46–53.
19. Newman SP, Morén F, Trofast E, Talace N, Clarke SW. Deposition and clinical efficacy of terbutaline sulphate from Turbuhaler, a new multi-dose powder inhaler. Eur Respir J 1989; 2:247–252.
20. Smaldone G, Perry R J, Bennett W D, Messina M S, Zwang J, Ilowite J. Interpretation of "24 hour lung retention" in studies of mucociliary clearance. J Aerosol Med 1988; 1:11–20.
21. Agnew JE, Lopez-Vidriero MT, Pavia D, Clarke SW. Functional small airways defense in symptomless cigarette smokers. Thorax 1986; 41:524–530.
22. Newman SP, Hirst PII, Pitcairn GR, Clark AR. Understanding regional lung deposition data in gamma scintigraphy. In: Respiratory Drug Delivery VI. Hilton Head, SC, 1998:19–26.
23. International Commission on Radiological Protection. Human respiratory tract model for radiological protection. 1994. ICRP Publication 66. Ann ICRP, 24, nos 1–3.
24. Borgström L, Nilsson M. A method for determination of the absolute bioavailability of inhaled drugs. Pharm Res 1990; 7:1068.
25. Richards R, Dickson C, Renwick A, Lewis R, Holgate S. Absorption and disposition

kinetics of cromolyn sodium and the influence of inhalation technique. J Pharmacol Exp Ther 1987; 241(3): 1028–1032.
26. Biddiscombe M. The radiolabelling of salbutamol with technetium-99m and its application to the study of salbutamol deposition in the human respiratory tract. Ph. D. thesis, University of London, 1994.
27. Borgström L, Newman S P, Weisz AA, Moren F. Pulmonary deposition of inhaled terbutaline: Comparison of scanning gamma camera and urinary excretion methods. J Pharm Sci 1995; 81:753–755.
28. Finlay WH, Stapleton KW. The effect on regional lung deposition of coupled heat and mass transfer between hygroscopic droplets and their surrounding phase. J Aerosol Sci 1995; 26:655–670.
29. Portstendörfer J, Gebhart J, Robig G. Effect of evaporation on the size distribution of nebulized aerosols. J Aerosol Sci 1977; 8:371–380.
30. Smaldone GC, Diot P, Groth M, Ilowite J. Respirable mass: vague and indefinable in disease. J Aerosol Med 1998; 11(1): S105–S111.
31. Finlay W, Stapleton K. Undersizing of droplets from a vented nebulizer caused by aerosol heating during transit through an Anderson impactor. J Aerosol Sci 1999; 30(1): 105–109.
32. Clark AR. MDIs: physics of aerosol formation. J Aerosol Med 1996: 9(suppl 1): S 19.
33. Clark AR. Medical aerosol inhalers: past, present, and future. Aerosol Sci Tech 1995; 22: 374–391.
34. Clark A, Hollingworth A. The relationship between powder inhaler resistance and peak inspiratory conditions in healthy volunteers—implications for in vitro testing. J Aerosol Med 1993; 6(2):99–110.
35. Price A, Rowland M, Aarons L, Pritchard J, Falcoz C. The use of LUDEP, as a tool, in the prediction of total and regional deposition: advantages, limitations and possible developments of the package. In: Drug Delivery to the Lungs IX, The Aerosol Society, 1998:51–55.
36. Newman S. P. How well do in vitro particle size measurements predict drug delivery in vitro. J Aerosol Med 1998; 11(1):S97–S103.
37. Olsson B. Borgström L, Asking L, Bondesson E. Effect of inlet throat on the correlation between measured fine particle dose and lung deposition. In: Respiratory Drug Delivery V. Phoenix AZ: 1996.
38. Swift DL. The oral airway—a conduit or collector for pharmaceutical aerosols? In: Respiratory Drug Delivery IV. Richmond, VA: 1994.
39. Thiel CG. Can in vitro particle size measurements be used to predict pulmonary deposition of aerosol from inhalers? J Aerosol Med 1998; 11(1):S43–S51.
40. Clark AR, Newman SP, Dasovich N. Mouth and oropharyngeal deposition of pharmaceutical aerosols. J Aerosol Med 1998; 11(1):S116–S121.
41. Pritchard J, Burnell P. Interpretation of in vitro particle size data from dry powder inhalers. In: Respiratory Drug Delivery VI. Hilton Head, SC, 1998: 401–404.
42. Pritchard J, Layzell G, Miller J. Correlation of cascade impactor data with measurements of lung deposition for pharmaceutical aerosols. In: Drug Delivery to the Lungs VII, The Aerosol Society, 1996: 101–104.

43. Borgström L, Asking L, Beekman O, Bondesson E, Kallen A, Olsson B. Discrepancy between in vitro and in vivo variability for a pressurized metered dose inhaler and a dry powder inhaler. J Aerosol Med 1998; 11(1):S59–S64.
44. Melchor R, Biddiscombe M, Mak V, Short M, Spiro S. Lung deposition patterns of directly labelled salbutamol in normal subjects and in patients with reversible airflow obstruction. Thorax 1993; 48:506–511.

5

Factors Affecting the Clinical Outcome of Aerosol Therapy

ERIC DEROM

Ghent University Hospital
Ghent, Belgium

LARS THORSSON

AstraZeneca R&D
Lund, Sweden

I. Introduction

The major advantage of topical administration of a drug is the possibility to achieve high local concentrations and to avoid high systemic concentrations. In clinical practice, the decision of a physician to initiate a treatment with inhaled β_2-agonists or glucocorticosteroids in patients with asthma or chronic obstructive pulmonary disease (COPD) is easy, as their efficacy is beyond any discussion. Adverse reactions to aerosolized drugs are rare (1) and may be circumvented by choosing an alternative formulation or an alternative drug. To deposit in the airways, the drug must be aerosolized, for which an inhalation system is necessary. Pressurized metered dose inhalers (pMDIs), dry-powder inhalers (DPIs), and nebulizers are the currently used delivery systems. Health care providers involved in aerosol therapy should be critically informed about these systems in order to make appropriate comparisons and intelligent choices for their patients. Indeed, each formulation is a unique combination of a drug and a device, and it is that combination, rather than the drug itself, that causes a portion of the emitted dose drug to be deposited in the airways to elicit the clinical effect.

Depending on the device used, a more or less important portion of the inhaled drug will impact on the tongue or back of the pharynx (Fig. 1). This portion will be swallowed down (unless the patient rinses his or her mouth) and will either in part or totally be absorbed from the gastrointestinal (GI) tract. Part of this will be inactivated by first-pass metabolism in the liver. Only the fraction escaping this inactivation will contribute to systemic effects. Thus, as currently prescribed drugs are not inactivated in the lung, a major fraction of the systemically available drug emanates from absorption via the lungs and another fraction from the GI tract. In addition to pulmonary and extrathoracic deposition, a large number of other factors will influence the success of a treatment with an aerosolized drug. In this chapter, the main focus is on DPIs and pMDIs as used in outpatients. Some of the issues mentioned in some sections of this chapter also apply to nebulizers. These devices are, however, discussed in Chap. 8.

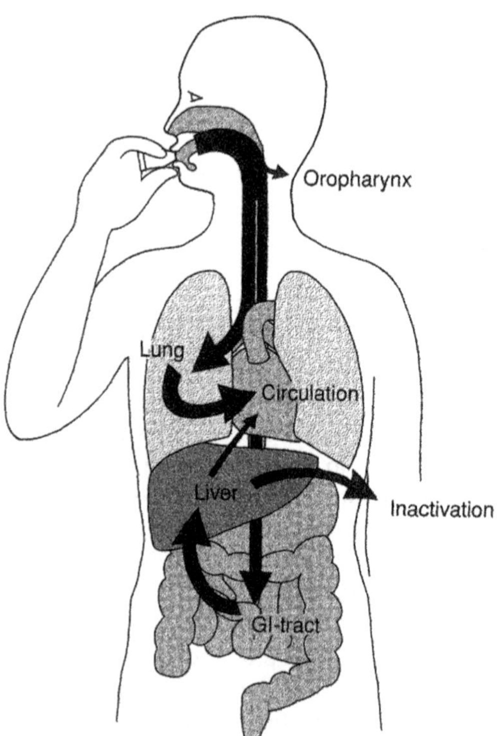

Figure 1 The fate of an inhaled drug. The total amount of drug in the systemic circulation is the sum of the systemic absorption via the lungs and via the GI tract.

II. In Vitro Performance of the Formulation

A. Background

Measurements of the quantity and quality of the aerosolized drug allow characterizing the dosing properties of inhalation devices in vitro. Multistage impactors are used to assess particle mass and mass distribution of an aerosol, and methods are available to estimate the mass median aerodynamic diameter (MMAD) of the aerosol as well as the dose of delivered from and retained within an inhalation system.

B. Current Use of In Vitro Measurements

Measurements of the total amount of drug emitted as well as its size properties were originally developed to estimate the quality of a manufactured aerosol. In vitro measurements have also been used to investigate whether a generic formulation is equivalent to the originator in terms of dose and size properties. In addition, such measurements make it possible to assess whether the addition of a radiolabel to the drug alters its composition or particle size distribution and to examine the potential effects of handling or mishandling of a device on aerosol output and quality.

In recent years, attempts have been made to predict the in vivo behavior and clinical effect of aerosolized drugs by comparing in vitro measurements of emitted dose and size properties delivered via different devices (2). Fine particle dose is, however, not the only variable influencing pulmonary deposition. Inertia of the particles, the applied negative pressure and inhalation flow, breathing pattern, and alterations in flows within the respiratory tract caused by disease-related changes in local geometry of the airways will inevitably modify aerodynamic behavior and pulmonary deposition of aerosolized drugs.

For pMDIs, in vitro studies do not take hygroscopic growth in the airways or the differences in plume geometry into account. The ability of the cascade impactor to predict the behavior of aerosolized drugs in vivo in a reliable way has been recently questioned. Indeed, it has been demonstrated that several generic pMDIs with fine particle fractions comparable to the original formulation (as measured in vitro) appeared to behave differently in vitro once attached to a large-volume spacer (3–5).

C. Clinical Relevance

It is generally accepted that in vitro measurements are important in monitoring the production process of aerosolized drugs, as they allow an estimation of reproducibility of dose and particle size distribution of the aerosol delivered by a given formulation. The clinical relevance of specific in vitro measurements has to be evaluated for each parameter. For instance, recent data show that the variability in pulmonary deposition of terbutaline inhaled via Turbuhaler is lower than with the corresponding pMDI in healthy volunteers and in patients with asthma (6), despite the fact that the in vitro dose variability is greater with Turbuhaler than with the pMDI formulation (7).

A good description of the particle size properties of an aerosolized drug may give some predictive information on its gross behavior within the tracheobronchial tree. Pulmonary deposition studies will, however, always be necessary to bridge between in vitro measurements and the clinical effect. Therefore, determinations of therapeutic equivalence of different formulations should not rely on in vitro measurements alone. Pharmacokinetic measurements of the systemic absorption are used to evaluate whether two formulations are equivalent. In addition, therapeutic equivalence, pharmacodynamic investigations, and, in some instances, in vivo radiolabel deposition studies should be taken into account (8–10).

It is generally accepted that in vitro studies may be informative in two particular areas. First, the interpretation of pulmonary deposition studies, as determined by gamma scintigraphy, is difficult if the radiolabeled formulation has not been properly validated in vitro (11). Second, in vitro studies have provided useful information in the assessment of the impact of inappropriate handling of a device on aerosol delivery. For instance, in vitro studies have demonstrated the importance of storing devices at different temperatures and humidity (12), the relevance of priming or shaking the pMDI canister before actuation (13), and the effects of delay, multiple actuations, and spacer electrostatic charge on drug output from a spacer device (14,15).

III. Patient Preference

A. Background

The development of new devices has generated a number of studies in which preference is assessed.

B. Possible Impact on Clinical Outcome

Most studies do not provide relevant information on patient preference and patient compliance, as study periods rarely exceed 7 weeks (16–19).

C. Clinical Relevance

Although it is reasonable to assume that preference for one or another device may affect patient compliance, the clinical significance of this phenomenon remains difficult to value. Furthermore, studies looking at patient's preference that are sponsored by the pharmaceutical industry often tend to have a biased questionnaire in favor of their own products, and new products tend to be preferred over old. As patient's preference is one of the determinants of compliance, long-term comparative studies on the effect of a drug inhaled via different devices on compliance are probably more informative than studies on patient preference.

IV. Patient Compliance

A. Background

Compliance to treatment is defined as adherence to treatment by the patient, as prescribed by the physician. Various causes of noncompliance may be identified: (1) patient-related causes, e.g., the patient does not understand the processes behind the disease or the aim of the treatment, a problem that might be more specifically encountered with inhaled glucocorticosteroids than with β_2-agonists, as the immediate effects of inhaled corticosteroids are not perceived; (2) inhaler-related causes, e.g., inhalers that are impractical, not portable, or difficult to use; (3) financial causes, e.g., insufficient reimbursement of the treatment, an issue that may vary from one country to another.

B. Possible Impact on Clinical Outcome

Poor compliance has detrimental effects, as the occasional or systematic omission of a dose excludes the patient to benefit from the expected effects. Lack of compliance in patients who need a chronic treatment with inhaled glucocorticosteroids or inhaled long-acting β_2-agonists may result in a less optimal control of the disease and persistent morbidity from asthma (20). It is also a major cause of apparent treatment failure (21) and causes excess in mortality (22).

C. Clinical Relevance

Self-reported compliance and canister-weight measures of adherence suggested an overall compliance of 70% over a 2-year follow-up period in patients participating in the Lung Health Study, in which a pMDI containing an anticholinergic was prescribed (23). Other clinical studies, in which inhalers equipped with electronic monitoring systems were used, have indicated that up to 40% of the patients tend to underuse (24) and about 20% to overuse their medication despite adequate study supervision (25). Whether the characteristics of the device may affect compliance remains to be investigated. Retrospective data from New Zealand indicate that for inhaled glucocorticosteroids, the mean daily inhaled dose was significantly higher for DPIs than for pMDIs (26).

It has been shown that compliance may be improved by regular instruction and education (27–29) as well as by a reduction of the number of daily inhalations (30). In this context, it is likely that the combination of a glucocorticosteroid with a long-acting β_2-agonist in one formulation may improve compliance and control of asthma, as a fixed combination of a glucocorticosteroid with a short-acting β_2-agonist has been shown to do so (31).

V. Pharmacodynamic and Pharmacokinetic Properties of the Inhaled Drug

A. Background

Drugs are generally characterized by their pharmacodynamic and pharmacokinetic properties, such as receptor binding affinity, retention in lung tissue, distribution volume, and clearance. Important differences in pharmacokinetic properties do exist for different drugs within a specific drug class—e.g., β_2-agonists and glucocorticosteroids. Aerosol therapy is also influenced by device-, drug-, and formulation-related factors, which determine pulmonary and systemic bioavailability and hence clinical and systemic effects.

Pharmacodynamic Aspects: Selectivity, Agonism, and Antagonism

β_2-Agonists

These drugs exert their effects on airway function by mediation of β_2-receptors located on the surface of the smooth muscle and other tissues of the airways. β_1- and β_2-receptors are, however, distributed throughout the body. Stimulation of these receptors are considered to be responsible for side effects, such as tachycardia, arrhythmias, prolongation of the Q-Tc interval, tremor, and decrease in serum potassium, and become generally apparent when higher than conventional doses are inhaled (32–34). The relationship between increase in FEV_1 and the inhaled dose of a β_2-agonist is not linear but consists of a steep part followed by a "plateau" (34).

Some β_2-agonists, such as isoprenaline and fenoterol, behave as full agonists of the β_2-receptor, whereas salbutamol and terbutaline are partial antagonists. Moreover, fenoterol is less selective than salbutamol or terbutaline for β_2-receptors (35). These differences have important clinical consequences. For example, fenoterol has greater cardiovascular effects than salbutamol and greater intrinsic myocardial effects than terbutaline in healthy volunteers and in patients with asthma (32). It also appears that the maximum response elicited by fenoterol in terms of reduction in plasma potassium, increase in heart rate and inotropy is greater than that by salbutamol, and that the dose required to reach 50% of maximum response is substantially lower for fenoterol than for salbutamol (35).

Glucocorticosteroids

Glucocorticosteroids exert their effects by binding to glucocorticosteroid receptors, which are localized in the cytoplasm of target cells. There is only one single class of glucocorticosteroid receptors, with no evidence of subtypes of differing affinity in different tissues (36). Glucocorticosteroid receptors are widely distributed within the human lung, in particular in airway epithelial cells and bronchial vascular endothelial cells. Glucocorticosteroids may control airway inflammation in asthma by inhibiting many aspects of the inflammatory process, such as increasing the transcription of anti-inflammatory genes and decreasing the transcription of inflammatory genes.

In general, dose-response studies show marked and statistically significant differences between treatment with different doses and placebo, but most often fail to show statistically significant differences between adjacent doses, unless these differ by a factor of more than 4 in dose (36). This makes it difficult to use clinical effect as an outcome measurement to discriminate between different drugs or devices, even if the true difference would be as large as two- to threefold. As with β_2-agonists and other drugs, the dose-response curve flattens once higher doses are used (36).

Potency and Receptor Affinity

β_2-Agonists

A good knowledge of the in vivo potency of β_2-agonists is important, as this allows determining the therapeutic equivalence of the bronchodilating dose for inhalation on a weight for weight basis for a given device. Moreover, it helps the clinician to adapt the dose when switching from one drug to another. Caution is, however, necessary toward equivalence studies in which different inhalation devices are used. Indeed, if the comparison is not performed on the steep part of the dose-response curve, a failure to discriminate between the two formulations may be due to the fact that the response measured is on the flat part of the dose-response curve.

Glucocorticosteroids

Glucocorticosteroids also differ in their receptor affinity and potency. Relative to dexamethasone, fluticasone has he highest affinity (22.0), followed by beclamethasone monopropionate (BMP) (13.0), the active metabolite of beclamethasone diproprionate (BDP), and budesonide (9.4). Conversely, triamcinolone and flunisolide exhibit much lower affinities (36,37). In vitro studies on receptor binding affinity of different glucocorticosteroids suggest that fluticasone is at least twice as potent than BDP and budesonide. The in vivo potency is, however, heavily dependent on the drug delivery to the site of action (the airways), and different formulations have been shown to vary severalfold in this respect (38). A lower receptor binding affinity can thus be compensated by an increase in pulmonary deposition or by an increase in dose. In addition, a drug with higher receptor affinity is likely to be more potent with regard to systemic effects (36,37).

Local Retention

β_2-Agonists

β_2-agonists have been characterized as those that directly activate the receptor, such as salbutamol; those that are taken up into a membrane depot, such as formoterol; and those that interact with a receptor-specific auxiliary binding site, such as salmeterol (39). These differences in retention are reflected in the kinetics of airway smooth muscle relaxation and bronchodilatation. Indeed, in vitro studies have shown that, in the guinea pig trachea, salmeterol produces relaxation that is longer than that of salbutamol and persists significantly after washout. Similar data have been reported with formoterol (40). For salmeterol, it appears that in patients with asthma, the enhanced retention in lung tissue is at the expense of the onset of action, which is slower than that of salbutamol (41) or formoterol (42,43).

Glucocorticosteroids

Retention in lung tissue of inhaled glucocorticosteroids has not been studied extensively. It appears that differences between glucocorticosteroids exist in terms of tissue binding and lipophilicity. Association with intracellular formation of long-chain fatty acid esters has been reported with budesonide (44), whereas prolonged retention of fluticasone in central lung tissue has been reported (45). Data obtained in experimental conditions are, however, not necessarily predictive for duration of action in vivo, and clinical studies will always be required to confirm their relevance.

Volume of Distribution

After inhalation, a fraction of the drug is deposited in lungs, the major fraction of which is rapidly absorbed and reaches the systemic circulation. Plasma concentrations thus reflect pulmonary absorption as well as the fraction of the drug that is absorbed from the GI tract, escaping the hepatic first-pass inactivation. Volume of distribution allows an estimation of the distribution of a drug into plasma and other tissues. A large volume of distribution indicates a high degree of distribution into body tissues other than plasma.

β_2-Agonists

Distribution volume of the currently prescribed β_2-agonists is similar for salbutamol and terbutaline, and slightly higher for fenoterol. Side effects, associated with β_2-agonists, such as increase in heart rate and tremor, appear to be correlated with plasma concentrations, although a great variability among patients has been reported (46).

Glucocorticosteroids

The volume of distribution has been reported to differ markedly between inhaled glucocorticosteroids and to be positively correlated with the lipophilicity of the drug. Although plasma concentrations and systemic effects correlate for a given drug, the magnitude of their concentration is in itself not predictive of systemic effects. Indeed, high doses of inhaled fluticasone results in greater cortisol suppression than comparable doses of budesonide in healthy volunteers (47–49) and patients with asthma (50,51), despite the fact that fluticasone plasma concentrations are up to six times lower than those of budesonide (52).

Clearance and Elimination Half-Life

Elimination half-life is a function of both volume of distribution and clearance. It affects the amount of drug present in the body at steady state as well as the rate and extent of accumulation. Accumulation is more likely to occur if the dosing interval is of the same magnitude as or shorter than the elimination half-life of the drug in question.

β_2-Agonists

All β_2-agonists are cleared rapidly, such that drug accumulation does not occur (46).

Glucocorticosteroids

Although clearance is similar for most currently used inhaled glucocorticosteroids, vast differences in elimination half-life between inhaled glucocorticosteroids appear to exist. Fluticasone, for which volume of distribution averages 12 L/kg and half-life ranges between 8 and 14 h has been shown to accumulate (52). The half-life of fluticasone is substantially longer than that of triamcinolone or budesonide, having a half-life of only about 2 to 3 h (53). This difference in half-lives may explain the aforementioned difference in suppression of cortisol secretion between fluticasone and budesonide in healthy volunteers and in asthmatic patients observed after 3–5 days of treatment.

B. Clinical Relevance

Physicians often overlook pharmacodynamic and pharmacokinetic properties of aerosolized drugs. Differences in β_2-selectivity and the presence of a partial antagonistic activity make that salbutamol and terbutaline, are thought to be less associated with disturbing side effects and asthma mortality than fenoterol (54).

Increased potency has sometimes been claimed to be an advantage, as smaller amounts of drug will lead to a similar therapeutic effect. It should be emphasized that the maximal effect, elicited by inhaled β_2-agonists or glucocorticosteroids, is not affected by the potency of the drug. Prolonged pulmonary retention of an inhaled drug, however, may represent an advantage, as is now clear from studies with long-acting β_2-agonists in asthmatic patients (55). Although differences in lung retention between inhaled glucocorticosteroids appear to exist, the potential clinical relevance of this finding—less systemic exposure, reduced dosing frequency, and hence a better therapeutic compliance—remains to be investigated. Prolonged elimination half-life is, however, of some relevance, as it causes accumulation of the drug and may lead to measurable systemic effects. The clinical relevance of a measurable systemic effect, such as a suppression of adrenal function or an alteration in serum markers of bone metabolism, remains unknown. However, the relationship between a measurable systemic effect and the development of a clinically relevant side effect—such as cataract, osteoporosis, or reduced growth—remains to be established. In fact, only the relationship between inhaled glucocorticosteroids and skin thinning or easy bruising is generally accepted to be causal of nature (56,57).

VI. Handling and Maintenance of the Inhaler

A. Background

Handling and mishandling of the inhaler involves all the different actions or the omission of these actions needed to cause optimal delivery of an aerosol from the inhaler. The number and the complexity of the actions or steps patients must undertake to deliver the aerosol differ from one device to another. Incorrect handling is more likely to occur with systems that require a high number of complex actions (e.g., nebulizers) than with less complex systems, such as a pMDI and even simpler devices, such as a DPI. The use of an inappropriate inhalation flow will not affect the amount and characteristics of drug emitted from a pMDI but is of relevance for a DPI, since the deaggregation of the powder into fine particles is highly dependent on the negative pressure applied by the patient (58,59). Incorrect handling of nebulizers includes the use of an incorrect flow setting or of a wrong dilution of drug in the solvent.

DPIs and pMDIs do not require any maintenance, whereas nebulizers do. Poor maintenance may lead to contamination of the wet parts of a nebulizer and cause bacterial respiratory tract infections (60). For spacers and add-on devices, the amount of electrostatic charge present may depend on how much the device has been used and on washing procedures (8,61,62) (see Chap. 12).

B. Possible Impact on Clinical Outcome

Incorrect handling affects the efficacy of the treatment to a lesser extent than noncompliance. For example, in vitro studies have shown that omission to shake the pMDI before use reduced total and fine particle dose by 25 and 36%, respectively, while two actuations separated by 1 s decreased fine particle dose by 16% (13). The same authors also demonstrated that storing the pMDI stem down reduced total and fine particle dose of the next actuations by at least 23%. New spacers with high electrostatic charge deliver 23% less salbutamol particles of < 6.8 μm than used ones, whereas washing them with an anionic or cationic detergent resulted in an increase of 55–70% in small particle delivery compared to delivery from new spacers (14,63).

Experimental data indicate that when Turbuhaler was inadequately stored with the cap off, a humid environment decreased the fine particle fraction (64). In addition, exhaling into Turbuhaler perturbed the fine particle fraction for three subsequent shots (64). For another DPI, salmeterol/fluticasone Diskus/Accuhaler, storage at humid conditions also decreased the delivered fine particle fraction (65). In this case, there is no cap to protect against moisture ingress and the device must be packed in an aluminum foil bag when marketed in the United States.

C. Clinical Relevance

The way the patient should handle the device should be taught, practiced, and checked regularly. Patients should also receive clear instructions about maintenance of inhalers. Indeed, inappropriate use of inhalers and mistakes in the inhalation technique occur frequently. In a study of 281 patients with asthma or COPD using either pMDIs or DPIs, it was demonstrated that 88% made at least one mistake (66). Follow-up studies indicate that problems with device handling may reappear as soon as 2 weeks after initial instruction, thereby mandating the prescribing physician to reinstruct patients periodically (67). As it has been shown that patients unable to use one device tend to do better with another system, physicians should develop a rational inhaler strategy, taking various factors such as age, ability to learn the correct use, and patient preference into account (68).

Inappropriate use of inhalers or mistakes in inhalation technique reduces the dose delivered and compromises the efficacy of the treatment. For example, it was demonstrated that the increase in FEV_1 was 80% of maximum achievable after inhalation from the unprimed pMDI, compared to 92% after inhalation from the primed one (69). In one study with plastic spacers, priming of the spacer by actuating the pMDI a few times increased pulmonary deposition of glucocorticosteroids in asthmatic patients by 40–50% (70), whereas in another study, pulmonary deposition of salbutamol was doubled if the spacer was coated with benzalkonium chloride (71). For Turbuhaler, pulmonary deposition decreased by 50% if the flow applied to inhale was reduced from a normal flow of 60 L/min to a suboptimal flow of 30 L/min (72), whereas in others studies, the bronchodilating effect was similar at 30 and 60 L/min in both children and adults (73,74).

VII. Relationship Between Pulmonary Deposition and Clinical Effect

A. Definitions

In order to inhale an aerosolized drug, the patient should activate the inhaler, from which a dose is subsequently emitted (Table 1.). Some of this metered dose is retained in the inhaler, adapter, spacer, or mouthpiece (retained dose). Only a fraction of the delivered dose will reach the airways, since some of it may be lost into the air or on the face, another fraction will be deposited in the oropharynx, and a small part of the drug will be exhaled (Fig. 2).

In clinical studies, pulmonary deposition of a drug delivered from a given formulation is generally expressed as a fraction of a reference dose, which may be the

Table 1 Dose Definitions

Expression	Definition
Nominal dose	Dose written on the package label; also called labeled dose
Metered dose	Amount of drug leaving or contained in the metering unit
Delivered dose	Amount of drug leaving the device
Fine particle dose	Amount of drug contained in particles < 5 μm
Retained amount	Amount of drug retained in the device
Inhaled dose	Amount of drug entering the subject through inhalation
Exhaled amount	Amount exhaled
Recovered amount:	Amount recovered from, e.g., wiping the face and hands with a tissue
Dose to subject	Inhaled dose minus the amount of drug leaving the subject through exhalation and mouth rinsing
Lung dose	Amount of drug deposited in the lungs

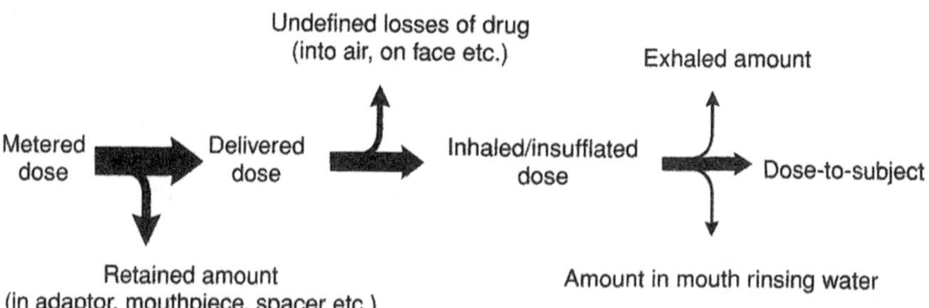

Figure 2 Illustration of dose definitions and drug losses of an inhaled formulation on its way to the lung.

metered or delivered dose. The nominal dose can be based on either the metered or the delivered dose. This issue is important, as, for example, budesonide delivered via a pMDI attached to a Nebuhaler, with a high retention in the spacer, has a pulmonary deposition of 34% with reference to the normal metered dose, compared to 76% with reference to the dose delivered from the spacer (75, 76). In this section, nominal dose will be used as dose reference, unless otherwise mentioned.

B. Background

The amount of topically available drug, relative to the nominal dose, is determined by a number of factors: delivery characteristics of the inhaler, handling of the device, inhalation technique of the patient, and patient-related physiological factors, such as airway narrowing, airway closure, and mucus plugging. The mechanisms by which handling of the inhaler and inhalation technique critically determine drug delivery (and hence, pulmonary deposition) are outlined in a previous section of this chapter. This section will focus on the relationship between pulmonary deposition and clinical effect and the clinical relevance of differences in pulmonary deposition between inhalers containing the same drugs.

It is also possible to estimate regional deposition of drugs within the tracheobronchial tree, and differences between devices have been shown to exist in this regard (38). The clinical relevance of regional deposition and targeting drugs to certain areas of the tracheobronchial tree are beyond the scope of this chapter; they are discussed in Chap. 7.

C. Relationship Between Inhaled Dose and Clinical Effect

The relationship between the pulmonary deposition and the airway effects of inhaled β_2-agonists and glucocorticosteroids consists of an initial slope followed by a plateau. The existence of a sigmoid dose-response relationship has two important consequences. First, a higher dose of drug inhaled by the patient and deposited in the lung will induce a higher response only if the lower dose of the drug yielded a response that was still on the slope of the dose response curve. Second, once the plateau or level of maximal response is reached, further increases in dose will not add to the pulmonary effects but could contribute to the development of systemic side effects, as pulmonary deposited drugs will be absorbed and reach the systemic circulation.

At appropriate doses, a twofold increase in dose of an inhaled β_2-agonist has been shown to result in a statistically significant increase in bronchodilating effect (11). Conversely, it appears to be much more difficult to assess this relationship for inhaled giucocorticosteroids, as an at least fourfold increase in dose is necessary to obtain a statistically significant difference in effect (36). The next paragraphs of this section therefore focus mainly on the relationship between pulmonary deposition and clinical effects of β_2-agonists.

D. Pulmonary Deposition and Inhalation Technique

In a study with pMDIs containing radiolabeled Teflon particles, Newman demonstrated that pulmonary deposition was markedly improved by the use of a longer breath-holding time (10 versus 4 s), a low inhalation flow (30 versus 80 L/min), and by actuating at the beginning of inspiration (77,78). Others have subsequently confirmed these findings (79). Flow-dependent deposition of pMDIs was further demonstrated in studies showing that the use of a breath-actuated pMDI increased pulmonary deposition in "poor" coordinators (80).

In patients with reversible airway obstruction (81), the greatest bronchodilatation was obtained when the pMDI containing terbutaline was actuated during a slow inhalation (25 to 30 L/min) and actuation is followed by a breath-hold lasting 10 s. A significant correlation between mean bronchodilator response for the different inhalation modes and pulmonary deposition of labeled Teflon particles obtained in the aforementioned studies was reported (77). Studies with other β_2-agonists inhaled via pMDI have given similar results (82) and confirmed the clinical relevance of flow dependency of pulmonary deposition for pMDIs.

The inhalation flow affects pulmonary deposition but not the properties of the aerosol delivered by a pMDI Conversely, the intrinsic properties of the aerosol emitted from a DPI—a breath-actuated device—are highly dependent on the inhalation effort of the patient (83), and the inhalation flow must always be sufficiently high to produce an aerosol containing the optimal amount of fine particles (72,84)

The impact of flow-dependency on pulmonary deposition has been assessed for Rotahaler in healthy volunteers using the charcoal block method: the use of a low and high inhalation flow resulted in a pulmonary deposition of 3.6 and 7.0%, respectively of the nominal dose (85). Studies with Turbuhaler have yielded depositions ranging from 16.8% in a first study and between 20 and 27% in later studies, when an inhalation flow of approximately 60 L/min was applied (72,86,87). Pulmonary deposition was reduced by half once the inhalation flow fell below 30 L/min (72).

Although, in one study with children, a significantly greater increase in FEV_1 was obtained when salbutamol was inhaled via Rotahaler at a higher flow of 90 to 120 L/min that at an inhalation flow of 30 to 50 L/min (31), most studies in which the effects of terbutaline inhaled via Turbuhaler were assessed showed that at a low inhalation flow of 30 L/min, a less pronounced improvement of expiratory flow was obtained than at a higher inhalation flow (60 L/min) (88). In another study, it could be shown in children who inhaled terbutaline via Turbuhaler at flows of 13, 22, 31, and 60 L/min that the bronchodilating action was flow-dependent once the inhalation flow was below the critical value of 30 L/min (74). It should, however, be underlined that even an extremely low flow, 13 L/min, resulted in a bronchodilating effect.

E. Differences in Pulmonary Deposition Between Devices

Differences in pulmonary deposition between devices have been reported. The pulmonary deposition varies from 5% for Spinhaler and 20–30% for Turbuhaler (11) to 38% for pMDIs with large-volume spacers (38) or Respimat (89,90) if the optimal inhalation technique is used for each of the devices. Numerous studies have been conducted in which the efficacy of inhalers containing the same drug has been compared and their relative effectiveness established. Both cumulative and noncumulative dose designs have been used, and clinical response tends to be higher after the same total dose has been given as a cumulative dose rather than a single dose. Noncumulative dose designs seem to be more sensitive (11). The best way to establish the relationship between pulmonary deposition and clinical effect is to measure both variables at the same time point. This has been done in only a small number of studies. In two studies, terbutaline was administered via Turbuhaler and pMDI in patients with mild to moderate asthma. For Turbuhaler, a peak inspiratory flow of 60 L/min was aimed for, whereas patients were asked to generate a flow of 90 L/min for the pMDI. In these studies, inspiratory volume and breath-holding time were also standardized. In the first study, the effect of 0.5 mg of terbutaline inhaled via Turbuhaler or pMDI on the increase in FEV_1 was similar (91). Pulmonary deposition was 22.6% of the nominal dose after Turbuhaler and 8.8% after pMDI. As the discrepancy between the difference in deposition and the similarity of the bronchodilating effect might have been caused by the administration of too high doses, a second study was conducted (92); it also included a 0.25-mg terbutaline dose. In that study, pulmonary deposition was similar to that obtained in the first study. The 0.25-mg terbutaline dose given by Turbuhaler resulted in a significantly higher FEV_1 response than 0.25 mg inhaled via pMDI. The increase in FEV_1 after the 0.5-mg dose given via pMDI and the 0.25-mg dose inhaled via Turbuhaler were similar, indicating that the amount of drug reaching the effector site, the lungs, determined the clinical effect. In addition, the difference in clinical effect between 0.25 and 0.5 mg given by Turbuhaler did not reach statistical significance, indicating that 0.25 mg terbutaline administered via Turbuhaler already resulted in a close to maximum effect.

Several clinical studies have focused on the bronchodilating effects of salbutamol inhaled via pMDI and via Diskhaler, Rotahaler, and Turbuhaler. Conflicting results have appeared for multidose comparisons between Rotahaler and pMDI, as in some studies identical dose-response curves were obtained (93,94), whereas the difference was in favor of the pMDI in other studies (95). For Diskhaler and Autohaler, only inconclusive single-dose studies have been published, whereas at equal nominal doses, salbutamol delivered via Turbuhaler generally gave responses that were superior to those from Diskhaler (96) and pMDI (97).

F. Clinical Relevance

A good knowledge of the two most important factors affecting pulmonary deposition of inhaled drugs is of clinical relevance, because the eventual pulmonary deposition rather than the delivered dose determines the clinical effect of inhaled bronchodilators. For years, improper inhalation technique has been recognized as a frequent cause of treatment failure (98). Lack of insight of the deposition characteristics of the prescribed formulation is, however, at least as important. Inhalers characterized by a high pulmonary deposition may represent an advantage, as a switchover from "device A" with low pulmonary deposition to "device B" with high pulmonary deposition might lead to an improvement in symptoms. Conversely, if a device with a higher pulmonary deposition is used, attempts should always be made to reduce the prescribed dose of the drug in patients whose disease is well under control in order to avoid unnecessary exposure of the patient to intrapulmonary and hence systemic concentrations of the drug.

Most of the work on the relationship between pulmonary deposition and clinical effect has been done with β_2-agonists, since the immediate effect these drugs is easy to measure. Although it is more difficult to conduct comparative studies with inhaled glucocorticosteroids and anticholinergics, it is very likely that the same concepts also hold true for these drugs, as some studies clearly suggest (99,100).

VIII. Extrathoracic Deposition, Local Side Effects, and Systemic Effects

A. Background

The major fraction of the drug delivered by an inhaler will deposit in the oropharynx (Fig. 1) This extrathoracic fraction may contribute to local side effects and, if swallowed, to systemic effects. Indeed, although most of drug will be metabolized and inactivated in the gut and/or in the liver by the first-pass metabolism, some of the swallowed drug may reach the systemic circulation. The extrapulmonary fraction will, however, contribute to systemic effects for inhaled drugs that are only incompletely inactivated by the first-pass metabolism. Conversely, systemic effects of inhaled drugs, which are almost completely inactivated by the first-pass metabolism, will result almost entirely from the fraction of the drug that is deposited in the airways and subsequently absorbed from them.

B. Clinical Relevance of the Extrathoracic Fraction for Local Side Effects

As β_2-agonists do not exert local side effects of any clinical significance whereas the local side effects of anticholinergics are mainly bad taste and mouth dryness, extrapulmonary deposition does not represent a clinically relevant issue that should affect the choice of an inhalation system. Conversely, it has been shown that oral candidiasis, one of the local side effects of inhaled glucocorticosteroids, occurs in 5% of the patients using a pMDI and is somewhat related to the dose deposited in the oropharynx. Indeed, reduction of the deposition by use of large-volume spacers (101) or a Turbuhaler (102) results in a decreased incidence of candidiasis. Hence, systems characterized by a high pulmonary and a low pharyngeal deposition of inhaled glucocorticosteroids, such as the combination of a pMDI with a large-volume spacer or the recently developed Respimat (89), could represent an advantage in this regard.

C. Clinical Relevance of Extrathoracic Fraction for Systemic Effects

β_2-Agonists

Systemic absorption of the extrapulmonary fraction through the GI tract has been reported for β_2-agonists. Only 7% of a nominal dose of terbutaline delivered via a pMDI reaches the systemic circulation via the GI tract (103), whereas approximately 35% of a dose of salbutamol (104) reaches the systemic circulation by GI absorption. These differences in GI absorption may well explain differences in systemic concentrations between β_2-agonists, but the clinical relevance of this difference is minimal, in particular since there is no clear relationship between systemic concentration of β_2-agonists and side effects

Inhaled Glucocorticosteroids

Extrathoracic deposition of inhaled glucocorticosteroids may contribute to the development of systemic effects if these are not completely inactivated by the first-pass metabolism. For that reason, the extrathoracic fraction of fluticasone, which is inactivated for 99% by first-pass metabolism, does not contribute to the development of systemic effects. It may, however, be expected that the extrathoracic fraction of budesonide and even more of beclomethasone may lead to systemic effects, as 11% (53) and 20% (105) of the respective drugs eventually reaches the systemic circulation through GI absorption. Reductions in systemic effects with high doses of inhaled BDP have been documented if the pMDI was attached to a large-volume spacer (106). Rinsing the mouth and blocking the GI uptake with charcoal reduced plasma concentrations of budesonide inhaled via Turbuhaler in children by approximately 20% (107) The observation that systemic bioavailability of budesonide inhaled via a pMDI attached to a spacer was virtually not affected by administration of activated charcoal (75) indicates that, for this formulation, the main contribution to the system originates from the pulmonary, and not from the extrathoracic, fraction.

IX. Lung Versus Total Bioavailability Ratio (L/T Ratio)

A. Background

The amount of aerosolized drug reaching the effector site, the lung, determines the elicited effect. The systemic effect will be caused by the drug deposited in the lungs (pulmonary bioavailability) and the fraction deposited in the oropharynx that will be absorbed in the GI tract but not inactivated by the first-pass metabolism (oral bioavailability). Each combination of active drug and device is unique in terms of division of delivered drug between lungs and oropharynx and hence of balance between the desired local activity and undesired systemic activity.

B. Possible Impact on Clinical Outcome

It is possible to evaluate the balance between pulmonary bioavailability and systemic bioavailability if the following data are known: retention of the drug in the inhaler, the percentage pulmonary and oropharyngeal deposition of the drug, the degree of GI absorption, and the inactivation by the first-pass metabolism. From these data the L/T ratio (L = local bioavailability; T = systemic bioavailability) can be derived.

Calculations have shown that for terbutaline, the L/T ratio averages 0.55 for a pMDI and 0.81 for Turbuhaler (108). For salbutamol, the L/T ratio averages 0.35 for pMDI, 0.15 for Rotahaler, 0.24 for Diskhaler, and 0.45 for Turbuhaler (108). The differences in value between salbutamol and terbutaline are a reflection of inherent differences in GI absorption and first-pass metabolism between these drugs.

For budesonide, similar calculations have yielded 0.59 for pMDI, 0.84 for Turbuhaler, and 0.95 for pMDI with Nebuhaler (109).

A higher L/T ratio will always indicate a more favorable ratio with respect to the balance between desired and undesired effect resulting from a good targeting ability of the combination of substance and device, or from a low contribution of the GI tract. It may be a guide in the choice between devices containing the same the substance. A high L/T ratio also implies that it is the pulmonary bioavailability that determines the systemic activity.

C. Clinical Relevance

The clinical relevance of L/T ratio, a theoretical concept, is, however, less clear. Indeed, the L/T ratio is useful only in comparing the same drug substance in different inhaler devices. Comparisons between drugs should not be made, as different substances may differ in terms of relative activities in lungs and systemic circulation. For example, inhaled glucocorticosteroids, such as fluticasone, with minimal GI bioavailability and hence a very high L/T ratio, have been shown to exert systemic effects (51). The L/T ratio should thus always be verified clinically. The L/T ratio informs the physician about the potential for dose reduction if a switch to a device with a higher L/T ratio is made. The L/T ratio helps to explain why cortisol suppression is less pronounced if BDP is inhaled via pMDI attached to a large-volume spacer (106). It also explains why pulmonary deposition of budesonide via Turbuhaler is approximately twice that via a pMDI, whereas the systemic bioavailability is only increased by approximately 50% (75). From a theoretical point of view, a treatment provided via a device with a higher L/T ratio is more cost-effective, in particular for formulations containing expensive medications. The savings induced by dose reduction may, however, be counterbalanced by a more expensive device or by a decrease in patient compliance.

X. Studies in Healthy Volunteers

A. Background

Sometimes data on side effects or on pulmonary or extrapulmonary deposition obtained in healthy volunteers are used to make predictions about what may occur in patients with asthma or COPD, in particular if such studies in patients are not available. There is, however, some evidence that differences may exist between the behavior of an aerosolized drug in healthy volunteers and that in a patient with airflow obstruction. Although total pulmonary deposition seems to be comparable in normal subjects and asthmatic patients, pharmacokinetics (P. J. Anderson, personal communication) and regional distribution may differ (109). Indeed, recent scintigraphic studies indicate a more central distribution in patients after inhalation of budesonide via Turbuhaler (38) or of sodium cromoglycate administered via pMDI attached to a spacer (110).

Another discrepancy between asthmatic patients and healthy volunteers is the difference in systemic effects of inhaled glucocorticosteroids. High doses of inhaled glucocorticosteroids (budesonide 1600 μg/day via Turbuhaler, fluticasone 2000 μg/day via Diskhaler) for 4 to 7 days suppressed cortisol secretion by 34 and 55%, respectively, in healthy volunteers (47) and by 16 and 34%, respectively, in patients with mild to moderate asthma (51). This difference, which may be related to the disease itself, previous treatment with corticosteroids, or interactions with other treatments remains to be elucidated. Healthy normal subjects are preferred over asthmatic patients for safety testing in order to obviate the potentially confounding effects of past or current steroid therapy in the degree of airways inflammation and obstructive impairment, which could act to reduce the power of the assay (111)

B. Clinical Relevance

Although it is much easier to assess a number of aspects that pertain to aerosol therapy in healthy volunteers, extrapolation of these results to patients should be made with caution. For example, the systemic activity of different formulations and drugs may very well be compared in healthy volunteers, but the clinical relevance of these should always be verified in pulmonary patients.

XI. Cost-Effectiveness

A. Definition and Causes

In the past, attention has always been focused on the efficacy of a therapy and its ability to modify the physiological alterations caused by the disease. In recent years, the economic impact of the disease itself as well as its treatment has received increased attention. In such an analysis, it is essential to consider both direct costs (medication, hospitalizations, and use of the emergency department) as well as indirect costs (time off work or school, early retirement). The high prevalence of asthma and COPD makes that this economic issue is of increasing relevance for society. For asthma, several studies have shown that treatment with inhaled drugs is cost-saving in terms of direct health care costs (22,112). In order to determine which asthma treatment with inhaled glucocorticosteroids and inhaled β_2-agonist is cost-effective, not only the drugs but also the inhalation devices should be taken into consideration.

B. Possible Impact on Clinical Outcome

Several studies have performed an economic evaluation of the different methods to deliver aerosolized drugs in hospitalized patients (113). Conversely, data on efficacy and cost-effectiveness of two equivalent treatments, administered via different devices to outpatients with asthma are scarce. Efficacy, measured as the total number of exacerbations, days with exacerbations and hospitalizations, and healthcare utilization were measured over a period of 52 weeks in 445 patients, treated either via pMDI or via Turbuhaler in Canada (114). In this study, effectiveness of treatment and cost differences were in favor of the DPI.

C. Clinical Relevance

Trials in which cost-effectiveness of treatments are compared provide extremely useful information, but a study period of several months or years is needed to obtain a realistic estimation of overall health care expenses. Indeed, such trials provide an integrated view on efficacy of the treatment provided, since efficacy takes factors such as patient compliance, efficacy of the drug, preference, acceptance, handling, and ease of use of the device into account. However, differences in cost and patient preference (often related to cultural background) make it difficult to extrapolate data obtained in one specific country.

XII. General Conclusions

Although it has sometimes been claimed that variety of factors may affect the clinical outcome of aerosol therapy, only a limited number of these are of real clinical relevance. Differences in reproducibility of delivered dose, geometric characteristics, and fine particle mass between devices may be detected in vitro. It is, however, difficult if not impossible to extrapolate in vitro findings directly to clinical relevance. Patient compliance is undoubtedly of great importance, as clinical improvement cannot be expected in patients who do not take the prescribed medicines. Conversely, the impact of patient preference for one or the other device is less clear, as this variable is difficult to assess. Each formulation is a unique combination of a drug and a device, and the pharmacodynamic and pharmacokinetic performance of the drug is of a great clinical relevance. This is a complex area, as not only one by one but also a whole spectrum of variables—such as receptor affinity, drug retention, and pulmonary deposition—should be compared. Handling and maintenance is another clinically relevant factor that may affect the outcome of the treatment, as this can lead to a several-fold variability in drug output. Clinicians should have a good knowledge of the existing differences in pulmonary deposition between devices, as it may range between 5 and 50% of the nominal dose. This is an issue of particular interest if different formulations for a given drug are available. There is a good relationship between pulmonary deposition and clinical efficacy, as long as the maximum effect has not been reached. For most currently available drugs and formulations, extrathoracic deposition contributes minimally to the development of systemic effects and is thus a matter of lesser importance. Low oropharyngeal deposition of inhaled glucocorticosteroids is, however, an issue of some clinical relevance in patients suffering from oral candidiasis. The L/T ratio may be useful to compare different formulations of an inhaled glucocorticosteroid with a relatively low first-pass inactivation. Studies in healthy volunteers are useful to compare drugs and devices with regard to differences in pulmonary deposition or systemic effects and to bridge between in vitro findings and clinical studies in patients. The clinical relevance of the different outcomes has to be systematically verified in patients, since differences in sensitivity to systemic effects and in regional distribution within the lungs may exist between healthy subjects and patients with pulmonary disease. Finally, it is difficult to make general statements from comparisons between cost-effectiveness of different formulations because of large differences in terms of cost and general acceptance of formulations from one country to another.

References

1. Snell NJ. Adverse reactions to inhaled drugs (editorial). Respir Med 1990; 84:345–348.
2. Borgström L. In vitro, ex vivo, in vivo veritas. Allergy 1999; 54: 88–92.
3. Derom E, Pauwels R. Bioequivalence of inhaled drugs (editorial) Eur Respir J 1995; 8:1634–1636
4. Miller MR, Bright P. Differences in output from corticosteroid inhalers used with a volumatic spacer. Eur Respir J 1995; 8:1637–1638.
5. Barry PW, O'Callaghan C. In vitro comparison of the amount of salbutamol available for inhalation from different formulations used with different spacer devices. Eur Respir J 1997; 10:1345–1348.
6. Borgström L, Bengtsson T, Derom E, Pauwels R. Variability in lung deposition of inhaled drug, within and between asthmatic patients with a pMDI and a dry powder inhaler, Turbuhaler. Int J Pharm 2000 193:227–230.
7. Borgström L, Asking L, Beckman O, Bondesson E, Kallen A. Olsson B. Discrepancy between in vitro and in vivo dose variability for a pressurized metered dose inhaler and a dry powder. J Aerosol Med 1998; 11:S59–S64.
8. Pierart F, Wildhaber JH, Vrancken I, Devadason SG, LeSouef PN. Washing plastic spacers in household detergent reduces electrostatic charge and greatly improves delivery. Eur Respir J 1999; 13:673–678.
9. Rogers DF, Ganderton D. Determining equivalence of inhaled medications. Consensus statement from a workshop of the British Association for Lung Research, held at Royal Brompton National Heart & Lung Institute, London 24 June 1994. Respir Med 1995; 89:253–261.
10. Snell NJ, Ganderton D. Assessing lung deposition of inhaled medications. Consensus statement from a workshop of the British Association for Lung Research, held at the Institute of Biology, London UK on 17 April 1998. Respir Med 1999; 93:123–133.
11. Pauwels R, Newman S, Borgström L. Airway deposition and airway effects of antiasthma drugs delivered from metered-dose inhalers. Eur Respir J 1997, 10:2127–2138.
12. Meakin BJ, Cainey J, Woodcock PM. Effect of exposure to humidity on terbutaline delivery from turbuhaler dry power inhalation devices (letter; comment). Eur Respir J 1993; 6:760–761.
13. Everard ML, Devadason SG, Summers QA, LeSouef PN. Factors affecting total and "respirable" dose delivered by a salbutamol metered dose inhaler. Thorax 1995; 50:746–749.
14. Wildhaber JH, Devadason SG, Eber E, Hayden MJ, Everard ML, Summers QA Effect of electrostatic charge, flow, delay and multiple actuations on the in vitro delivery of salbutamol from different small volume spacers for infants. Thorax 1996; 51:985–988.
15. Barry PW, O'Callaghan C. The effect of delay, multiple actuations and spacer static charge on the in vitro delivery of budesonide from the Nebuhaler. Br J Clin Pharmacol 1995; 40:76–78.

16. Boe J, Stiksa G, Svensson K, Asbrink E. New method of evaluating patient preference for different inhalation delivery systems. Ann Allergy 1992; 68:255–260.
17. Zellweger JP, Anderhub HP, Longloh P. Efficacy and tolerance of terbutaline and budesonide administered via a pressurized aerosol inhaler or a Turbuhaler in asthmatic patients. Schweiz Rundsch Med Prax 1993; 82:561–564.
18. Vilsvik JS, Ringdal N, Albrektsen T, Holthe S Comparison of the acceptability of the Ventolin metered-dose inhaler and the Bricanyl Turbuhaler Ann Allergy. 1993; 70:300–304
19. van der Palen J, Klein JJ, Schildkamp AM. Comparison of a new multidose powder inhaler (Diskus/Accuhaler) and the Turbuhaler regarding preference and ease of use. J Asthma 1998; 35:147–152.
20. Horn CR, Clark TJ, Cochrane GM. Compliance with inhaled therapy and morbidity from asthma. Respir Med 1990; 84:67–70.
21. Gillies J. Overview of delivery system issues in pediatric asthma. Pediatr Pulmonol (suppl) 1997; 15:55–58.
22. Barnes PJ. Efficacy of inhaled corticosteroids in asthma. J Allergy Clin Immunol 1998; 102:531–538.
23. Rand CS, Nides M, Cowles MK, Wise RA, Connett J Long-term metered-dose inhaler adherence in a clinical trial. The Lung Health Study Research Group. Am J Respir Crit Care Med 1995; 152:580–588.
24. Milgrom H, Bender B, Ackerson L, Bowry P, Smith B, Rand C. Noncompliance and treatment failure in children with asthma. J Allergy Clin Immunol 1996; 98:1051–1057.
25. Mawhinney H, Spector SL, Kinsman RA, Siegel SC, Rachelefsky GS, Katz RM. Compliance in clinical trials of two nonbronchodilator, antiasthma medications. Ann Allergy 1991; 66:294–299.
26. Frost GD, Penrose A, Hall J, MacKenzie DI. Asthma-related prescribing patterns with four different corticosteroid inhaler devices. Respir Med 1998; 92:1352–1358.
27. Allen RM, Jones MP, Oldenburg B. Randomised trial of an asthma self-management programme for adults. Thorax 1995; 60:731–738.
28. Cote J, Cartier A, Robichaud P, Boutin H, Malo JL, Rouleau M. Influence on asthma morbidity of asthma education programs based on self-management plans following treatment optimization. Am J Respir Crit Care Med 1997; 155:1509–1514.
29. Cochrane GM. Compliance and outcomes in patients with asthma. Drugs 1996; 52 (suppl 6): 12–19.
30. Mann M, Eliasson O, Patel K, ZuWallack RL. A comparison of the effects of bid and qid dosing on compliance with inhaled flunisolide. Chest 1992; 101:496–499.
31. Barnes PJ, O'Connor BJ. Use of a fixed combination beta 2-agonist and steroid dry powder inhaler in asthma. Am J Respir Crit Care Med 1995; 151:1053–1057.
32. Wong CS, Pavord ID, Williams J, Britton JR, Tattersfield AE. Bronchodilator, cardiovascular, and hypokalaemic effects of fenoterol, salbutamol, and terbutaline in asthma (see comments). Lancet 1990; 336:1396–1399.
33. Rahman AR, McDevitt DG, Struthers AD, Lipworth BJ Sex differences in hy-

pokalaemic and electrocardiographic effects of inhaled terbutaline. Thorax 1992; 47:1056–1059.

34. Lipworth BJ, Clark RA, Dhillon DP, Brown RA, McDevitt DG. Beta-adrenoceptor responses to high doses of inhaled salbutamol in patients with bronchial asthma. Br J Clin Pharmacol 1988; 26:527–533.
35. Burgess C, Beasley R, Crane J, Pearce N. Adverse effects of beta2-agonists. In Pauwels R, O'Byrne PO, eds. Beta2-Agonists in Asthma Treatment. New York: Marcel Dekker, 1997:257–282.
36. Barnes PJ, Pedersen S, Busse WW. Efficacy and safety of inhaled corticosteroids: new developments. Am J Respir Crit Care Med 1998; 157 S1–S53.
37. Hochhaus G, Mollman H, Derendorf H, Gonzalez-Rothi RJ. Pharmacokinetic/pharmacodynamic aspects of aerosol therapy using glucocorticoids as a model. J Clin Pharmacol 1997; 37:881–892.
38. Thorsson L, Kenyon C, Newman S, Borgström L. Lung deposition of budesonide in asthmatics a comparison of different formulations. Int J Pharm 1998; 168:119–127.
39. Johnson M. The beta-adrenoceptor. Am J Respir Crit Care Med 1998; 158 S146–S153.
40. Anderson P, Lötvall J, Linden A. Relaxation kinetics of formoterol and salmeterol in the guinea pig trachea in vitro. Lung 1996; 174:159–170.
41. Ullman A, Svedmyr N. Salmeterol, a new long acting inhaled beta 2 adrenoceptor agonist: comparison with salbutamol in adult asthmatic patients. Thorax 1988; 43:674–678.
42. Derom EY, Pauwels RA. Time course of bronchodilating effect of inhaled formoterol, a potent and long acting sympathomimetic. Thorax 1992; 47:30–33.
43. Palmqvist M, Persson G, Lazer L, Rosenborg J, Larsson P, Lötvall J. Inhaled dry-powder formoterol and salmeterol in asthmatic patients: onset of action, duration of effect and potency (see comments). Eur Respir J 1997; 10: 2484–2489.
44. Miller-Larsson A, Mattsson H, Hjertberg E, Dahlback M, Tunek A, Brattsand R. Reversible fatty acid conjugation of budesonide. Novel mechanism for prolonged retention of topically applied steroid in airway tissue. Drug Metab Dispos 1998; 26:623–630.
45. Esmailpour N, Hogger P, Rabe KF, Heitmann U, Nakashima M, Rohdewald P. Distribution of inhaled fluticasone propionate between human lung tissue and serum in vivo. Eur Respir J 1997; 10:1496–1499.
46. Morgan DJ. Clinical pharmacokinetics of beta-agonists. Clin Pharmacokinet 1990; 18:270–294.
47. Lönnebo A, Grahnén A, Jansson B, Brundin RM, Ling-Andersson A, Eckernas SA. An assessment of the systemic effects of single and repeated doses of inhaled fluticasone propionate and inhaled budesonide in healthy volunteers. Eur J Clin Pharmacol 1996; 49:459–463.
48. Grahnén A, Eckernas SA, Brundin RM, Ling AA. An assessment of the systemic activity of single doses of inhaled fluticasone propionate in healthy volunteers. Br J Clin Pharmacol 1994; 38: 521–525.
49. Boorsma M, Andersson N, Larsson P, Ullman A. Assessment of the relative systemic potency of inhaled fluticasone and budesonide. Eur Respir J 1996; 9:1427–1432.

50. Clark DJ, Lipworth BJ. Adrenal suppression with chronic dosing of fluticasone propionate compared with budesonide in adult asthmatic patients. Thorax 1997 52:55–58.
51. Derom E, Van Schoor J, Verhaeghe W, Vincken W, Pauwels R. Systemic effects of inhaled fluticasone propionate and budesonide in adult patients with asthma. Am J Respir Crit Care Med 1999; 160:157–161.
52. Thorsson L, Dahlstrom K, Edsbacker S, Kallén A, Paulson J, Wiren JE. Pharmacokinetics and systemic effects of inhaled fluticasone propionate in healthy subjects. Br J Clin Pharmacol 1997; 43:155–161.
53. Ryrfeldt A, Andersson P, Edsbacker S, Tonnesson M, Davies D, Pauwels R. Pharmacokinetics and metabolism of budesonide, a selective glucocorticoid. Eur J Respir Dis 1982; 63(suppl 119):86–95.
54. Beasley R, Pearce N, Crane J, Burgess C. Beta-agonists: what is the evidence that their use increases the risk of asthma morbidity and mortality? J Allergy Clin Immunol 1999; 104:18–30.
55. Woolcock A, Lundback B, Ringdal N, Jacques LA. Comparison of addition of salmeterol to inhaled steroids with doubling of the dose of inhaled steroids. Am J Respir Crit Care Med 1996; 153:1481–1488.
56. Mak VH, Melchor R, Spiro SG. Easy braising as a side-effect of inhaled corticosteroids. Eur Respir J 1992; 5:1068–1074.
57. Roy A, Leblanc C, Paquette L, Ghezzo H, Cote J, Cartier A. Skin bruising in asthmatic subjects treated with high doses of inhaled steroids: frequency and association with adrenal function. Eur Respir J 1996; 9:226–231.
58. Richards R, Sounders M. Need for a comparative performance standard for dry powder inhalers. Thorax 1993; 48:1186–1187.
59. Olsson B, Asking L. Critical aspects of the function of inspiratory flow driven inhalers. J Aerosol Med 1994; 7:S43–S47.
60. Cobben NA, Drent M, Jonkers M, Wouters EF, Vaneechoutte M, Stobheringh EE. Outbreak of severe Pseudomonas aeruginosa respiratory infections due to contaminated nebulizers. J Hosp Infect 1996; 33:63–70.
61. O'Callaghan C, Lynch J, Cant M, Robertson C. Improvement in sodium cromoglycate delivery from a spacer device by use of an antistatic lining immediate inhalation, and avoiding multiple actuations of drug. Thorax 1993; 48:603–606.
62. Wildhaber JH, Devadason SG, Hayden MJ, Eber E, Summers QA, LeSouef PN. Aerosol delivery to wheezy infants: a comparison between a nebulizer and two small volume spacers. Pediatr Pulmonol 1997, 23:212–216.
63. Wildhaber JH, Devadason SG, Hoyden MJ, James R, Duffy AP, Fox RA Electrostatic charge on a plastic spacer device influences the delivery of salbutamol. Eur Respir J 1996; 9:1943–1946.
64. Meakin BJ, Cainey JM, Woodcock PM. Drug delivery characteristics of Bricanyl Turbohaler dry powder inhalers. Int J Pharm 1995; 119:91–102.
65. Daniels GF, Ashurst IC, Malley TR, Walker S, Noble R, Gillet B. Simulated patient in-use testing at extreme environmental conditions of a dry powder inhaler device containing a combination of salmeterol and fluticasone propionate (abstr). Eur J Respir 1999; 14 (suppl 30): 2284.

66. van Beerendonk I, Mesters I, Mudde AN, Tan TD. Assessment of the inhalation technique in outpatients with asthma or chronic obstructive pulmonary disease using a metered-dose inhaler or dry powder device. J Asthma 1998; 35:273–279.
67. Kesten S, Elias M, Cartier A, Chapman KR. Patient handling of a multidose dry powder inhalation device for albuterol. Chest 1994; 105:1077–1081.
68. Pederden S. Inhalers and nebulizers: which to choose and why? Respir Med 1996; 90:69–77.
69. Blake KV, Harman E, Hendeles L. Evaluation of a generic albuterol metered-dose inhaler: importance of priming the MDI. Ann Allergy 1992; 68:169–174.
70. Kenyon CJ, Thorsson L, Borgström L, Newman SP. The effects of static charge in spacer devices on glucocorticosteroid aerosol deposition in asthmatic patients. Eur Respir J 1998; 11:606–610.
71. Anhoj J, Bisgaard H, Lipworth BJ. Effect of electrostatic charge in plastic spacers on the lung delivery of HFA-salbutamol in children. Br J Clin Pharmacol 1999; 47:333–336.
72. Newman S, Moren F, Trofast E, Talaee N, Clarke S. Terbutaline sulphate terbutaline: effect of inhaled flow rate on drug deposition and efficacy. Int J Pharm 1991; 74:209–213.
73. Engel T, Scharling B, Skovsted B, Heinig JH. Effects, side effects and plasma concentrations of terbutaline in adult asthmatics after inhaling from a dry powder inhaler device at different inhalation flows and volumes. Br J Clin Pharmacol 1992; 33:439–444.
74. Pedersen S, Hansen OR, Fuglsang G. Influence of inspiratory flow rate upon the effect of a Turbuhaler. Arch Dis Child 1990; 55:308–310.
75. Thorsson L, Edsbacker S. Lung deposition of budesonide from a pressurized metered-dose inhaler attached to a spacer. Eur Respir J 1998; 12:1340–1345.
76. Thorsson L, Edsbacker S, Conradson TB. Lung deposition of budesonide from Turbuhaler is twice that from a pressurized metered-dose inhaler P-MDI. Eur Respir J 1994; 7:1839–1844.
77. Newman S, Pavia D, Garland N, Clarke SW. Effects of various inhalation modes on the deposition of radioactive presurized aerosols. Eur J Respir Dis 1982; 63(suppl 119) 57–65.
78. Newman S, Steed K, Hooper G, Kallén A, Borgström L Comparison of gamma scintigraphy and a pharmacokinetic technique for assessing pulmonary deposition of terbutaline sulphate delivered by pressurized metered dose inhaler. Pharm Res 1995; 12:231–236.
79. Farr SJ, Rowe AM, Rubsamen R, Taylor G. Aerosol deposition in the human lung following administration from a microprocessor controlled pressurised metered dose inhaler. Thorax 1995; 50:639–644.
80. Newman SP, Weisz AW, Talaee N, Clarke SW. Improvement of drug delivery with a breath actuated pressurised aerosol for patients with poor inhaler technique. Thorax 1991; 46:712–716.
81. Newman S, Pavia D, Clarke S. Simple instructions for using pressurized aerosol bronchodilators. J R Soc Med 1980; 73:776–779.

82. Lawford P, McKenzie D. Pressurized aerosol inhaler technique: how important are inhalation from residual volume, inspiratory flow rate and the time interval between puffs? Br J Dis Chest 1983; 77:276–281.
83. Dolovich M. Inhalation technique and inhalation devices. In: Pauwels R, O'Byrne PO, eds. Beta$_2$-Agonists in Asthma Treatment. New York: Marcel Dekker, 1997:229–256.
84. Pitcairn G, Lunghetti G, Ventura P, Newman S. A comparison of the lung deposition of salbutamol inhaled from a new dry powder inhaler, at two inhaled flow rates. Int J Pharm 1994; 102:11–18.
85. Olsson B, Borgström L, Asking L, Bondesson E. Effect of inlet troat on the correlation between fine particle dose and lung deposition. In: Dalby RN, Byron PR, Farr SJ, eds. Respiratory Drug Delivery V. Buffalo Grove, IL: Interpharm Press, 1996:273–281.
86. Borgström L, Newman S, Weisz A, Morén F. Pulmonary deposition of inhaled terbutaline: comparison of scanning gamma camera and urinary excretion methods. J Pharm Sci 1992; 81:753–755.
87. Borgström L, Bondesson E, Morén F, Trofast E, Newman SP. Lung deposition of budesonide inhaled via Turbuhaler: a comparison with terbutaline sulphate in normal subjects. Eur Respir J 1994; 7:69–73.
88. Dolovich M., Vanziegelheim M, Hidinger K. Influence of inspiratory flow rate on the response to terbutaline sulphate inhaled via the Turbuhaler (abstr). Am Rev Respir Dis 1988; 137:433.
89. Newman SP, Steed KP, Reader SJ, Hooper G, Zierenberg B. Efficient delivery to the lungs of flunisolide aerosol from a new portable hand-held multidose nebulizer. J Pharm Sci 1996; 85:960–964.
90. Newman SP, Brown J, Steed KP, Reader SJ, Kladders H. Lung deposition of fenoterol and flunisolide delivered using a novel device for inhaled medicines: comparison of (RESPIMAT with conventional metered-dose inhalers with and without spacer devices. Chest 1998; 113:957–963.
91. Pauwels R, Derom E. Deposition and pharmacodynamics of terbutaline inhaled via Turbuhaler (abstr). J Aerosol Med 1991; 4:A187.
92. Borgström L, Derom E, Ståhl E, Wåhlin-Boll E, Pauwels R. The inhalation device influences lung deposition and bronchodilating effect of terbutaline. Am J Respir Crit Care Med 1996; 153:1636–1640.
93. Svedmyr N, Löfdahl C, Svedmyr K. The effect of powder aerosol compared to pressurized aerosol. Eur J Respir Dis 1982; 63(suppl 119):81–88.
94. Duncan D, Paterson I, Harris D, Crompton G. Comparison of the effects of salbutamol inhaled as a dry powder and by conventional pressurized aerosol. Br J Clin Pharmacol 1977; 4:669–671.
95. Hetzel MR, Clark TJ. Comparison of salbutamol Rotahaler with conventional pressurized aerosol. Clin Allergy 1977; 7:563–568.
96. Carlsson LG, Arwestrom E, Friberg K, Kallén A, Lunde H, Löfdahl CG. Efficacy of cumulative doses of salbutamol administered via Turbuhaler or Diskhaler in patients with reversible airway obstruction. Allergy 1998; 53:712–715.

97. Löfdahl CG, Andersson L, Bondesson E, Carlsson LG, Friberg K, Hedner J. Differences in bronchodilating potency of salbutamol in Turbuhaler as compared with a pressurized metered-dose inhaler formulation in patients with reversible airway obstruction. Eur Respir J 1997; 10:2474–2478.
98. Goodman DE, Israel E, Rosenberg M, Johnston R, Weiss ST, Drazen JM. The influence of age, diagnosis, and gender on proper use of metered-dose inhalers (see comments). Am J Respir Crit Care Med 1994; 150:1256–1261.
99. Bollert FG, Matusiewicz SP, Dewar MH, Brown GM, McLean A, Greening AP. Comparative efficacy and potency of ipratropium via Turbuhaler and pressurized metered-dose inhaler in reversible airflow obstruction. Eur Respir J 1997; 10:1824–1828.
100. Gross G, Thompson PJ, Chervinsky P, Vanden Burgt J. Hydrofluoroalkane-134a beclomethasone dipropionate, 400μg, is as effective as chlorofluorocarbon beclomethasone dipropionate, 800 μg, for the treatment of moderate asthma. Chest 1999; 115:343–351.
101. Salzman GA, Pyszczynski DR. Oropharyngeal candidiasis in patients treated with beclomethasone dipropionate delivered by metered-dose inhaler alone and with Aerochamber. J Allergy Clin Immunol 1988; 81:424–428.
102. Selroos O, Backman R, Forsen KO, Löfroos AB, Niemisto M, Pietinalho A. Local side-effects during 4-year treatment with inhaled corticosteroids—a comparison between pressurized metered-dose inhalers and Turbuhaler. Allergy 1994; 49:888–890.
103. Borgström L, Nilsson M. A method for determination of the absolute pulmonary bioavailability of inhaled drugs: terbutaline. Pharm Res 1990; 7:1068–1070.
104. Morgan DJ, Paull JD, Richmond BH, Wilson-Evered E, Ziccone SP. Pharmacokinetics of intravenous and oral salbutamol and its sulphate conjugate. Br J Clin Pharmacol 1986; 22:587–593.
105. Lipworth BJ. New perspectives on inhaled drug delivery and systemic bioactivity (editorial) [published erratum appears in Thorax 1995 May; 50(5):592]. Thorax 1995; 50:105–110.
106. Brown PH, Matusiewicz SP, Shearing C, Tibi L, Greening AP, Crompton GK. Systemic effects of high dose inhaled steroids: comparison of beclomethasone dipropionate and budesonide in healthy subjects. Thorax 1993; 48:967–973.
107. Pedersen S, Steffensen G, Ohlsson SV. The influence of orally deposited budesonide on the systemic availability of budesonide after inhalation from a Turbuhaler. Br J Clin Pharmacol 1993; 36:211–214.
108. Borgström L. Local versus total systemic bioavailability as a means to compare different inhaled formulations of the same substance. J Aerosol Med 1998; 11:55–63.
109. Thorsson, L. Studies on the deposition, bio-availability and systemic activity of glucocorticoids in man. Ph.D. thesis. Lund, Sweden: Lund University, 1998.
111. Newman SP, Hirst PH, Pitcairn GR. Understanding regional lung deposition data in gamma scintigraphy. In: Dalby RN, Byron PR, Farr SJ, eds. Respiratory Drug Delivery VI. Buffalo Grove, IL: Interpharm Press, 1998:9–16.
112. Boulet LP, Cockcroft DW, Toogood J, Baskerville JR., Hargreave FE. Comparative

assessment of safety and efficacy of inhaled corticosteroids, report of a committee of the Canadian Thoracic Society. Eur Respir J 1998; 11:1194–1210.

113. Barnes PJ, Jonsson B, Klim JB. The costs of asthma. Eur Respir J 1996; 9:636–642.
114. Turner MO, Gafni A, Swan D, FitzGerald JM. A review and economic evaluation of bronchodilator delivery methods in hospitalized patients. Arch Intern Med 1996; 156:2113–2118.
115. Liljas B, Ståhl E, Pauwels RA. Cost-effectiveness analysis of a dry powder inhaler (Turbuhaler) versus a pressurised metered dose inhaler in patients with asthma. Pharmacoeconomics 1997; 12:267–277.

6

In Vivo Measurements of Lung Dose

MARK L. EVERARD

Sheffield Children's Hospital
Sheffield, England

MYRNA B. DOLOVICH

McMaster University
Hamilton, Ontario, Canada

I. Introduction

Over recent years there has been increasing interest in the in vivo assessment of drug delivery to the lungs when using aerosolized therapy. This surge of interest has resulted from a desire to understand the strengths and limitations of current aerosol systems and a wish on the part of some to understand basic mechanisms in order to develop improved delivery systems in the future. It should be remembered that current aerosol delivery systems utilize technology that has been around for many decades and that these devices were brought to market long before direct assessment of drug delivery to the lung was attempted. Jet nebulizers first appeared more than 60 years ago, pressurized metered-dose inhalers (pMDIs) more than 40 years ago, and dry-powder systems 30 years ago. Spacers and holding chambers were first produced some 20 years ago to try and overcome many of the problems known to be associated with the use of pMDIs. All these devices were brought to market on the basis of pharmacodynamic studies which suggested that useful therapeutic effects could be obtained. Nominal or prescribed doses were chosen empirically without any need to assess the likely lung dose in vivo.

A. Aerosols for the Treatment of Pulmonary Disease

The results of in vivo deposition studies undertaken in the past decade have highlighted the high intersubject variability in lung dose and the operator-dependent nature of these devices. Such studies have, along with pharmacodynamic and in vitro studies, provided information that allows us to compare delivery systems and to make recommendations regarding optimization of inhalation technique and strategies to minimize potential side effects (1–3). However, they have not altered the only effective guide to choosing the prescribed drug dose when using one of the current delivery systems, which is to use the lowest dose that produces the desired therapeutic response (2)—an approach that maximizes the "therapeutic index" by ensuring efficacy while reducing the chance of systemic side effects. We currently do not know what *lung* dose is required in treating an asthmatic patient with inhaled steroids or the optimal lung dose in administering nebulized antibiotics to a patient with cystic fibrosis. Furthermore, we cannot accurately predict the lung dose that will be achieved when an individual patient uses a particular delivery system.

Despite all these uncertainties, we know that valuable therapeutic effects can be obtained using the inhaled route, and it is worth recalling the reasons that the inhaled route has been used for many centuries to treat pulmonary disease (4).

For drugs such as β-agonists, the onset of action is much more rapid when they are given by inhalation and bronchodilation is achieved within minutes compared with several hours when administered orally (5). Portable inhalers were developed to provide patients, wherever they are, with rapid relief of symptoms.

Furthermore, by administering drugs "directly to their site of action," the systemic exposure can be reduced, resulting in an improved the "therapeutic ratio" for a variety of drugs including corticosteroids, sympathomimetic agents, and antibiotics such as aminoglycosides. However, it should be remembered that the pattern of distribution via the inhaled route is likely to be much less uniform than if drug is delivered via the systemic route. In addition, drugs that cannot be delivered via the GI tract, such as sodium cromoglycate, must be delivered via the inhaled route.

By necessity, the respiratory tract excludes foreign material, in contrast to the GI tract, which is adapted to take in large foreign bodies. The challenge for aerosol scientists has been to produce devices that generate aerosols containing sufficient drug in "respirable particles" to produce a therapeutic effect. This challenge was met in part many decades ago but, in contrast to almost all other areas in medicine, the technology used to deliver therapeutic aerosol has evolved little over recent decades. Current devices remain generally inefficient but, more importantly, remain difficult to use effectively, in large part because the method of use is not obvious.

Devices currently available are able to generate aerosols that will deliver therapeutic doses of drugs into the lungs. However, because they are so operator-dependent, coupled with the interindividual variability in airways geometry and the distribution of airways disease, it is not possible to accurately predict lung doses in individual patients. Though this lack of precision may seem far from ideal, it should be remembered, for example, that we do not know the likely intrapulmonary concentrations achieved in using oral antibiotics. However, clinical studies have demonstrated efficacy and safety with empirically chosen doses. Indeed, there has probably been as much or more time and effort invested in in vivo assessment of delivery to the target organ using the inhaled route as there has been in most other therapeutic areas. The reasons that this work has not translated into improved delivery systems are that current devices have, on the whole, proven to been adequate in terms of efficacy and safety (when used as effectively) and because of the focus by many pharmaceutical companies on the drug rather than the delivery system.

Though it is well known that most current devices are difficult to use optimally and are frequently misused, useful therapeutic effects are still obtained, and therefore there has been relatively little pressure to produce devices appropriate to the twenty-first century. This may change due to developments in other therapeutic areas.

B. Novel Agents

People have been interested in using the respiratory tract as a route for delivering systematically acting drugs for many years (6–9). Indeed, it was proposed that insulin could be delivered via the respiratory tract soon after the arrival of both jet nebulizers in the 1930s and pMDIs in the mid 1950s, though this approach was soon abandoned in both cases because of the unacceptable variability in delivery to the lung. The advent of novel systems with much lower variability is set to change this situation. It is, in many ways, easier to produce reproducible drug delivery to the lungs for systematically acting drugs such as insulin, as these drugs are targeted at the distal airways. By producing an aerosol containing particles between 1 and 3 μm in diameter, variability in deposition in the upper airways is greatly reduced. However, more importantly, the manufacturers have concentrated on developing devices that will deliver reproducible doses and that can be used effectively by patients with little or no training.

It has been proposed that a variety of peptides can be administered as aerosols. Furthermore, novel therapies for pulmonary disease—including gene therapy, immunomodulatory therapies such as gamma interferon (10) surfactant, and chemotherapeutic agents—are being formulated for inhalation. However, it will not be possible to exploit such approaches until we have a better understanding of how to manipulate the aerosol to achieve these ends. In vivo assessment of drug delivery has now become a vital part of device/drug combination development for both traditional therapeutic areas and, more importantly, for the novel forms of therapy.

C. Surrogates for In Vivo Data

Accurate predictions of in vivo lung dose using in vitro data obtained from multistage impingers and laser diffraction (11–13) has not been successful, though there is a reasonable correlation between some parameters and lung dose (14–17). In vitro work has been of value in device development and in quality control during manufacture but has been much less valuable in producing meaningful information regarding deposition of drug from a given device within the respiratory tract of patients even when delivery occurs under optimal conditions. Improved in vitro techniques using approaches such as anatomically correct upper airways and inspiratory profiles derived from patients (18) will mean that in vitro modeling information should become increasingly valuable, particularly if these techniques can be validated against results obtained in vivo. However, while this may reduce the need for extensive in vivo studies, it is unlikely that they will ever completely replace the need for well-designed in vivo assessment of delivered dose.

D. Techniques for In Vivo Assessment of Drug Delivery Systems

This chapter focuses on techniques available for measuring aerosolized drug delivery to the respiratory tract from therapeutic devices. These are essentially radiolabeled deposition studies and pharmacokinetic studies. Other approaches, such as the aerosol bolus technique (19–22) and the administration of monodispersed therapeutic aerosols (23), are used for assessing the behavior and deposition of particles in the respiratory tract, but these cannot be applied to standard delivery systems. Attempts to directly quantify drug in the lung have involved assaying drug concentrations in resected lung tissue (24), bronchoalveolar lavage (BAL), and sputum (25). Interpretation of data, particularly from studies involving the latter two methods, is fraught with difficulty, as the inherent heterogeneity associated with BAL and sputum production introduces considerable variability.

II. Imaging and Pharmacokinetic Approaches

The two basic approaches to the direct assessment of lung dose are pharmacokinetic techniques and imaging techniques. The former is divided into classical pharmacokinetic techniques and indirect measurements, such as the urinary or plasma salbutamol techniques, while the latter is divided into 2D planar gamma scintigraphy or 3D single photon emission computed tomography (SPECT) and positron emission tomograpy (PET).

Information that can be obtained from such studies includes

Total lung dose
Extrapulmonary delivery
Distribution within the airways
Total systemic exposure
The influence of factors such as disease and inhalation technique on deposition throughout the respiratory tract
Clearance of particles from the lungs
Intra- and intersubject variability
Relationship between lung dose and therapeutic effects

The information that is actually obtained from a study will depend upon the design of the study and the quality of information or data obtained from the study.

A. What Value Are Such Studies?

There is currently no ideal technique that will provide all of the above information. In vivo studies are clearly of interest in that they improve our understanding of aerosol therapy in general and may contribute to the development of improved delivery systems. Undoubtedly they have highlighted the weaknesses of current devices and they have emphasized that these devices are inefficient, with high intra and intersubject variability even when used by trained volunteers.

In addition to providing information that satisfies scientific curiosity and contributes to product development, such studies are increasingly been undertaken to provide information required by regulatory authorities, though the regulatory authorities' interpretation of such studies does not appear to take into account the difference between results obtained in a controlled environment and those obtained in the "real world," where patient issues such as cognition and beliefs play a major role. These issues are partly and indirectly addressed in clinical trials. It has also been suggested that one of the advantages of undertaking studies using gamma-emitting nucleotides is that they provide "visually striking images for promotional material" (26), though whether this can be justified as the principal reason for a study involving radionuclides is debatable.

It is also important to realize that gamma camera images can be extremely misleading, since the image can be changed significantly by altering the gain on the camera. Two apparently completely different images can be produced from the same data, and therefore no image should be interpreted without first calculating doses in the separate compartments.

B. Limitations of In Vivo Assessment of Lung Dose

It should be remembered that results from such studies must not be overinterpreted. Methodologies vary significantly between laboratories performing apparently similar studies, and there may be highly significant differences in their approaches to radiolabeling the drug, validating the effectiveness of the radiolabel, and analyzing the data, including factors such as tissue attenuation of activity and definition of lung regions. It has been estimated that, under ideal circumstances, planar imaging can achieve an accuracy of approximately 10% for lung dose, provided that drug is uniformly distributed and that all the methodological problems are addressed (27). Ideally, in comparing devices or techniques, this should be done within individual patients and not using results obtained from different studies from different centers, as variation in techniques will significantly affect the accuracy of results.

Clinicians and patients wish to have a delivery system/drug combination that reliably delivers a therapeutic dose to the site of action while minimizing side effects. Interpretation of deposition studies cannot alone predict the therapeutic index. For instance:

A given device may increase the amount of drug delivered to the lung compared with another device and therefore appear "safer." If the quantity of drug delivered on both occasions is on the steep part of the dose-response curve, improved therapeutic effects may be see and indeed the therapeutic index will have improved; but if the doses are on the "plateau," increased side effects resulting from increased pulmonary absorption may be observe for little increase in therapeutic effect.

A device may appear to have a good "therapeutic index" when used optimally, but when used suboptimally it may have a very poor index. For example, a pMDI utilizing a steroid with only partial first-pass matabolism may have good therapeutic index when used optimally, but if a patient actuates the device in the mouth but does not inhale, the index will be very poor. In vivo studies in trained volunteers do not address this issue.

The debate over the value of developing a solution based beclomethasone pMDIs highlights the fact that we understand even less about the how altering the pattern of drug deposition within the lung will affect the therapeutic index. The pattern of drug delivery is altered using this solution, based the pMDI increasing the proportion of drug in the periphery of the lung. Whether this alters the therapeutic index significantly, either positively or negatively remains unclear and can be determined only in pharmacodynamic studies (28,29).

Gamma scintigraphy can provide visually striking pictures, an idea of total lung dose, and an indication of the likely intrapulmonary distribution when using one device compared with different formulations, and this is of undoubted interest. However, the results cannot tell clinicians what they really want to know, which is:

For a given therapeutic effect, which device is likely to be safer in clinical practice? and

Are any differences noted in the results from scintigraphic studies of any clinical relevance given the need to use the lowest dose that works with whichever device is chosen?

Such problems should not detract from the value of in vivo assessment of drug delivery. But in considering designing a study or interpreting a study, such limitations must be borne in mind. Such studies will never replace clinical studies assessing safety and efficacy but will provide useful and often interesting complementary information and are likely to be increasingly important in product development as our understanding and interpretation of such studies improves.

C. Summary

Both pk and imaging studies have limitations for the measurement of delivered lung dose and response. In the former, no direct information is provided for distribution within the airways, while with the latter technique, the assessment of lung dose is foremost dependent on the accurate radiolabeling of the drug and sensitive imaging of the lung.

Comparisons between devices and/or inhalation techniques should be undertaken in the same group of subjects.

No standards for imaging techniques have been established.

Differences in techniques between centers mean that direct comparisons between studies is rarely possible.

Changes in lung dose may translate into alterations in clinical response and therapeutic index, depending on the position on the dose-response curve.

The effect of altering the penetration index is poorly understood.

While pk and imaging studies in normals can provide benchmark data, measurement should be undertaken in the intended population for the therapy being evaluated.

D. Choice of Technique

The choice of technique is influenced by factors such as the strengths and limitations of each approach, the expertise available, and the type of question that needs to be answered. At present there is no "gold standard," with all pharmacokinetic and imaging techniques having advantages and disadvantages.

III. Imaging

As noted above, there are three main imaging methodologies:

Planar gamma scintigraphy
Single photon emission computed tomography (SPECT)
Positron emission tomograpy (PET)

Advantages of Using Imaging

The first approach provides a 2D image, the latter two, 3D information. The first two approaches utilize gamma-emitting radionuclides, while positron emitters utilize isotopes. Such approaches have a number of advantages over pharmacokinetic studies but inevitably have important limitations and cannot be viewed as superior to pharmacokinetic techniques. Their greatest strength lies in the ability to localize deposition within compartments of the respiratory tract. Pharmacokinetic studies can generally identify the contribution to the total systematic load that can be attributed to pulmonary deposition and that entering via the GI tract but does not provide more precise localization of deposition. In many circumstances, this is probably not a problem; indeed, some argue that these data are more than adequate for most purposes (28). However, there are undoubtedly examples of information being provided by gamma scintigraphy that could not be provided in other ways. These include the observation that drug delivery to areas of the lung most severely affected by a disease process is reduced compared with less affected areas (30,31) and the nonhomogeneous distribution when a drug is inhaled with the patient in an upright position (32). Again the clinical significance of these observations remains to be: determined (33). In children, such studies have highlighted the poor delivery to the lungs when very young children are upset (34,35), but this has also been demonstrated using an indirect pharmacokinetic study (36).

Disadvantages at Imaging Techniques

All imaging techniques utilize radionucleotides, which pose a health risk to the subjects, the radiopharmacist preparing the formulation, and the individual administering the device. Indeed, it is likely that for most studies the risk is greater for those preparing the formulation than those inhaling it, as most aerosol devices contain multiple doses requiring high doses to be manipulated during formulation. Planar imaging can generally be achieved with a lung dose of 1–4 MBq. The doses required increase significantly for SPECT, often requiring up to 30 MBq to be deposited in the lungs, and exposure is increased further if computed tomography (CT) is employed to provide precise localization of lung borders (37). Doses for PET scanning are higher still, but because of the much shorter half-lives of the positron emitters, the overall risk is probably comparable (38). Though studies need to pass stringent safety regulations, there is still a finite risk, with all of these studies, that an untoward consequence will be manifest many decades later. The risk for most planar studies appears to be very low and often comparable to the radiation received in a 12-h flight or from a few weeks' background radiation. However, oropharyngeal and tracheal doses and the presence of "hot spots" of deposition within the lungs will have a significant impact on the level of risk (39). Because the effects may not be manifest for many decades, the risks are relatively greater in children than in older subjects. Moreover, though adverse genetic effects in the children of subjects exposed to radiation for research purposes have not been observed, this remains a further source of concern in studying children and young adults. The issues surrounding the risks of using radiation for in vivo assessment have been discussed previously (40,41). *In essence it is essential to conduct studies in a manner that will minimize risk and to limit the use of this approach to studies that will provide answers that cannot be obained in other ways.* The design of the study should ensure that administered doses adhere to the ALARA principle (as low as reasonably achievable) and exposure be within the annual effective aggregate dose (42). The minimum number of subjects should be used to answer a specific question unequivocally.

Methodological Challenges

All the imaging techniques involve a number of methodological problems, including the need to correct for attenuation of radiation by body tissues and the need for correction due to both natural decay of activity and biological decay with time. The latter represent absorption of the radionuclide from the airways. The half-life of TcO_4 once separated from the drug is in the order of 11 min while that in the oropharynx may be as high as 25 min.

The activity of the radionuclide will decline with time and it will also be cleared from the lung through absorption and mucociliary clearance. The former is relevant in that there may be a delay of some hours between formulating the radiopharmaceutical and administering it to a subject. Since the physical rate of decay of the isotope is known, this effect can be quantified. As noted above, some radionuclides are absorped very rapidly from the lungs, and this is of particular relevance when using SPECT, which may require acquisition times of 5–20 min. To date there is no entirely satisfactory method for correcting for this problem, particularly as the radionuclide present in the bronchial and pulmonary circulations will contribute to the image as time passes. However, defining an area of tissue away from the lung field (e.g., the thigh) can provide information on circulating levels of radioactivity. The $t_{1/2}$ obtained from this data can be applied to calculate the biological $t_{1/2}$ lung and the $t_{1/2}$ effective. It is this latter $t_{1/2}$ value that is applied to the deposition counts from the camera to correct for decay and absorption but not mucociliary clearance.

It is important to recognize that, other than when using PET emitters very few radiolabeling studies involve directly labeling the drug. Most studies utilize gamma-emitting isotopes, such as 99m technetium ($^{99m}T_c$) that are associated with but not part of the drug particle in suspension or drug in solution (43). As such, useful information from these studies will be obtained only if the label accurately follows the drug during inhalation. Unless firmly bound, the label and drug rapidly dissociate after being deposited and the label no longer provides a marker for the drug. $^{99m}T_c$ has a short half life, on the order of 6 h (44), and—more importantly—when inhaled as pertechnatate (TcO_4^-), it is also cleared very rapidly from the lungs, with a half-life on the order of 10–15 min (44). PET permits direct labeling of drugs, but the very short half-life of the label may preclude lengthy imaging to determine drug redistribution. For imaging studies to be in any way an accurate representation of the behavior of the drug, the techniques used must be precise and validated. Many studies have been published in the past without clear evidence that the label did indeed follow the drug accurately or that correction for factors such as tissue attenuation, effective decay of the isotope, and background radiation were made.

In assessing a radiolabeled study, it is necessary to review:

The radiolabel used

The validity of the label as assessed by in vitro testing, using particle sizing techniques to ensure that the distribution of drug and label are the same, thus indicating that the label provides a useful surrogate for drug distribution

Measurement of dose-to-dose reproducibility in terms of drug and radioactivity

The labeling process must not affect the properties of the drug formulation; that is, the labeled drug must behave in the same way as the standard unlabeled formulation when tested both in vitro and in vivo

Tissue and device attenuation corrections

Definition of lung borders and lung regions

Correction for background radiation as applied to the images

The issue of rapid clearance from the lungs of certain radionuclides is considered, particularly for techniques such as SPECT, which require relatively longer acquisition times than planar imaging

Total accountability of dose or “mass balance” (rarely attempted)

Expression of the results of lung dose as a percentage of the emitted or nominal dose

Information regarding the sensitivity and resolution of the gamma camera

Time required to acquire the image

Various approaches to these issues are discussed below.

A. Planar Gamma Scintigraphy

This is the most widely used approach for assessing the deposition of aerosols from drug delivery systems. Its advantages over the other imaging modalities are that it is relatively cheap and analysis of the data is relatively straight forward. Time to acquire the images can be short (1–4 min), minimizing the problem associated with the very short biological half life within the lungs of the most commonly used label, $^{99m}TcO_4^-$. Techniques have been developed for labeling drug solutions (but not suspensions), pMDI and dry powder formulations so that this approach can be applied to many drug formulations dispensed from these delivery devices.

Doses used can be relatively low and striking 2D images can be produced; familiarity with such images engenders confidence that valuable information is being provided. This is undoubtedly true provided that the information is interpreted within the limits of the technique. Many such studies have now been published involving a range of subjects, including preterm ventilated and nonventilated infants (46), young children (47), adults, and the elderly (30,31) and have included a variety of disease states such as bronchopulmonary dysplasia, asthma, chronic obstructive pulmonary disease, and cystic fibrosis. However, the majority of such studies involve relatively young, healthy volunteers.

Such studies have frequently been used to compare one device with another with the object of claiming benefits of one over another. This needs to be borne in mind in considering extrapolating from such studies to routine clinical practice.

Though planar imaging does permit some quantification of aerosolized drug distribution within the lungs, it provides only a 2D representation of an extremely complex 3D structure, and it is inevitable that a considerable amount of the drug depositing in the "central zone" will be resident in the distal airways and alveoli (48,49).

B. Single Photon Emission Computed Tomography (SPECT)

SPECT imaging is more complex than planar imaging in that, rather than obtaining anterior and posterior images of the thorax, the gamma camera rotates through a full 360 degrees and subsequent manipulation of the data using computers permits 3D images to be constructed (37,50). This approach has potential advantages in that it may improve the accuracy of assessing the pattern of deposition within the lungs. However, it has the associated disadvantages of long acquisition times and relatively high doses. Newer, multihead dual and triple cameras are now available but are not widely used for these studies. The per-pixel resolution is similar to or greater than that of the gamma camera (8–10 mm).

At least one study has shown that SPECT scanning, with its 3D resolution, gave a statistically significant improvement in the accuracy of assessing central and peripheral deposition (51). This has not been universal, though in each study there was a tendency toward improved resolution (52–54). SPECT scanning currently requires higher doses and much greater imaging time, usually 15–20 min (50), compared with the 1–4 min that is usual for planar imaging. Even in those few units with multiheaded gamma cameras specially designed for this purpose, imaging times are still on the order of 5–10 min (50).

Over recent years the techniques has been refined using either computed tomography (CT) or magnetic resonance imaging (MRI) to improve anatomic definition of lung borders. When combined with complex mathematical models and computers, SPECT can provide much more sophisticated information regarding the pattern of radionuclide deposition in the airways (55,56). However, because the CT or MRI image is obtained on a separate machine, the images must be aligned with the SPECT ones, and this may introduce further errors in the analysis.

Expressing the deposited dose per airways generation has highlighted the fact that, with most current devices, the bulk of drug is deposited beyond generation 16—that is, beyond the conducting airways (48,49,55,56). However, because of the enormous surface area peripherally, the concentration of deposited drug is greater in the central regions of the lung, and this has been borne out in studies involving lung resection (24). Again, such information is of considerable interest, though for current drugs the significance of these observations is often unclear.

The cost, complexity, and radiation doses involved currently limits this more sophisticated approach to the analysis of SPECT data to a relatively small number of centers.

C. Positron Emission Tomography (PET)

Positron emmission tomography (PET) is a 3D functional imaging technique, providing accurate and highly specific information about the dose and distribution of an inhaled or injected PET tracer in the lung (57,58). A series of transaxial slices through the lungs are obtained, comparable to a CT scan. The transaxial information is used to reconstruct, postimaging, the lung activity for the other two planes, enabling coronal and sagittal images of the lungs to be viewed. PET resolution is approximately 4–6 mm per slice (twice that of SPECT), enabling upto 120 slices per plane to be obtained. Because of the nature of the emmissions and the use of coincidence counting, scatter is minimal and location of the pixels or voxels (volume unit) containing the radioactivity is precise.

Correction for the natural decay of the PET isotope used is incoporated into the software protocols; correction for tissue attenuation of the radioactivity is made directly using PET and following each procedure by acquiring a transmission scan with an external source of radioactivity. The advantages are that the

(A)

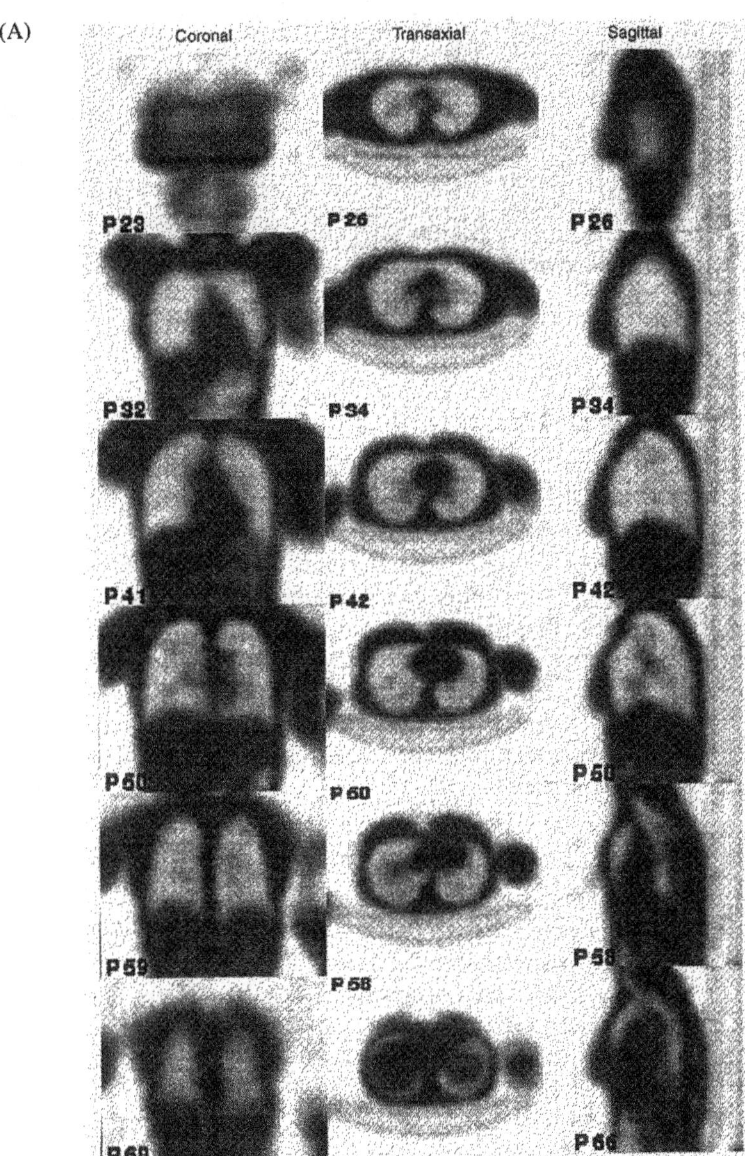

Figure 1 (A) Selection of PET transmission scans from the coronal, transaxial, and sagittal planes in a subject with cystic fibrosis. Each slice is 6 mm thick. As shown, lung geometry changes with lung depth. (B) The emission (aerosol) data are overlaid on its specific transmission slice and corrected for attenuation voxel by voxel, thus resulting in a more accurate calculation of delivered dose. Regional lung data are calculated for each slice based on the area of the specific transmission slice.

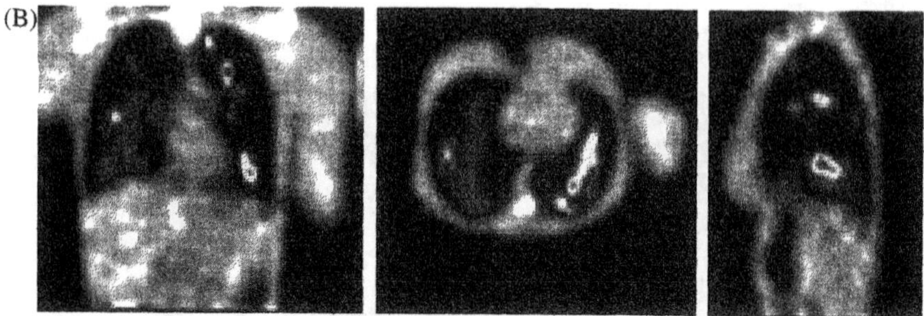

Figure 1 Continued

geometry is constant, as the patient remains in the same position under the scanner as for the original investigation, and that the corrections are applied to each voxel in each slice of each plane. Applying attenuation correction to the deposition data allows absolute amounts of radioactivity to measured per cubic millimeter of lung tissue, giving the actual topographic distribution of drug throughout the lung. The transmission image is also used to define the lung borders, providing landmarks from which to regions of interest. When the lungs are imaged over time, the kinetics of the drug can be described for the whole lung as well as for specific regions. As with SPECT, multiple regions of interest, concentric about the hilum, can be defined and the deposition data per region of interest, reconstructed in all three planes.

D. Labeling

PET emitters that are used in the lungs are the short-lived isotopes of carbon, oxygen, nitrogen, fluorine, and neon, with physical half-lives ranging from 2 to 110 min. Positron emitters are produced in a cyclotron, usually situated in close proximity to the PET scanner. The isotopes can be inhaled directly, for example, to compare the 3D distribution of therapeutic aerosols (69,60), or incorporated into other molecules, such as albuterol. Thus, a number of drug molecules used to treat lung diseases can be labeled directly with ^{18}F or ^{11}C and the isotope then incorporated to complete the synthesis of the drug. Once completed, the pharmaceutical formulation to be tested must be manufactured, incorporated into the inhaler being tested (pMDI, DPI, or nebulizer), and the emitted dose and particle size validated. Given the short half-lives of the PET isotopes, this is clearly not a simple process. Positron emitters can also be inhaled as solution aerosols or gases for assessing lung physiology (62,63) PET permits accurate 3D imaging and could potentially be used for investigations into a wide range of topics related to disease processes, biological function, and drug action within the respiratory tract (62). Hence PET might prove to be a very valuable and informative mode of imaging, but currently its applications are limited by the very short half-life of the positron-emitting nuclei and the limited number of centers with access to this form of technology.

E. Labeling Drugs or Drug Surrogates for Planar and SPECT Imaging

Nebulizers

The traditional method for labeling drug solutions delivered from both jet and ultrasonic nebulizers has been the so called "soup" method, in which a drug solution is mixed with a gamma-emitting radionuclide. This approach has been used for more than a quarter of a century (61) and it has been assumed, quite reasonably, that the droplets generated by the nebulizer contain drug and radiolabel in proportions determined by the solution from which they are generated. Since the particle size characteristics of the aerosol are largely determined by the design of the nebulizer and the driving gas flow used, it is also reasonable to assume that the particle size characteristics will be little altered by the addition of most radionuclides. Relatively few studies have attempted to determine whether these assumptions are valid for a particular combination of drug and radionuclide, but those that have found that the drug did follow the label (62,63) and the radioisotope had little effect on the particle size characteristics of the aerosol (62,64). As the radiolabel travels with the drug in droplets but is not bound to the drug, information on deposition can be obtained. If a nonabsorbable tracer is used e.g., ^{99m}Tc-albumin or ^{99m}Tc-sulfur colloid, imaging can occur over a longer period of time, enabling both deposition and mucocilary clearance to be measured (64). However, if drug and label dissociate rapidly after deposition, these studies will not provide any information regarding clearance of the drug following deposition. It is possible to directly label some drugs such as pentamidine (65), and hence the fate of drug once inhaled can be assessed (provided that the labeling involves isotope substitution), but it is doubtful if information relating to the pattern of deposition can be improved.

Technetium-labeled compounds such as human serum albumin (HSA) can be inhaled from nebulizers to measure deposition and clearance in disease and pre- and post–drug therapy (66). They can also be used to compare delivery systems, but no clinical outcomes can be assessed if the drug is not included.

The "soup method" is of course not suitable for drug suspensions, such as the steroid preparations for use with nebulizers, since the drug may not be uniformly distributed in either the suspension or the droplets generated by the nebulizer. However, radioactive particles whose characteristics are similar to the drug particle may be useful surrogates for suspension aerosols inhaled from nebulizers (67).

Studies utilizing jet nebulizers should take into account the great variation in nebulizer output and particle size that can occur between nebulizers of the same make, even those from the same batch (68–70). Some manufacturers have started to address this problem by using improved molding techniques. Another potential problem, ignored in many studies, has been the use of inappropriate methods for obtaining particle size measurements. It is frequently not realized that marked drying of wet aerosols occurs when cascade impactors are used, resulting in much finer droplet sizes than would be obtained with laser particle sizing systems (13), which can measure the size characteristics of the aerosol droplets as they leave the nebulizer. Thus laser particle sizing is the method of choice for measuring the output from nebulizers containing drugs in solution, as the information obtained using this approach may permit more accurate prediction of the site of deposition (13).

Laser particle sizing cannot be used for suspensions as it does not distinguish between drug and carrier. The potential for aerosols to change in size due to hygroscopic growth or drying also means that the characteristics of an aerosol can be significantly altered if a length of tubing is introduced between the nebulizer and patient (71).

It is well known that intersubject variation can be very large when studying deposition of aerosol from a nebulizer. It should be remembered that intrasubject variability is also significant when studies utilizing nebulizers are repeated, and this must be taken into account in deciding upon subject numbers (72). Much of this variability probably stems from differences in inhalation patterns (73), hence variability may be reduced to some extent by using predetermined patterns of inhalation, but this does not mimic the clinical situation.

Pressurized Metered-Dose Inhalers and Dry-Powder Inhalers

During the past decade there has been a relative explosion of deposition studies using "direct" labeling techniques, though other approaches have been used. One involved direct labeling of the ipratropium bromide molecule using ^{77}Br for the bromide moiety (74), while others have utilized labeled monodisperse Teflon particles to replace drug particles (75,76) or spray-dried uniform particles of cromoglycate (77). However, the chemical and physical properties of a system utilizing Teflon rather than drug are almost certainly different from those of a system containing active drug. In 1988, Kohler et al. described a method in which ^{99m}Tc was added to a pMDI canister together with propellants, surfactant, and drugs (78). Subsequent workers (79–83) have modified and improved the technique such that no alterations to the contents of the canister are required other than the addition of the radiolabel. These methods are not applicable to all pMDI products; hence careful in vitro validation is essential before undertaking deposition studies.

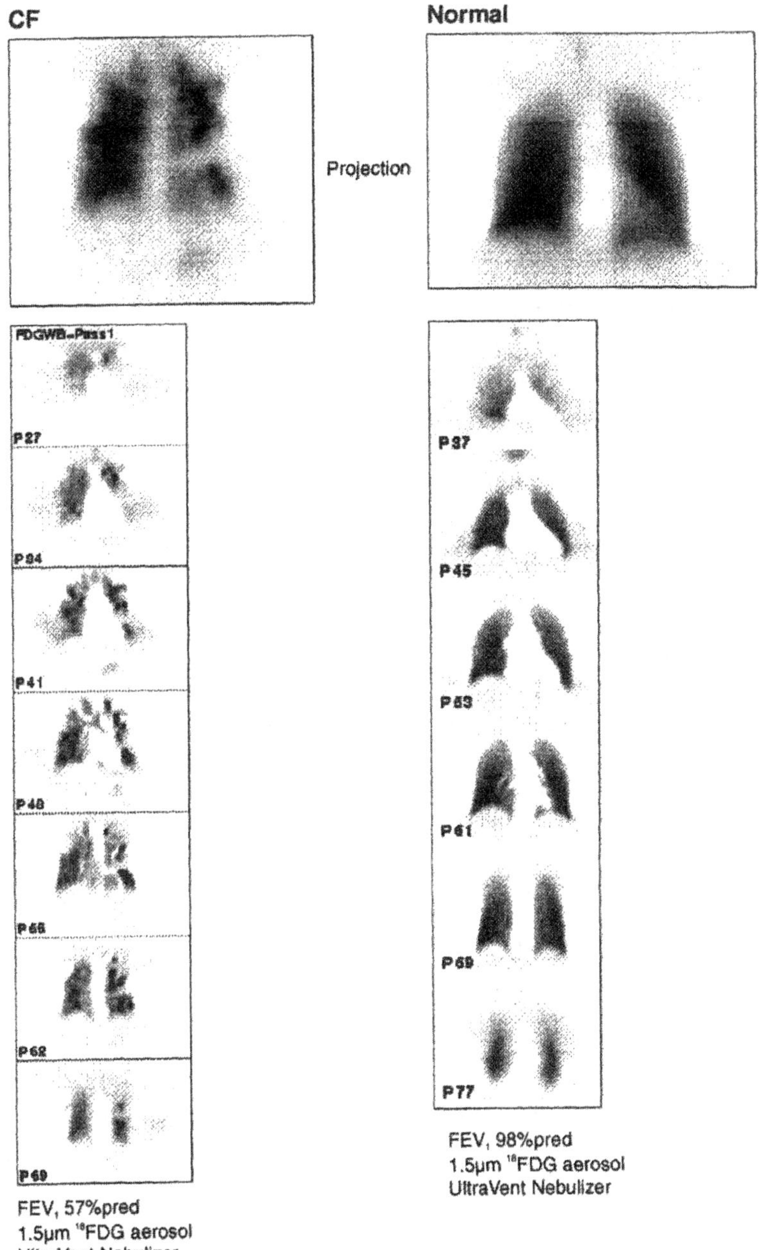

Figure 2 Coronal slices and projection view obtained after inhaling a 1.5 μm aerosol of ^{18}FDG from the Ultravent jet nebulizer (Mallinckrodt, St. Louis, MO). Slices are shown from the anterior, midsection, and posterior lung for a normal subject (right) and a subject with cystic fibrosis (left). Greater detail of lung distribution of the aerosol is provided by the PET scan. The cumulative or projection scan (all the coronal slices summed) would be comparable visually to 2D images obtained with a gamma camera.

The term *direct labeling* is misleading in that the radiolabel is not part of the drug structure but is associated either with the micronized drug particles or the surfactant coating, depending upon the drug/surfactant combination used (81). Many studies utilizing this approach have been performed during the last decade. Similar techniques have been used for labeling powders (47,83,84), though for some powders particular adaptations are required.

Validation of Labeling

As noted above, essential to these techniques is in vitro verification of the accuracy of the labeling techniques (85), and details of this have frequently been omitted in publications. Accuracy of labeling should be confirmed by means of a cascade impactor or similar particle sizing device using assays for both drug and radioactivity. It should be shown that:

The radiolabel follows the drug—that is, they are deposited in equal proportions on each impactor stage.
The radiolabeling procedure does not alter the dose and particle size distribution of the aerosol in comparison to the unlabeled drug.
The labeling procedure does not alter the dose delivered.

Published data show that the particle size distribution may be affected to some extent by the process and that there is frequently a difference between the distribution of the radiolabel and drug. These differences are often small but may have a significant effect on the results obtained in vivo.

As with jet nebulizers, inhalation patterns can be prescribed or spontaneous. For example, subjects using powder inhalers may inhale at maximal inspiratory flows, as advocated in the clinical setting, or taught to aim for a predetermined inspiratory flow(86). Deposition results will vary depending upon the inspiratory flow used (87,88).

F. Assessment of Deposition

In any experiment, a number of parameters should be assessed. These include:

The dose of radioactivity deposited within the respiratory tract of the subject.
The distribution of radioactivity within the body.
The distribution of radioactivity within the lungs.

In addition it is desirable where possible to assess the clinical response to an administered radiolabeled drug, but this will be valid only if the drug is unaltered by the labeling process.

Total Delivered Dose of a Radiolabeled Drug

In the measurement of deposition of aerosolised drugs using radioactivity, it is the radioactivity and not the drug that is being measured directly. Accurate quantification requires addressing all the issues noted above, including corrections for attenuation in various parts of the body, background radiation, and camera sensitivity.

Dose Accountability (Mass Balance)

It should be noted that the delivered dose can vary from dose to dose due to the way devices are handled (47,88,90) and to a lesser extent due to innate variability of the device. Therefore, one cannot be entirely confident that the dose delivered during previous in vitro testing accurately reflects the dose to a subject during a deposition study. A calibration routine to measure emitted doses, in terms of radioactivity and drug, from a number of individual actuations from the pMDI of DPI should be standard practice. Moreover, attempting to account for all of the dose, including that retained within the devices and that exhaled, is *essential* to minimize potential errors resulting from unrecognized variability in delivered dose.

If all the correction factors were valid, then the total dose delivered during a study—that is, the dose retained in the actuator, the dose in the upper airway, that swallowed, the dose in the lungs, and the dose exhaled—should, when summated, come to very close to the "total dose" or nominal dose of radioactivity. Unfortunately, few studies use this approach to validate their results, with most authors simply preferring to express the lung dose as a percentage of the body dose and then expressing this, in turn, as a percentage of the dose of drug and not radioactivity they believe had been delivered, so that there is no internal check that the device has performed as expected during dosing.

What is detected by the imaging system is radioactivity; therefore, the topical radioactivity data should be related only to the dispensed and measured emitted dose of radioactivity.

It is important to recognize that the exhaled dose when inhaling from nebulizers and indeed some pMDIs without breath-holding may be as high as 20%; therefore an exhalation filter is essential to obtain an accurate mass balance.

Some investigators have tried to quantify the total dose deposited by using a controlled pattern of breathing and drug collection on filters (25) or by modifying the aerosol bolus/photometric method to quantify the dose deposited (91).

For studies using dry powders and pMDIs, the predicted emitted dose of activity can be obtained by collecting a dose onto a filter, applying a suction flow comparable to what would be used during the study. It must be remembered that as much as 20% of the nominal dose can be retained within the actuator when using pMDIs (80); similarly, for DPIs, significant amounts of drug remain within the device (45,47). It is also important to remember that the retained dose will vary depending upon the inspiratory flow being applied (47).

Distribution of Deposited Radioactivity Within the Body

Planar Imaging

A large number of methods for analyzing data and presenting the results have been used in lung deposition studies. As a result it is frequently difficult to compare the results obtained from different laboratories in any meaningful way.

Depth of Source. The measurement of the absolute quantity of radioactivity within the respiratory tract is complicated by attenuation and scatter of gamma rays within the body. In addition, for planar imaging, correction must be made for the effect of distance of activity from the gamma camera, as deposition occurs in 3D. If a simple anterior image were obtained, activity deposited posteriorly would generate fewer counts per second than an equal quantity deposited anteriorly. To correct for this, the geometric mean of counts obtained from anterior and posterior images of the chest is calculated. This measurement is largely independent of lung depth (92).

Attenuation. Several methods have been devised in an attempt to correct for attenuation when using 2D planar imaging and 3D SPECT. These include the administration of a known dose of radiadation intravenously in the form of microaggregates, which are assumed to be entirely trapped within the pulmonary circulation (91,93–95); the use of "phantoms," in which a radiation source is placed within a block of material which is designed to simulate the chest wall (96,97); calculations based upon reference values for different chest thicknesses (98,99); body-mass index (99); and the use of "flood sources" (100,101) to obtain transmission images for each subject. Attenuation of activity in the stomach and oropharynx is significantly greater than that for the chest, and different correction factors for these areas must be included. Indeed, attenuation from central and peripheral regions of the lung differs significantly, though local corrections are rarely applied.

The microaggregate method is often regarded as the gold standard for determining attenuation within the chest but there are inevitably some differences between the distribution of injected microaggregates of albumin (MAA) and radiolabeled therapeutic aerosols (94). More importantly, this method may be unsuitable for most studies because of the increased radiation dose required. However, a decreased dose of Tc-MAA can be used along with longer imaging time to reduce this dose. Little work has been done to assess the accuracy of the other methods until recently. Forge and colleagues (101) showed that phantom methods significantly underestimated the dose within the lung in adults. Perhaps more importantly, the same correction factor is often used for all subjects, which can introduce significant nonsystematic inaccuracies (92). Calculation of an attenuation factor using a "flood source" tended to slightly overestimate the dose within the lungs but was considerably more accurate. This method involves recording an image of a source of gamma rays, usually ^{99m}Tc, using a gamma camera. The subject is then placed between the gamma camera and the flood source and a second image is recorded. The attenuation factor for each subject is calculated for each subject from the difference in counts and is specific for the individual gamma camera. Further advantages of this method are that the lung outlines can be defined and attenuation factors for both head and stomach can be calculated, though this is rarely done. The additional radiation exposure using this method is low. The study found that two "buildup factor" methods, which have not been used in deposition studies, were the most accurate, but these are more complicated than the geometric mean/flood source method which was felt to be sufficiently accurate (101).

Fok et al. (85) compared amounts of radioactivity detected in intact right and left rabbit lungs by the gamma camera to the absolute amount of radioactivity in the same excised lungs measured by a gamma counter. The gamma-camera counts were converted to microcuries using a tissue attenuation factor obtained from perfusion scanning. The results from both methods were the same.

More recently Pitcairn and Newman (98) attempted to assess the validity of a range of correction factors in 10 healthy young adults and found that failure to use a method for correcting for attenuation significantly underestimated lung dose. However, they found relatively little difference in the results obtained with transmission scans, using a method based on chest wall thickness and a perfusion technique with *mean* lung doses being estimated as being in the range 24.8–29.7% with one inhaler and 10.2–12% for a second. In all cases the same data was used and differences resulted from the attenuation correction factor used. For the two inhalers the mean calculated lung dose without correction factor being applied were 19.6 and 6.5%. A more recent study still using simulation to calculate lung dose noted again that for a limited number of healthy males, the chest-wall-thickness method gave good approximation to the actual value(99). The authors noted that body mass index provided better precision but also commented that as they had used data from healthy adults, the general applicability of these techniques will still require testing in a wider population.

The attenuation of gamma rays from the stomach is approximately twice that from the lungs while attenuation of signal from the oropharynx and mouth can be quite variable. It should be remembered that inhalation from a pMDI or DPI results in high oral deposition with much less in the oropharynx. Attenuation correction factors (ACFs) will be different for these two regions of the upper airway as indeed it will be for different areas of the chest. It is unclear whether more precise calculation of ACFs within regions of the chest will be of significant benefit given the approximations required during labeling and in imaging. However, failure to apply local ACFs can influence calculation of the "penetration index," and it has been suggested that in this respect the transmission scan or correction based on a perfusion scan (99) or the use of corrections based on the distribution of inhaled xenon (102) may prove superior.

Deposition within the upper airways is frequently assumed to be the difference between the calculated lung dose and the delivered dose and is frequently not directly quantified. As noted above, this can introduce significant inaccuracies, particularly if the lung dose is expressed as a percentage of the body dose.

Scatter. It appears that for isotopes such as ^{99m}Tc, ignoring the effects of scatter does not lead to excessive errors(27).

Distribution Within the Lungs. For planar studies, it has been conventional to divide the images into central and peripheral regions of the lung, with the implication that central regions contain predominantly large airways and the peripheral regions predominantly alveoli. However, because of the 2D nature of the image, there is inevitably much overlap of conducting airways and alveoli, particularly in the central region (48). Consequently the "penetration index"—that is, the ratio of peripheral to central deposition, obtained from planar images—is relatively intensive to changes in patterns of deposition (99,102). Moreover, there has been no standard method of defining central and peripheral regions, and many arbitrary methods for dividing the lung into central and peripheral regions have been used. This makes it extremely difficult to compare results from different investigators.

Calculation of penetration index can be greatly influenced by minor misalignment of regions of interest. The use of a transmission scan, or, better still, a ventilation scan to define the lung margins can significantly reduce errors due to misalignment and the use of arbitrary regions of interest based on the deposition image (99,102). The use of a ventilation scan permits the central to peripheral (C/P) ratio to be corrected for ventilation using counts derived from the ventilation scan (102,103).

In an attempt to define the dose deposited in nonciliated peripheral regions, formulations such as ^{99m}Tc HSA, which are absorbed very slowly from the alveoli, have been used. Images obtained immediately after delivery are compared with those 24 h later allowing for decay of activity. The assumption has been that residual activity lies within the alveoli, the activity within the conducting airways having been removed by mucociliary clearance (27,66,104). This assumption is an oversimplification and clearance of such products is probably more complex than previously assumed (27,99). This technique also greatly increases the residence time of the radionuclide within the lung, resulting in an increase radiation dose to the target organ and the body.

Perhaps more importantly, it is frequently unclear what the significance of a "good" penetration index is. For a drug like pentamidine, good peripheral deposition is obviously desirable, as its site of action is the alveoli. For drugs such as steroids and antibiotics in cystic fibrosis, their site of action is likely to be the conducting airways (106); hence alveolar deposition is probably undesirable. However the surface area of distal airways is much greater than that of earlier generations and in order to deliver adequate doses to smaller conducting airways, significant deposition beyond the conducting airways is likely since current devices, which produce polydisperse aerosols, cannot accurately target specific regions. Indeed as noted above, current devices deliver the majority of the drug to distal airways. For highly soluble drugs such as bronchodilators, redistribution of drug from central to more peripheral regions through the bronchial circulation may obviate the need for good peripheral deposition, but this is unproven. The influence of disease on deposition is also a major factor. Any significant airflow obstruction has a major impact on the pattern of deposition of conventional polydispersed aerosols. Airways disease results in much greater central deposition, and indeed such trends can be observed before significant spirometric changes are detectable in groups such as smokers (30,31).

SPECT and PET

As mentioned previously, the use of SPECT scanning has, in some studies, improved resolution when compared with conventional planar scanning but the increased dose and complexity involved makes it debatable whether these techniques can be justified routinely in children. This may change with improved equipment. A further technical problem with SPECT is that the relatively long acquisition time causes problems with radionuclides such as ^{99m}Tc–sodium pertechnetate that are rapidly cleared from the lungs and subsequently appear in the pulmonary circulation.

The major advances reported by Fleming and Martonen in SPECT image analysis greatly increase the power of this approach but the complexity of the techniques have prevented widespread use of this technique to date.

G. Summary of Issues for Imaging Studies

Radiolabeling

The validity of the labeling should be assessed in vitro using a multistage device such as the Andersen cascade impactor (ACI), which is able to detect clinically significant changes. It has been suggested that for a DPI, method 1 of the European Pharmacopoeia should be used employing a five-stage high-precision liquid impinger operated at a flow corresponding to a pressure drop of 4 kPa through the device and pulling 4 L of air through the device (105). However, the resolution is not as good as with the ACI, which can also be operated at 60 L/min with corrections to the stage cutoff diameters.

In particular, the labeling procedure should not alter the total amount of drug delivered or the particle size distribution of the drug when aerosolized. Furthermore, the distribution of drug and label should be the same when assessed in vitro. Validation data should include total dose delivered from both standard delivery systems and labeled devices together with a detailed description of the particle size distribution of the standard formulation, the labeled drug, and the distribution of label most conveniently presented as a histogram. Data relating to dose retained within the delivery system should also be included.

The suggestion that the labeling is satisfactory provided that the ratio of fine-particle fraction of radiolabeled drug to unlabeled drug is +/– 20% emphasizes that this is not a precise technique, particularly as labeling is only one source of potential error (105).

Such validation should be undertaken using the amount of activity to be used in studies as there are instances where the procedure appears to be effective during validation using low doses, but the labeling has been shown not to be satisfactory using the full dose.

Validation on Study Day

The validation procedure should be undertaken for each study device. The data for the drug will not be available during the study day as the drug will still be "hot" and therefore not available to be assayed, but this will ensure that any anomalies are identified. An assessment of the unit-emitted dose and the distribution of label will provide some reassurance that the labeling procedure is likely to have been adequate prior to administering the radiopharmaceutical to subjects.

Dose of Radioactivity to Be Used

Administered dose will depend upon the technique in question. The lowest dose compatible with adequate data should be used to minimize radiation exposaure.

Correction for Attenuation and Background Activity

Transmission scans provide a means of obtaining individualized correction factors for attenuation though there is evidence that chest wall thickness will provide a guide to attenuation correction, at least in relatively fit young adults. Attenuation varies significantly between sites in the body with that for activity deposited in the lungs being significantly less than for the stomach, mouth and oropharynx. Even within the lung attenuation varies significantly. A transmission scan has the additional advantage that it will also permit the edges of the lungs to be identified. Alternatively, an inhaled gas such as krypton or xenon can be used to outline the edges of the lungs and can be used to correct for both attenuation and volume.

Studies are still being published without any attempt at correcting for attenuation (107). In such cases the results should not be expressed as an absolute figure though intra-subject comparisons of devices can be undertaken using the same subjects.

Presenting Data

Attempts should be made to account for all the activity administered including that retained within the device. That is, drug in the lungs, upper airways, stomach, exhalation filter, and device must be quantified. Failure to do so can lead to spurious conclusions. If correction factors are accurate, then the sum of all the calculated lung dose, upper airways, and swallowed dose together with the exhaled dose should match the expected delivered dose. Simply expressing data as a percentage of the body dose as occurs in most publications permits inaccuracies in the method to be obscured.

A mass balance is essential if the accuracy of the results are to be valid and images obtained from such studies should be viewed with suspicion as the "message" contained in and image can be altered be manipulated very simply. It is vital to present the calculated dose to each compartment.

Correction for Decay and Absorption

The activity of the radionuclide will decline with time and it will also be cleared from the lung through absorption and mucocilary clearance. The former is relevant in that there may be a delay of some hours between formulating the radiopharmaceutical and administering it to a subject. Since the physical rate of decay of the isotope is known this effect can be quantified. As noted above, some radionuclides are absorped very rapidly from the lungs and this is of particular relevance when using SPECT, which may require acquisition times of 5–20 min. To date there is no entirely satisfactory method for correcting for this problem particularly as the radionuclide present in the bronchial and pulmonary circulations will contribute to the image as time passes.

Intrapulmonary Distribution

No standardized approach has been devised, and again only conclusions drawn from studies comparing results within the same subject can be used with any confidence.

IV. Pharmacokinetic Studies

There have been fewer pharmacokinetic studies than imaging studies involving inhaled therapy largely due to difficulties involved in measuring the small quantities of drug delivered to the patient and in obtaining complete sample collection. This problem has largely been overcome by the improved analytical techniques currently available and the use of analysis of sparse data. The pharmacokinetics of variety of inhaled drugs have been studied in many patient groups, including very young children and health volunteers (36,90,108–121).

Imaging has gained popularity because of the visual representation of drug deposition. However it can be argued that more clinically relevant data maybe obtained from pharmacokinetic studies in that they permit investigators to quantify the total systemic exposure to a drug. They also quantify the total amount of drug absorbed from the lungs, and it is argued that this may provide a valuable index of the quantity of drug likely to reach it site of action, since most current drugs are almost entirely absorbed into the systemic circulation once they reach the epithelium. It has been argued that some drug deposited centrally in the airways is removed by mucociliary clearance and that this fraction accounts for some of the differences in results obtained using imaging and pharmacokinetic approaches. This drug will be quantified as "pulmonary" using imaging techniques but will not contribute to the therapeutic effect (28). The magnitude of such an effect is the subject of much debate. If imaging times are kept short, mucociliary clearance is less of a problem. However, pK samples are collected over much longer time intervals.

Pharmacokinetic techniques have provided information that cannot be obtained through conventional imaging. This includes the observation that pulmonary clearance of terbutaline is increased in smokers (122) and by exercise (123). Further advantages derived from using pharmacokinetic techniques include the ability to avoid the use of radiation and for some techniques the ability to repeat the studies several times in the same subject. Moreover, standard formulations can be used avoiding the risk of altering the formulation during labeling (124).

A. Methods

There are currently no techniques that will directly quantify local concentrations within the target organ, the lungs, but it is possible to determine pulmonary dose indirectly by measuring drug concentrations in the circulation or more indirectly still, the urine. Techniques available include:

The use of drugs not absorbed from the GI tract
Charcoal-block methods
Correction for drugs of known bioavailability
Indirect methods, such as 30-min urinary excretion

The biggest single challenge is to distinguish drug reaching the systemic circulation via the lungs from drug reaching the systemic circulation via the GI tract. Certain drugs such as sodium cromoglycate (36,108,109) and fluticasone proprionate (116–118) are either not absorbed from the GI tract or essentially fully metabolized by the liver after absorption. If no drug reaches the systemic circulation from the GI tract, it can be assumed that the quantity of drug reaching the systemic circulation represents the lung dose when inhaling through the mouth provided that there is no drug metabolism within the lungs. For patients inhaling from a face mask via the nose this may not be the case, as significant absorption via the nasal mucosa can occur (125).

For other drugs, GI absorption can be blocked using activated charcoal (110–115), and this approach can used for a number of drugs. To use this approach, drug must be fully absorbed from the lungs and not metabolized during transit. A reference intravenous dose is also required. In the method described by Borgstrom et al. subjects urine was collected for 48 h after inhalation and a reference formulation of deuterium-labeled analogue of terbutaline was administered intravenously.. In these studies, higher pulmonary doses were found using the gamma scintigraphy method. The reason for this is unclear and may reflect inaccuracies in one or both methods or perhaps the lower values achieved in the pharmacokinetic studies reflect mucociliary clearance of drug from central airways. In contrast studies using inhaled steroids have generally noted higher pulmonary values using pharmacokinetic techniques than imaging techniques. The reasons are unclear.

In order to avoid the need for activated charcoal, some investigators calculate the lung dose by correcting for the GI contribution, using oral bioavailability data (90). This can be applied only to drugs administered to subjects in whom the oral bioavailability has been clearly established in the subject group.

B. Indirect Technique

The charcoal-block method attempts to collect all drug absorbed through the lungs. The 30-min urinary salbutamol method has been used in a number of studies to compare devices and inhalation techniques (126–128). The method is based on the observation that, in the majority of subjects, little if any of the swallowed drug is excreted in the urine in the first 30 min after administering the drug. It should be noted, however, that a proportion approximately (approximately 10%) of subjects do excrete significant amounts of orally administered drug in the first 30 min. In those in whom this is not the case, the amount of drug excreted in 30 min reflects the pulmonary dose.

A similar approach has been to measure plasma salbutamol levels at 30 min (129–132). These studies have often included pharmacokinetic components, such as the effect of the beta agonist on heart rate tremor and serum potassium. A major problem with this approach is that multiple doses are required, with as many as 12 doses being used in the studies involving plasma levels to detect both the drug and the pharmacodynamic responses, while the urinary salbutamol method generally involves four inhalations.

The results from these type of studies do not provide an absolute lung dose but do allow comparison between devices when used by individuals. The technique appears relatively robust with intrasubject variability being reported as around 10%, results similar to data from other types of studies. Whether these techniques can be applied to other drugs is unclear.

V. Choice of Subjects

The choice of subjects clearly has a major influence on the validity of a study. Most studies attempting to assess the delivery of therapeutic aerosols using imaging or pharmacokinetic studies involve relatively few subjects. This is largely influenced by the cost and logistical difficulties involved, though obviously it is desirable to use the lowest number of subject compatible with a clear answer to a given question.

In some studies specific patient groups have been included. Clearly there is no way of substituting for a ventilated infant or for cystic fibrosis patients with severe pulmonary damage. Such studies provide valuable information regarding the performance of a given device in clinical practice. Many more studies have utilized well-trained healthy volunteers to assess the performance of a device. These studies are performed under carefully controlled conditions, which, on occasion, go as far as controlling the inhalation flow using pneumotachographs and flow profiles. The results obtained using these well-trained, supervised volunteers inhaling under optimal conditions are of interest, but the results do not necessarily reflect use in the real world. The pattern of deposition will be quite different to that in an individual with significant airflow obstruction, while even apparently minor deviations from standard operating procedures can have a major impact on the results. For instance, a recent study found a 48% reduction in lung dose in a carefully controlled study during which the investigator forgot to shake the pMDI before use (90).

Because of concerns regarding the potential for late effects in using radionuclides, females of childbearing age should be screened to ensure that they are not pregnant, and in general such techniques should only be used in children if the information is likely to add significantly to our knowledge and contribute to improved therapy in the future.

Previous studies have indicated that intersubject variability is high with current devices even under controlled conditions. This can be attributed to a variety of causes, including anatomic differences, but the largest single cause is likely to be variation in inhalation technique. There has been far less work looking at intrasubject variability. The high intra- and intersubject variability causes problems when trying to compare results from different studies particularly where different techniques have been employed. Ideally crossover designs should be used to compare devices.

VI. Relationship Between Drug Delivery and Effect

To date there has been relatively little work correlating the pattern of deposition with the therapeutic outcome or pharmacodynamic effects (118,124, 133–135). This perhaps is not too surprising, as most β-agonists are administered at or close to supramaximal doses and therefore generally administered close to the plateau of the dose response curve, while the therapeutic effects of inhaled steroids are observed over weeks and indeed for bronchial hypersresponsiveness further benefits are still being observed after a couple of years of therapy.

VII. Summary

Aerosol therapy has, to date, been used almost exclusively to treat pulmonary disease, but the era of using the respiratory tract to deliver potent systemic drugs and novel agents for pulmonary disease is dawning.

Most drug delivery systems currently used to treat pulmonary disease were developed and introduced into clinical practice long before assessments of pulmonary drug delivery were undertaken. The pharmaceutical companies have seen little reason to improve on the current devices, utilizing technology that is many decades old, because the current systems do produce useful therapeutic responses and are relatively safe ("therapeutic index") if used effectively.

Measuring deposition under controlled conditions will provide an upper limit of deposition from that particular delivery device in the population studied.

Studies have indicated that, even in tightly controlled settings, current systems are highly operator-dependent, and that it is not possible to predict pulmonary doses in clinical practice. Pharmaceutical companies—and, perhaps more importantly, regulatory authorities—have not addressed this issue of operator dependence and intrasubject variability. The advent of novel delivery systems that do address these issues will force the pharmaceutical companies and regulators to consider these issues in some detail in the future.

Assessment of airways deposition alone does not provide us with an index of the therapeutic ratio for a given drug, as the therapeutic index will change dramatically if the device is used inappropriately. For instance, actuating a pMDI but not inhaling will result in extremely high oral deposition with no therapeutic effect.

The approach chosen to determine the in vivo lung dose achieved with a given device in a given patient group will be influenced by the resources available and the information required. A variety of approaches are possible, all of which have advantages and disadvantages.

Imaging can be chosen if information regarding distribution of drug within the airways is required. The amount of information available increases with the complexity of the method chosen. However, such information comes at a cost in terms of expense, complexity, and radiation exposure. Pharmacokinetic techniques provide an index of total lung dose and systemic exposure, and it could be argued that for many studies this approach would be appropriate. For more complex studies designed to further our understanding of the fate of drugs, sophisticated techniques such as PET may be required.

References

1. Pedersen S. Inhalers and nebulisers: which to choose and why? Respir Med 1996; 90:69–77.
2. Everard ML. Assessment of aerosol delivery systems. Pediatr Pulmonol 1997; 16:186–187.
3. Dolovich M. Aerosol delivery to children: what to use, how to choose. Pediatr Pulmonol 1999; 18 (suppl):79–82.
4. Sakula A. A history of asthma. J R Coll Phys Lond 1988; 22:36–44.
5. Webb J, Rees J, Clark TJ. A comparison of the effects of different methods of administration of beta 2 sympathomimetics in patients with asthma. Br J Dis Chest 1982; 76:351–357.
6. Byron PR, Patton JS. Drug delivery via the respiratory tract. J Aerosol Med 1994; 7:49–75.
7. Wolff RK. Safety of inhaled proteins for thrapeutic use. J Aerosol Med 1998; 11:197–219.
8. Laube BL. Time to peak insulin level, relative bioavailability, and effect of site of deposition of nebulized insulin in patients with non-insulin dependent diabetes mellitus. J Aerosol Med 1998; 11:153–173.
9. Farr SJ, Gonda I, Licko V. Physicochemical and physiological factors influencing the effectiveness of inhaled insulin. In: Respiratory Drug Delivery VI. Buffalo Grove, IL: Interpharm Press, 1988:25–33.
10. Virgolini I, Kurtaran A, Leimer M, Smith-Jones P, Agis II, Angelberger P, Kletter K, Valent P, Linkesch W, Eichler H-G. Inhalation scintigraphy with iodine 123-labeled interferon gamma-1 b: Pulmonary deposition and dose escalation study in healthy volunteers. J Nucl Med 1997; 38:1475–1481.
11. Dolovich M. Measurement of particle size characteristics of metered dose inhaler (MDI) aerosols. J Aerosol Med 1991; 4:251–253.
12. Dolovich M. In vitro measurement of medications from MDIs and spacers devices. J Aerosol Med 1996; 9(supp 1):S49–S58.
13. Clark AR. The use of laser diffraction for evaluation of the aerosol clouds generated by medical nebulizers. Int J Pharm 1994.
14. Thiel C. Can in vitro particle size measurements be used to predict pulmonary deposition of aerosol from inhalers? J Aerosol Med 1998; 11(suppl 1):S43–S52.
15. Clark AD, Gonda I, Newhouse MT. Towards meaningful laboratory tests for evaluation of pharmaceutical aerosols. J Aerosol Sci 1998; 11(suppl 1): S1–S7.
16. Newman SP. J Aerosol Med 1998; 11: S97–S104.

17. Egan M, Clark AR. Modelling the deposition of inhaled powdered drug aerosols. J Aerosl Sci 1994; 25: 175–86
18. Burnell P, Malton A, Reavill K, Ball M. Design, validation and initial testing of the electronic lung. J Aerosol Sci 1998; 29:1011–1025.
19. Stahlhofen W, Gebhart J, Heyder J. Experimental determination of regional deposition of aerosol particles in the human respiratory tract. Am Ind Hyg Assoc J 1980; 41: 38–98.
20. Schulz A, Tuch T, Brand P. Schulz H, Mutius E, Erdl R, Reinhardt D, Heyder J. Aerosol bolus dispersion during breathing in healthy children. J Aerosol Med 1993; 6 (suppl): 65–69.
21. Blanchard JD. Aerosol bolus dispersion and aerosol-derived airway morphometry: Assessment of lung pathology and response to therapy. Part 1. J Aerosol Med 1996; 9:183–206.
22. Bennett WD, Zeman KL, Kim C. Variability of fine particle deposition in healthy adults: effects of age and gender. Am J Crit Care Med 1996; 153:1641–1647.
23. Zanen P, Go LT, Lammers J-W. Optimal particle size for 132 agonist and anticholinergic aerosols in patients with severe airflow obstruction. Thorax 1996; 51:977–980.
24. Esmailpour N, Hogger P, Rabe K, Heitmann U, Nakashima M, Rohdewald P. Distribution of inhaled fluticasone propionate between human lung tissue and serum in vivo. Eur Respir J 1997; 10:1496–1499.
25. Ilowile JS, Gorvoy JD, Smaldone GC. Quantitative deposition of aerosolised gentamicin in cystic fibrosis. Am Rev Respir Dis 1987; 136:1445–1449.
26. Newman S. Scintigraphic assessment of therapeutic aerosols. Crit Rev Ther Drug Carrier Syst 1993; 10:65–109.
27. Gonda I. Scintigraphic techniques for measuring in vivo deposition. J Aerosol Med 1996; 9:S59–S67.
28. Chrystyn II. Is total dose more important than particle distribution? Respir Med 1997; 91 (suppl A):17–19.
29. Thompson PJ, Davies RJ, Young WF, Grossman AB, Donnell D. Safety of hydrofluoroalkane-134a beclomethasone diproprionate extrafine aerosol. Respir Med 1998; 91(suppl A):33–39.
30. Dolovich MB, Sanchis J, Rossman C, Newhouse MT. Aerosol penetration: a sensitive index of peripheral airways obstruction. J Appl Physiol 1976; 40:468–471.
31. Itoh H, Ishii Y, Maeda H, Toso G, Torizuka K, Smalldone G. Clinical observations of aerosol deposition in patients with airways obstruction. Chest 1981; 80(suppl):837–840.
32. Baskin M, Abd A, Ilowite J. Regional deposition of aerosolised pentamidine: effects of body position and breathing pattern. Ann Intern Med 1990; 113:677–683.
33. Smaldone GC. Deposition patterns of nebulised drugs: is the pattern important? J Aerosol Med 1994; 7:S25–S32.
34. Murakam, G., Igarashi T, Adachi Y. Measurement of bronchial hyperactivity in infants and preschool children using a new method. Ann Allergy 1990; 64:383–387.
35. Tal A, Golan H, Aviram M. Deposition pattern of radiolabeled salbutamol inhaled from a metered-dose inhaler by means of a spacer with mask in young children with airway obstruction. J Pediatr 1996; 128:479–484.

36. Iles R, Lister P, Edmunds AT. Crying significantly reduces absorption of aerosolised drug in infants. Arch Dis Child 1999; 81:163–165.
37. Conway J, Fleming J, Holgate S. Three-dimensional imaging of inhaled aerosols. Eur Respir Rev 1997; 7:44,180–183.
38. Dolovich M, Nahmias C, Coates G. Unleashing the PET: Applying 3D functional imaging to the lung. In: Byron P, Daly R, Farr SJ, eds. Proceedings of Respiratory Drug Delivery VII. Buffalo Grove, IL: Interpharm Press, 2000.
39. Bailey MR, Dorrian M-D, Birchall A. Implications of airway retention for radiation doses from inhaled radionulides. J Aerosol Med 1995; 8:373–390.
40. Everard ML. The use of radiolabelled aerosols for research purposes in paediatric patients: ethical and practical aspects. Thorax 1994; 49:1259–1266.
41. Makrigiorgos GM, Adelstein SJ, Kassis AI. Limitations of conventional internal dosimetry at the cellular level. J Nucl Med 1989; 30:1856–1864.
42. Use of ionizing radiation and radionuclides on human beings for medical research, training and non-medical pruposes. World Health Organization WHO Technical Series Report 611, Geneva 1977.
43. Farr SJ. The physico-chemical basis of radiolabelling metered dose inhalers with 99m TC. J Aerosol Med 1996; 9(suppl 1):S27–S36.
44. Atkins HL, Weber DA, Susskind H, Thomas SR. MIRD dose estimate report No. 16: Radiation absorbed dose from technetium -99m diethylenetriaminepentaacetic acid aerosol. J Nucl Med 1992; 33:1717–1719.
45. Melchor R, Biddiscombe MF, Mak VHM, Short MD, Spiro SG. Lung deposition patterns of directly labelled salbutamol in normal subjects and in patients with reversible airflow obstruction. Thorax 1993; 48:506–511.
46. Fok TF, Monkman S, Dolovich M, Gray S, Coates G, Paes B, Rashid F, Newhouse M, Kirpalani H. Efficiency of aerosol medication delivery from a metered dose inhaler versus jet nebulizer in infants with bronchopulmonary dysplasia. Pediatr Pulmonol 1996; 21:301–309.
47. Devidason S, Everard ML, MacErlean C, Summer Q, Rollo C, Swift P, Borgstrom L, Le Souef PN. Lung deposition from the Turbuhaler in children with cystic fibrosis. Eur Respir J 1997; 10:2023–2028.
48. Martonen TB, Yang Y, Dolovich M. Definition of airway composition within gamma camera images. J Thorac Imaging 1993; 9:188–197.
49. Martonen TB, Yang Y, Dolovich M, Guan X. Computer simulations of lung morphologies within planar gamma camera images. Nucl Med Commun 1997; 18:861–869.
50. Chan HK. Use of single photon emission computed tomography in aerosol studies. J Aerosol Med 1993; 6:23–32.
51. Phipps P, Gonda J, Bailey D, Borham P, Bautovich G, Anderson S. Comparison of planar and tomographic gamma scintigraphy to measure the penetration index of inhalation aerosols. Am Rev Respir Dis 1989; 139:1516–1523.
52. Logus JW, Trajan, M Hooper HR, Lentle BC, Mann SFP. Single photon emission tomography of lungs imaged with Tc-labelled aerosol. J Can Assoc Radiol 1984; 35:133–138.
53. Perring S, Summers QA, Fleming JS, Nassim MA, Holgate ST. A new method of quantification of the pulmonary regional distribution of aerosols using combined

CT and SPECT and its application to nedocromil sodium administered by metered dose inhaler. Br J Radiol 1994; 67:46–53.

54. Chua HL, Collis GG, Maxwell L, Chan K, Langford JH, Newbury AM, Bower GD, Le Souef PN. The effect of age and method of delivery on aerosol deposition in children Am Rev Respir Dis 1991; 143:
55. Fleming JS, Hashish AH, Conway JH, Nassim MA, Holgate ST, Halson P, Moore E, Bailey AG, Martonen TB. Assessment of deposition of inhaled aerosol in the respiratory tract of man using three dimensional multi-modality imaging and mathematical modelling. J Aerosol Med 1996; 9:317–327.
56. Fleming JS, Hashish AH, Conway JH, Hartley-Davis R, Nassim MA, Guy MJ, Coupe J, Holgate ST, Moore E, Bailey AG, Martonen TB. A technique for simulating radionuclide images from the aersool deposition pattern in the airway tree. J Aerosol Med 1997; 10:199–212.
57. Schuster DP. Positron emission tomography: theory and its application to the study of lung disease. Am Rev Resp Med 1989; 139:818–840.
58. Rhodes CG, Hughes JMB. Pulmonary studies using positron emission tomography. Eur Respir J 1995; 8:1001–1017.
59. Dolovich M, Nahmias C, Thompson M, Uki S, Freitag A, Coates G. Positron emission tomographic PET) imaging of the lung in cystic fibrosis: 3D assessment of the distribution of inhaled therapy. AJRCCM 1999; 59(part 2):A687.
60. Dolovich M, Inman M, Wahl L, Nahmias C, Hargreave F, Coates G. 3D imaging of the lung: PET scanning and aerosols. Am J Resp Crit Care Med 1998; 157:A78.
61. Alderson PO, Secker-Walker RH, Strominger DB, Markham J, Hill RL. Pulmonary deposition of aerosols in children with cystic fibrosis. J Pediatr 1974; 84:479–484.
62. Thomas SHL, O'Doherty MJ, Graham A, Blower PJ, Geddes DM, Nunan T O. Pulmonary deposition of nebulised amiloride in cystic fibrosis: comparison of two nebulisers. Thorax 1991a; 46:717–721.
63. Witten ML, Bowers MC, Hall JN, Quan SF, Shen Q, Lemen RJ. A rapid analytical method for measuring drug distribution in aerosols. Radiopharmacy 1992; 20:155–158.
64. O'Doherty MJ, Thomas, S, Page C, Clark AR, Mitchell D, Heduan E, Nunan TO, Bateman NT. Does $^{99m}T_c$ human serum albumin alter the characteristics of nebulised pentamidine isethionate? Nucl Med Commun 1989; 10:523–529.
65. O'Doherty MJ, Thomas SHL, Page CJ, Blower PJ, Bateman NT, Nunan TO. Disposition of nebulized pentamidine measured using direct radiolabel 123 iodopentamidine. Nuc Med Commun 1993; 14:8–11.
66. Svartengren K, Svartengren M, Philipson K, Barck C, Bylin G, Camner P. Clearance in small ciliated airways in allergic asthmatics after bronchial provocation. Respiration 1999; 66:112–118.
67. Cheung D, Bowen B, Rashid F, Rhem R, Dolovich M. Preparation of microaggregated human serum albumin labelled with ^{99m}Tc to enable in vivo evaluation of suspension aerosols. Am J Resp Crit Care Med 1998; 157:A638.
68. Newman SP, Pellow PGD, Clarke SW. Droplet size distributions of nebulised aerosols for inhalation therapy. Phys Physiol Meas 1986; 7:139–146.

69. Sanchis J, Dlovich M, Chalmers R, Newhouse MT. Quantitation of regional aerosol clearance in the normal lung. J Appl Physiol 1972; 33:757–762.
70. Alvine GF, Rogers P, Fitzsimmons KM, Ahrens RC. Disposable nebulizers. How reliable are they? Chest 1992; 101:316–319.
71. Watterberg KL, Clark AR, Kelly HW, Murphy S. Delivery of aerosolized medication to intubated babies. Pediatr Pulmonol 1991; 10:136–141.
72. Thomas SHL, O'Doherty MJ, Page CJ, Nunan TO. Variability in the measurement of nebulized aerosol deposition in man. Clin Sci 1991; 81:767–775.
73. Bennett WD. Aerosolized drug delivery: fractional deposition of inhaled particles. J Aerosol Med 1991; 4:223–227.
74. Spiro SG, Singh CA, Tolfree SE, Partridge MR, Short MD. Direct labelling of ipratropium bromide aerosol and its deposition pattern in normal subjects and patients with chronic bronchitis. Thorax 1984; 39:432–435.
75. Newman SP, Millar AB, Lennard-Jones TR, Moren F, Clarke SW. Improvement of pressurised aerosol deposition with Nebuhaler spacer device. Thorax 1984; 39:935–941.
76. Zainudin BMZ, Biddiscombe M, Tolfree SEJ, Short M, Spiro SG. Deposition patterns of salbutamol inhaled from a pressurised metered dose inhaler, as a dry powder, and as a nebulised solution. Thorax 1990; 45:469–473.
77. Vidgren P, Vidgren M, Paronen P, Vainio P, Karjalainen P, Nuutinen J. Removal of inhaled 99mTc-labelled particles of disodium cromoglycate from the lungs. Acta Pharm Nord 1991; 3:155–158.
78. Kohler D, Fleischer W, Matthys H. New method for easy labelling of β-agonists in metered dose inhalers with technetium 99m. Respiration 1988; 53:65–73.
79. Summers QA, Clark AR, Hollingworth A, Fleming J, Holgate ST. The preperation of a radiolabelled aerosol of nedocromil sodium for administration by metered dose inhaler that accurately preserves particle size distribution of the drug. Drug Invest 1990; 2:90–98.
80. Newman SP, Clark AR, Talee N, Clarke SW. Pressurised aerosol deposition in the human lung with and without an "open" spacer. Thorax 1989; 44:706–710.
81. Clarke JG, Farr SJ, Wicks SR. Technetium-99m labelling of suspension type pressurised metered dose inhalers comprising various drug/surfactant combinations. Int J Pharm 1992; 80:R1–R5.
82. Vidgren M, Paronen P, Vidgren P, Nuutinen J, Vainio P. Effect of the new spacer-device on the deposition of the inhaled metered dose aerosol. Pharmazie 1990; 45:922–924.
83. Zainudin BMZ, Biddiscombe M, Tolfree SEJ, Short M, Spiro SG. Comparison of bronchodilator responses and deposition patterns of albutamol inhaled from a pressurised metered dose inhaler, as a dry powder, and as a nebulised solution. Thorax 1990; 45:469–473.
84. Newman SP, Moren F, Trofast E, Talee N, Clarke SW. Deposition and clinical efficacy of terbutaline sulphate from Turbuhaler, a new multi-dose powder inhaler. Eur Respir J 1989; 2:247–252.
85. Dolovich M. In vitro measurements of delivery of medications from MDIs and spacer devices. Proceedings of in vitro/in vivo standards of measurement for MDIs Workshop, Atlanta GA. J Aerosol Med 1996; 9(suppl 1):S49–S58.

86. Borgström L, Derom E, Stahl E, Wahlin-Boll E, Pauwels R. The inhalation device influences lung deposition and bronchodilating effect of terbutaline. Am J Respir Crit Care Med 1996; 153:1636–1640.
87. Dolovich M, Ruffin R E, Roberts R, Newhouse M. Optimal delivery of aerosol from metered dose inhalers. Chest 1981; 80S:911–915.
88. Everard ML, Devidason S, Le Souef PN. Effect of multiple actuations on total and respirable dose delivered by metered dose inhalers. Thorax 1995; 50:746–749.
89. Newman SP, Pavia D, Garland N, Clarke SW. Effects of various inhalation modes on the deposition of radioactive pressurized aerosols. Eur J Respir Dis 1982; 63(suppl 119):57–65.
90. Thorsson L, Edsbacker S. Lung deposition froma pressurised metered dosc inhaler attached to a spacer. Eur Respir J 1998; 12:1340–1345.
91. Smaldone GC, Fuhrer J, Steigbigel RT, Mc Peck M. Factors determining pulmonary deposition of aerosolized Pentamidine in patients with human immunodeficiency virus infection. Am Rev Respir Dis 1991; 143:727–737.
92. Gonda I. Absolute and and relative quantification of deposition by scintigraphy. J Biopharm Sci 1992; 3:191–197.
93. Messina MS, Smaldone GC. Evaluation of quantitative aerosol techniques for use in bronchoprovocation studies. J Allergy Clin Immunol 1985; 75:252–257.
94. Cross CE, Hornof WJ, Koblik PD, Fisher PE. Aerosol deposition: practical considerations of methodology for direct measurement of aerosol delivery to the lung bronchiolar-alveolar surfaces. J Aerosol Med 1992; 5:39–45.
95. Fok TF, Al-Essa M, Kirpalani II, Monkman Sm, Bowen B, Coates G, Dolovich M. Estimation of pulmonary deposition of aerosol using gamma scintigraphy. J Aerosol Med 1999; 12:9–15.
96. Asmundsson T, Johnson RF, Kilburn KH, Goodrich JK. Efficiency of nebulizers for depositing saline in human lung. Am Rev Respir Dis 1973; 108:506–512.
97. Ruffin RE, Dolovich MB, Wolff RK, Newhouse MT. The effects of preferential deposition of histamine in the human airway. Am Rev Respir Dis 1978; 117:485–492.
98. Pitcairn GR, Newman SP. Tissue attenuation corrections in gamma scintigraphy. J Aerosol Med 1997; 10:187–198.
99. Fleming JS, Conway JH, Holgate ST, Moore E A Hashish AH, Bailey AG, Martonen TB. Evaluation of the accuracy and precision of lung aerosol deposition measurements from planar radionulcide imaging using simulation. Phys Med Biol 1998; 43:2423–2429.
100. Macey DJ, Marshall R. Absolute quantification of radiotracer uptake in the lungs using a gamma camera. J Nucl Med 1982; 23:731–735.
101. Forge NI, Mountford PJ, O'Doherty MJ. Quantification of technetium-99m lung radioactivity from planar images. Eur J Nucl Med 1993; 20:10–15.
102. Agnew JE. Characterizing lung aerosol penetration. J Aerosol Med 1991; 3:237–249.
103. Dolovich M, Sanchis J, Rossman C, Newhouse MT. Aerosol penetrance: a sensitive index of peripheral airways obstruction. J Appl Physiol 1976; 40(3):468–471.
104. Bennett WD, Ilowite JS. Dual pathway clearace of 99m Tc-DTPA from the bronchial mucosa. Am Rev Respir Dis 1989; 139:1132–1138.

105. Assessing lung deposition of inhaled medication. Consensus statement from a workshop of the British Association for Lung Research. Respir Med 1999; 93:123–133.
106. Hamid Q, Song Y, Kotsimbos TC, Minshall E, Bai T. Hegele RG. Inflammation in small airways in asthma. J Allergy Clin Immunol 1997; 100:44–51.
107. Leach CL, Davidson PJ, Boudreau RJ. Improving airway targeting with the CFC-frec HFA-beclomethasone metered dose inhaler compared with CFC-beclomethasone. Eur Respir J 1998; 12:1346–1353.
108. Richards R, Simpson S, Renwick A, Holgate S. The absorption and distribution kinetics of cromolyn sodium and the influence of inhalation technique. J Pharmacol Exp Ther 1987; 241:1028–1032.
109. Auty RM, Brown K, Neale MG, Snashall PD. Respiratory tract deposition of sodium cromoglycate is highly dependent upon technique of inhalation using the spinhaler. Br J Dis Chest 1987; 81:371–380.
110. Edsbacker S, Szefler S. Glucocorticoid pharmacokinetics: principles and applications. In: Schleimer RP, Busse WW, O'Byrne P, eds. Inhaled Glucocorticoids in Asthma: Mechanisms and Clinical Actions. New York: Marcel Dekker, 1997:381–445.
111. Pedersen, Steffensen G, Ohlsson S. The influence of orally deposited budesonide on the systemic availability of budesonide after inhalation from a Turbuhaler. Br J Clin Pharmacol 1993; 36:211–214.
112. Thorsson L, Edsbacker S, Conradson T-B. Lung deposition of budesonide from Turbuhaler is twice that from a pressurised metered-dose inhaler. Eur Respir J 1994; 7:1839–1844.
113. Borgstrom L, Newman S, Weisz A, Moren F. Pulmonary deposition of inhaled terbutaline: comparison of scanning gamma camera and urinary excretion methods. J Pharm Sci 1992; 81:753–755.
114. Newman S, Steed K, Hooper G, Kallen A, Borgstrom L. Comparison of gamma scintigraphy and pharmacokinetic technique for assessing pulmonary deposition of terbutaline sulphate delivered by pressurised metered dosc inhaler. Pharm Res 1995; 12:231–266.
115. Beckman O, Bondesson E, Asking L, Kallen A, Borgstrom L. Intra- and interindividual variations in pulmonary deposition via Turbuhaler and pMDI. Drug Delivery to the Lungs VI. The Aerosol Society, 1995.
116. Johnson M. Fluticasone proprionate: pharmacokinetics and pharmacodynamic implications of different aerosol delivery systems. In: Byron PR, Farr SJ, eds. Proceedings of RRD VI. Hilton Head, SC, 1998.
117. Thorsson L, Dahlstrom K, Edsbacker S, Kallen A, Paulson J, Wiren J-E. Pharmacokinetics and systemic effects of inhaled fluticasone proprionate in healthy subjects. Br J Clin Pharmacol 1997; 43:155–161.
118. Mollman H, Wagner M, Meibohm B, Hocchaus G, Barth J, Stockman R, Kreig M, Weisser H, Falcoz C. Darendorf H. Pharmacokinetic and pharmacodynamic evaluation of fluticasone proprionate after inhaled administration. J Clin Pharmacol 1998; 53:459–467.
119. Agertoft L, Pedersen S. Systemic availability and pharmcokinetics of nebulised budesonide in pre-school children with asthma. Arch Dis Child 1998; 79:0–6.

120. Derendorf H, Hochhaus G, Rohatagi S, Mollmann H, Barth J, Sourgens H, Erdmann M. Pharmakokinetics of triamcinolone acetonide after intravenous, oral and inhaled administration. 1995; 35:302–305.
121. Falcoz C, Mackie AE, Moss J, Norton J, Ventresca GP, Brown A, Field E, Harding SM, Wire P, Bye A. Pharmacokinetics and systemic exposure of inhaled beclomethasone diproprionate. Eur Respir J 1996; 9(suppl 23):162S.
122. Schmekel B, Borgstrom L, Wollmer P. Differences in pulmonary absorption of inhaled terbutaline in healthy smokers and non-smokers. Thorax 1991; 46:225–228.
123. Schmekel B, Borgstrom L, Wollmer P. Exercise increase the rate of pulmonary absorption of inhaled terbutaline. Chest 1992; 101:742–745.
124. Pauwels R, Newman S, Borgstrom L. Airway deposition and airway effects of anti-asthma drugs delivered from metered-dose inhalers. Eur Respir J 1997; 10:2127–2138.
125. Lipworth BJ, Seckl JR. Measures for detecting systemic bioactivity with inhaled and intranasal corticosteroids. Thorax 1997; 52:476–482.
126. Hindle M, Newton DAG, Chrystyn H. Investigations of an optimal inhaler technique with the use of urinary salbutamol excretion as a measure of relative bioavailability to the lung. Thorax 1993; 48:607–610.
127. Chenge JK, Chrystyn H. Volumatic usage: some generic salbutamol metered dose inhalers can be used. Thorax 1994; 49:1162–1163.
128. Hindle M, Newton DAG, Chrystyn H. Dry powder inhalers are bioequivalent to metered-dose inhalers: a study using a new urinary albuterol (Salbutamol) assay technique. Chest 1995; 107:629–633.
129. Newnham DM, McDevitt DG, Lipworth BJ. Comparison of the extrapulmonary β_2-adrenorecptor responses and pharmacokinetics of salbutamol given by standard metered dose inhaler and modified actuator device. Br J Clin Pharmacol 1993; 36:445–450.
130. Newnham DM, Lipworth BJ. Nebuliser performance, pharmacokinetics, airways and systemic effects of salbutamol given via a novel nebuliser delivery system (Venstream). Thorax 1994; 49:762–770.
131. Clark DJ, Gordon-Smith J, McPhate G, Clark G, Lipworth BJ. Lung bioavailability of generic and innovator salbutamol metered dose inhalers. Thorax 1996; 51:325–326.
132. Lipworth BJ. Pharmacokinetics of inhaled drugs. Br J Clin Pharmacol 1996; 42:697–705.
133. Johnson MA, Newman SP, Bloom R, Talaee N, Clarke SW. Delivery of albuterol and ipratropium bromide from two nebulizer systems in chronic stable asthma. Chest 1989; 96:1–10.
134. Derom E, Pauwels R. Relationship between airway deposition and effects for inhaled bronchodilators. In: Respiratory Drug Delivery VI. Buffalo Grove, IL: Interpharm Press, 1998.
135. Dolovich M. New propellant-free technologies under investigation. J Aerosol Med 1999; (suppl 1):S9–S17.

7

Targeting the Lungs with Therapeutic Aerosols

PIETER ZANEN

Heart Lung Centre Utrecht
Utrecht, The Netherlands

BETH L. LAUBE

Johns Hopkins University School of Medicine,
Baltimore, Maryland

I. Introduction

For inhaled medications to be efficacious, an adequate dose of the drug must deposit in the lungs. This means minimizing losses in the oropharynx. Minimizing drug losses in the oropharynx should also enhance the therapeutic index of some drugs (i.e., the ratio of benefit to adverse effects). In addition, it is likely that targeting the inhaled mass for deposition in regions of the lungs that contain the drug's effector cells and/or receptors will also improve efficacy. For example, a bronchodilator aerosol will probably be most efficacious when targeted to deposit in the tracheobronchial region of the lungs compared to deposition in the alveolar region, which lacks smooth muscle and thus will be unaffected by the drug's bronchodilatory action. On the other hand, drugs that are administered to the lungs for systemic delivery will probably benefit from targeted deposition in the alveolar region, compared to the conducting airways, because of the larger surface area for absorption and minimal mucociliary clearance and proteolytic enzymes.

To achieve effective targeting within the lungs, known factors that govern aerosol deposition—including particle size, inspiratory flow rate, lung volume at the time of inhalation and breath-holding time—must be understood. Each of these factors interacts with several mechanisms of deposition. A short review of these mechanisms of deposition is presented below. For a more detailed review, we refer the reader to Chap. 2.

II. Polydisperse Versus Monodisperse Aerosols

Many of the basic principles of aerosol deposition theory have been validated with laboratory-generated monodisperse aerosols, which means that the particles are all the same size. A perfectly monodisperse aerosol has a geometric standard deviation (GSD) of 1.0, but an aerosol is said to be acceptably monodisperse if the GSD is less than 1.22 (1).

Unlike laboratory-generated aerosols, aerosolized drugs are almost invariably polydisperse, which means that the particles cover a wide range of sizes. They may be irregular in shape as well. In 1966, the Task Group of the International Committee on Radiological Protection (IRCP) suggested that the size distribution of a polydisperse aerosol is best described by its mass median aerodynamic diameter (MMAD) and GSD. The Task Group defined aerodynamic diameter as the diameter of a unit-density sphere that has the same settling velocity as the particle in question. Settling velocity was defined as a constant speed of settling that occurs when the force of gravity equals the air resistance. Redefining particle size in this way made it possible to compare irregularly shaped polydisperse particles by normalizing them in terms of their settling velocities (2).

III. Mechanisms of Deposition

In 1935, Findeisen published his "Uber das Absetzen kleiner in der Luft suspendierter Teilchen in der mensliche Lunge bei der Atmung," which was the first attempt to calculate the deposition of aerosols (3). The Findeisen model included four mechanisms for deposition of particles. These were (1) impaction, (2) sedimentation, (3) Brownian diffusion, and (4) interception. This review focuses only on the first two mechanisms proposed by Findeisen, because Brownian diffusion affects particles <1 μm; these are usually too small for therapeutic purposes and interception is normally insignificant except for elongated particles such as fibers. For more information about diffusion and interception, we refer the reader to Chap. 2.

Electrostatic precipitation is another mechanism for particle deposition; it is important when aerosols are administered from holding chambers or spacers. We refer the reader to Chap. 12 for more information about electrostatic charge and aerosol delivery systems.

A. Impaction

The predominant mechanism for deposition of particles >3 μm is inertial impaction. Inertial impaction occurs primarily in the oropharynx, trachea, and larger conducting airways. This is because these particles cannot follow the sudden airflow changes in these airways, and they collide with the airway wall.

Impaction in the Oropharynx

We said above that successful targeting of inhaled medications assumes minimal losses of drug in the oropharynx. The major determinant of losses of inhaled drug within the oropharynx is particle impaction as a result of inertial forces. Impaction of particles within the oropharynx occurs primarily at the 90-degree bend in the posterior oral cavity and at the larynx. Newman et al. used gamma camera imaging technology to show the effect of particle size on aerosol impaction in the oral cavity (4). Seven patients with cystic fibrosis (CF) inhaled radiolabeled aerosols of the antibiotic carbenicillin on two different occasions. Aerosols were generated by two different nebulizers and were characterized as having mass median diameters (MMDs) of 7.3 or 3.2 μm. Although the GSD for each aerosol was not reported, it is likely that the GSDs were similar, since each was generated from a liquid, using standard nebulizer systems.

Figure 1 shows the gamma camera images of the lungs of one CF patient after inhaling the two aerosols. The contour lines represent lung outlines at 15 and 30% of the maximum count rate, respectively. Dose deposited within the lungs was expressed as a percent of the dose deposited in the lungs and oropharynx combined. Dose deposited within the lungs was greatest for the 3.2-μm aerosol (right image), whereas a larger fraction of the 7.3-μm aerosol was retained in the oropharynx (left image) and was swallowed (visualized as stomach activity).

Impaction of aerosols within the oropharynx occurs not only because of large particle size but also because of high aerosol velocity, either due to some feature of the delivery system, such as the use of a pressurized propellant, or as a result of inhalation at a high inspiratory flow rate. Figure 2 shows the effect of high aerosol velocity associated with a pressurized propellant on the deposition of 3-μm monodisperse Teflon particles in a patient with chronic obstructive pulmonary disease (COPD). Newman et al. quantified the fraction of particles labeled with technetium 99m (^{99m}Tc) in the mouth, lungs, and stomach with a gamma camera (5). Average deposition within the lungs ($n = 8$), expressed as a percentage of the inhaled dose, was only 8.8%, while 80% was deposited in the mouth. These high losses in the oropharynx were due to a combination of factors. First, incomplete evaporation of the propellants that coated the particles led to a large particle size. Second, the high aerosol velocity attributed to the particles by the propellant increased the probability of particles impacting on the airway surface.

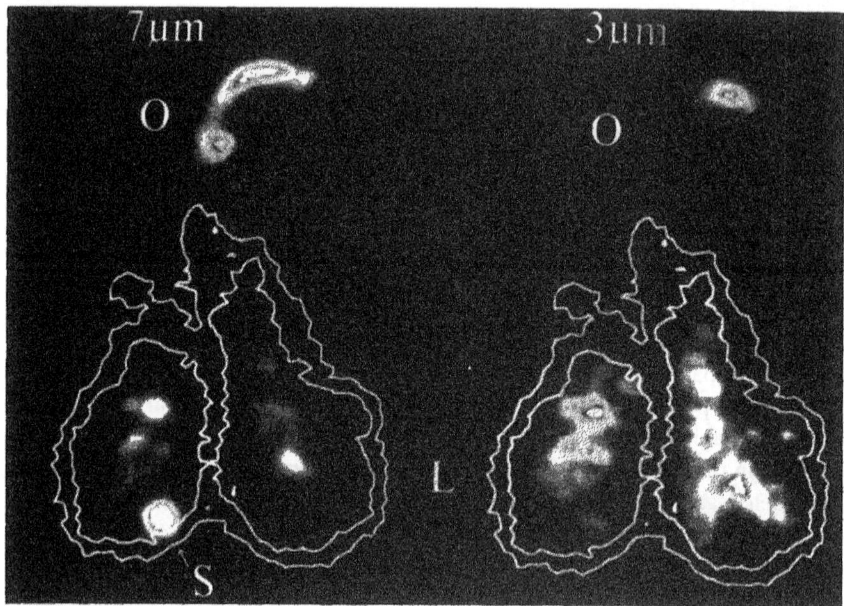

Figure 1 Gamma camera scans of aerosol deposited in the lungs (L), oropharynx (O), and stomach (S) of a CF patient after inhaling radioaerosols composed of 7.3- (left) or 3.2-μm (right) particles. (From Ref. 4.)

The patient's inspiratory flow rate also affects impaction of aerosol particles in the oral cavity. Data from a study by Anderson et al. show the effect of increasing inspiratory flow rate on oropharyngeal deposition of an aerosol with 3.0-μm MMAD (6). In that study, the authors increased flow rate from 0.4 to 1.2 L/s in a group of normal subjects. The aerosol was generated by nebulizer, so there was no additional effect of pressurized propellant. As inspiratory flow rate increased, average deposition in the oral cavity increased from 20 to 38%.

Laube et al. (7) compared oropharyngeal deposition over a narrower range of inspiratory flow rates. Three normal subjects inhaled a radiolabeled aerosol, generated by nebulizer (MMAD = 2.3 μm), at increasing inspiratory flow rates. Single-probe gamma detectors, collimated to record counts only from the bronchopulmonary region (below the larynx) or the oropharynx, were used to quantify total deposition fraction. Counts within the oropharynx region were expressed as a percentage of total deposition. Fractional deposition in the oropharynx was reproducibly minimized when patients inhaled between 13 and 35 L/min, averaging from 10 to 20% of the total activity

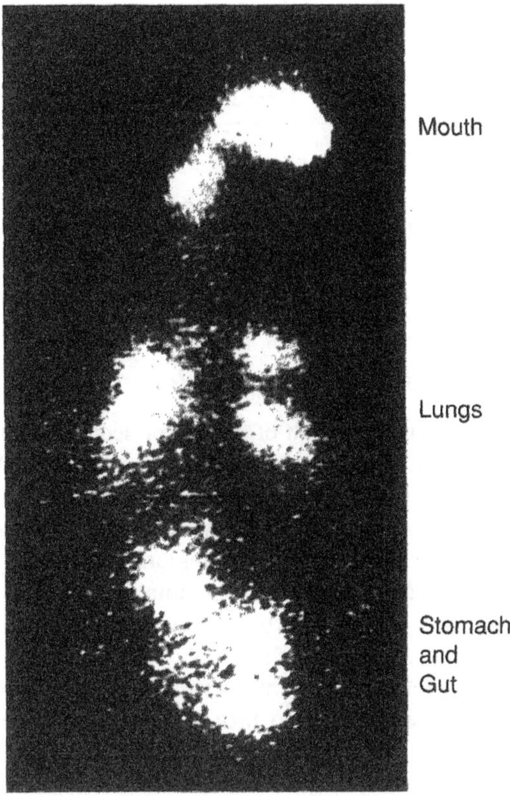

Figure 2 Gamma camera image of the head, lungs, and stomach of a patient following inhalation of radiolabeled Teflon particles from a pressurized canister. (From Ref. 5.)

deposited. Above 35 L/min, there was a dramatic increase in oropharyngeal deposition.

Farr et al. also examined the effect of inspiratory flow rate on deposition. For those experiments, they measured the lung deposition of a radiolabeled aerosol delivered by metered-dose inhaler (MDI) using the Smartmist device, which detects inspired volume and flow rate. With this device, a trigger point can be established for a predefined flow rate and volume. A microprocessor gives a signal to an electromechanical device, which then actuates the MDI. Table 1 summarizes their results. For the same lung volume, the investigators found that lung-deposition was higher when inspiratory flow rate was 30 L/min as opposed to 270 L/min (8). This increase in lung deposition meant that oropharyngeal deposition was reduced at the lower flow rate as compared with the higher rate.

Table 1 Fractional Deposition as a Function of Inspiratory Flow Rate

Trigger point	Lung deposition (% dose)
Firing flow: 30 L/min Volume at time of firing: 300 mL	14.1
Firing flow: 270 L/min Volume at time of firing: 300 mL	8.4

Source: Adapted from Ref. 8.

B. Sedimentation

Smaller particles deposit as a result of gravity or sedimentation. However, this process requires enough residence time for completion. In the larger airways of the tracheobronchial region of the lungs, where the air velocity is high, residence time is at a minimum. However, air velocity slows in the smaller airways of the tracheobronchial region and in the alveolar region, resulting in greater residence time. For this reason, sedimentation is the predominant deposition mechanism in the smaller airways and alveoli, affecting particles smaller than 3 μm and larger than 0.5 μm.

Clearly, any increase in residence time will enhance the probability that smaller particles will sediment. Two factors that enhance residence time and thereby increase the probability of deposition in the smaller airways are an increase in the lung volume during inhalation and an increase in breath-holding time. Landahl modeled the effect of inhalation volume on total deposition. He revised the Findeisen model of deposition by adding the influence of lung volume and showed that larger inhaled volumes would lead to increased total deposition within the lungs (9). Landahl validated his model by administering monodisperse 0.11- to 6.3-μm particles to healthy volunteers. Inhalation volumes increased from 450 to 1350 mL. Inspiratory flow rate was constant at 300 mL/s. Total deposition was quantified as the difference between the number of inhaled particles and the number exhaled (10). Table 2 shows that increasing the volume of inhaled particles air resulted in enhanced total deposition for all particles, presumably because of increased residence time.

Newman et al. showed similar results in patients with lung disease. They incorporated 3.2-μm Teflon particles labeled with the radioisotope ^{99m}Tc into MDIs. Then they asked a group of patients with COPD to actuate the MDI while they inhaled at 30 L/min, starting from different lung volumes: 20, 50, and 80% of the vital capacity (VC). After inhalation, patients held their breaths for 4 s. Measurement of lung, alveolar, and conducting airway deposition fractions revealed that when actuation started at the lowest volume (i.e., 20% VC), signifi-

Table 2 Effect of Changes in Inhalation Volume on Total Deposition (% of inhaled)

	Inhalation mode (flow and volume)		
Particle Size (μm)	300 mL/s, 450 mL	300 mL/s, 900 mL	300 mL/s, 1350 mL
0.11	34	36	46
0.25	32	32	41
0.55	17	23	33
1.4	26	53	65
2.9	52	69	82
3.8	59	72	89
6.3	86	93	96

Source: Adapted from Ref. 10.

cantly more particles deposited in the lungs than when actuation began at the higher volumes (11). These findings are shown in Table 3. They demonstrate that under these breathing conditions, the deeper inspiration (starting from 20% VC) resulted in higher total and regional lung deposition fractions compared to more shallow inspirations starting from 50% and 80% VC.

Newman et al. (12) repeated the same experiments in another group of patients with COPD who were told to hold their breaths for 10 s after completing the inhalation maneuver. Under those conditions, the investigators found that the deposition fraction for the whole lung was the same whether patients began their inhalation at the low or higher lung volumes. Similar results were reported for deposition fraction in the conducting airways and alveoli. These findings are due to the increase in breath-holding time (10 s), which enhanced the residence time and resulted in increased deposition by sedimentation, regardless of the lung volume at the time of inhalation.

Table 3 Effect of Changes in Lung Volume at the Time of Inhalation on Deposition Fraction (% of dose)

	Lung volume at actuation		
Deposition fraction	20% VC	50% VC [a]	80% VC
Conducting airways	7.4	5.0	4.2
Alveoli	3.0	1.9	2.0
Whole lung	10.4	6.9	6.2

[a] Vital capacity.
Source: Ref. 11.

IV. Factors That Affect Aerosol Targeting

Particles that penetrate beyond the oropharynx and enter the lower airways may deposit in two broad regions of the lungs: the tracheobronchial zone and the pulmonary zone, as shown in Fig. 3 (13). Anatomically, it is assumed that the tracheobronchial zone is composed of the trachea and the larger conducting airways, whereas the pulmonary zone contains the smaller airways and alveoli. The extent to which particles deposit in either region is dependent on particle size, inspiratory flow rate, and lung volume at the time of inhalation (14). Whether a particle will impact or sediment also depends on the value of these parameters. For example, a small particle can deposit by impaction mechanisms when inhaled fast or by sedimentation when inhaled slowly.

A. Particle Size

Several investigators have modeled deposition within the lung as a function of particle size. Gerrity related particle size and regional deposition on a per airway generation basis, as shown in Fig. 4 (15). His calculations took into account the Landahl equations (9) and the Weibel-A lung model (16). This model

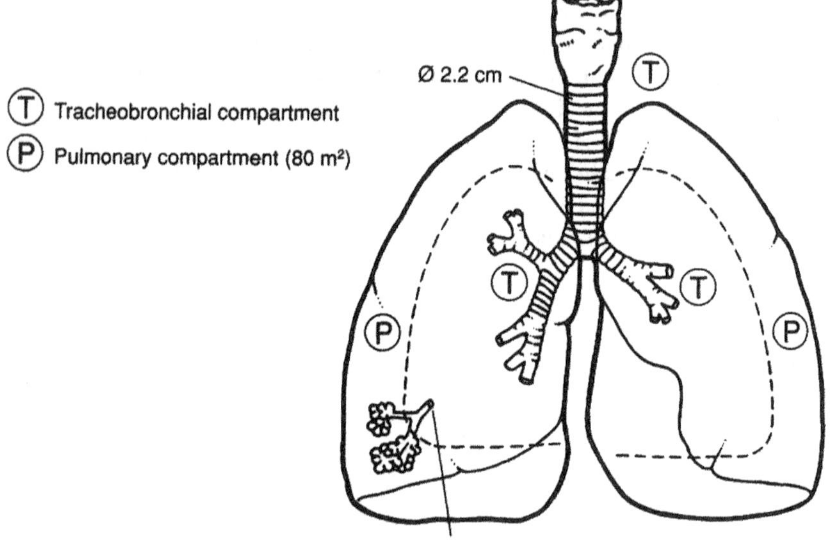

Figure 3 Tracheobronchial and pulmonary regions of the lower respiratory tract. (From Ref. 13.)

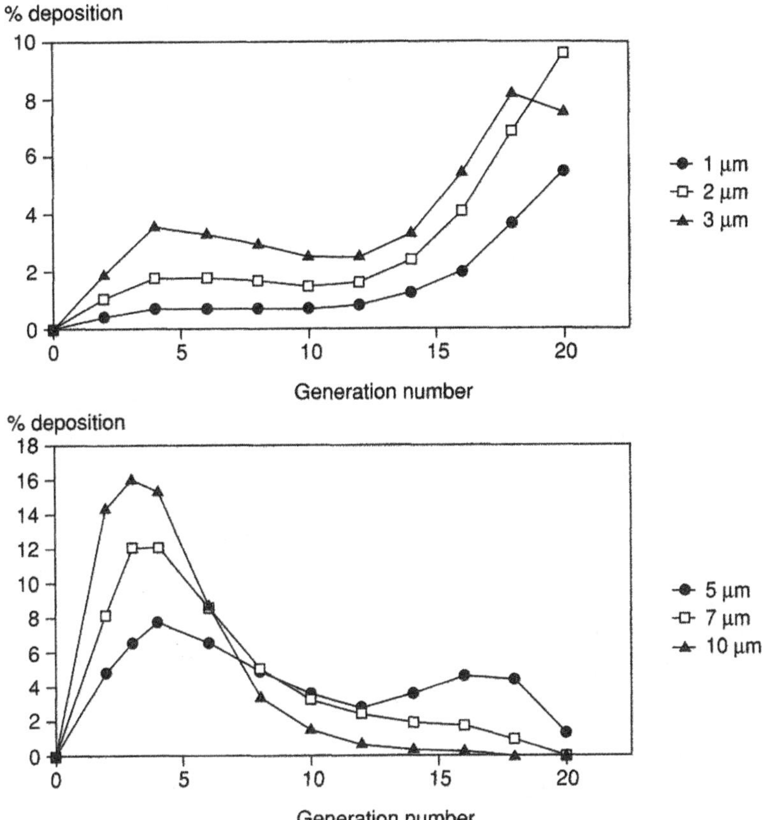

Figure 4 Regional deposition of 1-, 2-, 3-, 5-, 7-, and 10-μm nonhygroscopic particles. (From Ref. 15.)

predicts that large monodisperse particles will deposit in the proximal airways, while smaller ones will deposit in the distal airways. This model also predicts that deposition will be spread over many airway generations. This "spread" in deposition will be enhanced with polydisperse aerosols. In addition, according to the model, large particles may reach the distal airways in low numbers. So when an abundant number of large particles are inhaled, the burden to the alveoli may be significant.

Yeh and Shum developed a model for regional deposition on a per lobe basis instead of per airway generation. Airway dimensions to the terminal bronchioles were obtained from measurements of the cast of the lungs from a human cadaver. Information for generations beyond the terminal bronchioles was estimated from the Weibel lung model (16). Regional deposition was defined as tracheobronchial (TB) and pulmonary (P) in each of five lobes. According to this model, total and regional deposition in each of the lobes will increase with increasing particle size (i.e., between 1 and 3 μm). These data are shown in Table 4.

The model also predicts that regional deposition in the tracheobronchial region will be greatest in the lower left lobe for 1-, 2-, and 3-μm particles; whereas deposition in the pulmonary region will be greatest in the lower right lobe for these same particles (17).

B. Inspiratory Flow Rate

Studies by Laube et al. (18) and Farr et al. (8) show the effect of changes in inspiratory flow rate on regional deposition in human subjects. Figure 5*A* and *B*, taken from Laube et al. (18), shows the change in deposition pattern within a human lung following fast (~60 L/min, *A*) and slower (~12 L/min, *B*) inspirations of an aerosol (MMAD = 1.5 μm) that was radiolabeled with ^{99m}Tc and generated by jet nebulizer. The distribution of radioaerosol within the lungs was quantified with a gamma camera. The amount of radioactivity detected in an inner (large conducting airways) and outer lung zone (smaller airways and alveoli) was expressed as an inner versus outer zone ratio (I/O ratio). Higher I/O ratios indicated increased deposition in the larger, central airways. In nine subjects, I/O ratios averaged 2.91 after the fast inspiratory maneuver. This was reduced to 1.84 after the slower inspiration, indicating enhanced deposition in the smaller airways.

Similarly, using the Smartmist device described earlier, Farr and associates (8) reported that, for a given lung volume of 300 mL, the central/peripheral ratio (an indicator of deposition in the larger airways versus the lung

Table 4 Percent Deposition Per Lung Lobe

d (μm)	Region	UR	MR	LR	UL	LL
1	TB	0.32	0.14	0.62	0.33	0.68
	P	1.91	1.01	3.40	1.69	0.32
2	TB	0.56	0.25	1.12	0.57	1.21
	P	2.85	1.50	5.17	2.57	5.02
3	TB	0.79	0.37	1.61	0.80	1.74
	P	3.09	1.63	5.66	2.83	5.50

Key: UR, upper right; MR, middle right; LR, lower right; UL, upper left; LL, lower left; TB, tracheobronchial; P, pulmonary; d, aerodynamic particle size.
Source: Ref. 17.

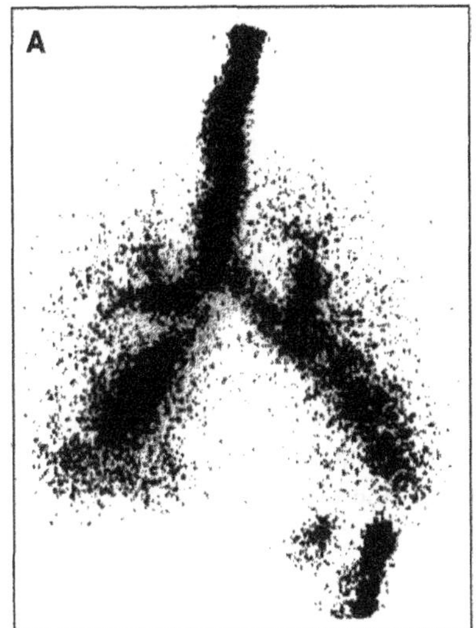

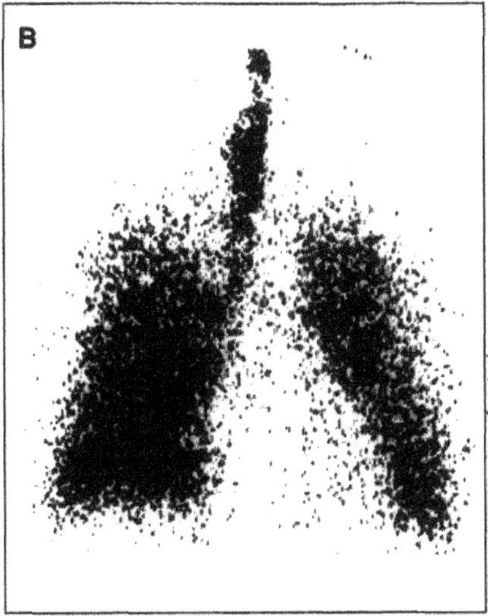

Figure 5 Gamma camera scans of lungs and trachea of an asthma patient after rapid (A) and slow (B) inhalation of radiolabeled aerosol. (From Ref. 18.)

periphery) was significantly enhanced when inspiratory flow rate was 270 L/min versus 30 L/min.

C. Inhalation Volume

Pavia et al. randomly assigned inhalation volumes ranging from 0.11 to 0.88 L to 44 patients with airways obstruction and measured the alveolar deposition of radiolabeled polystyrene particles (5 ± 0.7 μm) generated from an MDI. The patient's FEV_1 and inspiratory flow rate were also measured. A multiple regression analysis of the alveolar deposition, inhalation volume, FEV_1 and inspiratory flow rate revealed that for every liter increase in inhalation volume and for every liter increase in FEV_1, the alveolar deposition rose by 40 and 11%, respectively. In contrast, alveolar deposition decreased by 0.75% for every 1 L/min increase in inspiratory flow rate (19).

D. Conclusions

The data presented above suggest the following:

Targeted delivery of aerosolized medications to broad regions of the lungs (i.e., large, central airways versus smaller airways and alveoli) can be achieved by manipulating particle size, inspiratory flow rate, and inhalation volume.

Targeting of therapeutic aerosol particles to specific airway generations is not possible because both monodisperse and polydisperse aerosols will deposit over several generations.

For particles that deposit by impaction mechanisms (i.e., particles > 3 μm), high inspiratory flow rates (>30 L/min) lead to enhanced losses of drug in the oropharynx and increased deposition in the trachea and larger central airways. Slower inspirations should enhance deposition of these particles in the lung periphery.

For particles that deposit by sedimentation mechanisms (i.e., particles > 0.5 μm and < 3 μm), an increase in inhalation volume and the use of a breath-hold will enhance deposition in the distal lung as a result of increasing the residence time.

V. Therapeutic Aerosols and Their Targets

To optimize the efficacy of an inhaled drug, it is necessary to deliver an adequate dose beyond the oropharynx and, if possible, to direct deposition to a specific broad region(s) of the lung that contains the target cells and receptors. In the sections below, we discuss various sites and/or cell populations to which different classes of inhaled drugs should be directed when the lung is the target organ (e.g., bronchodilators and anti-inflammatory drugs) and when the lung is an alternative route for delivery to the systemic circulation (e.g., insulin). We review the available data for the location of the target cells and/or receptors for each type of drug as follows:

Bronchodilators: smooth muscle cells and β-adrenergic/cholinergic receptors
Steroidal anti-inflammatory drugs: eosinophils and glucocorticoid receptors
Nonsteroidal anti-inflammatory drugs: eosinophils and mast cells
Histamine: H_1 and H_3 receptors
Methacholine: smooth muscle cells and muscarinic (M_3) receptors
Drugs intended for systemic delivery: the alveolar region

A. Bronchodilators

Bronchodilators have a clear target in the lungs. Smooth muscle β_2-agonists, such as albuterol, relax smooth muscle by occupying β_2-receptors, while anticholinergic drugs, such as ipratropium bromide, prevent constriction of smooth muscle by occupying cholinergic receptors. It is clear that for optimal effect, these drugs should be directed to those regions of the lung where the amount of smooth muscle and the populations of these receptors are highest.

Smooth Muscle Distribution

During autopsy, Hossain et al. determined the amount of smooth muscle in the airway walls of patients who died of asthma. She then compared her findings to the amount of smooth muscle found in the airways of healthy controls. She found that the amount of smooth muscle decreased from the larger airways toward the lung periphery in the controls. In the asthmatics, there was an increase in the amount of smooth muscle in all airways compared to the controls and less of a decrease in the amount of muscle toward the lung periphery (20).

Another group of researchers found that patients with asthma can be subdivided into two types based on the amount of muscle present in the airways at autopsy. Their data are presented in Table 5. Lungs were selected from patients with or without bronchial asthma. Type 1 patients showed an increase in the amount of muscle in the larger airways, whereas type 2 patients demonstrated an increase in the amount of muscle in large and smaller airways (21).

β-Receptor and Cholinergic-Receptor Location

In experiments in ferret lungs, Barnes et al. showed that β-receptors were located near airway smooth muscle and their numbers increased in the smaller airways. They also found that a large number of these receptors was present in the alveoli (22). In other experiments, they found an increase in both α- and β-receptors in peripheral airways and a decrease in cholinergic receptors (23). These investigators have also shown that a similar distribution pattern for β-receptors is found in the human lung (Table 6) (24).

B. Anti-Inflammatory Drugs

Steroidal and nonsteroidal anti-inflammatory drugs such as corticosteroids, sodium cromoglycate, and nedocromil sodium, respectively, are used to treat asthma and COPD. In the sections below, we present potential targets for these

Table 5 Thickness (μm) of Airway Smooth Muscle in Various Patients with Disease and in Control Subjects

Group	Large bronchi 2<R<3 mm	Small bronchi 0.3<R<0.4 mm
Controls	12.4	5.6
Asthma, type 1	64.6	5.6
Asthma, type 2	32.8	11.5
Emphysema	26.8	6.6

Source: Ref. 21.

Table 6 Location of β-Receptors in Human Airways

	Grain count/1000 μm^2	β_1 (%)	β_2 (%)
Bronchial epithelium	213	0	100
Bronchiolar epithelium	129	0	100
Bronchial smooth muscle	28	0	100
Bronchiolar smooth muscle	92	10	90
Alveolar wall	513	30	70

Source: Ref. 24.

drugs in patients with asthma because their usefulness in treating asthma is clear and well established.

In delivering aerosolized steroidal and nonsteroidal anti-inflammatory drugs to patients with asthma, one cell population that should be targeted is the eosinophil. This is because asthma is generally believed to involve an eosinophilic type of inflammatory reaction (25). Steroids reduce the number of eosinophils in circulation, the recruitment of eosinophils to local tissue sites, the survival of eosinophils in the presence of cytokines, and the production of cytokines responsible for or involved in all of these processes (25). Cromolyn inhibits the ability of eosinophils to kill complement-coated schistosomula organisms and to express, upon stimulation, complement C3b and Fcγ receptors (26). Nedocromil inhibits the release of proteins from eosinophil granules and leukotriene (LTC_4) formation by eosinophils (27,28).

Eosinophil Cell Distribution

Faul et al. (29) sampled the cellular contents in proximal and distal airways from five patients who died of an asthma attack within an hour after onset. Table 7 summarizes the results of that study, which indicate a heavier cellular infiltrate in

Table 7 Number of Cells (×10^4/μm^2) Present in Proximal and Distal Airways of Asthmatic Patients Who Died Within 1 h After the Onset of Symptoms

	Proximal airways	Distal airways
T cells	10.9	7.7
Macrophages	9.7	3.4
Eosinophils	1.7	0.3
Activated eosinophils	1.14	0.3

Source: Ref. 29.

the proximal airways for all cell types including eosinophils. These data suggest that inflammation was centrally located in these patients.

Azzawi et al. reported similar results (30). They compared the number of leukocytes, T cells, B cells, and eosinophils in a 115-μm deep layer beneath the lamina reticularis of intrapulmonary bronchi in healthy people who died of drowning or in road accidents and in those who died of an asthma attack lasting for several hours. These data are summarized in Table 8.

From this table, it is clear that the asthmatics differed from the healthy subjects in the number of leukocytes, T cells, and eosinophils in these larger airways. Azzawi and colleagues also correlated the number of eosinophils present and the duration of the terminal episode, which ranged from a few hours to several days. The longer the duration, the higher the eosinophil count in the airways (30).

Synek et al. counted and compared the number of inflammatory cells (mast cells, activated and resting eosinophils, monocytes/macrophages, neutrophils, and $CD3^+/CD8^+$ T cells) in the large (diameter >2 mm) and smaller (diameter <2 mm) airways of subjects who died of asthma and in those who died of nonasthmatic causes. The results showed that for the smaller (<2-mm) airways, the cell count did not differ, indicating that the severity of inflammation in these airways was similar in the two groups. However, in the larger airways, some differences were present. In the airway wall but not in the epithelium, a greater number of eosinophils were present in the subjects who died of asthma. The $CD3^+/CD8^+$ T-cell count, on the other hand, was lower in the large-airway epithelium (31).

The combined data from the above studies suggest that there may be a greater cellular infiltrate of eosinophils in the larger central airways than in the smaller airways of patients who die of asthma. However, most asthma patients do not die of their disease, so it is not clear how these findings pertain to those patients. Hamid et al. addressed this question by obtaining lung tissue from asth-

Table 8 Number of Cells per Millimeter Length of Epithelial Basement Membrane Present in Intrapulmonary Bronchi of Asthmatic Patients and Controls

	Asthma	Controls
Leukocytes	96.9	41
T cells	72.8	27.9
B cells	12.4	13.0
Eosinophils	62.7	1.0
Activated eosinophils	35.7	0

Source: Ref. 30.

matics who needed surgery for concomitant lung carcinoma. Comparing large and small airways within the asthmatic group revealed a slight increase of activated but not total eosinophils in the small airways ($p<0.05$) (32). They then compared cell counts from these samples with those from nonasthmatic carcinoma patients. Sample airways were divided into <2 mm (small airways) and >2 mm diameter (large airways). Mast cells, activated and resting eosinophils, macrophages, neutrophils, and T cells were counted. With the exception of the macrophages and neutrophils, the asthmatic airways showed an increase in cellular content. Mast cells were most abundant in the larger airways of the asthmatic patients.

Carroll et al. divided the airways into three classes: <6 mm, 6–16 mm, and >16 mm (membranous, small, and large cartilaginous, respectively). Eosinophils and lymphocytes were counted in all three classes of airways in subjects, who (1) died of asthma; (2) were asthmatics but died of other causes; and (3) controls. For lymphocytes, the number decreased toward <6 mm airways, and no significant differences were noted between fatal and nonfatal asthmatics. Eosinophils were most abundant in the large airways of those who died of asthma. This was also true for those with nonfatal asthma, but the difference in numbers for the classes of airways was less dramatic (33).

Kraft et al. (34) studied the distribution of eosinophils in transbronchial (alveolar tissue) and endobronchial (fourth and fifth airway generations) biopsies from patients with nocturnal and nonnocturnal asthma. They found that the number of eosinophils was slightly higher in the alveoli for both groups of patients. However, as lung function deteriorated during the night for the patients with nocturnal asthma, Kraft noted that the number of eosinophils increased.

Glucocorticosteroid Receptor Location

Another approach to targeting aerosolized steroids is to target the glucocorticosteroid receptor. Adcock et al. examined the distribution of glucocorticosteroid receptors in 3 asthmatics who were undergoing heart transplantation and in 15 nonasthmatic controls. Glucocorticosteroid receptor mRNA was found in every cell type in the lungs. But the highest concentrations were recovered from the alveolar walls, endothelium, and smooth muscle cells of the bronchial and pulmonary vessels. Lower amounts were found in airway epithelium and smooth muscle. There were no differences between asthmatics and controls. Visualization of glucocorticosteroid receptor protein by antibody staining revealed that most protein was found in the alveolar walls, endothelium, and smooth muscle cells of vessels. Again, no difference was found between asthmatics and controls (35). Vachier et al. confirmed these results. They also reported no difference in receptor mRNA or protein for healthy subjects and asthmatics (36).

Mast-Cell Location

As mentioned above, nonsteroidal anti-inflammatory drugs, such as sodium cromoglycate and nedocromil sodium, inhibit various aspects of eosinophil expression and secretion. It is also assumed that this class of drugs stabilizes the membrane of the mast cell, thereby preventing cell degranulation and the release of inflammatory facilitating compounds. For this reason, the mast cell also appears to be a good candidate for targeting this class of inhaled drugs.

The two distinct types of mast cells in humans are distinguished by differences in their secretory granule protease constituents. MC_{TC} cells contain chymase, carboxypeptidase, cathepsin G-like protease and tryptase. They are the predominant type of mast cells found in the skin and in the gastrointestinal submucosa. MC_T cells contain only tryptase and are the predominant type of mast cell found in the lung, particularly in the alveoli, and in the small intestinal mucosa (37,38). Although one of these mast cell types often predominates in a given tissue, smaller amounts of the other mast cell type are also usually present. In addition, the relative amount of each type of mast cell within the tissue may change with tissue inflammation or fibrosis (39).

C. Histamine

H_1- and H_3-Receptor Location

Histamine plays a central role in immunologic and anti-inflammatory responses, particularly in the immediate hypersensitivity response. Three subclasses of histamine receptors have been identified: H_1, H_2, and H_3 receptors. H_1 receptors are involved in mediating increased vascular permeability, pruritus, contraction of smooth muscle in the respiratory and gastrointestinal tracts, release of mediators of inflammation, and recruitment of inflammatory cells. Among other effects, H_3 receptors mediate the negative feedback control of histamine synthesis and release and may play some defensive role against excess bronchoconstriction. H_1 and H_3 receptors are both found primarily in bronchial smooth muscle in the human respiratory tract (40).

D. Methacholine

M_3-Receptor Location

Methacholine acts through muscarinic (M_3) receptors to contract smooth muscle. It is often aerosolized and delivered in increasing concentrations during bronchoprovocation challenge. Asthma patients typically respond to inhaled methacholine at lower doses than do subjects who do not have asthma. Thus, it is often used to differentiate between asthmatic patients and non asthmatic subjects. It is also used to determine the effectiveness of inhaled medications that act to prevent smooth muscle contraction. The degree of its effectiveness, in terms of bronchoconstriction, is probably related to the distribution of smooth muscle and the location of M_3 receptors within the airways.

We have discussed what is known about the distribution of smooth muscle in human airways earlier in this section, under bronchodilators. As for muscarinic receptors, in general, radioligand binding and autoradiography studies reveal that they are present in high density in the human lung. The distribution of these receptors is greatest in the large airways and least in the peripheral airways. More specifically, M_3 receptors are found in large and some peripheral airways as well as in submucosal glands (41,42). Given the distribution of these receptors, it is not surprising that a muscarinic antagonist has been shown to cause selective dilation of large, central airways when given as an aerosol (43).

E. Drugs for Systemic Delivery

Alveolar Region

One of the most important determinants for optimizing treatment outcome with drugs that are administered to the lung by inhalation, as an alternative route of delivery to the systemic circulation, is the site of deposition within the lungs. This is because the bioavailability of these drugs is dependent upon absorption of the drug across the epithelial and endothelial membranes, and absorption in the alveolar region of the lungs is probably superior to that in the larger conducting airways.

The mucosa of the lung constitutes one of the largest resorptive surfaces of the human body (i.e., approximately 75 m^2), and most of this surface area is found in the alevolar region of the lungs (16). For this reason alone, the alveolar region of the human lung is the ideal region for targeting deposition of inhaled drugs for systemic delivery. Several other features make this region the best target for systemic delivery of inhaled drugs. First, mucociliary clearance mechanisms are minimized in this region (44), so drugs remain on the mucosal surface for a longer period of time. This should enhance absorptive mechanisms. Second, this region of the lungs provides an extremely thin (0.1-μm) and vesiculated cell barrier, which further promotes absorption (16,44–46). Quantitation of individual cell size and number of vesicles reveals that in both endothelial and epithelial cells, more than 70% of the total plasma membrane is located in vesicles that may function as a transcellular shuttle for proteins (46).

F. Conclusions

We have summarized the possible targets for various classes of aerosolized drugs below. Some targets are clearer than others.

Bronchodilators: β_2 Agonists

Based on observed differences in the distribution of smooth muscle cells in patients at autopsy, some asthmatics may profit from a more diffuse deposition pattern including both large and smaller bronchi, while the optimal deposition pattern for others may be the larger bronchi.

Based on the distribution of β_2 receptors, the optimal target appears to be the smaller airways in patients with asthma.

Steroidal and Nonsteroidal Anti-Inflammatory Drugs That Target Eosinophils

Data obtained from asthma patients who have died from their asthma suggest that there may be a greater infiltrate of eosinophils in the larger airways than in the smaller airways.

Data from living subjects do not support these findings. Therefore, it is unclear where drugs should be deposited in the lungs if they are designed to target eosinophils.

Steroidal Anti-Inflammatory Drugs That Target Glucocorticosteroid Receptors

Since high concentrations of glucocorticosteroid receptor mRNA have been reported in the alveolar walls, endothelium, and smooth muscle cells of bronchial and pulmonary vessels, these may be possible targets for steroidal anti-inflammatory drugs.

Nonsteroidal Anti-Inflammatory Drugs That Target Mast Cells

The alveolar region of the lung may he a possible target, since MC_T cells are the predominant mast cell found in the lung and are found primarily in the alveolar region.

H_1 and H_3 Receptors

Since H_1 and H_3 receptors are both found primarily in bronchial smooth muscle in the human respiratory tract, this region of the lungs appears to be the best target for the delivery of H_1- and H_3-receptor antagonists.

Muscarinics and Antimuscarinics

Based on the distribution of M_3 receptors, inhaled muscarinics and antimuscarinics should be targeted to the larger central airways of patients with asthma.

Inhaled Drugs for Systemic Delivery

The alveolar region of the human lung is the ideal region for targeting deposition of inhaled drugs for systemic delivery.

VI. The Clinical Effects of Targeting

Since aerosol deposition can be targeted to several broad regions of the lungs—as a result of alterations in particle size, inspiratory flow rate, and inhalation volume—it is logical to review the clinical effects of targeting as a function of these parameters. We emphasize changes in clinical measures such as increased bronchodilatation or a reduction in bronchial reactivity. Experiments in which changes in deposition pattern are directly measured using a gamma camera are also presented. But changes in deposition pattern alone cannot predict changes in clinical effects. Ideally, the two approaches should be combined such that improvement in the clinical effect is demonstrated when deposition pattern is altered in a particular way. Results from the few studies that utilize this combination approach are also presented.

A. Altering Particle Size Distribution

Bronchodilators (β_2 Agonists)

The clinical effect of alterations in the particle size of bronchodilators has been studied by several investigators. Clay et al. (47) compared the efficacy of terbutaline aerosol composed of particles with an MMAD of 10.3, 4.6, or 1.8 μm in terms of improving pulmonary function in patients with asthma. Aerosols were generated by three different nebulizers. Eleven asthmatics inhaled a fixed volume of 700 mL at 14 breaths per second. The dose was estimated to be 2.5 mg terbutaline. All three aerosols elicited significant and similar FEV_1, FVC and peak-flow changes with respect to baseline. Nevertheless, the smallest aerosol was more potent than the other two aerosols in terms of improving the MEF_{50}, and MEF_{25}. This difference in the effect on MEF_{50} and MEF_{25} may have been due to a greater dose being deposited in the smaller airways with the 1.8-μm aerosol compared to the others. This is because Clay later showed, in a different set of patients, that 80% of the 1.8-μm aerosol particles deposited in the lung, compared to 60 and 44% of the 4.6- and 10.3-μm aerosols, respectively (48).

Other data indicate that bronchodilator particles that are ≤5.6 μm are more efficacious than larger particles. Rees et al. (49) incorporated terbutaline crystals into standard MDIs and generated polydisperse aerosols characterized by three different MMADs: 5.6, 9.1, and 13.6 μm. In 10 patients with asthma, they found that only the smallest aerosol (5.6 μm) significantly improved the FEV_1, sG_{aw}, and MEF_{50}. Since the two other aerosols had no significant bronchodilating effect, the investigators concluded that the efficacy of this bronchodilator could be enhanced if the aerosol particles were ≤5.6 μm.

Johnson et al. (50) also found that particles <5.6 μm appear to be more potent than larger particles. In that study, 8 patients with chronic, stable asthma inhaled albuterol aerosols composed of 3.3- or 7.7-μm particles. They found that the percent improvement in FEV_1 was significantly higher after inhalation of the aerosol consisting of the smaller particles compared to the aerosol with larger particles. Radiolabeling studies did not show significant differences in the ratio of peripheral-to-central deposition for the two aerosols but did show a higher total lung dose for the aerosol with the smaller particle size. This finding indicated that the 3.3-μm aerosol penetrated beyond the oropharynx to a greater extent than the 7.7-μm aerosol, and this difference in deposition fraction could explain its increased potency.

The importance of the mass of aerosol that is deposited in the lung was also shown by Persson et al. (51), who modified the mouthpiece of terbutaline Turbuhalers so that they delivered either 90, 40, or 5 μg as <5-μm particles. When pulmonary function was measured before and after administration of these three aerosols in a group of patients with asthma, the FEV_1 was least improved when the low dose (i.e., 5 μg) was delivered. The two higher doses did not differ from each other.

Ruffin et al. (52) investigated the effect of altering particle size below the 5.6-μm cutoff, as suggested by Rees (49) and others. They compared changes in pulmonary function after administering isoproterenol aerosols with MMADs of 3.3 and 1.5 μm to six asthmatics. The isoproterenol was admixed with the radioisotope ^{99m}Tc, so that the dose and distribution of each aerosol could he quantified from analyses of gamma camera lung scans obtained after inhalation of the radioaerosol. Lung distribution was quantified in terms of an inner/outer (I/O) ratio. Higher ratios indicated enhanced deposition in the larger, central airways. Radiolabeled isoproterenol was administered in increasing doses, followed by gamma scintigraphy of the lungs and pulmonary function testing. Drug administration continued until the patient complained of tremor, the heartbeat increased by more hart 40 beats per minute, or changes in the patient's FEV_1 indicated a predetermined maximum response.

I/O ratios for the 1.5-μm aerosol ranged from 2.1:1 to 3.2:1. In contrast, the I/O ratio for the 3.3-μm aerosol ranged between 3.4:1 to 8.0:1. In 3 of 6 patients, Ruffin found that the cumulative dose-response curves and the ED_{50} for the 3.3-μm aerosol were significantly shifted to the left of the 1.5-μm aerosol curves. ED_{50} is the effective dose that caused 50% of the maximum possible response. An example of this shift in the dose-response curve for one of the subjects is shown in Fig. 6.

These patients also demonstrated large differences in their I/O ratios for the two aerosols. The aerosol with the larger particles resulted in higher I/O

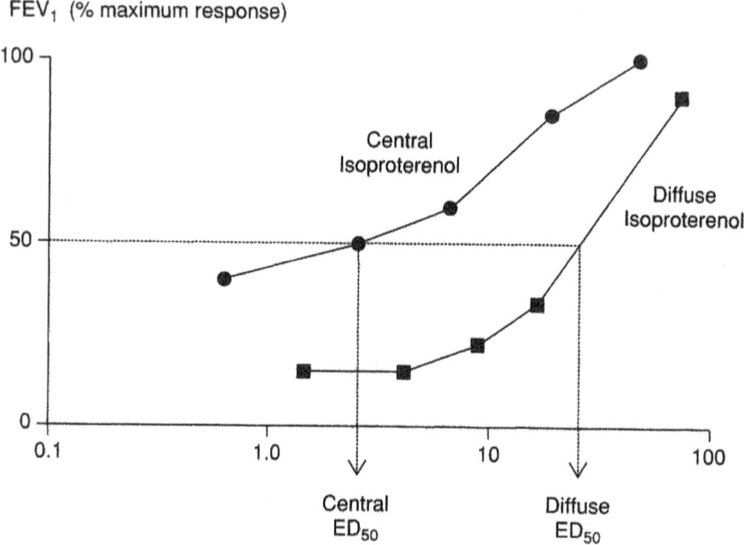

Figure 6 Cumulative right lung isoproterenol dose (μg) after inhalation of 1.5- and 3.3-μm aerosols. (From Ref. 52.)

ratios, indicating a more central deposition pattern compared to the aerosol with smaller particles. These results suggested that the 3.3-μm aerosol was more potent than the 1.5-μm aerosol in terms of bronchodilatation in these three patients, and this change in potency appeared to be related to a difference in the site of deposition for the two aerosols. In the other three patients, there was little difference in the I/O ratio or the FEV_1 response for the two aerosols.

Patel and coworkers (53) used a spinning-top generator to manufacture monodisperse isoproterenol aerosol composed of 2.5- and 5-μm particles. In patients with mild asthma, dose-response curves for all lung function parameters were shifted to the left for the aerosol with the 2.5-μm particles compared to that with the 5-μm particles, indicating a higher potency for the former aerosol. The authors concluded that this increase in potency could be due to an increase in the dose of drug delivered. These results were similar to those of Ruffin et al. (52) and Johnson et al. (50), because they also indicated that bronchodilator particles appear to be most effective when formulated in the 2.5- to 3.5-μm range.

In contrast to these findings, Mitchell et al. (54) found that altering particle size below ≤5.6 μm did not change the bronchodilator effect. They generated 1.4- and 5.5-μm salbutamol aerosols using two different nebulizers. Deposition fraction within the lung periphery was quantified by radiolabeling the aerosols and quantifying deposition with a gamma camera. In 8 patients with chronic severe but stable asthma, the authors found that peripheral lung deposition was similar for both aerosols (i e., 60%). Mean increases in FEV_1 were also similar for the two aerosols.

Hultquist et al. (55) reported similar results. They compared the efficacy of 1.5- and 4.8-μm bronchodilator particles generated by two different nebulizers and could not show an advantage for the smaller aerosol. Sixteen patients with chronic, moderately severe but stable asthma inhaled the two aerosols. Neither the cumulative FEV_1 dose-response curves nor parameters for gas exchange showed significant differences.

The data on the relationship between alterations in particle size and the clinical efficacy of β_2-aerosols are summarized in Table 9. From this table, it is clear that, for a β_2-agonist aerosol, most studies indicate that particles should be ≤5.6 μm. Some studies indicate that the actual particle size below 5.6 μm is irrelevant (54,55). Other researchers found that differences in the particle size below 5.6 μm affected the degree of bronchodilatation (47,50,52,53).

These contradictions may be due to the experimental design of the studies. Most of the studies used different nebulizers to generate smaller or larger polydisperse aerosols. However, differentiating between the effects of different polydisperse aerosols can be confounded by considerable overlap in size distributions and the possibility that total and regional deposition for these aerosols may not be different. Another confounder could be differences in nebulizer output. It is well known that different types of nebulizer have different mass outputs (56,57). Thus, a nebulizer that generates an aerosol composed of large particles but has a high mass output could be more efficacious than a nebulizer that produces an aerosol with smaller particles and a lower output. This is especially important in comparing the effects of an aerosolized drug such as a bronchodilator, which has a broad window of dosing efficacy.

Zanen and coworkers (58) avoided the above confounders by generating

Table 9 Summary of the Relationship Between the Potency of β_2-Aerosols and Particle Size

Reference	MMAD of aerosol (μm)			Most potent Aerosol
52	1.5	3.3		3.3
49	5.6	9.1	13.6	5.6
47	1.8	4.6	10.3	1.8
54	1.4	5.5		No difference
50	3.3	7.7		3.3
53	2.5	5		2.5
55	1.5	4.8		No difference

β_2-aerosols that were monodisperse and by controlling the inhaled dose and breathing maneuvers. Aerosols were generated by a spinning-top generator, while the particle size distribution and the aerosol mass were constantly monitored. In one experiment, eight stable asthmatics inhaled three salbutamol aerosols composed of 1-, 2.8-, or 5-μm particles and a placebo. They inhaled doses of 5-, 10-, 20-, and 40-μg salbutamol with each aerosol, and after each dose, the improvement in lung function was quantified. The findings of Zanen et al. are summarized in Table 10.

The resulting dose-response curves showed a clear difference from placebo for all three of the salbutamol aerosols. For measurements of FEV_1, MEF_{75}, MEF_{50}, and MEF_{25}, the 2.8-μm aerosol was significantly more efficacious than the 5-μm aerosol. For measurements of PEF, the 2.8-μm aerosol was significantly more efficacious than the 1.5-μm aerosol. These results suggest that, in mild asthmatics, the particle size of choice for a β_2-aerosol should be close to 2.8 μm. These results are similar to the previous findings of Ruffin et al. (52), Johnson et al. (50), and Patel et al. (53).

Corticosteroids

The reformulation of beclomethasone MDI formulations using HFA propellants has provided us with some insight as to the relationship between the particle size and the aerosol velocity of corticosteroids delivered by MDI and their clinical effect. Particles generated from an HFA-MDI containing the newly formulated beclomethasone aerosol primarily are composed of 1.1- to 2.1-μm particles, compared to 3.3- to 4.7-μm particles generated by the older CFC-MDI (59). At the same time,

Table 10 Mean (SD) Improvement in Lung Function (Percent Predicted) After Inhalation of Salbutamol Aerosols with Different Particle Sizes

Lung function parameter	Particle size			Significantly different aerosols
	1.5 μm	2.8 μm	5 μm	
VC	7 (7.8)	8.1 (9.4)	6 (8.9)	NS
R_{tot}	–27.6 (93)	–84.3 (92)	–52.7 (62.1)	NS
FVC	8.9 (5.6)	9.6 (9.3)	7.9 (6.6)	NS
FEV_1	12.8 (4.3)	14.6 (6.5)	10.1 (4)	2.8 vs. 5
MEF_{25}	12.1 (6.6)	14.9 (9.5)	9.2 (7.9)	2.8 vs. 5
MEF_{50}	15.2 (6.7)	18.5 (9.4)	12.1 (6.2)	2.8 vs. 5
MEF_{75}	17 (4.4)	21.4 (9)	14.6 (5.6)	2.8 vs. 5
PEF	9 (7.1)	15 (7)	13.1 (7.9)	2.8 vs. 1.5

Source: Ref. 58.

the velocity of the aerosol particles generated by the HFA-MDI is significantly slower than that of the CFC-MDI (59).

Such changes in particle size distribution and aerosol velocity are likely to affect the amount of drug that penetrates beyond the oropharynx and deposits in the lungs. This hypothesis was confirmed by Leach et al., who added a radiolabel to a CFC- and HFA-beclomethasone MDI and quantified lung deposition in healthy volunteers as a percent of the dose that deposited in the lungs and oropharynx combined. Deposition patterns for the two formulations are shown in Fig. 7A and B. For the HFA-MDI, 55–60% of the dose deposited in the lungs (Fig. 7B, right), while 29–33% deposited in the oropharynx. In contrast, only 4–7% of the CFC-MDI aerosol deposited in the lungs (Fig. 7A, left), while ≥90% deposited in the oropharynx (60). These differences in dose deposited for the two formulations need to be confirmed in other, independent laboratories.

A change in particle size and aerosol velocity as a result of the HFA reformulation could also lead to an alteration in the site of deposition of beclomethasone (BDP) within the lung compartment, perhaps favoring the lung periphery to a greater extent than the CFC formulation. Such a change in the site of deposition is suggested from data by Seale et al., who showed that the area under the curve (AUC) of 200 μg of the HFA formulation of BDP was similar to that of 400 μg of the CFC formulation in patients with mild to moderate asthma (61). C_{max} was higher for the HFA formulation. These results suggest that more of the HFA formulation was being absorbed into the systemic circulation compared to the CFC-formulation, perhaps because more of the HFA-formulation was depositing in the alveolar region than the CFC-formulation. These results are summarized in Table 11.

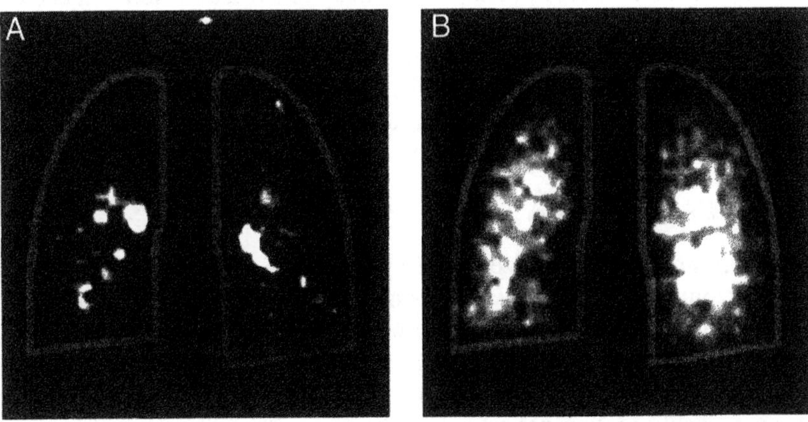

Figure 7 Lung deposition with CFC-MDI (A) and HFA-MDI (B). (From Ref. 60.)

Table 11 Summary of Pharmacokinetics for HFA-BDP and CFC-BDP

	200 μg HFA-BDP	400 μg HFA-BDP	400 μg CFC-BDP
C_{max} (pg/mL)	590	1191	410
T_{max} (h)	3	3	4
AUC (pg × h/mL)	2339	4962	2092

Source: Ref. 61.

A comparison of the therapeutic efficacy of the 800-μg/day HFA and 1500-μg/day CFC formulations of beclomethasone has shown that the two preparations have similar clinical effects (62). In that study, patients with asthma were randomized to use the HFA or CFC preparation for 12 weeks. Peak flow and FEV_1 were measured at regular intervals. Statistical analysis showed that the two formulations were equivalent in terms of improvement in these two parameters. Another study showed equivalence for the HFA formulation compared to the CFC formulation in terms of possible adverse effects—measured as acute tolerability, urinary free cortisol, and adrenal responsiveness (63).

It is not clear why half the daily dose of beclomethasone administered as an HFA formulation was not more effective than the full dose administered as the CFC formulation, since the deposited dose appears to be 7–8 times greater than the CFC formulation (60). One explanation may involve differences in the site of deposition for the two aerosols: lung parenchyma for the HFA formulation versus the conducting airways for the CFC formulation. Such a difference in the site of deposition for the two aerosols is supported by the AUC data, which indicate that the smaller particles and slower velocity associated with the HFA formulation resulted in increased absorption and loss of drug into the systemic circulation compared to the CFC formulation. If airway deposition is key to the clinical response to this drug, a peripheral deposition pattern could lead to a decrease in the effectiveness of the HFA formulation and possibly more systemic side effects, due to enhanced absorption, compared to the CFC-formulation.

Sodium Cromoglycate

Using a spinning-disk nebulizer, Godfrey et al. (64) generated 2- and 11.7-μm sodium cromoglycate particles. Approximately 30 mg of drug was inhaled by patients with exercise-induced bronchospasm (EIB). Subsequent exercise testing showed that the therapeutic effect of the 11.7-μm aerosol was no different from that of placebo. Only the smaller 2-μm aerosol was effective in reducing EIB. This is probably because not enough of the drug with the larger particles penetrated beyond the oropharynx to provide protection.

Methacholine

Schmekel et al. (65) examined the effect of altering particle size on the clinical effect of methacholine (muscarinic-receptor agonist) in eight patients with mild asthma and documented airway hyperresponsiveness to methacholine. In these experiments, two different nebulizers were used to generate and administer similar doses of methacholine as small particles (MMAD = 2 μm) or larger particles (MMAD = 9 μm). The radioisotope ^{99m}Tc was added to the methacholine solutions so that the deposition patterns of each aerosol could be quantified using gamma camera imaging technology. The specific airway conductance (sG_{aw}) was measured at baseline and immediately after each challenge to assess any changes in lung function. Analyses of the lung images showed that the methacholine aerosol composed of the larger particles deposited predominantly in the larger, central airways, whereas deposition of the aerosol with the smaller particles favored the more peripheral airways. Decreases in sG_{aw} from baseline values were also significantly different for the two aerosols in the two cases, with the most pronounced decreases associated with the aerosol composed of the larger particles and the central airway deposition pattern. These findings suggest that the pulmonary response to inhaled methacholine can be significantly augmented by targeting the aerosol to deposit in the larger, central airways, perhaps because of an increase in muscarinic receptors in that lung region.

Ipratropium Bromide

Zanen et al. (66) investigated the optimal particle size for ipratropium bromide (a muscarinic receptor antagonist). Using a protocol that was similar to the one they followed for salbutamol (see β-receptors, above), they found ipratropium bromide aerosols comprising 1.5- or 2.8-μm monodisperse particles resulted in significantly greater improvements in FEV_1, MEF_{50}, and MEF_{25} as compared with an aerosol composed of 5-μm particles. Results from that study are summarized in Table 12.

It is unknown if these findings were the result of superior targeting to the site of muscarinic receptors by the aerosols with the smaller particles or if the smaller particles were more potent because more drug penetrated beyond the oropharynx compared to the larger particles. This is because imaging of the deposition pattern for the three aerosol particles was not included in the experimental protocol.

Insulin

Pillai and colleagues (67) evaluated the importance of differences in aerosol particle size on the observed therapeutic effect of inhaled insulin in rhesus monkeys. They compared the performance of two nebulizer systems, an ultrasonic nebulizer

Table 12 Mean (SD) Improvement in Lung Function (Percent Predicted) After Inhalation of Salbutamol Aerosols with Different Particle Sizes

Lung function parameter	Particle size			Significantly different aerosols
	1.5 μm	2.8 μm	5 μm	
VC	13.6 (13)	11.5 (12.5)	7.7 (7.8)	NS
R_{tot}	−74.4 (73.2)	−114.8 (97.1)	−104.5 (135.9)	NS
FVC	12.4 (12.4)	13 (12.1)	9.4 (10.8)	NS
FEV_1	20.3 (8.7)	23.7 (12.1)	15.6 (9.8)	1.5/2.8 vs. 5
MEF_{25}	23.7 (15)	19.3 (14.7)	15.3 (12.7)	1.5/2.8 vs. 5
MEF_{50}	24.7 (10.7)	24.7 (12.1)	17.7 (10.3)	1.5/2.8 vs. 5
PEF	21 (7.2)	22 (13.2)	16.6 (12.4)	NS

Source: Ref. 66

(MMAD = 4.2 μm; GSD = 2.0) and a jet nebulizer (MMAD = 0.81 μm; GSD = 1.8), in terms of their effectiveness in lowering blood glucose levels. The mass of insulin deposited below the trachea was quantified by admixing the radioisotope ^{99m}Tc with the insulin solution to be aerosolized and imaging the lungs with a gamma camera after inhalation. The average dose of insulin that deposited in the lungs using the ultrasonic nebulizer was 0.38 U/kg body weight versus a dose of 0.14 U/kg body weight for the jet nebulizer.

Although the lung dose was higher for the ultrasonically nebulized aerosol, the bioavailability of insulin, determined from area under the insulin concentration-time curves, was lower when compared to the jet nebulizer. The efficacy of the ultrasonically nebulized aerosol in terms of lowering blood glucose levels was also less, averaging only a 40–45% decrease compared to a 50–55% decrease with the jet nebulized aerosol.

These differences in bioavailability and efficacy were probably due to differences in the site of deposition of the aerosols within the lungs. Lung images obtained after inhalation of aerosol generated by the ultrasonic nebulizer showed distinct hot spots at the carina and bronchi, suggesting significant deposition in the larger airways, whereas the jet nebulizer resulted in a uniform deposition pattern and increased deposition in the alveolar region of the lungs.

B. Altering Inspiratory Flow Rate

Sodium Cromoglycate

Laube et al. (68) conducted a study to determine the effect of altering inspiratory flow rate on the efficacy of sodium cromoglycate (SC). On two different days, eight patients with asthma underwent an allergen challenge 30 min after pretreatment with SC that was generated by an MDI into a large-volume holding chamber and inspired fast (70 L/min) or slowly (30 L/min). MMAD averaged 4.3 μm (GSD = 1.7) for aerosol that was inhaled slowly. Percent decreases in FEV_1 at a common dose of allergen on the two challenge days were compared. Figure 8 shows the allergen-induced decreases in FEV_1 after inspiring drug using the two breathing maneuvers.

FEV_1, at a common dose of allergen, decreased an average of 5.4% after slow inhalation of SC versus a decrease of 12.6% after faster inhalation of the drug, indicating an increase in the protective effect of SC when inhaled at the slower rate (~30 L/min). Since these averages may have been affected by the extreme data, the protective effect of inhaling SC at the slower rate may be more clinically important in some patients than in others.

Distribution of SC within the lungs was quantified in 7 of 8 patients who inhaled SC admixed with the radioisotope ^{99m}Tc during the slow or faster inspiratory maneuvers. Distribution was quantified in terms of (1) an I/O ratio, an indicator of deposition in the larger, central airways (inner zone) versus the

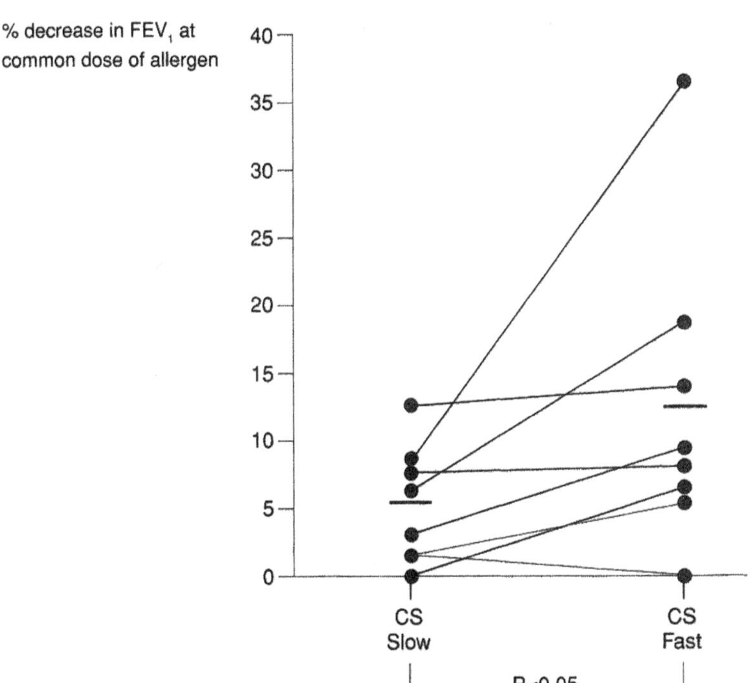

Figure 8 Mean percent decrease in FEV_1 at common dose of allergen after pretreatment with slow inspiration of SC versus faster inspiration. (From Ref. 68.)

smaller airways and alveolar region (outer zone), and (2) skew, an indicator of distribution uniformity.

Mean I/O ratios and skew values were also significantly decreased after slow inspiration of SC, indicating that the slow inspiratory maneuver distributed the drug more uniformly throughout the lungs. Differences in the decreases in FEV_1 and skew values for the two breathing maneuvers were significantly correlated, suggesting that protection against the allergen exposure was enhanced when distribution uniformity of the drug within the lungs was also enhanced (Fig. 9).

Histamine

Anderson et al. examined the effect of altering inspiratory flow rate on the regional lung deposition of inert particles and on the pulmonary response to histamine aerosol. In one experiment, six healthy nonsmokers inhaled 6-μm Teflon particles that were labeled with the radioisotope indium 111 (^{111}In) at 0.04 and 0.5 L/s. Tracheobronchial deposition averaged 50% after inhaling at 0.04 L/s, compared to 30% after inhaling at 0.5 L/s. Alveolar deposition increased from 1 to 28% with the lower inspiratory rate (69).

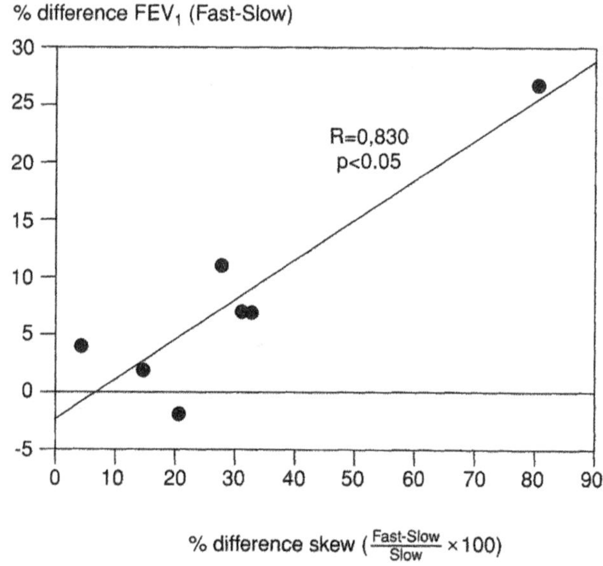

Figure 9 Linear regression analysis for percent difference in decrease in FEV_1 with slow versus faster inhalation of SC and percent difference in the skew values for the two inspiratory maneuvers. (From Ref. 68.)

In another experiment, the investigators instructed volunteers to inhale histamine aerosol that was generated by jet nebulizer at 0.6 and 0.055 L/s. They reported that airway resistance was increased after the slower inhalation maneuver (i.e., 2.83 × baseline) compared to that recorded after the faster inhalation (i.e., 2.23 × baseline) (p <0.05). Based on their first experiment, the investigators concluded that the enhanced potency in histamine aerosol, observed during the slower inhalation maneuver, could be due to reduced oropharyngeal deposition and increased penetration of drug into the lungs (70).

Methacholine

Laube et at. (18) examined the effect of altering inspiratory flow rate on the pulmonary response to inhaled methacholine. On two study visits, nine patients with asthma inhaled a saline solution containing the radioisotope ^{99m}Tc that was generated by jet nebulizer (MMAD = 1.5 μm; GSD = 2.47) during a slow inspiratory maneuver (12 L/min) or faster inspiration (60 L/min). Distribution of the radioaerosol after each inspiratory maneuver was quantified from gamma camera images of the lungs. The faster inspiration resulted in a more central deposition pattern with hot spots of radioactivity. After the slower inhalation, aerosol deposition was more uniform with greater penetration to the lung periphery (see Fig. 5A and B). The deposition pattern was characterized in terms of the inner outer zone ratio (I/O ratio) and skew, as described above under sodium cromoglycate.

On two additional visits, the same patients inhaled increasing concentrations of methacholine aerosol during the same fast or slower inspiratory maneuvers until they demonstrated a 20% decrease in their FEV_1 (PD_{20}). Methacholine aerosol was generated by the same jet nebulizer used to generate the radioaerosol. I/O ratios and skew values were significantly higher after fast inhalations of the radioaerosol (averaging 2.91 and 1.12, respectively), compared to the slower inhalations (averaging 1.84 and 0.74, respectively). This indicated enhanced deposition of the radioaerosol in the larger, central airways with the faster inspirations. Methacholine PD_{20} averaged 5.9 cumulative units when the drug was inhaled rapidly versus 15.7 cumulative units with the slower breathing maneuver, indicating an increase in the potency of methacholine when it was inhaled at faster inspirations. Since these averages may have been affected by the extreme data, the observed increase in potency at 60 L/min may be more clinically important in some patients than in others.

Differences in the values of skew following the two breathing maneuvers were inversely correlated with differences in methacholine PD_{20}, such that PD_{20} decreased as skew values, or deposition heterogeneity, increased (Fig. 10).

These studies extend the work of Schmekel et al. (65) who reported similar results with methacholine that was targeted to the larger, central airways or

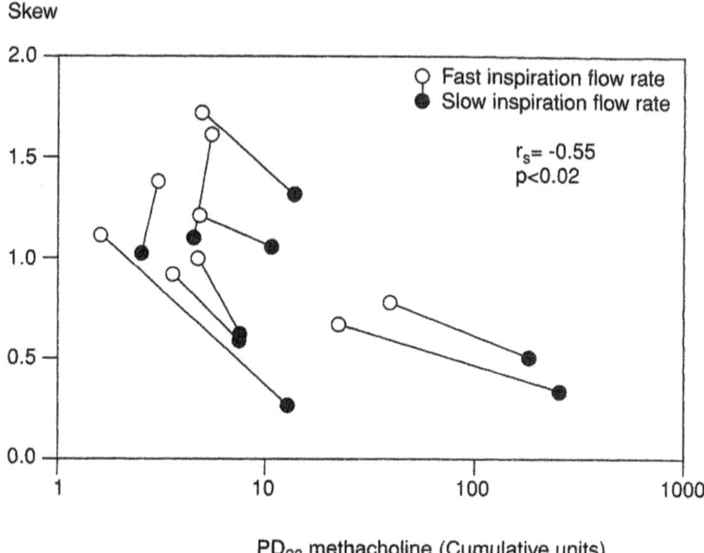

Figure 10 Spearman rank correlation analysis of the differences in skew values and PD_{20} values for methacholine after rapid and slow inhalation. (From Ref. 18.)

lung periphery by manipulating aerosol particle size. Together, these two studies clearly show that the site of deposition within the lungs significantly affects the pulmonary response to inhaled drugs that affect muscarinic receptors and/or airway smooth muscle, with the larger, central airways being the more sensitive target for this class of drugs.

C. Altering Inhalation Volume

Insulin

Farr and coworkers studied the effects of altering lung volume on the effectiveness of inhaled insulin in terms of lowering blood glucose levels. They found that a deep inhalation maneuver (inhaled volume 4.1 L) led to a rapid increase in insulin plasma levels (T_{max} 7 ± 6 min) and high C_{max} values (30 ± 11 U/mL). Subcutaneous injection in the same volunteers showed considerably slower absorption. When insulin was inhaled using a shallow maneuver (inhaled volume 2.2 L), the pharmacokinetic profile resembled that of the subcutaneous injection (71). It is not known how the larger inhalation volume affected the pulmonary absorption of insulin. However, previous studies of the effect of inhalation volume on particle deposition indicate that larger inhalation volumes result in an increase in the total amount of drug deposited (see "Factors That Affect Regional Aerosol Deposition," above).

Laube et al. (72) quantified the regional deposition pattern of radiolabeled insulin diluent aerosol during a slow, deep breathing maneuver in seven patients with type II diabetes, using gamma camera imaging technology. Then, they related the deposition pattern, expressed as the ratio of aerosol particles deposited in apical versus basal regions of the lung (A/B ratio), to the maximum decrease in blood glucose levels for each of the patients. They found that both A/B ratio (range = 0.5–1.2) and maximum percent decrease in glucose (range = 27–70%) varied considerably between patients. They also noted that these two parameters were significantly related, such that lower A/B ratios (indicating increased deposition of aerosol in the lung base) were associated with greater percent decreases in blood glucose levels. This relationship is shown in Fig. 11.

These results suggest that, in patients with type II diabetes, enhanced distribution of insulin to the base of the lungs may lower glucose levels to a greater extent than distribution that favors the lung apex. One explanation for this finding could involve the larger surface area for absorption in the base of the lungs. Another explanation could involve the greater total blood flow per unit volume in the base of the lung compared to the apices. Both explanations

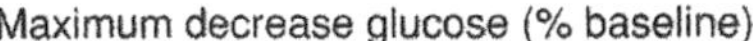

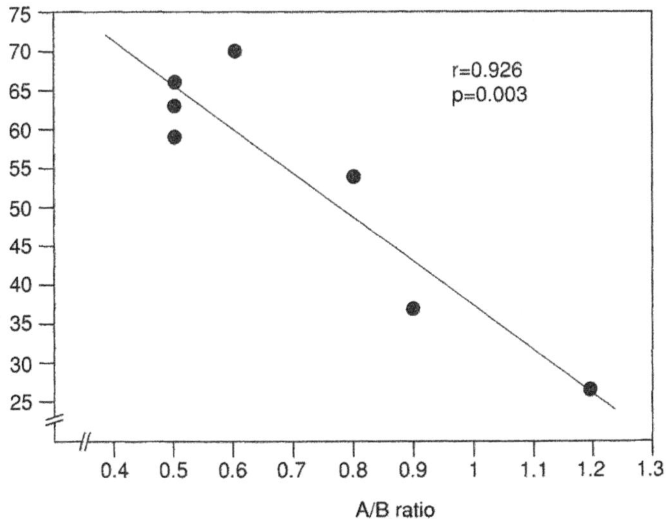

Figure 11 Linear regression analysis of maximum percent decrease in glucose after inhalation of insulin aerosol and A:B ratios after radioaerosol inhalation. (From Ref. 72.)

could increase the bioavailability of insulin by leading to a more rapid transfer of insulin to the blood.

D. Using a Spacer with a Metered-Dose Inhaler

Reducing Drug Losses in the Oropharynx

It is well known that only about 10–20% of the dose that is generated by a metered-dose inhaler (MDI) penetrates beyond the oropharynx and deposits in the lungs (5, 73–75). This is because there is not enough time for the propellant to evaporate, so particle size is large, and there is only a small distance between the patients's mouth and the aerosol actuator, so aerosol velocity remains high. Both these features enhance impaction and loss of aerosolized medications in the oropharynx, as discussed previously in this chapter. One way to slow down the high initial droplet speed and allow liquid propellant to evaporate is to actuate the aerosol into a holding chamber or spacer device.

Currently many such devices are available. In general, the use of these devices leads to less deposition of drug in the oropharynx, but it does not necessarily improve lung deposition. This is because a large percentage of the drug deposits in the spacer. A few examples of how spacers reduce oropharyngeal deposition and their effect on lung deposition are provided below.

Dolovich et al. reported that oropharyngeal deposition was reduced from 65% of the emitted dose to 6.5% in a group of patients with varying degrees of airflow obstruction who inhaled aerosol from an MDI alone and an MDI used in combination with the small volume Aerochamber spacer, respectively. Total and regional lung deposition fractions were unaltered by the addition of the spacer (76).

Newman studied the effect of using a larger-volume spacer (Nebuhaler) in combination with an MDI. In nine patients with obstructive lung disease, they found that oropharyngeal deposition decreased from 80.9% with the MDI alone to 16.5% with the MDI/spacer. Lung deposition increased from 8.7 to 20.9% (77).

The reduction in oropharyngeal deposition by using a spacer with an MDI is especially important in the case of inhaled steroids because it also reduces the incidence of candidiasis. Thus, using a spacer with an inhaled steroid is a good example of how the therapeutic index of this class of drug can be enhanced. Nevertheless, there is little evidence to suggest that spacers improve the clinical outcome of inhaled medications. For more details about spacers, we refer the reader to Chap. 12.

E. Using Dry-Powder Inhaler Aerosols

Dry-powder inhalers (DPIs) lack the actuation/inhalation coordination problems of MDIs and are therefore easier to use. The powder formulation is usually composed of a blend of lactose and micronized drug. The lactose acts as a bulking agent and prevents the micronized drug from agglomerating. During inhalation, the inspired air aerosolizes the blend and separates the drug crystals from the lactose.

In general, DPIs show lower total lung deposition percentages than MDIs. Melchor et al. (75) radiolabeled pure salbutamol and incorporated it into both an MDI and a DPI and then measured total lung deposition as a percentage of the nominal dose. In healthy volunteers, 22% of the MDI dose was detected in the lungs, compared to 12.5% of the DPI dose. In asthmatics, these figures were 18.2 and 11.4%, respectively. Others have reported similar results (78).

Although total lung deposition is usually less with a DPI versus an MDI, alveolar deposition sometimes appears to be enhanced with the DPI. This was shown by Thorsson et al., who measured the systemic uptake of budesonide that was inhaled by healthy volunteers from a Turbuhaler DPI and an MDI. They reported that the systemic availability was 32% for the Turbuhaler and 15% for the MDI (79). This was also shown for terbutaline delivered by the Turbuhaler DPI (80).

The efficiency of DPI devices, in terms of lung and alveolar deposition, varies with the type of inhaler, the drug formulation, and the inspiratory flow rate (81). The effect of these factors are discussed briefly in the following paragraphs.

Type of Inhaler

Deposition is dependent on the type of DPI. This has been shown by Vidgren et al., who manufactured a radiolabeled sodium cromoglycate/lactose blend and compared deposition of this "standard" formulation when inhaled from an ISF inhaler and a Rotahaler. They found that deposition within healthy lungs was 16.4% for the ISF inhaler and 6.2% with the Rotahaler (82). Similar findings have been reported by Broadhead (83).

Drug Formulation

Other experiments have shown that the drug formulation affects the aerosol particle size distribution of a powder. Using the same DPI (i.e., Easyhaler), Steckel et al. reported that 19.9% of the mass of beclomethasone aerosol was <6.4 μm, while 36% of the mass of salbutamol was <6.4 μm (84).

Inspiratory Flow Rate

In general, efficient delivery of powder from a DPI depends on the inspiratory flow rate generated by the patient. This requires that the patient overcome a certain amount of resistance inherent in the DPI. Clark et al. determined the resistance of several DPIs; their data are depicted in Table 13 (85). In addition, Ross

Table 13 Resistance of Six Commercial DPIs

Device	Resistance ($cmH_2O^{1/2}$/L/min)
Rotahaler	0.040
Spinhaler	0.051
ISF inhaler	0.055
Diskhaler	0.067
Turbuhaler	0.100
Inhalator	0.180

Source: Ref. 85.

et al. also showed that an increase in the flow through a DPI inhaler leads to a reduction in the MMAD and an increase in the mass <5 μm (86).

Bronchodilators

The clinical effects of varying inspiratory flow rate or drug formulation for a bronchodilator delivered by a DPI delivery system have been studied by a few investigators. Engel et al. taught patients with asthma to inhale at increasing peak flow rates through a Turbuhaler (87). They found that the highest flow of 84 L/min led to the release of 86% of a 5-mg terbutaline dose, whereas the lowest flow of 34 L/min resulted in the release of only 58% of the same dose. Nevertheless, no significant differences in terms of bronchodilatation or side effects were reported. Zanen et al. reported similar results. They found equivalent bronchodilator effects when patients inhaled a salbutamol/lactose blend from an ISF inhaler at 40 or 80 L/min (88).

Varying the drug formulation may affect the clinical response. Nielsen and coworkers compared absolute changes in FEV_1 in 16 children with exercise-induced asthma, who inhaled a formoterol/lactose blend (instead of salbutamol/lactose), generated by an Aerolizer inhaler, prior to exercise challenges at 3 and 12 h. Patients inhaled drug at different inspiratory flow rates (60 versus 120 L/min) on two different study days (89). The investigators reported that the effect of the formoterol was dependent on the inspiratory flow rate with the lower flow rate resulting in a reduced clinical response compared to the higher flow rate. They attributed this difference to a reduction in the fine particle fraction when the aerosol was inhaled at the lower flow rate.

These experiments were based on changing the peak flow through the inhaler. However, it has recently become clear that peak flow may not be the best parameter to measure. Both de Boer et al. and Everard et al. have shown that the rise in flow (i.e., the acceleration in flow rate) through the inhaler just after the start of inspiration may be a better parameter to measure. Using a Pulmicort 200

Turbuhaler DPI, de Boer et al. showed that an increase of 0.5 L/s^2 produced a fine particle fraction of approximately 20%, while a rise of 12 L/s^2 led to a fine particle fraction of approximately 50%. The latter results were independent of the peak flow reached, which varied between 40 and 60 L/min (90). These data have been confirmed by Everard et al. who used a 400-μg budesonide Turbuhaler DPI (91).

F. Using a Nebulizer

Particle Size

It is well known that the particle size distribution of aerosols generated by various nebulizers differs widely. For more information on nebulizers and particle size, we refer the reader to Chap. 8. It should not be surprising that these differences in particle size also affect deposition within the lung. Matthys et al. compared several nebulizers and reported a wide range of MMADs, with the smallest being 2.8 μm and the largest 24 μm. Radiolabeled saline was administered to 10 normal subjects using these same nebulizers. Gamma camera images of the respiratory tract showed that nebulizers that generated particles with an MMAD >10–15 μm failed to deliver significant amounts of aerosol to the lungs. Most of the aerosol deposited in the extrapulmonary airways (92).

Botha et al. (93) measured the lung deposition of an aerosol containing ^{99m}Tc-labeled macro-aggregates that was generated by six different nebulizers. They reported a minimum deposition of 0.3% and a maximum of 4.2% after 3 min of nebulization.

Mass Output

Nebulizers also vary in terms of their mass output. Smith and coworkers measured the size distribution and the mass output of 23 nebulizer/compressor combinations. Like Matthys et al. (92), they found a wide range in MMADs: 2.6–16.2 μm. They also reported a broad range in mass output: minimum output was 47% of a 2.5-mL fill; maximum output was 81%. Figure 12 shows that there was a weak correlation between the percentage of particles <5 μm and the volume output over a fixed amount of time (94).

Compressor Flow

Others have investigated the effect of changing the compressor flow on the particle size distribution of various nebulizers. Using a Cirrhus nebuliser, Everard et al. increased compressor flow from 4 to 8 L/min. This resulted in decreasing the MMAD from 7 to 3.7 μm, whereas the percentage of the droplet mass <5 μm increased from 26.8 to 70.8% (95). These data are similar to those reported by

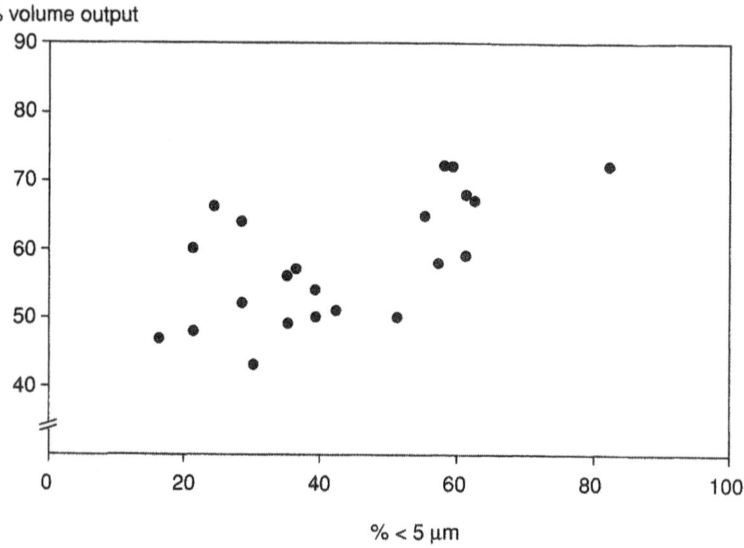

Figure 12 Correlation between percent particles <5 μm and percent volume output for 23 nebulizer systems. (Adapted from Ref. 94.)

Newman et al., who demonstrated that the relationship between increasing driving flow and droplet size <5 μm is valid for many jet nebulizers (96).

Viscosity and Surface Tension

McCallion et al. studied the relationship between viscosity and surface tension and MMAD. Results from that work showed that there was no significant relationship between these parameters for jet nebulizers. They did show a weak correlation between MMAD and viscosity for ultrasonic nebulizers, such that higher viscosity values were associated with larger MMADs (97).

It is not clear how the differences in MMAD and mass output between nebulizers affect the site of deposition of aerosolized medications or if changes in deposition site affect the clinical response to various inhaled drugs. This is because nebulizers have until recently been used primarily to deliver bronchodilators, which may be less sensitive to changes in deposition site than other classes of drugs.

G. Conclusions

In this section, we have reviewed the clinical effects of altering the site of deposition of various classes of aerosolized drugs. Clinical effects have been reported in terms of changes in pulmonary function tests or bronchial reactivity to specific and nonspecific stimuli. Alterations in deposition site were accomplished by manipulating aerosol particle size, inspiratory flow rate, and lung volume at the time of inhalation. In many cases, it was not possible to directly confirm that alterations in deposition site were achieved. Nevertheless, clinical measurements were often significantly affected by manipulations of these determinants of aerosol deposition, suggesting the following preliminary conclusions. Additional studies that combine measurements of changes in clinical effects with a method for quantifying changes in deposition pattern are necessary to confirm these findings.

β_2-Agonist

Nebulizer studies and monodisperse aerosol experiments in mild asthmatics suggest that pulmonary function measurements are most improved when particle size is approx. 2.5 μm. It is not clear if these improvements are the result of targeting the larger, central airways or because of increased deposition beyond the oropharynx.

Corticosteroids

Studies with beclomethasone suggest that HFA-MDI formulations produce smaller particles than CFC-MDI formulations, which may lead to a reduction in the dosage necessary to control asthma symptoms.

Sodium Cromoglycate

Smaller particles (i.e., 2 μm) appear to be more effective in preventing EIB than larger particles (i.e., 11.7 μm). But it is not known if this is because the smaller-particle drug is better targeted to eosinophil and/or mast cell locations than the larger particle or if oropharyngeal losses are reduced.

When delivered by MDI into a large holding chamber (MMAD = 4.3 μm), inhalation at ~30 L/min appears to be more effective in preventing the acute effects of allergen challenge than inhaling drug at ~70 L/min. This clinical improvement appears to be related to targeting the drug to the smaller airways.

Histamine

When delivered by nebulizer, slow inhalation (i.e., 0.055 L/s) is more effective than faster inhalation (i.e., 0.6 L/s) in terms of increasing airway resistance; this enhanced potency could be due to increased deposition beyond the oropharynx.

Methacholine

For nebulized methacholine, two studies suggest that bronchoconstriction is enhanced when methacholine is targeted to the larger, central airways by inhaling large particles (i.e., 9 µm), or inspiring at a high flow rate (i.e., ~60 L/min).

Ipratropium bromide

In one study, 1.5- and 2.8-µm monodisperse aerosols were more effective in improving pulmonary functions than 5.0-µm particles. It is unknown if this was the result of superior targeting of the site of muscarinic receptors with the smaller particles or if the smaller particles were more potent because more drug penetrated beyond the oropharynx.

Insulin

Systemic bioavailability and the efficacy of nebulized insulin, in terms of lowering blood glucose levels, appear to be enhanced when aerosol is targeted to the alveolar region of the lungs by generating small aerosol particles.

Enhanced deposition in the base of the lungs, compared to deposition in the lung apex, also appears to increase drug efficacy.

A deep inhalation of the drug versus a shallow inhalation appears to increase the rate of absorption of insulin.

MDI/Spacer Combinations

The use of a spacer device with an MDI reduces drug losses in the oropharynx. It also reduces the adverse effects associated with inhaled steroids (i.e., candidiasis). However, it does not appear to improve the clinical response to inhaled drugs.

DPIs

The use of a DPI may result in less total drug deposited in the lungs compared to an MDI, but alveolar deposition may be enhanced. It is not known if this difference in deposition site leads to any clinical benefit.

Nebulizers

Nebulizers vary significantly in terms of their particle size and mass output. However, it is not clear how these differences effect the deposition pattern and the clinical response to various inhaled drugs, because, until recently, nebulizers have been used primarily to deliver bronchodilators, which may be less sensitive to changes in deposition site than other classes of drugs.

VII. Targeting the Lungs During Nose Breathing

Pediatricians are frequently faced with small children or babies who need to be treated with inhaled drugs. But babies (< 1-yr-old) are obligatory nose breathers and will not breathe through the mouth, while small children frequently cannot be motivated to mouth breathe or may have difficulty inhaling at high inspiratory flow rates, which appear to be necessary for proper dosing with some DPIs. For these reasons, many pediatricians have wondered if it is possible to use nose breathing for pulmonary drug delivery.

A. Modeling Nasopharyngeal Deposition

The Task Group on Lung Dynamics of the International Radiological Protection Commission (2) developed a lung/deposition model, which included a nasopharyngeal region. This region began at the anterior nares and ended with the larynx. To calculate nasopharyngeal deposition, the Task Group used the empirical equation derived by Pattle (98): $N = -0.62 + 0.475\ D^2_a F$, where N is the fraction of particles of diameter D_a which deposit in the nose during an inhalation of F L/min. They then calculated nasopharyngeal deposition at various flow rates. These data are summarized in Table 14. The data suggest that a high percentage of small particles (<3 μm) inhaled at low flows are capable of bypassing the nasopharynx.

B. Total and Regional Deposition After Nose Breathing

Experimental data on total and regional deposition during nose breathing were obtained by Heyder et al. (99) in healthy adult volunteers who inhaled monodisperse particles with increasing particle diameter through the nose at a fixed flow

Table 14 Nasopharyngeal Deposition of Unity Spheres as a Percent of Particles Entering the Nose

Tidal volume	Diameter of spheres (μm)						
	0.6	1	2	3	4	6	10
750 cm^3	0	3.6	40.6	55.2	65.4	79.9	99.2
1450 cm^3	0	27.5	52.2	66.5	77.3	92.3	100
2150 cm^3	6.8	37.1	60.7	73.6	84.4	100	100

Source: Ref. 2.

and volume. Volunteers breathed through airtight nose masks with teeth and lips closed. Fig. 13 summarizes their results.

Heyder et al. found that particles <3 μm do penetrate beyond the nose and deposit primarily in the alveolar region. However, the number of particles that bypass the nose appears to be lower than what is predicted from the model (i.e., ~20%). In addition, only about 3% of 1- to 5-μm particles deposit in the bronchial airways during nose breathing. Therefore, if one is interested in targeting those airways, it will be necessary to administer large amounts of aerosol to compensate for the losses in the nose.

The above data were obtained in healthy adult volunteers. Chua et al. (100) quantified the deposition of a polydisperse aerosol in the lungs of eight children with cystic fibrosis (median age = 10.8 years; range = 6.3–18.0 years), who breathed via the nose with a face mask and closed mouth on one occasion and via the oral route with a mouthpiece on another. Aerosol was generated by nebu-

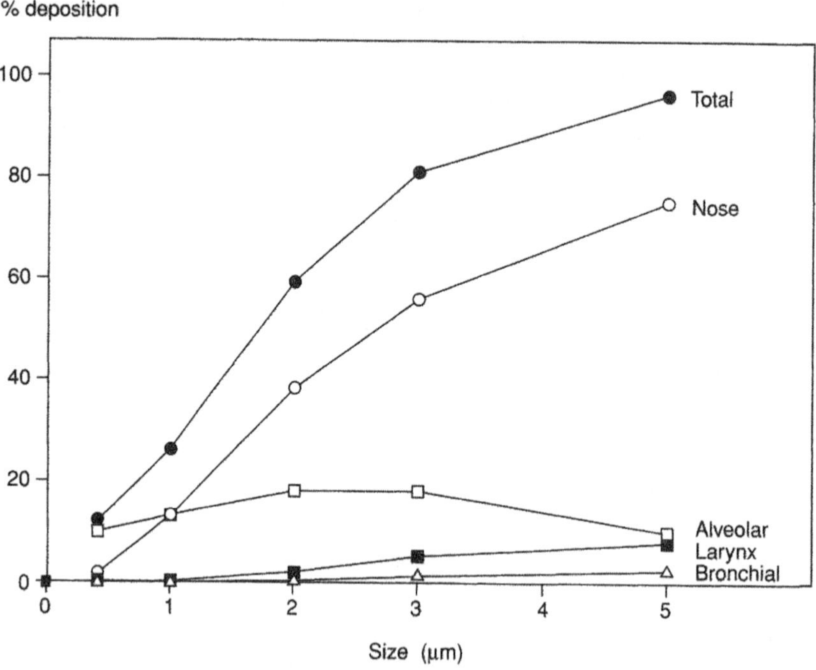

Figure 13 Total and regional deposition after nose breathing (flow rate = 250 cm^3/s; tidal volume = 500 cm^3). (Adapted from Ref. 99.)

lizer from a saline solution containing the radioisotope ^{99m}Tc (MMAD = 2.3 μm; GSD = 2.3). Planar lung images were used to record radioactivity in the lungs with both routes of administration. Activity deposited in the lungs was expressed as a percent of the activity emitted by the nebulizer. Chua et al. reported that median lung deposition for nasal inhalation was 2.7% (range = 1.6–4.4%) in these children. The median increased to 6.0% (range = 4.9–9.1%) when they breathed by mouthpiece.

C. Conclusions

In adults and children, the majority of aerosol particles that are inhaled through the nose deposit in the nose.

Targeting the bronchial airways is difficult, since only about 3% of 1- to 5-μm particles deposit in those airways during nose breathing.

Targeting the alveolar region appears more feasible, since ~20% of particles <3 μm that are inhaled at low flows bypass the nasopharynx and deposit in that region during nose breathing.

VIII. Targeting Constricted Airways

In diseased lungs, the airways are often more constricted relative to healthy lungs, so one might expect significant differences in lung deposition fraction and deposition pattern (101). The impact of constriction on aerosol deposition is discussed below. We present deposition data based on models of constricted airways as well as experimentally derived data, taken from healthy subjects in which constriction was induced by methacholine provocation, and from patients who are constricted in their baseline state.

A. Mathematical Models of Deposition in Constricted Airways

Kim et al. developed a lung model based on the Weibel-A model in which they decreased airway diameter by 25 or 40% in both the peripheral and central airways (102). Then they calculated the increases in resistance and deposition. Their results are presented in Fig. 14A and B. The upper graph represents the situation after a diameter reduction of 25%, the lower one after a 40% reduction. It is clear from the graphs that there is no simple one-to-one relationship between the increase in resistance and deposition. This is to be expected, because resistance relates to airway diameter raised to the fourth power, while deposition does not. Nevertheless, from both graphs, it is clear that the model predicts that as resistance increases, the increase in deposition will occur mainly in the larger airways (generations 0–7). Deposition in generations 8–16 will be less affected by the increase in resistance.

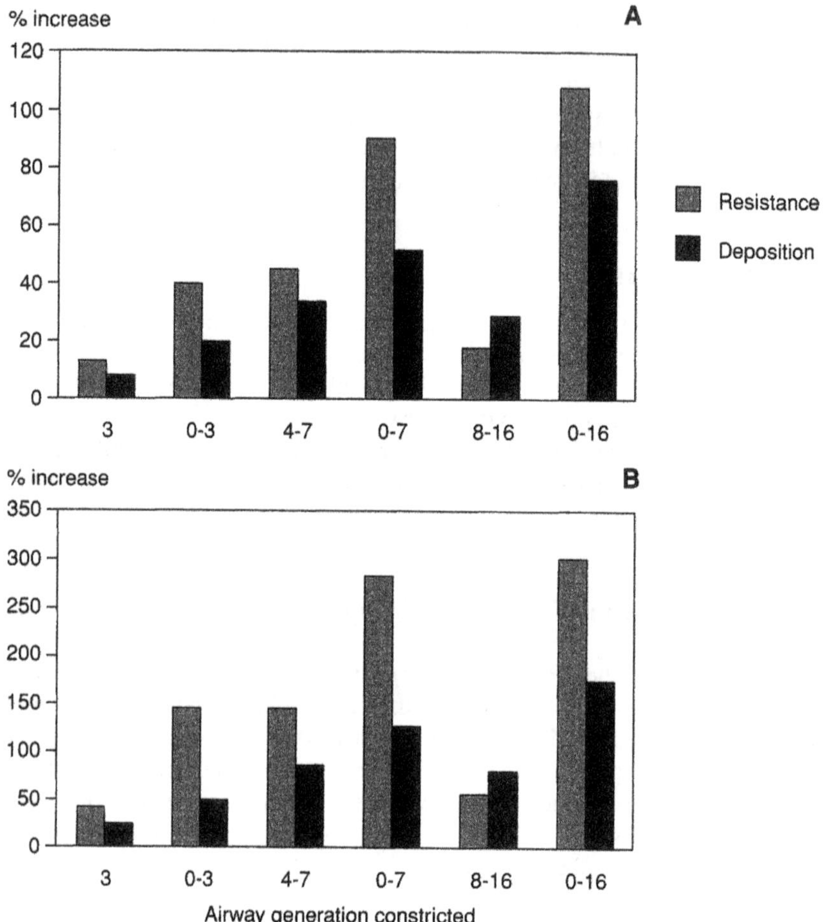

Figure 14 Percent increase in resistance and deposition of 3-μm particles after reducing airway diameter by 25% (A) and 40% (B). (From Ref. 102.)

B. Measurements of Deposition in Constricted Airways

Induced Constrictions: Healthy Subjects

Svartengren and coworkers (103) quantified deposition in eight healthy subjects under control conditions and after constriction was induced by methacholine challenge. In both situations, inspiratory flow rate was regulated at 0.5 L/s. Under control conditions, alveolar deposition of 6-μm-labeled Teflon particles labeled with ^{111}In ranged from 38 to 68% in these subjects. At the same time, alveolar deposition correlated significantly with resistance (R_{aw}) ($r = -0.72$, $p<0.05$). Methacholine-provocation increased R_{aw} by a factor of two to three in these subjects, and this resulted in a further decrease in the alveolar deposition of the Teflon particles. During induced constriction, alveolar deposition ranged from 12–24% and was no longer correlated with R_{aw}.

In another experiment by the same group, inhalation flow was reduced to 0.2 L/s. At that flow rate, R_{aw} and alveolar deposition were no longer correlated under control conditions. However, during induced constriction, alveolar deposition was still reduced when compared to control conditions (104).

Constriction in the Baseline State: Patients with COPD and Asthma

Many investigators have used gamma camera imaging of the lungs following the inhalation of a radioaerosol to identify ventilation abnormalities. For example, Lin et al. imaged the lungs of COPD patients using a ^{99m}Tc–colloid aerosol and found that the aerosol showed a patchy deposition pattern. Hyperdense and hypodense areas were found to be next to each other. In addition, penetration of the aerosol into the smaller airways was often severely limited. Lin and colleagues also showed that the lower the FEV_1/FVC ratio or maximum midexpiratory flow (MMEF), the lower the alveolar deposition, quantified as the amount of radioactivity that was present 24 h after aerosol administration ($r = 0.82$ and $r = 0.76$, respectively) (105).

In 1979, Santolicandro et al. confirmed and expanded the findings of Lin et al. (104). They reported a centrally oriented deposition pattern for 0.5–1.5 μm ^{99m}Tc–labeled particles in patients with asthma. In COPD patients, they found a patchy, nonuniform deposition pattern (106).

Anderson et al. asked five asthmatic volunteers (mean FEV_1 40% of predicted) to inhale NaCl particles ranging from 0.02–0.24 μm. Total deposition of these particles was measured as the difference between the inhaled fraction and the exhaled fraction. When they compared total deposition fraction in the asthma patients to that observed in a group of normal subjects, they found that the deposition fraction was higher in the patients with asthma. Anderson concluded that this was partly due to the patients' constricted airways, but it may also have been due to a longer residence time for particles in the asthmatic airways, since the asthmatic volunteers breathed more slowly than the healthy volunteers (6).

Schiller-Scotland et al. (107) measured total deposition of 1- to 3-μm particles in healthy and asthmatic volunteers. The results of that comparison are shown in Fig. 15. Although deposition fraction for the two groups was different when 1- and 2-μm particles were inhaled, there was no difference in deposition fraction for 3-μm particles (inspiratory flow = 250 mL/s; no breath-holding). A second finding was that the deposition of 1-μm particles was inversely correlated to the FEV_1/IVC ratio and to the MEF_{50} values. These correlations could

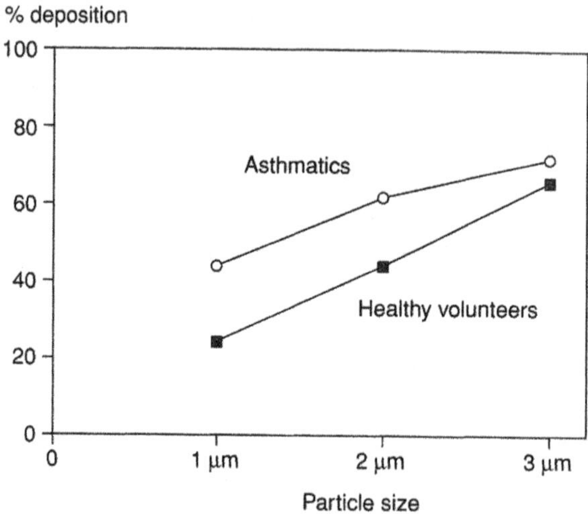

Figure 15 Total airway deposition of nonhygroscopic particles in healthy and asthmatic subjects. (Adapted from Ref. 107.)

not be demonstrated for the larger particles. When the experiments were repeated with the addition of a 6-s breath-hold, the differences in deposition fraction for the 1- and 2-µm particles disappeared, probably as the result of the increase in residence time.

Greening et al. (108) further examined the possibility that the deposition pattern of inhaled aerosols can be related to the degree of airway constriction. They asked a group of normal subjects and a group of patients with varying degrees of chronic airflow obstruction to inhale a 1.2-µm aerosol labeled with ^{99m}Tc. Afterward, the deposition pattern within the lungs was quantified by gamma camera and expressed in terms of a penetration index, with a higher index indicating greater deposition in the lung periphery. They found that this index was significantly correlated to FEV_1%predicted ($r=0.91$, $p<0.001$), such that lower indices were associated with lower FEV_1 values. In addition, the index was correlated to the residual volume ($r=-0.88$, $p<0.001$), such that high RV values were associated with lower indices. Similar findings were later reported for 1- and 3.6-µm particles and inhaled dry powders (109–111).

Constriction in the Baseline State: Patients with Cystic Fibrosis

Laube et al. administered a ^{99m}Tc-labeled aerosol (MMAD = 1.12 µm; GSD = 2.04), generated by a jet nebulizer, on two different study days to five patients with cystic fibrosis (CF) who had a mean FEV_1 of 35% of predicted (112). Distribution of the aerosol within the lung compartment was quantified from gamma camera scans of the lungs following aerosol inhalation and was expressed in terms of skew (an indicator of distribution uniformity). Gamma camera scans for the 2 study days are shown in Fig. 16.

Skew values for the CF group averaged 0.95 and 0.80 for the 2 study days, respectively, which were significantly higher than the average skew values of 0.39, previously measured in nine normal subjects. Images that were obtained on the 2 study days in the CF group were highly reproducible for each of the patients because the degree of airways obstruction at the time of aerosol inhalation

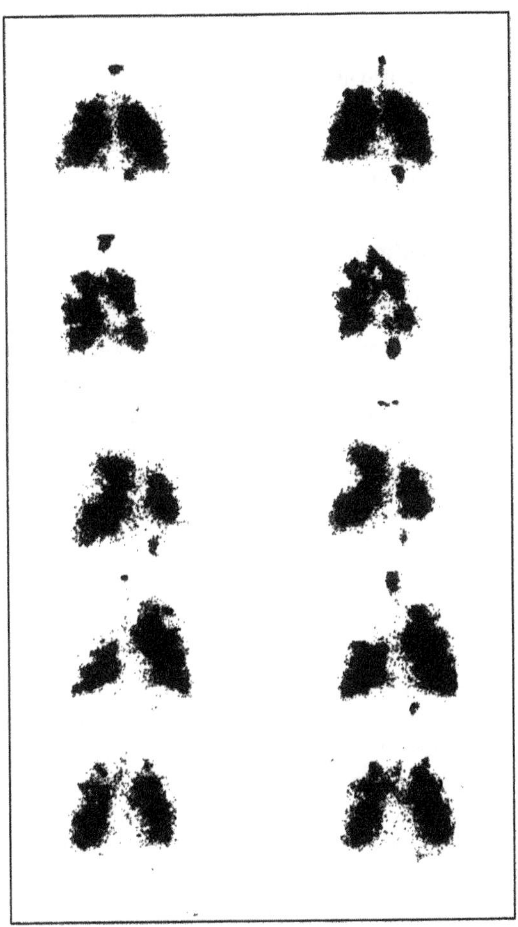

Figure 16 Images of cystic fibrosis patients. (From Ref. 112.)

was well matched and other factors known to affect deposition, such as inspiratory flow rate and aerosol particle size, were also controlled.

Anderson et al. (113) administered 70-cm^3 boluses of 1-μm monodisperse particles to 11 normal volunteers and 11 patients with cystic fibrosis. In measuring the spreading of the bolus at expiration and particle deposition, they found that bolus spreading and particle deposition were increased in the CF patients compared to the normal subjects. Among the patients with CF, pulmonary function parameters indicating obstruction (i.e., FEV_1/FVC ratios expressed as a percent of predicted) were significantly correlated with spreading and aerosol deposition.

C. Conclusions

The impact of constricted airways on aerosol deposition appears to be as follows:

Increases in central airway deposition
Reduces penetration to the smaller, peripheral airways and alveoli
Deposition pattern is patchy or nonuniform, with regions of both high and lower deposition concentration

IX. Targeting Different Age Groups

A. Deposition in Adults

As long as we remain healthy, it is likely that total deposition within the lungs does not change significantly with age. This hypothesis was partly confirmed by Bennett et al. (114), who asked 62 healthy volunteers of various ages to inhale 2 μm carnauba wax particles and measured total deposition as the difference between the inhaled and exhaled fraction. They found no influence on total deposition as a result of increasing age. Mean deposition in the group aged 18–49 years was 29%, while in subjects >60 years, it was 30%.

B. Deposition in Children

Compared to adults, three parameters are different in young children: (1) the diameter of the airways is reduced; (2) the inhalation volume is reduced; and (3) the breathing frequency is increased. Hofmann et al. (115) designed a mathematical deposition model, based on airway morphometry as reported by Phalen et al. in children ranging from 11 days to 21 years (116). A set of tidal volumes and breathing frequencies was adopted, which simulated the age-specific patterns. These sets were chosen such that they represented an activity range of low to maximal. For the small child, the model predicts that tracheobronchial deposition will be higher for all particle sizes compared to the adult. The largest differences are predicted to be between 7-month-old babies and adults. A higher tracheobronchial deposition could have a profound effect in terms of dose per airway generation. For example, Hofmann calculated that the dose of a 1-μm aerosol to the fourth airway generation of a 7-month-old baby is 2.2 times higher than that of an adult. This increase in dose was based on a small increase in deposition and a significant reduction in surface area, such that the small increase in deposition is augmented several times (117).

The model also predicts that total deposition (tracheobronchial plus pulmonary deposition) will be lower in children than in adults. Experimentally derived data support this prediction. Tal et al. (118) quantifed the deposition of salbutamol aerosol admixed with ^{99m}Tc in the lungs of 15 children (mean age = 21 months; range = 3 months to 5 years) with airway obstruction, using gamma camera imaging technology. Aerosol was generated during one actuation of an MDI into a spacer with face mask (Aerochamber). Deposition in the lungs of the children was compared to that measured in the lungs of two healthy adults, aged 46 and 40 years. On average, 1.97% of the initial dose of salbutamol deposited in the lungs of the children, whereas 19% deposited in the lungs of the adults.

Lung deposition in children may be further reduced by administering aerosols with large particle-size characteristics. This was demonstrated by Mallol et al. (119), who studied the effect of aerosol particle size on the deposition of polydisperse aerosols in the lungs of 10 unsedated infants with cystic fibrosis who breathed via a face mask. Five infants breathed a saline aerosol with MMD = 7.7 μm (GSD = 1.6). Five other infants breathed an aerosol with MMD = 3.6 μm (GSD = 2.2). Both aerosols were generated by nebulizer and contained the radioisotope ^{99m}Tc. Deposition in the lungs was quantified with a gamma camera and expressed as a percent of the initial nebulizer dose. The amount of aerosol deposited in the lungs of the infants who breathed the larger particles averaged 0.76%, which was significantly less than the 2.0% deposited in the lungs of the infants who breathed the smaller particles. These findings illustrate that, in children as well as in adults, it is important to generate aerosols with small particles when drugs are administered by inhalation.

C. Conclusions

In healthy adults > 18 years of age, total lung deposition (tracheobronchial and pulmonary) does not appear to change with age.

Models and experimental data indicate that total deposition will be significantly reduced in babies and young children compared to older children and adults.

This difference suggests that adult doses of aerosolized medications should not be reduced when administered to babies and young children, because the dose that deposits is already significantly reduced as a result of decreased airway diameter and inhalation volume and increased breathing frequency.

For the small child compared to the adult, models predict that tracheobronchial deposition will be higher for all particle sizes, with the largest differences predicted to be between 7-month-old babies and adults. These differences need to be confirmed in vivo.

Such differences could lead to a significant increase in dose of drug on a per-airway-generation basis in the larger, central airways of babies compared to adults.

X. Summary

Inhalation therapy is currently the cornerstone of the treatment for a variety of lung diseases. Changing from oral to inhalation therapy has resulted in a significant improvement in the ratio of beneficial to adverse effects. This ratio could be further improved by (1) delivering an adequate dose of the inhaled medication to the lungs; (2) directing deposition to specific regions of the lung that contain the drug's target cells and receptors; and (3) reducing losses in those regions where the drug has little or no effect.

In this chapter, we have reviewed the state of the art in terms of what is known about how to improve total and regional delivery of various classes of aerosolized drugs to the lungs of children and adults in health and disease, with the targets being either the specific cells and receptor populations within the lung or the systemic circulation. We have also presented results from studies that have investigated the clinical effects of targeting broad regions of the lungs known to contain specific cells and receptors for different classes of inhaled drugs. Many of these studies examined the clinical effects by quantifying changes in the pulmonary response to specific drugs when the site of deposition within the lungs was presumably changed by manipulating the major determinants of aerosol deposition (i.e., particle size, inspiratory flow rate, and inhalation volume). Other studies quantified changes in deposition after altering these major determinants with gamma camera imaging technology and related deposition changes to alterations in the pulmonary response to various specific and nonspecific stimuli. However, these studies are only preliminary in nature. Further research is necessary in at least three broad areas:

First, extensive research is needed to clearly identify and map the location of specific drug receptors and cell targets within the lungs. It is likely this will require new imaging modalities as well as new aerosol-generation and delivery technologies.

Second, research is needed to quantify the clinical effect of altering the delivery of drugs to previously identified specific targets within the lungs. This will require studies that combine technologies for the quantification of the delivery of drugs to site-specific locations, with measurements of changes in the clinical response associated with alterations in deposition.

Third, research is needed that focuses on quantifying total and regional deposition of aerosolized medications in the lungs of babies and young children. This is because intervention in a disease process at the earliest time point is now considered to be critical to future clinical outcome. By understanding aerosol deposition in this age group, it will be possible to properly dose babies and young children with aerosolized medications and to develop new aerosol delivery systems for early targeting of cells associated with lung pathologies.

References

1. Fuchs NA, Sutugin AG. Aerosol Science. New York: Academic Press, 1966.
2. Task Group on Lung Dynamics. Deposition and retention models for internal dosimetry of the human respiratory tract. Health Phys 1966; 12:173–207.
3. Findeisen W. Uber das Absetzen kleiner in der Luft suspendierten Tailchen in der menslichen Lunge bei der Atmung. Pflügers Arch Ges Physiol 1935; 236:367–379.
4. Newman SP, Woodman G, Clarke SW. Deposition of carbenicillin aerosols in cystic fibrosis: effects of nebulizer system and breathing pattern. Thorax 1988; 43:318–322.
5. Newman SP, Pavia D, Morèn F, Sheahan NF, Clarke SW. Deposition of pressurised aerosols in the human respiratory tract. Thorax 1981; 36:52–55.
6. Anderson M, Svartengren M, Philipson K, Camner P. Deposition in man of particles inhaled in air or helium-oxygen mixture at different flow rates. J Aerosol Med 1990; 3:209–216.
7. Laube BL, Swift DL, Adams GK III. Single-breath deposition of jet nebulized saline aerosol. Aerosol Sci Tech 1984; 3:97–102.
8. Farr SJ, Rowe AM, Rubsamen, Taylor G. Aerosol deposition in the human lung following administration of a microprocessor controlled metered dose inhaler. Thorax 1995;50:639–644.
9. Landahl HD. On the removal of airborne droplets by the human respiratory tract: I. The lung. Bull Math Biophys 1950; 12:43–56.
10. Landahl HD, Tracewell TN, Lassen WH. On the retention of air-borne particulates in the human lung: II. Ind Hyg Occup Med 1951; 3:359–366.
11. Newman SP, Pavia D, Morèn F, Clarke SW. Improving the bronchial deposition of pressurised aerosols. Chest 1981; 80(suppl):909–911.
12. Newman SP, Pavia D, Garland N, Clarke SW. Effects of various inhalation modes on the deposition of radioactive pressurized aerosols. Eur J Respir Dis 1982; 63(suppl 119):57–65.
13. Simonsson BG. Anatomical and pathophysiological considerations in aerosol therapy. Eur Respir Dis 1982; 63(suppl 119):7–14

14. Heyder J, Armbuster L, Gebhart J, Grein E, Stahlhofen W. Total deposition of aerosol particles in the human respiratory tract for nose and mouth breathing. J Aerosol Sci 1975; 6:311–328.
15. Gerrity TR, Lee PS, Hass J, Marinelli A, Werner P, Lourenco RV. Calculated deposition of inhaled particles in the airway generations of normal subjects. J Appl Physiol 1979; 47:867–873.
16. Weibel ER. Morphometrics of the lung. In: Ferm WO, Rahn H, eds. Handbook of Physiology. Sec. 3. Respiration Washington, DC: American Physiological Society, 1964:284–307.
17. Yeh HC, Shum GM. Models of human lung airways and their application to inhaled particle deposition. Bull Math Biol 1980; 42:461–480.
18. Laube BL, Norman PS, Adams GK III. The effect of aerosol distribution on airway responsiveness to inhaled methacholine in patients with asthma. J Allergy Clin Immunol 1992; 89:510–518.
19. Pavia D, Thompson ML, Clarke SW, Shannon HS. Effect of lung function and mode of inhalation on penetration of aerosol into the human lung. Thorax 1977; 32:194–197.
20. Hossain S. Quantitative measurement of bronchial muscle in men with asthma. Am Rev Respir Dis 1973; 107:99–109.
21. Ebina S, Yaegashi H, Chiba R. Takahashi T, Motomiya M. Tanemura M. Hyperreactive site in the airways tree of asthmatic patients revealed by thickening of bronchial muscles. Am Rev Respir Dis 1990; 141:1327–1332.
22. Barnes PJ, Basbaum CB, Nadel JA, Roberts JM. Localization of β-adrenoreceptors in mammalian lung by light microscopy autoradiography. Nature 1982; 299:444–447.
23. Barnes PJ, Basbaum CB, Nadel JA. Autoradiographic localization of autonomic receptors in airway smooth muscle. Am Rev Respir Dis 1983; 127:758–762.
24. Carstairs JR, Nimmo AJ, Barnes PJ. Autoradiographic visualization of beta-adrenoreceptor subtypes in human lung. Am Rev Respir Dis 1985; 132:541–547.
25. Schleimer RP. Glucocorticosteroids: their mechanisms of action and use in allergic disease. In: Middleton E, Jr, Reed CE, Ellis EF, Adkinson NF Jr, Yunginger JW, Busse WW, eds Allergy Principles and Practice. Vol 1. Baltimore: Mosby, 1993:893–925.
26. Kay AB, Walsh GM, Moqbel R, et al. Disodium cromoglycate inhibits activation of human inflammatory cells in vitro. J Allergy Clin Immunol 1987; 80:1–8.
27. Spry CJF, Kumaraswami V, Tai P-C. The effect of nedocromil sodium on secretion from human eosinophils. Eur J Respir Dis 1986; 69(suppl 147):241–243.
28. Bruijnzeel PLB, Hamelink ML, Kok PTM, et al. Nedocromil inhibits the A23187- and opsonized zymosan-induced leukotriene formation by human eosinophils but not by human neutrophils. Br J Pharmacol 1989; 96:631–636.
29. Faul JL, Tormey VJ, Leonard C, Burke CM, Farmer J, Horne SJ, Poulter LW. Lung immnopathology in cases of sudden death. Eur Respir J 1997; 10:301–307.
30. Azzawi M, Johnston PW, Majumdar S, Kay AB, Jeffrey PK. T lymphocytes and activated eosinophils in airway mucosa in fatal asthma and cystic fibrosis. Am Rev Respir Dis 1992; 145:1477–1482.

31. Synek M, Beasley R, Frew AJ, Goulding D, Holloway L, Lampe FC, Roche WR, Holgate ST. Cellular infiltration of the airways in asthma of varying severity. Am J Respir Crit Care Med 1996; 154:224–230.
32. Hamid Q, Song Y, Kotsimbos TC, Minshall E, Bai TR, Hegele RG, Hogg JC. Inflammation of small airways in asthma. J Allergy Clin Immunol 1997; 100:44–51.
33. Carroll N, Cooke C, James A. The distribution of eosinophils and lymphocytes in the large and small airways of asthmatics. Eur Respir J 1997; 10:292–300.
34. Kraft M, Djukanovic R, Wilson S, Holgate ST, Martin RJ. Alveolar tissue inflammation in asthma. Am J Respir Crit Care Med 1996; 154:1505–1510.
35. Adcock IM, Gilbey T, Gelder CM, Chung KF, Barnes PJ. Glucocorticoid receptor localization in normal and asthmatic lung. Am J Respir Crit Care Med 1996; 154:771–782.
36. Vachier I, Chiappara G, Vignola AM, Gagliardo R, Altieri E, Terouanne B, Bousquet J, Godard P, Chanez P. Glucocorticoid receptors in bronchial epithelial cells in asthma. Am J Respir Crit Care Med 1998; 158:963–970.
37. Irani AA, Schwartz LB. Neutral proteases as indicators of human mast cell heterogeneity. In Schwartz LB, ed. Neutral Proteases of Mast Cells. Basel: Karger, 1990:146.
38. Irani AA, Schechter NM, Craig SS, et al. Two types of human mast cells that have distinct neutral protease compositions. Proc Natl Acad Sci USA 1986; 83:4464.
39. Schwartz L, Huff T. Biology of mast cells and basophils. In: Middleton E Jr, Reed CE, Ellis EF, Adkinson NF Jr, Yunginger JW, Busse WW, eds. Allergy Principles and Practice. Vol 1. Baltimore: Mosby, 1993:140–141.
40. Simons FER, Simons KJ. Antihistamines. In: Middleton E Jr, Reed CE, Ellis EF, Adkinson NF Jr, Yunginger JW, Busse WW, eds. Allergy Principles and Practice. Vol. 1. Baltimore: Mosby, 1993:856–857.
41. Joad JP, Casale TB. [3H]-quinuclidinyl benzilate binding to the human lung muscarinic receptor. Biochem Pharmacol 1988; 37:973–976.
42. Casale TB, Ecklund P. Characterization of muscarinic receptor subtypes on human peripheral lung. J Appl Physiol 1988; 65:594–600.
43. De Troyer A, Yernault JC, Rodenstein D. Effects of vagal blockade on lung mechanics in normal man. J Appl Physiol 1979; 46:217–226.
44. Byron PR. Prediction of drug residence times in regions of the human respiratory tract following aerosol inhalation. J Pharm Sci 1986; 75:433–438.
45. DeFouw D. Ultrastructural features of alveolar epithelial transport. Am Rev Respir Dis 1983; 127(suppl):S9–S13.
46. Gil J. Number and distribution of plasmalemmal vesicles in the lung. Fed Proc 1983; 42:2414–2418.
47. Clay MM, Pavia D, Clacke SW. Effect of aerosol particle size on bronchodilation with nebulised terbutaline in asthmatic subjects. Thorax 1986; 41:364–368.
48. Clay MM, Clarke SW. Effect of nebulised aerosol size on lung deposition in patients with mild asthma. Thorax 1987; 42:190–194.
49. Rees PJ, Clark TJH, Morén F. The importance of particle size in response to inhaled bronchodilators. Eur J Respir Dis 1982; 119(suppl):73–78.

50. Johnson MA, Newman SP, Bloom R, Talaee N, Clarke SW. Delivery of albuterol and ipratropium bromide from two nebulizer systems in chronic stable asthma. Chest 1989; 96:6–10.
51. Persson G, Wirén JE. The bronchodilator response from inhaled terbutaline is influenced by the mass of small particles: a study on a dry powder inhaler (Turbuhaler). Eur Respir J 1989; 2:253–256.
52. Ruffin RE, Dolovich MB, Oldenburg FA, Newhouse MT. The preferential deposition of inhaled isoproterenol and propanolol in asthmatic patients. Chest 1981; 80:904–907.
53. Patel P, Mukai D, Wilson AF. Dose-response effects of two sizes of monodisperse isoproterenol in mild asthma. Am Rev Respir Dis 1990; 141:357–360.
54. Mitchell DM, Solomon MA, Tolfree SEJ, Short M, Spiro SG. Effect of particle size of bronchodilator aerosols on the lung distribution and pulmonary function in patients with chronic asthma. Thorax 1987; 42:457–461.
55. Hultquist C, Wollmr P, Eklund G, Jonson B. Effect of inhaled terbutaline sulphate in relation to its deposition in the lungs. Pulm Pharm 1992 5:127–132.
56. Loffert DT, Ikle D, Nelson HS. A comparison of commercial jet nebulizers. Chest 1994; 106:1788–1793.
57. Smith E, Dnyer J, Kendrick AH. Comparison of twenty-three nebulizer/compressor combinations for domiciliary use. Eur J Respir 1995; 8:1214–1224.
58. Zanen P, Go TL and J-WJ Lammers. The optimal particle size for beta-adrenergic aerosols in mild asthmatics. Int J Pharm 1994; 107:211–217.
59. June D. Achieving the change: challenges and successes in the formulation of CFC-free MDIs. Eur Respir Rev 1997; 41:32–34.
60. Leach CL, Davidson PJ, Boudreau RJ. Improved airway targeting with the CFC-free HFA-beclomethasone metered dose inhaler compared with CFC-beclomethasone. Eur Respir J 1998; 12:1346–1353.
61. Scale JP, Harrison LI. Effect of changing the fine particle mass of inhaled beclomethasone dipropionate on intrapulmonary deposition and pharmacokinetics. Respir Med 998; 92(suppl A):9–15.
62. Davies RJ, Stampone P, O'Connor BJ. Hydrofluoroalkane-134a beclomethasone dipropionate extrafine aerosol provides equivalent asthma control to chlorofluorocarbon beclomethasone dipropionate at approximately half the total daily dose. Respir Med 1998; 92(suppl A):23–31.
63. Thompson PJ, Davies RJ, Young WF, Grossman AB, Donnell D. Safety of hydrofluoroalkane-134a beclomethasone dipropionate extrafine aerosol. Respir Med 1998; 92 (suppl A):33–39.
64. Godfrey S, Zeidifard E, Brown K, Bell JH. The possible site of action of sodium cromoglycate assessed by exercise challenge. Clin Sci Mol Med 1974; 46:265–272.
65. Schmekel B, Hedenström H, Kämpe M, Lagerstrand L, Stålenheim G, Wollmer P, Hedenstierna G. The bronchial response, but not the pulmonary response to inhaled methacholine is dependent on the aerosol deposition pattern. Chest 1994; 106:1781–1787.

66. Zanen P, Go TL, J-WJ Lammers. The optimal particle size for parasympathicolytic aerosols in mild asthmatics. Int J Pharm 1995; 114:111–115.
67. Pillai RS, Hughes BL, Wolff RK, Heisserman JA, Dorato MA. The effect of pulmonary-delivered insulin on blood glucose levels using two nebulizer systems. J Aerosol Med 1996; 9:227–240.
68. Laube BL, Edwards AM, Dalby RN, Creticos PS, Norman PS. The efficacy of slow versus faster inhalation of cromolyn sodium in protecting against allergen challenge in patients with asthma. J Allergy Clin Immnunol 1998; 101:475–483.
69. Anderson M, Philipson K, Svartengren M, Camner P. Human deposition and clearance of 6 μm particles inhaled with extremely low flow rate. Exp Lung Res 1995; 21:187–195.
70. Anderson M, Svartengren M, Camner P. Human tracheobronchial deposition and effect of a histamine aerosol inhaled by extremely slow inhalations. J Aerosol Sci 1999; 30:289–297.
71. Farr SJ, Gonda I, Licko V. Physiochemical and physiological factors influence the effectiveness of inhaled insulin In: Byron PR, Dalby RN, Farr SJ, eds. Respiratory Drug Delivery VI. Buffalo Grove, IL: Interpharm Press, 1998:25–33.
72. Laube BL, Benedict G, Dobs A. Time to peak insulin level, relative bioavailability and effect of site of deposition of nebulized insulin in patients with non-insulin dependent diabetes mellitus. J Aerosol Med 1998; 11:153–173.
73. Morén F. Drug deposition of pressurised inhalation aerosols. Eur J Respir Dis 1982; 63(suppl 119):51–55.
74. Biddiscombe MF, Melchor R, Mak VHF, Marriot RJ, Taylor AJ, Short MD, Spiro SG. The lung deposition of salbutamol, directly labelled with technetium-99m, delivered by pressurized metered and dry powder inhalers. Int J Pharm 1993; 91:111–121.
75. Melchor R, Biddiscombe MF, Mak VHF, Short MD, Spiro SG. Lung deposition patterns of directly labelled salbutamol in normal subjects and in patients with reversible airflow obstruction. Thorax 1993; 48:506–511.
76. Dolovich M, Ruffin R, Newhouse MT. Clinical evaluation of a simple demand inhalation MDI aerosol delivery device. Chest 1983; 84:36–41.
77. Newman SP, Millar AB, Lennard-Jones TR, Morén F, Clarke SW. Improvement of pressurized aerosol deposition with Nabuhaler spacer device. Thorax 1984; 39:935–941.
78. Zainudin BMZ, Biddiscombe M, Tolfree SEJ, Short M, Spiro SG. Comparison of bronchodilator responses and deposition patterns of salbutamol inhaled from pressurized metered dose inhaler, as dry powder inhaler and as a nebulized solution. Thorax 1990; 45:469–473.
79. Thorsson L, Edsbäcker S, Conradson T-B. Lung deposition of budesonide from Turbuhaler is twice that from a pressurized metered dose inhaler P-MDI. Eur Respir J 1994; 7:1839–1844.
80. Borgström L, Derom E, Ståhl E, Wåhlin-Boll E, Pauwels R. The inhalation device influences lung deposition and bronchodilating effect of terbutaline. Am J Respir Crit Care Med 1996; 153:1636–1640.

81. Timsina MP, Martin GP, Marriott C, Ganderton D, Yianneskis M. Drug delivery to the respiratory tract using dry powder inhalers. Int J Pharm 1994; 101:1–13.
82. Vidgren M, Kärkäinen A, Karjalainen P, Paronen P, Nuutinen J. Effect of powder inhaler design on drug deposition in the respiratory tract. Int J Pharm 1998; 42:211–216.
83. Broadhead J, Edmond Rouan SK, Rhodes CT. Dry powder inhalers: evaluation of testing methodology and effect of inhaler design. Pharm Acts Helv 1995; 70:125–131.
84. Steckel H, Muller BW. In vitro evaluation of dry powder inhalers: I. Drug deposition of commonly used devices. Int J Pharm 1997; 154:19–29.
85. Clark AR, Hollingworth AM. The relationship between powder inhaler resistance and peak inspiratory conditions in healthy volunteers-implications for in vitro testing. J Aerosol Med 1993; 6:99–110.
86. Ross DL, Schultz RK. Effect of inhalation flow rate on the dosing characteristics of dry powder inhaler and metered dose inhaler products. J Aerosol Med 1996; 9:215–226.
87. Engel T, Scharling B, Skovsted B, Heinig JH. Effects, side effects and plasma concentrations of terbutaline in adult asthmatics after inhaling from a dry powder inhaler device at different inhalation flows and volumes. Br J Clin Pharmac 1992; 33:439–444.
88. Zanen P, van Spiegel PI, van der Kolk H, Tushuizen E, Enthoven R. The effect of the inhalation flow on the performance of a dry powder inhalation system. Int J Pharm 1992; 81:199–203.
89. Nielsen KG, Skov M, Klug B, Ifversen M, Bisgaard H. Flow-dependent effect of formoterol dry-powder inhaled from the Aerosizer. Eur Respir J 1997; 10:2105–2109.
90. Boer AH de, Bolhuis GK, Gjaltema D, Hagedoorn P. Inhalation characteristics and their effects on in vitro drug delivery from dry powder inhalers. Int J Pharm 1997; 153:67–77.
91. Everard ML, Devadason SG, LE Souëf PN. Flow early in the inspiratory manoeuvre affects the aerosol particle size distribution from a Turbuhaler. Resp in Med 1997; 91:624–628.
92. Matthys H, Köhler D. Pulmonary deposition of aerosols by different mechanical devices. Respiration 1985; 48:269–276.
93. Botha AS, Houlder AE, Wade L. Comparative study of lung deposition by different models SAMJ 1994; 84:63–68.
94. Smith EC, Denyer J, Kendrick AH. Comparison of 23 nebulizer/compressor combinations for domiciliary use. Eur Respir J 1995; 8:1214–1221.
95. Everard ML, Clark AR, Milner AD. Drug delivery from jet nebulizers. Arch Dis Child 1992; 67:586–591.
96. Newman SP, Pellow PGD, Clarke SW. Droplet size distributions of nebulized aerosols for inhalation therapy. Clin Phys Physiol Meas 1986; 7:139–146.
97. McCallion ONM, Taylor KNG, Thomas M, Taylor AJ. Nebulization of fluids of different physicochemical properties with air-jet and ultrasonic nebulizers. Pharm Res 1995; 12:1682–1688.

98. Pattle RE. In: Davies CN, ed. Inhaled particles and vapours. New York: Pergamon Press, 1961.
99. Heyder J, Gebhart J, Rudolf G, Schiller CF, Stahlhofen W. Deposition of particles in the human respiratory tract in the size range 0.005–15 μm. J Aerosol Sci 1986; 17:811–825.
100. Chua HL, Collis GG, Newbury AM, Chan K, Bower GD, Sly PD, LeSouef PN. The influence of age on aerosol deposition in children with cystic fibrosis. Eur Respir J 1994; 7:2185–2191.
101. Stahlhofen W, Gebhart J, Heyder J. Biological variability of regional deposition of aerosol particles in the human respiratory tract. Am Ind Hyg Assoc J 1981; 42:348–352.
102. Kim CS, Brown LK, Lewars GC, Sackner MA. Deposition of aerosol particles and flow resistance in mathematical and experimental airway models. J Appl Physiol 1983; 55:154–163.
103. Svartengren M, Philipson K, Linnman L, Camner P. Airway resistance and deposition of partcles in the lung. Exp Lung Res 1984; 7:257–269.
104. Svartengren M, Philipson K, Linnman L, Camner P. Regional deposition of particles in human lung after induced bronchoconstriction. Exp Lung Res 1986; 10:223–233.
105. Lin MS, Goodwin DA. Pulmonary deposition of an inhaled radioaerosol on obstructive pulmonary disease. Radiology 1976; 118:645–651.
106. Santolicandro A, Giuntini C. Patterns of deposition of labelled monodisperse aerosols in obstructive lung disease. J Nucl Med All Sci 1979; 23:115–127.
107. Schiller-Scotland CF, Gebhart J, Hochrainer D, Siekmeier R. Deposition of inspired aerosol particles within the respiratory tract of patients with obstructive lung disease. Toxicol Lett 1996; 88:255–261.
108. Greening AP, Miniati M, Fazio F. Regional deposition of aerosols in health and in airways obstruction: a comparison with kryton-81m ventilation scanning. Bull Eur Physiopathol Respir 1980; 16:287–298.
109. Kim CS, Kang TC. Comparative measurement of lung deposition of inhaled fine particles in normal subject and patients with obstructive lung disease. Am J Respir Crit Care Med 1997; 115:899–905.
110. Svartengren M, Anderson M, Bylin G, Philipson KL, Camner P. Regional deposition of 3.6 μm particles and lung function in asthmatic subjects. J Appl Physiol 1991; 71:2238–2243.
111. Yania M, Hatazawa J, Ojima F, Sasaki H, Itoh M, Ido T. Deposition and clearance of inhaled ^{18}FDG powder in patients with chronic obstructive pulmonary disease. Eur Respir J 1998; 11:1342–1348.
112. Laube BL, Links JM, LaFrance ND, Wagner HN, Rosenstein BJ. Homogeneity of bronchopulmonary distribution of ^{99m}Tc aerosol in normal subjects and in cystic fibrosis patients. Chest 1989; 95:822–830.
113. Anderson P, Blanchard JD, Brain JD, Feldman HA, McNamara JC, Heyder J. Effect of cystic fibrosis on inhaled aerosol boluses. Am Rev Respir Dis 1989; 140:1317–1324.

114. Bennett WD, Zeman KL, Kim C. Variability of fine particle deposition in healthy adults: effects of age and gender. Am J Respir Crit Care Med 1996; 153:1641–1647.
115. Hofmann W, Martonen TB, Graham RC. Predicted deposition of nonhygroscopic aerosols in the human lung as a function of age. J Aerosol Med 1989; 2:49–68.
116. Phalen RF, Oldham MJ, Beaucage CB, Crocker TT, Mortensen JD. Postnatal enlargement of human tracheobronchial airways and implications for particle deposition. Anat Rec 1985; 212:368–380.
117. Hofmann W, Graham RC, Martonen TB. Human subject age and activity level: factors addressed in a biomathematical deposition program for extrapolation modeling. Health Phys 1989; 57(suppl 1):49–59.
118. Tal A, Golan H, Grauer N, Aviram M, Albin D, Quastel R. Deposition pattern of radiolabeled salbutamol inhaled from a metered-dose inhaler by means of a spacer with mask in young children with airway obstruction. J Pediatr 1996; 128:479–484.
119. Mallol J, Rattray S, Walker G, Cook D, Robertson CF. Aerosol deposition in infants with cystic fibrosis. Pediatr Pulmonol 1996; 21:276–281.

8

Nebulization

The Device and Clinical Considerations

GERALD C. SMALDONE

State University of New York
Stony Brook, New York

PETER N. LeSOUEF

University of Western Australia
Perth, Australia

I. Nebulizers and the Clinician

An intellectual blow was struck against clinical aerosol science in the 1950s and 60s with the use of aerosolized antibiotics in the intensive care unit (ICU). The emergence of resistant organisms and the failure to reduce mortality resulted in a lack of interest in aerosol therapy among infectious disease specialists, surgeons, and the founders of the developing specialty of critical care (1). For routine aerosol therapy, pulmonologists and respiratory therapists relied only on aerosolized bronchodilators, which are extremely safe and easy to use. Compared with other drugs, bronchodilators are inexpensive; therefore, the costs of bronchodilator therapy are related to salary for personnel and the purchase of delivery devices (compressors, spacers, etc). As a result, the fundamental principles of aerosol delivery and dosing for clinically relevant aerosols were not well developed or well regulated by scientists and agencies such as the Food and Drug Administration in the United States.

Aerosolized pentamidine prophylaxis in the AIDS era kindled a new interest in topical therapy to the lung. Questions of dose to the lung were raised when treatment failures were analyzed. Competition between companies using different delivery devices led to the development of new techniques for the measurement of aerosol delivery. Aerosol dose and response in the lung, as well as systemic drug delivery to the body using the lung as a portal, have become important considerations for clinical researchers. In the last decade, a new industry has emerged reflecting exponential growth in concept and practice regarding development of clinically important aerosols. Companies are actively developing drugs for aerosol therapy in pulmonary inflammatory disease, aerosolized antibiotics, and systemic therapy; clinical trials are now under way designed to demonstrate the potential for aerosolized drugs as therapy for major diseases such as asthma, bronchitis, diabetes, and osteoporosis.

Three basic factors are important in the delivery of aerosolized agents to the lung: the aerosol itself, the pathophysiology of the human respiratory tract (e.g., breathing pattern and airway geometry), and the delivery device. The purpose of this chapter is to discuss the clinical aspects of drug delivery via nebulizers. Other reviews have approached the issues of aerosol distribution and airway physiology (2,3). The present chapter attempts to provide for the practicing clinician an overview of the factors important to an understanding of drug delivery via nebulization.

II. Principles

The construction and design of nebulizers is described elsewhere (4). In essence, to generate an aerosol, energy must be imparted to the medium that contains the drug. Usually, for a nebulizer, the medium is a liquid solution. Energy is supplied by the flow of a gas (often air or oxygen) supplied by a tank or compressor. The gas enters the nebulizer under pressure and is accelerated through an orifice. High-velocity air creates a low pressure within the nebulizer, and this draws liquid through a capillary tube into the gas stream. Here, the gas and liquid phases mix under highly turbulent conditions and shear forces create droplets that are suspended in the gas and carried off by the gas flow. With the distribution modified by internal baffles, a certain percentage of the original aerosol particles leave the nebulizer to be inhaled by the patient. The rest are recycled within the device. The important observation from this qualitative description is that the flow regime, encompassing an exchange of energy within the device, is chaotic and therefore difficult to describe by principles of fluid dynamics and physics. Thus, the design and function of nebulizers is largely empirical in nature. However, based on these considerations, the performance of a nebulizer will be affected to some degree by the cohesive forces of the liquid, such as surface tension, the internal baffle design and surface area of the device, the actual flow of gas entering the device, and—depending on the design—the flow of gas through the device created by the patient's own breathing.

III. Gravimetric Measurements and the "Standing Cloud"

The simplest method for measuring nebulizer function is the gravimetric method. By weighing the nebulizer during nebulization, the output can be defined as "change in weight per unit time." This process seems simple in concept but has certain fundamental assumptions: specifically, that the change in weight is related precisely to the delivery of aerosolized drug. Based on this assumption, many investigators have characterized nebulizers quantitatively for the purposes of standardizing drug delivery (5) or compared different nebulizers before clinical trials (6). While apparently straightforward, this method suffers from uncertainty regarding actual drug delivery due to differences in the amount of evaporation between different devices.

The uncertainty in gravimetric measurements has led to the development of other techniques designed to directly assess the quantity of drug actually aerosolized. Figure 1 illustrates the "standing cloud" technique, which captures particles leaving the nebulizer and thus measures aerosolized drug directly without any assumptions regarding the vapor losses. This technique is more complex, in that an assay is required to determine the quantity of drug captured on the filter. Standard curves can be generated relating aerosolized drug to a radioactive marker, or the quantity of drug in the aerosol can be measured directly using chemical assays. Recently, the standing cloud and gravimetric techniques have been compared by simultaneously weighing neb-

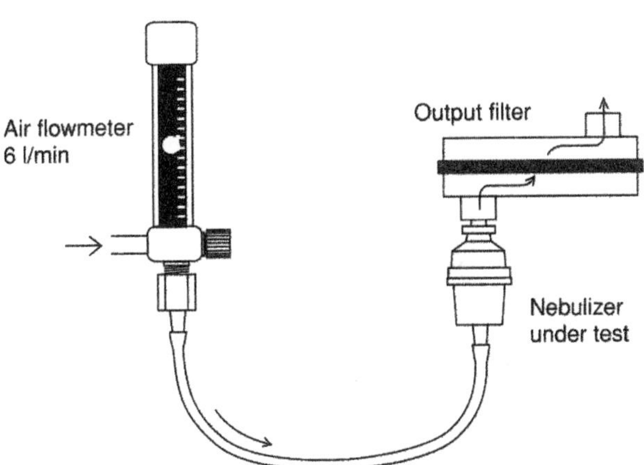

Figure 1 Sketch illustrating principles of the "standing cloud technique." Aerosol particles produced by the nebulizer are captured by the output filter, direct analysis of drug or a marker of the drug such as a radiolabel provides a quantitative estimate of nebulizer function. (Modified from Ref. 7.)

ulizers and capturing the aerosol produced (7). Figure 2 illustrates the results of that study. Aerosol particles produced during nebulization and captured on a filter were measured by radiolabel; for albuterol solution, there was a correlation between the percentage of the amount placed in the nebulizer (nebulizer charge) captured on the filter versus the percentage change in weight of the nebulizer. Surprisingly, for the conditions of the study, the slope of the correlation did not appear to be dependent on the brand of nebulizer (nine were tested) and, it did not seem to matter if the measurements were made early or late during nebulization (each data point represented a 2-min run). The slope of the line, however, was 0.62 and clearly demonstrated that there was not a one-to-one relationship between actual drug aerosolized versus change in weight. Further experiments carried out during the same study also demonstrated that the slope of the line would change significantly if the conditions of the experiment changed, particularly the nebulizer flow (Fig. 3). Thus it appears that for a large number of conventional devices, there is a correlation between production of aerosol and change in weight. On the bench, evaporation accounts for approximately 30–40% of the change in weight, and nebulizer flow and driving pressure are the most important variables that influence this relationship. The available data indicate that for screening pur-

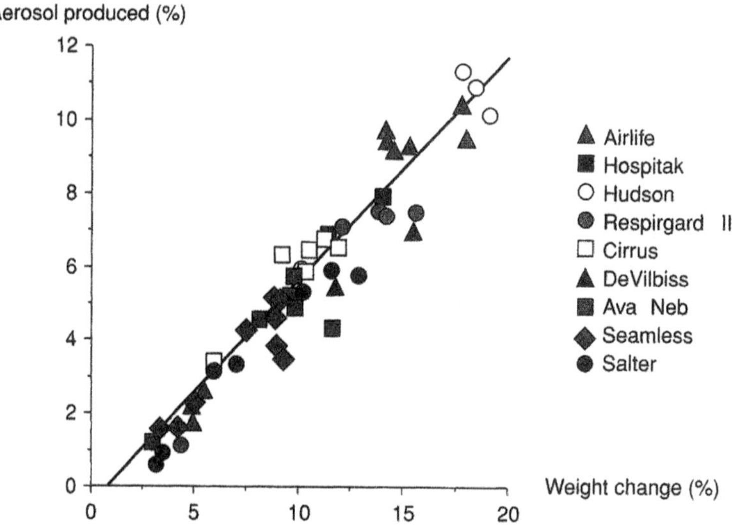

Figure 2 Relationship between aerosol measured by the standing cloud technique and weight change for a number of commercial nebulizers. There is a correlation between the two techniques ($r = 0.924$, $p < 0.0001$); slope of the line (0.619) is not equal to identity. (From Ref. 7.)

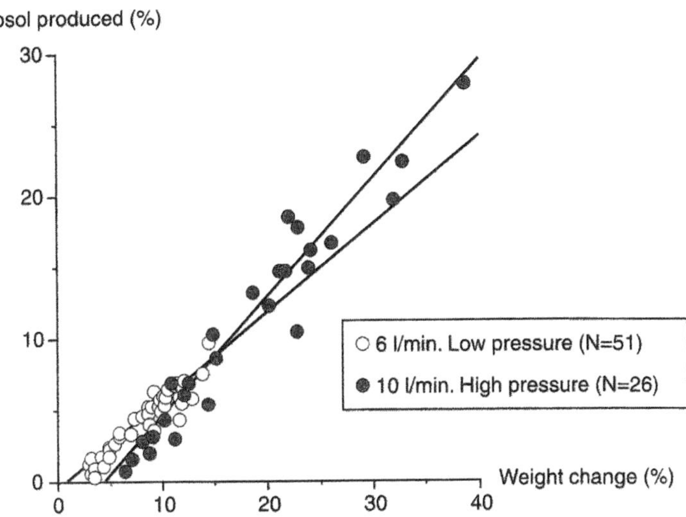

Figure 3 Influence of nebulizer flow on correlation between aerosol produced and weight change of nebulizer. (From Ref. 7.)

poses only, gravimetric analysis can be a satisfactory tool for comparing the function of conventional, continuously operating nebulizers. However, the widespread availability of drug assays and other important factors in drug delivery presented below preclude the use of gravimetric measurements in the final determination of suitable devices for clinical trials.

IV. Importance of Breathing Pattern

Inspection of Fig. 1, "the standing cloud technique," indicates that if a patient replaced the filter, it would be impossible for him or her to receive all of the nebulized particles, because the patient must exhale during continuous nebulization. Further, it is difficult to predict how many aerosol particles a patient would actually inhale depending on the source of the patient's tidal air—for example, if the patient breathed completely from the nebulizer or from a Y piece with inspiratory and expiratory valves. A common clinical scenario for describing an actual aerosol treatment is demonstrated in Fig. 4. On the left, the subject is inhaling from the nebulizer and a Y piece. This allows the flow regime within the nebulizer to remain constant as the patient breathes tidally, inhaling through the inspiratory port on the Y piece and exhaling through the expiratory limb. One-way valves control the direction of flow in the Y piece. On the right side of the figure,

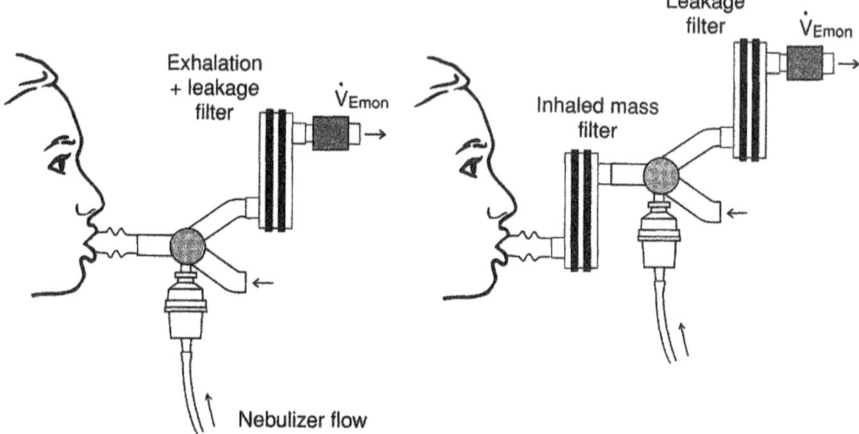

Figure 4 Cartoon depicting technique for quantification of nebulizer output and measurement of deposition. On the left, a patient inhales nebulized particles via a Y piece. The exhalation filter captures exhaled particles. On the right, the same patient performs a similar maneuver. The inhaled mass filter captures particles that would have been inhaled. Differences between filters measure deposition. Breathing pattern can be monitored using a pneumotachograph ($\dot{V}_{Emon}$ represents the sum of minute ventilation plus nebulizer flow leaving the expiratory arm of the Y piece). (From Ref. 9.)

a filter is placed just upstream to the patient's mouthpiece, allowing a direct sampling of particles that would have been inhaled during a standard treatment on the left. Figure 5 illustrates early data from two nebulizers generating aerosolized pentamidine (AeroTech II CIS-US, Bedford MA, and Respirgard II Marquest, Englewood, CO).

V. The Concept of Inhaled Mass and Lung Deposition

Aerosol terminology can be confusing, especially as applied to clinical drug delivery. This problem has been recognized and international meetings have been held to begin to determine standards and definitions (8). For example, as stated above, the amount of medication placed in the nebulizer is called the *nebulizer charge*. The volume of solution placed in the nebulizer is the *volume fill*. These definitions are important, because the amount of drug placed in the nebulizer is not the amount of drug actually deposited in the patient. Failure to recognize this fact has led to confusion regarding the "dose" of drug in clinical efficacy studies. To address this issue, the concept of *inhaled mass* has been proposed (8).

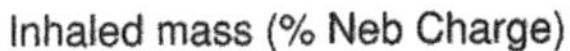

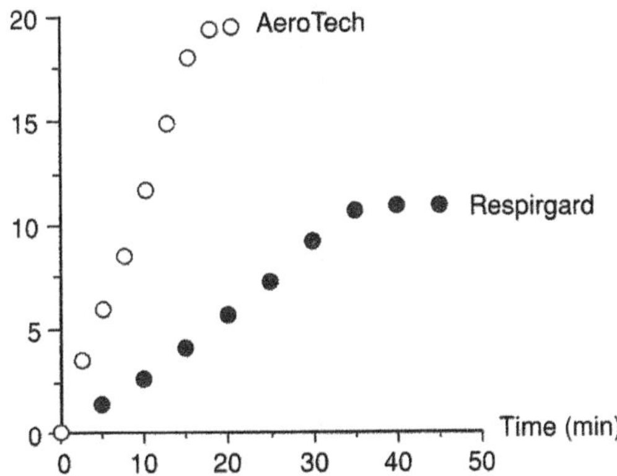

Figure 5 Inhaled mass of nebulized pentamidine as a percentage of the nebulizer charge for two commercially available nebulizers (AeroTech II CIS-US, Bedford, MA, and Respirgard II Marquest, Englewood, CO) plotted against time. (From Ref. 9.)

The actual amount of drug remaining in a patient after an aerosol treatment is expressed as "deposition" (Eq. 1).

$$\text{deposition} = \text{drug nebulized and inhaled} - \text{drug exhaled} \tag{1}$$

$$\text{drug nebulized and inhaled} = \text{inhaled mass} \tag{2}$$

The factors determining deposition are divided into two main components, the *inhaled mass* (Eq. 2), which reflects the characteristics of the specific delivery system (8), and the *deposition fraction* (DF, Eq. 3):

$$\text{deposition fraction} = \text{deposition} \div \text{inhaled mass} \tag{3}$$

which is simply a measure of the fraction inhaled that actually deposits. Then Eq. (1) can be rewritten as:

$$\text{deposition} = \text{inhaled mass} \times \text{DF} \tag{4}$$

The reason for this separation of terms is that the inhaled mass is a strong function of the type of delivery system utilized, and this term can often be measured by *in vitro* bench experiments. The DF is affected primarily by the physiology of the patient's respiratory tract and, for a given patient group, requires *in vivo* measurement. Failure to make a distinction between differences in drug delivery systems versus variation in human pathophysiology (i.e., Eq. 4) can lead to inappropriate conclusions regarding factors that ultimately determine the deposited dose in the lung. Depending on the device, and the disease, both the inhaled mass and the DF can be affected by the breathing pattern. Thus, breathing pattern is a common link between measurement of both factors and it should be taken into account in bench testing as well as in clinically based deposition experiments.

In the United States, federal regulation of aerosol "doses" varies with devices. The metered-dose inhaler (MDI) utilizes a metering valve that is highly regulated and functionally precise. Nebulizers as drug delivery systems are essentially unregulated.

For the same pattern of breathing, the quantity of aerosol inhaled over time is strongly dependent on the type of nebulizer utilized. As shown in Fig. 5, the AeroTech II produces aerosol at a rate approximately six times that of the Respirgard II (the difference in slopes). The plateau of each curve indicates the point at which the nebulizer runs dry and defines the amount of drug inhaled by the patient. For the AeroTech II, approximately 20% of the nebulizer charge is ultimately inhaled, versus 11% for the Respirgard II (9).

A. In Vitro Measurement of Inhaled Mass for Adult and Pediatric Aerosol Delivery

Using filters, the inhaled mass can be directly measured for a given patient; indeed, this technique can be expanded to measure the deposition of aerosol within the patient by comparing the amount inhaled versus the amount exhaled. The amount exhaled can be measured by filters on the expiratory line of the nebulizer (as shown in Fig. 4). *In vivo* filter measurements in patients can be cumbersome when different aerosol delivery devices are being screened in preclinical testing. Therefore, inhaled mass can be measured on the bench by substituting a mechanical ventilator for the patient (10). Figure 6 is a typical example. A piston pump (Harvard Pump, Harvard Apparatus, South Natick, MA) replaces the patient and the pump defines the pattern of breathing. The nebulizer mouthpiece is replaced by the inhaled mass filter, which captures all aerosol that would ordinarily be inhaled by a patient breathing with the specific breathing pattern set on the Harvard pump. To measure aerosol distribution, a cascade impactor can be interposed. Utilizing this scheme, many different devices can be tested on the bench without inconveniencing patients. In addition, variables that may affect nebulizer function, such as breathing pattern, are strictly controlled. European guidelines on the evaluation of nebulizer assessment have finally been drafted to take such factors into account and are mentioned briefly in the next chapter.

However, these approaches are best suited for studies pertaining to adults. Great care is needed in setting up and interpreting such studies in children, as

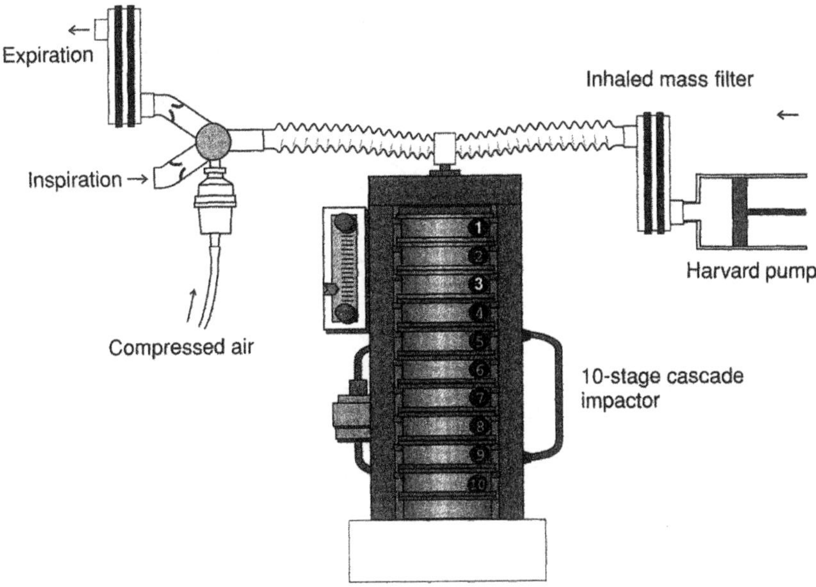

Figure 6 Sketch depicting technique for bench measurements of inhaled mass and particle distribution. Breathing pattern defined by settings on Harvard pump. Particles presented to "patient" are captured on the inhaled mass filter. In separate experiments, the cascade impactor measures inspired aerosol "isokinetically." (From Ref. 10.)

breathing pattern varies greatly with age (11). Breathing pattern can also be affected by the nebulizer itself, with factors such as resistance and dead space likely to be important. This may be particularly true in small children, with increased variability of breathing pattern being a likely cause of the high variability of data from younger children in aerosol studies using filters (12).

For continuously operating nebulizers, variables of importance appear to be tidal volume, duty cycle, and respiratory frequency. An example is shown in Fig. 7. The HEART nebulizer (Vortran Medical Technologies, Sacramento, CA) has a 200-mL reservoir so it "never" runs dry; thus, there is no plateau. The slopes are illustrated for two breathing patterns, adult versus pediatric. There is a significant difference in inhaled mass over time, all other things being equal except the pattern of breathing (13).

Other types of nebulizer modifications are linked to the breathing pattern and therefore can affect output. These include "breath actuation," in which the

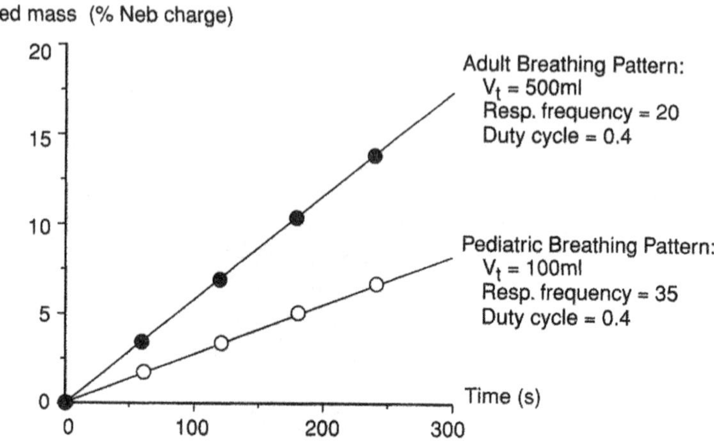

Figure 7 Influence of breathing pattern on inhaled mass during continuous nebulization. (From Ref. 13.)

nebulizer is activated only during inspiration. This modality can be utilized to minimize expiratory losses. A relatively recent development in nebulizer design includes the "breath-enhanced" nebulizer, which requires that the patient's inspiratory flow pass through the body of the nebulizer, collecting a greater number of the aerosol particles generated during inspiration than would normally be the case. The performance of these nebulizers is also likely to be more variable in young children due to the effects of their more irregular breathing patterns (Fig. 8) (12). Breath-actuated nebulizers can function efficiently at lower compressor flows and allow flexibility in design of compressor-driven systems. By definition, they are flow-dependent; therefore, the measurement of inhaled mass can be a strong function of breathing pattern.

B. Importance of Filter Dead Space

As mentioned above, dead space of the nebulizer can affect the breathing patterns of children receiving nebulizer therapy *in vivo* by stimulating their breathing. An independent problem exists in bench testing. Dead space, particularly of the sampling filter, can have a significant effect on the measurement of inhaled mass. For a fixed pattern of breathing, increasing filter dead space artifactually lowers inhaled mass. Errors can be detected as dead space exceeds 10% of the tidal volume. For small tidal volumes in the pediatric range, the errors are of considerable magnitude, but corrections can be made if tidal volume is adjusted for filter dead space (14).

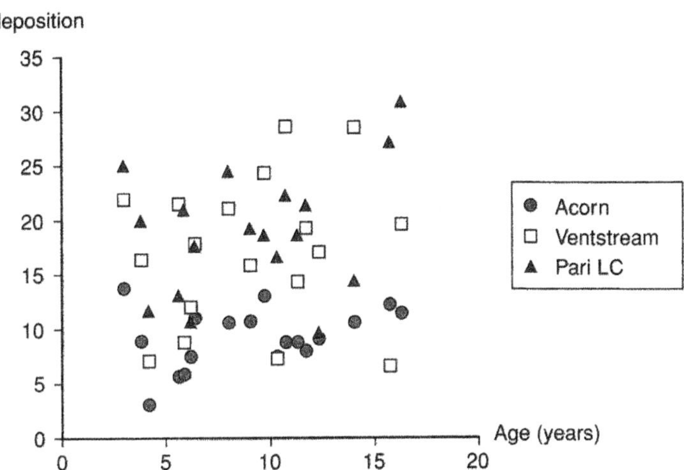

Figure 8 Comparison of filter deposition for a conventional nebulizer (Acorn Marquest Medical Products, Englewood, CO) and two inhalation enhanced nebulizers (Ventstream Medic-Aid, Sussex, UK, and Pari LC Pari Respiratory Equipment, Richmond VA) in children. Despite optimal laboratory conditions, there was high variability of deposition for all three nebulizers. (From Ref. 12.)

VI. Nebulizer Reproducibility

For a single AeroTech II or Respirgard II nebulizer, the slope and plateau illustrated in Fig. 5 describe its function during inhalation of aerosol by a patient. The slope describes the amount of aerosol produced over time, while the plateau depicts the ultimate efficiency of the nebulizer in terms of the quantity of aerosol produced before the nebulizer runs dry. To test nebulizer brands for interdevice variation, comparison studies have been performed on 10 examples of each device (9). Utilizing the slope and plateau as parameters, results for the 10 samples are plotted in Fig. 9. There is considerable variation between devices when measured under fixed laboratory conditions. As shown in Fig. 9, the AeroTech II and Respirgard II demonstrated similar degrees of variability about the mean with respect to the slope of the output curve. Variation in the plateau, however, was much reduced for the AeroTech II versus the Respirgard II. The variation in slope between individual devices is likely to reflect molding tolerances within the nebulizer orifice. In the examples of Fig. 9, the differences in variation in the plateau between brands of nebulizer may be related to the design of baffles. The AeroTech II has baffles within the body of the nebulizer, whereas the Respirgard II utilizes an extra one-way valve in the inspiratory line of the device to regulate

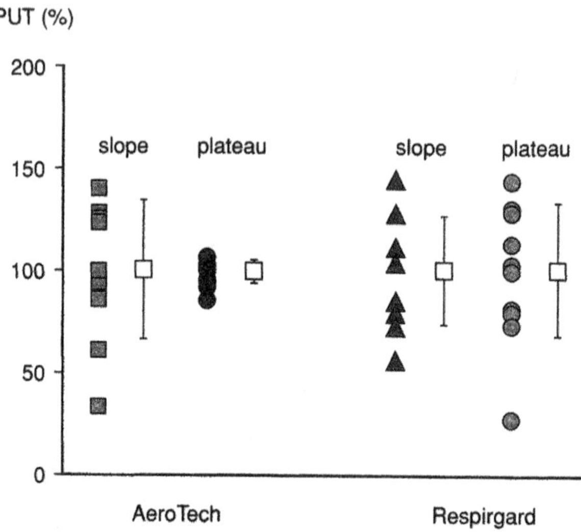

Figure 9 Reproducibility data from 10 examples of two commercially available nebulizers. Individual data points, mean, and standard deviation are illustrated for slope and plateau of the inhaled mass relationship depicted in Fig. 6. There is considerable scatter for both nebulizers, but the plateau of the AeroTech exhibits reduced variability. (From Ref. 9.)

particle distribution. Because that valve was outside the body of the nebulizer and upstream to the patient mouthpiece, it may have affected reproducibility. Reproducibility standards for nebulizer function are presently not defined by regulatory agencies.

VII. Components of the Nebulizer Charge

A. Solutions

As stated above, most drugs are nebulized as solutions—that is, the active principle is dissolved as a solute into a solution (usually aqueous), forming a continuous phase. Data from Fig. 5 represent typical nebulizer behavior for aqueous solutions. Other solvents have been used in rare circumstances. For example, cyclosporine, a drug with potential for topical therapy in lung transplant rejection is insoluble in water. The drug is readily dissolved in polar organic solvents such as alcohol or propylene glycol (15,16). Profound differences in nebulizer behavior have been observed for these different solvents. Figure 10 represents the output of an AeroTech II nebulizer filled with

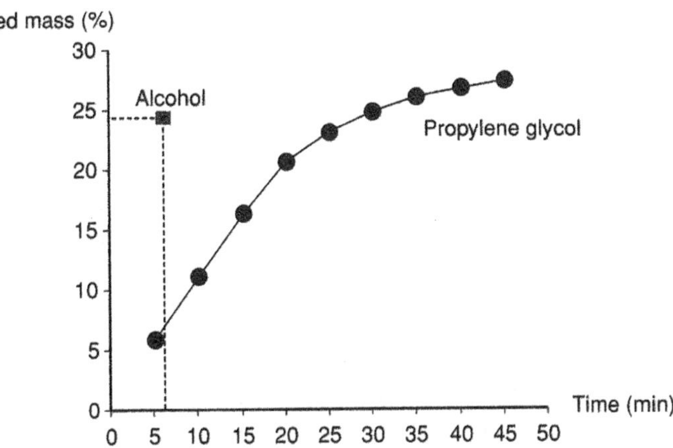

Figure 10 Influence of solvent on nebulizer function. Data represent inhaled mass versus time for cyclosporine dissolved in either ethanol or propylene glycol.

cyclosporine dissolved in either alcohol or propylene glycol represented as inhaled mass (as a percent of the nebulizer charge) versus time in minutes. This is the same representation seen in Fig. 5 for pentamidine. The volume fill of the nebulizer is 4.8 mL. For both solvents, similar amounts of cyclosporine were nebulized as indicated by an inhaled mass of approximately 24% for the alcohol and 27% for propylene glycol solution. There was a marked difference in the time of nebulization, however. The entire alcohol solution was nebulized in approximately 6 min, whereas the propylene glycol, which is much less volatile, is gradually nebulized with a plateau at approximately 40 min of nebulization. These observations have important clinical implications. Obviously, it is much more convenient to treat a patient in 6 versus 40 min. On the other hand, the entire nebulized mass of cyclosporine is delivered to the patient in 6 min via alcohol, indicating that the mass of drug per breath is significantly higher than when delivered over 40 min by propylene glycol. Therefore, for a constant breathing pattern, the concentration of cyclosporine in the gas phase inhaled into the respiratory tract is approximately 7 times higher for the alcohol than for propylene glycol. In early studies utilizing this drug, investigators found that the alcohol preparation appeared to be more irritating (15,17). More recent studies suggest that propylene glycol seems to be better tolerated (16). Other factors can be important in irritant responses that are unrelated to the nebulizer solution, such as the site of deposition in the airways and the distribution of irritant receptors. In clinical trials, it is difficult to separate all of these factors to clearly delineate the cause of airway irritation. While the reactive state of the patients' airways and sites of deposition are obvious variables, the points summarized in Fig. 10 can also be important and should be considered in the design of clinical trials.

B. Suspensions

Suspensions can be successfully nebulized. The fact that there are two phases in the nebulizer volume fill does not prevent carriage of suspended particles into the gas phase provided that the construction of the nebulizer accommodates the physical distribution of the suspended particles. Budesonide, a steroid used to treat asthma, has been available for some years as a suspension for nebulization. The influence of the physical state of the liquid on nebulizer function is evident from the data depicted in Figs. 11 and 12. Figure 11 is a standard graph representing inhaled mass from two experiments carried out on the same AeroTech II nebulizer with a fixed pediatric breathing pattern (tidal volume 200 mL frequency 25 breaths per minute, duty cycle 0.5). Two solutions were compared; the first being a conventional albuterol solution with a volume fill of 2 mL (1.67 mg drug). This simple aqueous solution was fully nebulized in approximately 9 min with an inhaled mass of 17%. Then the same nebulizer was filled with 2.0 mL budesonide suspension (1 mg drug) and nebulization ceased after 6 min with only 10% of the nebulizer charge captured on the inhaled mass filter. In Fig. 12 are shown the particle distributions measured by cascade impaction for the nebulized albuterol and budesonide. (The measurement of aerosol distributions is dis-

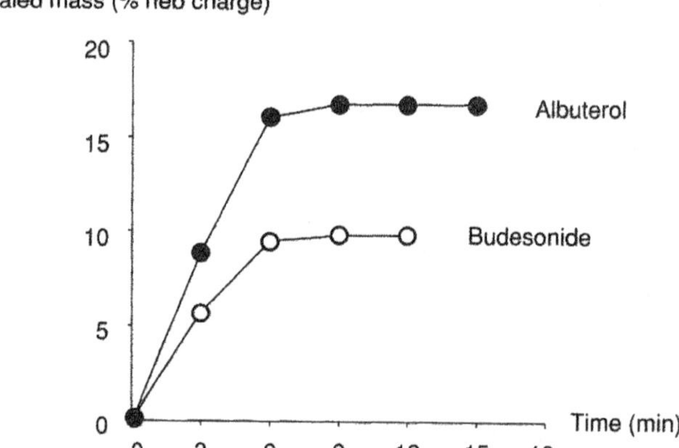

Figure 11 Inhaled mass versus time for a solution (albuterol) and a suspension (budesonide) using the AeroTech II nebulizer (tidal volume, 200 mL; frequency, 25 breaths per min; duty cycle, 0.5).

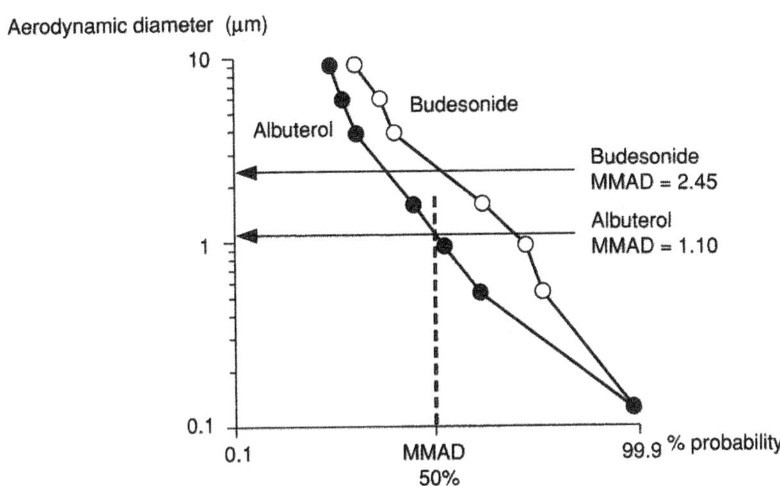

Figure 12 Aerosol distributions for the solutions produced in the experiments described in Fig. 11.

cussed formally below.) The figure clearly indicates that there was a significant difference between nebulized budesonide suspension [mass median aerodynamic diameter (MMAD) 2.45 μm] versus nebulized albuterol solution (MMAD 1.10 μm) captured in the cascade impactor from the same nebulizer at a fixed breathing pattern. In our experience, the AeroTech II nebulizer usually produces aerosols of approximately 1.0 μm when the liquid in the nebulizer is an aqueous solution. The nebulizer's relatively high efficiency, coupled with small particle distribution, reflects its internal baffling, which works well for typical aqueous solutions. For budesonide suspension, the internal baffles that are so important for the modification of the fine aqueous aerosol probably capture many of the larger nebulized particles. Milled budesonide has been reported to have a microscopically observed diameter of approximately 2.2–2.9 μm (18). Multiplying the microscopic diameter by the density of budesonide (1.26 g/mL) results in a range of MMAD (2.5–3.5 μm) reported for virtually all experimentally tested nebulizers for budesonide that emit relatively large particles (19).

VIII. The Lung Dose

Is there clinical evidence that the principles illustrated above are important determinants of treatment outcome in patients? To answer that question, a thorough understanding of the dose-response relationship for a given drug may be necessary. For aerosol therapy, this includes not just the inhaled mass but also the deposition in the lung, the regional distribution of the deposited drug, the retention of the drug within the lung, and, of equal importance, a realistic understanding of the response. In clinical studies, defining the appropriate response is often a major intellectual challenge. In bronchodilator trials, the FEV_1 or peak flow is easily measured. For aerosolized anti-inflammatory agents such as steroids or aerosolized antibiotics, the response is often vaguely defined and frequently reflects many variables besides the tested therapeutic regimen. For example, in the ICU, mortality is often the only endpoint that can be easily defined. It is not the purpose of this chapter to review clinical aerosol trials. However, examples that illustrate the problems and possible solutions are described below.

Monthly aerosolized pentamidine has been utilized as prophylactic therapy against *Pneumocystis carinii* pneumonia in high-risk patients with HIV infection. While effective, this therapy fails in a certain percentage of patients. In the large clinical trials defining the clinical efficacy of this mode of therapy, the dose-response curve was not determined. Whether patients who failed prophylaxis did so because of inadequate deposition of aerosolized pentamidine or other unknown factors remained uncertain. Figure 13 represents summary data from a study in 58 patients receiving directly supervised monthly therapy in

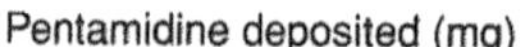

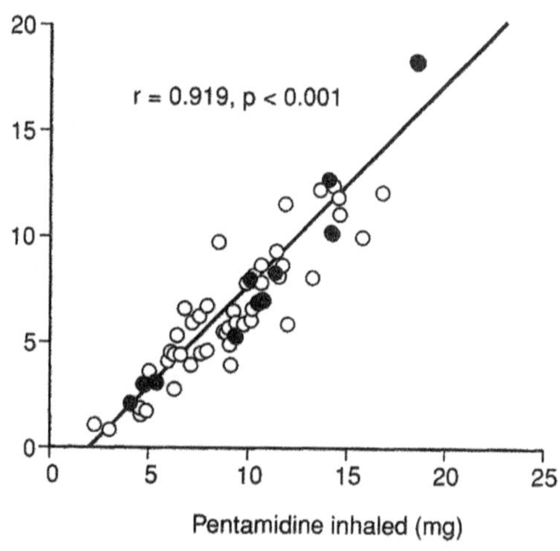

Figure 13 Pulmonary deposition of pentamidine plotted against the inhaled mass of pentamidine in patients receiving aerosolized prophylaxis. The filled circles describe those patients receiving prophylaxis who actually developed *Pneumocystis carinii* pneumonia. (From Ref. 20.)

which pentamidine deposition was actually measured and related to success or failure of aerosolized prophylaxis (20,21). The vertical axis represents pentamidine deposition measured by the mass balance filter technique plotted against the inhaled mass in milligrams. First, the graph indicates a wide range in deposition between individual patients. Superimposed on the overall relationship are data points that indicate which subjects failed prophylactic therapy. In spite of the wide distribution in individual values of deposition, there was a uniform distribution of prophylaxis failures throughout the group, suggesting that those patients who failed therapy did so because of factors unrelated to the pulmonary deposition of drug. An additional observation from Fig. 13 is the close correlation between pentamidine deposited versus pentamidine inhaled. This would indicate that patient-related factors such as the deposition fraction (DF, Eq. 4) were not major variables affecting deposition. Most patients treated with aerosolized pentamidine prophylaxis have relatively normal airways function. If disease is present, it is usually "restrictive" rather than obstructive. The nebulizer used, the AeroTech II (as shown above, Fig. 9), exhibits relatively good interdevice reproducibility, and variation between devices cannot account for the variation in inhaled mass seen on Fig. 13. These observations suggest that, for patients inhaling aerosolized pentamidine, differences in deposition were likely to be related to variation in breathing pattern between patients and that these latter factors (tidal volume, duty cycle) accounted for the changes in inhaled mass. In any event, as shown in the figure, failure of pentamidine prophylaxis was not related to differences in deposition of the drug (21,22). Recent studies would suggest that patients receiving aerosolized pentamidine failed because of other factors, such as a change in their immunological status or possible changes in the virulence of the organism (22).

The cyclosporine experience is a good demonstration of the potential usefulness of assessing dose and clinical response of an aerosolized medication before large-scale clinical trials are undertaken. As described above, cyclosporine is insoluble in aqueous solvents and the nebulized drug has been given to patients dissolved in either alcohol or propylene glycol. The nebulizer delivery system has been well characterized by bench studies, and these studies defined the clinical approach to therapy. Collaborating investigators have assessed the response to aerosol therapy in several ways—e.g., histologically from biopsies before and after therapy, levels of circulating mediators from bronchoalveolar lavage, and physiologically using pulmonary function testing (16,17). Figure 14 represents published changes that occurred in pulmonary function in lung transplant patients. FEV_1 versus time is shown for two groups of individuals who have received either a single or double lung transplant. The control group consisted of patients suffering from "persistent acute rejection"—a syndrome characterized by lack of response to any form of systemic immunosuppressive therapy designed to treat organ rejection. Over time, their pulmonary function

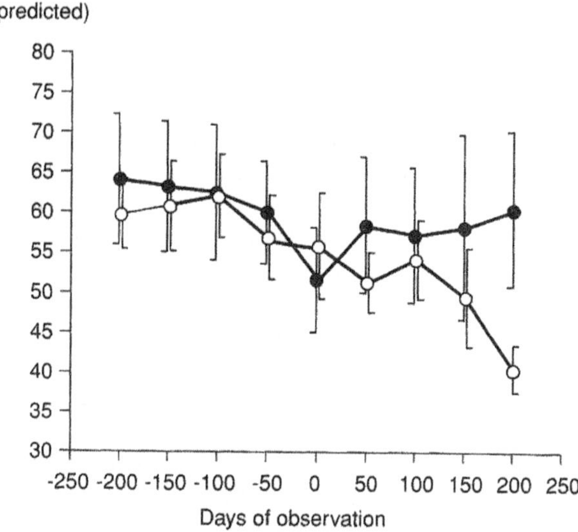

Figure 14 Spirometry over time from two groups of patients who have received lung transplants. Both groups are suffering from persistent acute rejection. The filled circles represent patients who were started on aerosolized cyclosporine at day 0 of observation. (From Ref. 16.)

declined; after approximately 450 days of observation, their FEV_1 averaged 40% of predicted (22 patients). A similar group of subjects (9 individuals) was identified with the same clinical syndrome (persistent acute rejection) and observed for 250 days (day –250 to day 0). As indicated on the figure, their decline in function was similar to that of the control group until they were started on aerosolized cyclosporine (day 0). At the end of the period of observation (200 days into therapy), there was a statistically significant increase in FEV_1 in the treated group. As indicated by the error bars, there was significant variation in FEV_1 among the treated patients. This variation is analyzed in Fig. 15. On this figure are compared the change in FEV_1 (day 0 to day 120 of aerosol therapy) versus deposited cyclosporine in the transplanted lung (7 of the 9 patients depicted in Fig. 14). Each of those individuals underwent a deposition study in which the quantity of cyclosporine actually deposited in the transplant (single or double lung) was determined by gamma camera imaging. While the numbers were small, patients who received the lower dose of aerosolized cyclosporine clearly had a reduced response as measured by FEV_1 (16). Prospective randomized controlled studies are being carried out in larger groups of patients.

The data from the pentamidine study, which indicated that the lung dose of

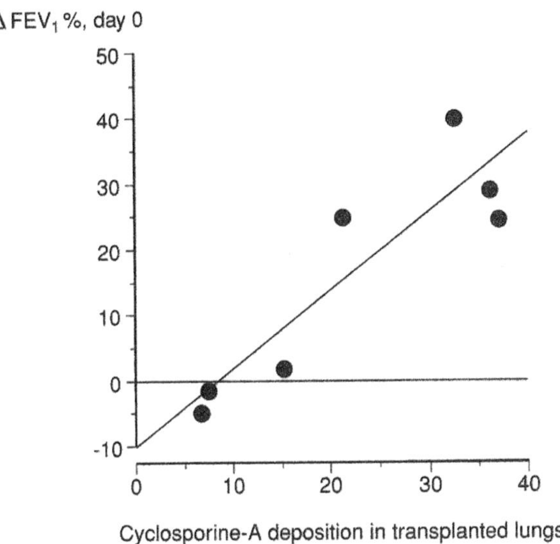

Figure 15 Change in spirometry (assessed by FEV_1) as a function of cyclosporine deposited in transplanted lung (s). (From Ref. 16.)

drug was not important in terms of the ultimate therapeutic response, are still extremely important because those data allowed investigators to contemplate other mechanisms of failure of therapy. Further, the pentamidine studies provided the stimulus for the development of many of the techniques described in this chapter and in this book that have helped to define modern concepts of aerosol therapy. The cyclosporine data serve as a model illustrating that the interaction between preclinical testing, knowledge of clinical airways pathophysiology, and measurement of deposition can define the behavior of a given aerosol before the design of expensive clinical trials.

IX. Measuring Particle Size During Nebulization

Figure 6 represents an *in vitro* simulation of a patient breathing an aerosol from a nebulizer and measurement of inhaled mass. An important additional goal is the assessment of the distribution of nebulized particles in a manner that represents as closely as possible the aeresol as it is actually inhaled by a patient. To measure the particle distribution investigators often use cascade impaction, described in principle in Fig. 16. The aerosol, which consists of particles suspended in a gas, enters the cascade impactor at a constant volumetric

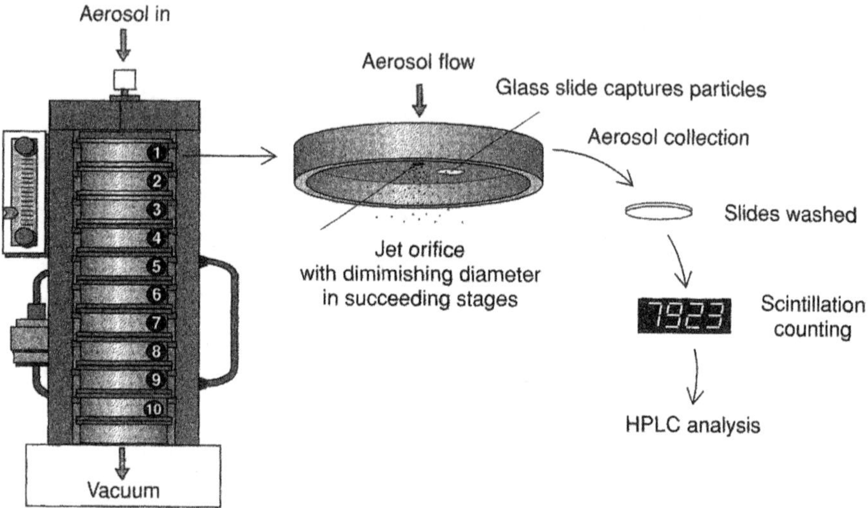

Figure 16 Diagram of 10-stage cascade impactor.

flow. The linear velocity of the carrier gas increases as the aerosol passes through a series of orifices within the impactor. At each stage, particles either impact on slides or pass on to the next stage, depending upon their inertia. In the impactor, particle inertia is determined by the aerodynamic diameter of the particle and its velocity through each orifice. Smaller particles are able to circumnavigate the slide and move to the next stage. Knowledge of the flow characteristics of each stage and control of the flow through the cascade impactor allows the aerodynamic distribution of diameters captured on the various stages to be quantified and plotted. A typical graphic analysis is called a *probability plot,* with the vertical axis representing the logarithm of the particle diameter and the horizontal axis probability. A typical log-normal aerosol distribution will be represented on this plot as a straight line. An example is shown in Fig. 12. Thus, for accurate measurement, the flow through the cascade impactor must be constant and carefully controlled. The advantages of cascade impaction are that the slides, which are removable, allow direct analysis of drug, and the graph depicted in Fig. 12 represents the aerodynamic behavior of the actual drug, budesonide. Other devices used to measure the behavior of aerosol particles primarily use light-scattering techniques and do not provide a direct measurement of drug behavior. Because of the importance of the drug analysis, regulatory agencies tend to favor cascade impaction in the description of an aerosol delivery system.

As stated above, nebulizer function may be dependent on flow through the nebulizer. To minimize the influence of the impactor on the function of the nebulizer during *in vitro* testing, "low flow" cascade impactors are often used. That is, the gas flow through the impactor required to carry the aerosol through the various stages is regulated by a pump running at 1–2 L/min. As shown in Fig. 6, placing the nebulizer in a "T" arrangement allows the vacuum pump to draw a constant flow through the nebulizer without perturbing nebulizer function. While flow through the nebulizer may resemble a sinusoidal breathing pattern, flow through the cascade impactor must be constant. This is called *isokinetic sampling*. By placing the filter in the inhaled mass position, particles entering the cascade impactor do so only during the inspiratory phase of the cycle, because all particles that pass the impactor heading toward the piston pump are captured by the filter and none are available during expiration. Under these circumstances, the flow regime in the nebulizer remains unperturbed and the particles entering the impactor are particles that have followed the same path as they would have if the patient were doing the breathing. Conditions of humidity and temperature are similar to the *in vivo* situation, because gases exhaled from the patient or the piston pump pass through the expiratory line on the Y piece. Other types of cascade impactors designed for quality-control measurement of aerosol plumes operate at high flows (20–30 L/min) and would obviously be unsuitable for the *in vitro* configuration demonstrated in Fig. 6.

A. Breathing Pattern and Changes in Aerosol Distribution

Nebulizers modify the aerosol as it is created, using internal baffles in a flow-dependent manner. If the patient modifies the flow through the nebulizer by breathing through it, the final aerosol distribution may be altered. This hypothesis was tested in bench studies evaluating different systems for the delivery of aerosolized pentamidine. This drug was delivered in early clinical trials via conventional jet nebulizers (AeroTech II, Respirgard II) and ultrasonic devices (e.g., Fisoneb, Fisons, NY). A major factor determining the particle distribution of ultrasonic systems is the vibrating frequency of the ultrasonic crystal. Most ultrasonic systems are expected to produce particles somewhat larger than those generated by small-volume nebulizers (i.e., greater than 3 μm). Figure 17 represents a sketch adapting the Fisoneb configuration to the *in vitro* bench testing system described previously for jet nebulizers depicted in Fig. 6. Experiments on this device were carried out in two configurations. In the first, a "standing cloud" configuration, the nebulizer was simply operated continuously, with a small internal fan conveying aerosol to the cascade impactor. The Harvard pump and the inspiratory filter were removed. The second configuration corresponds to the diagram in Fig. 17, in which the inspiratory filter and Harvard pump were attached with a

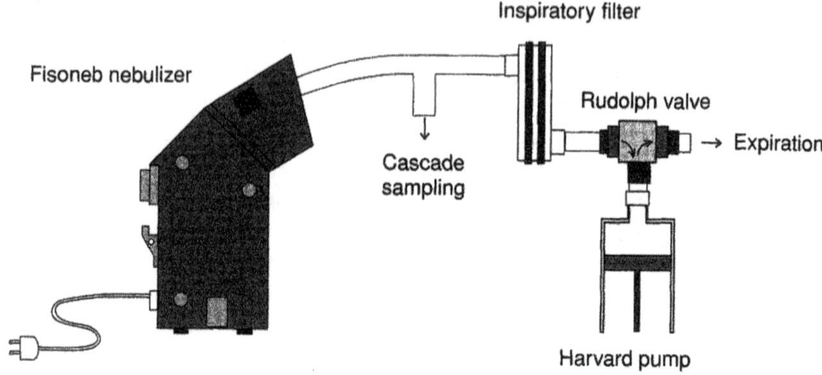

Figure 17 Schematic describing experiments measuring aerosol output from Fisoneb ultrasonic nebulizer. (From Ref. 10.)

Rudolph valve designed to separate inspiratory and expiratory gases. In that configuration, the Fisoneb was triggered only during inspiration and the inspiratory gases from the "patient's" breathing passed through the nebulizer. Thus, the flow regime within the nebulizer itself was different between the standing cloud experiment and the experiment when the system was actually ventilated by the Harvard pump. Cascade impaction experiments were carried out utilizing Technetium 99m (^{99m}Tc) as the radiolabel (Fig. 18). As shown in the figure, the particle distributions were different for the two experimental low configurations. The standing cloud MMAD of 5.3 μm was consistent with the excitation frequency of the Fisoneb crystal. However, when the device was ventilated with a typical adult breathing pattern (750 mL tidal volume, 20 breaths per minute, duty cycle 0.5) the MMAD decreased to 2.1 μm. The likely explanation for this phenomenon was the effect of baffles in the ultrasonic device, which behaved in a similar manner to the baffles in a jet nebulizer (10). These measurements emphasize the basic principle generally adopted by committees and agencies setting standards for aerosol characterization and regulation—that is, that the system be tested in a configuration that represents the circumstances under which it is to be used clinically.

B. Hygroscopic Considerations

Low-flow cascade impaction may have other technical advantages. The MMAD is often used to predict deposition in the human lung. However, many aerosols change their aerodynamic characteristics in real time after they are generated. For example, particles from MDIs may be mixed with volatile com-

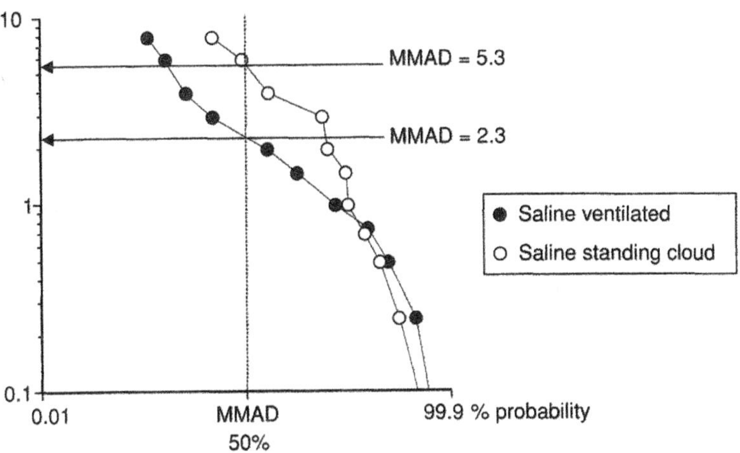

Figure 18 Aerosol distributions of saline particles produced by Fisoneb. Open circles, standing cloud aerosol-filled circles, saline aerosol following ventilation of nebulizer with Harvard pump. (From Ref. 10.)

ponents such as surfactant as well as volatile propellants. Further, the particle generating system may impart inertia to the particles, so that their behavior will reflect aerodynamic characteristics that are not fully predicted by MMAD alone. Finally, the particles themselves may undergo hygroscopic changes. In addition, devices designed to measure aerodynamic distributions often affect the aerosol or allow it to change its distribution because of the basic nature of their design. Light-scattering devices require dilution of aerosol to prevent coincidence effects and they do not measure drug directly, so the aerosol that is described may not be the same as that inhaled. Similar criticisms can be directed toward cascade impaction. High-flow cascade impactors, which are more suitable for quality-control measurements, will clearly perturb any system designed to function under conditions of tidal breathing. Low-flow cascade impactors do not capture all of the generated particles and there is the possibility that some particles may not be sampled. Cascade impactors are also not humidified or heated, so volatile aerosols may change when sampled and the reported results will not reflect body temperature and pressure. However, few studies have investigated the accuracy of these impressions. Often clinician/scientists are influenced by literature based on precisely controlled experiments performed with low-concentration test aerosols, such as dried salt particles. These aerosols allow the assessment of theories of particle growth and the effects of relative humidity on hygroscopic behavior, but they lack direct relevance to the clinical arena.

In fact, recent studies suggest that "wet aerosols" utilized in clinical environments are often relatively stable. For example, lung images obtained using aerosols characterized by low-flow cascade impaction seem representative of the MMADs reported (23,24). That is, smaller particles deposit more peripherally than larger ones. If aerosol droplets produced by wet nebulizers are indeed "stable," how can we account for this observation in terms of our knowledge of particle growth from studies of single particles or dry nuclei in humid atmospheres that tend to grow rapidly? Recent theories of hygroscopic growth involving "two-way coupled effects" have predicted stability of wet aerosols in nebulizers because of the interaction between the large number of particles within an aerosol cloud and their influence on stability of the vapor (25,26).

For nebulizers, one of the more important effects of two-way coupling may be its ability to partially or even completely prevent the evaporation of droplets. Because the mass of water carried by droplets is large, it is possible to predict stable water aerosols within nebulizer systems. Similar arguments can be applied to low-flow cascade impactors when they are attached to closed systems, and this may partially explain why MMAD measured by impactors appears to have some clinical relevance. More data are needed to further define the importance of this effect for both nebulizers and cascade impactors.

There are other unexpected "stabilizing effects" within wet nebulizers that may be related to two-way coupling. The concentration of solute in a continuously operating nebulizer is known to increase over time. This is related to the fact that solute is recycled within the nebulizer as water vapor is expelled. This observation implies that particles (droplets) emitted from the nebulizer late in the phase of nebulizer operation will contain a higher concentration of drug than particles emitted earlier during nebulization. On the other hand, data from inhaled mass experiments often demonstrate a linear output of drug from the nebulizer over time, as shown in Fig. 5. Because the quantity of drug being emitted from the nebulizer is constant and (from cascade impaction experiments) the MMAD of the aerosol over time is generally unchanged (9,10), the number of particles emitted in the aerosol must decrease during nebulization. Thus, MMAD and drug output over time remain constant in spite of the fact that solute concentration increases during nebulization.

X. Labeling Pharmaceutical Nebulizer Solutions for Bench Testing and Deposition Studies

A. Calibration via Cascade Impaction

Aerosol particles generated from nebulizer solutions containing drugs can be labeled with a short-acting isotope such as ^{99m}Tc. If particles of free technetium deposit in the lungs, they will be readily absorbed and cleared from the lungs by the circulation. To allow sufficient time to obtain a meaningful gamma camera image, the ^{99m}Tc should be bound to a substance such as sulfur colloid or human serum albumin.

The assumption should not be made that a drug and its radiolabel have similar aerodynamic properties. Preliminary bench testing of the pharmaceutical aerosol with and without the radiolabel is advised. These studies should confirm that the addition of radioactivity to the aerosol does not change the aerodynamic characteristics of the drug particles. In addition, the percentage of the drug inhaled should be shown to be equivalent to the percentage of radioactivity inhaled. This equivalence is necessary if the drug behavior in the aerosol is to be traced using radioactivity (e.g., using the mass balance technique or regional scanning with the gamma camera). Failure to test this relationship can lead to serious problems if the isotope is to be used to measure lung dose of the drug. For example, Fig. 19 demonstrates the quantitative relationship between an aerosolized drug (pentamidine) and a ^{99m}Tc radiolabel mixed with the solution in the nebulizer. Two experiments are shown, representing pentamidine in the aerosol (captured by cascade impaction) versus ^{99m}Tc bound to sulfur colloid (^{99m}Tc-SC) or human serum albumin (^{99m}Tc-HSA). Each relationship is well described by a straight line, but they have different slopes. The relationship for ^{99m}Tc-HSA is close to the line of identity,

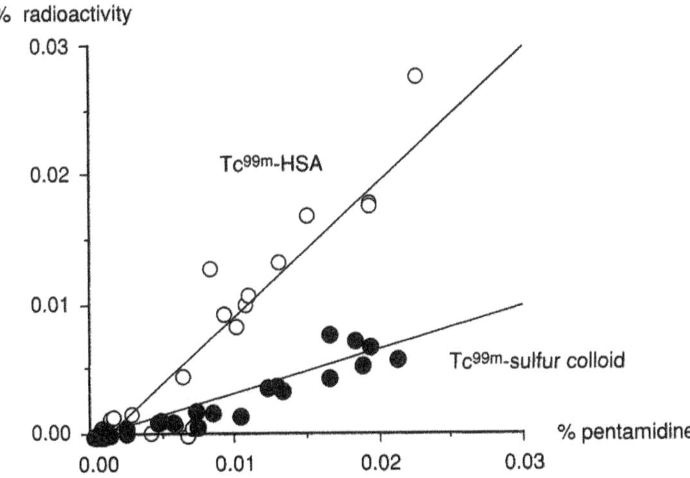

Figure 19 Relationship between radioactivity and drug activity for pentamidine aerosols. Open circles, particles labeled with ^{99m}Tc bound to human serum albumin (^{99m}Tc-HSA); filled circles, ^{99m}Tc bound to sulfur colloid. (From Ref. 27.)

indicating that for each 1% of drug deposited, 1% of radioactivity will be detected in the lung, whereas the slope of the ^{99m}Tc -SC/pentamidine relationship is only one-third that of ^{99m}Tc-HSA. This indicates that ^{99m}Tc-SC will underestimate pentamidine deposition by a factor of 3 to 1. Both isotope binding agents are suitable for deposition studies, but knowledge of the slope is necessary for accurate measurement of drug deposition (27).

B. Pediatric Considerations in Labeling Studies

Particular care is needed in designing aerosol deposition studies in children. Since children have a longer life expectancy than adults, the risk of a given radiation dose may be greater for them, and every effort must be made to minimize exposure (28). Minimal numbers of children should be used and doses of isotope should produce radiation levels that are only just enough above background levels to produce reliable data. In addition, only studies that are essential to improve and optimize aerosol delivery systems for children should use radioisotopes. For example, studies to assess different nebulizer setups should use *in vitro* bench testing rather than *in vivo* assessments of deposition.

XI. Route of Inhalation

The nose is an efficient filter, and patients should be encouraged to inhale aerosols through their mouths. Up to 300% more aerosol reaches the lungs if a nebulized aerosol is inhaled via the mouth rather then the nose (29). In infants and very young children, use of a mouthpiece is not usually possible, but from the age of 3 or 4 years, most children can tolerate a mouthpiece. How much the nose filters large particles and preserves smaller aerosol particles is not known. However, a deposition study that compared deposition using the two different routes in children did not show differences in the ratio of central to peripheral deposition, suggesting that there was no significant change in aerosol size distribution after nasal inhalation (29).

XII. Mechanical Ventilation

A. The Ventilator and Its Influence on Nebulization

Aerosol delivery via mechanical ventilation using nebulizers seems more complex than conventional nebulization. How should the nebulizer be powered? Where in the circuit should it be connected? Early studies in the ICU suggested that nebulized particles could be delivered to the lungs of intubated patients only with great difficulty. Compared to other devices such as MDIs, nebulizers were inefficient (30) and the endotracheal tube presented an additional barrier to the passage of particles into the respiratory tract (31). However, by taking the same approach to nebulization via the ventilator as shown above for spontaneous breathing, the factors important to aerosol delivery using mechanical ventilation can be defined.

The ventilator and its tubing (endotracheal tube etc.) can be viewed as an extension of the nebulizer, Further, the ventilator itself often includes an equivalent "compressor" providing the nebulizer flow, and the ventilator (like the Harvard pump) defines the breathing pattern. Therefore, in the intubated patient, inhaled mass can be measured *in vitro,* using filters, and deposition of particles can be measured *in vivo* using the gamma camera. Figure 20 illustrates these concepts. The nebulizer is inserted into a ventilator circuit and, in this example, is powered directly by the ventilator. The endotracheal tube is attached to a lung simulator (VT-1 Adult Ventilator Tester, Bio-Tek Instruments, Winooski, VT).

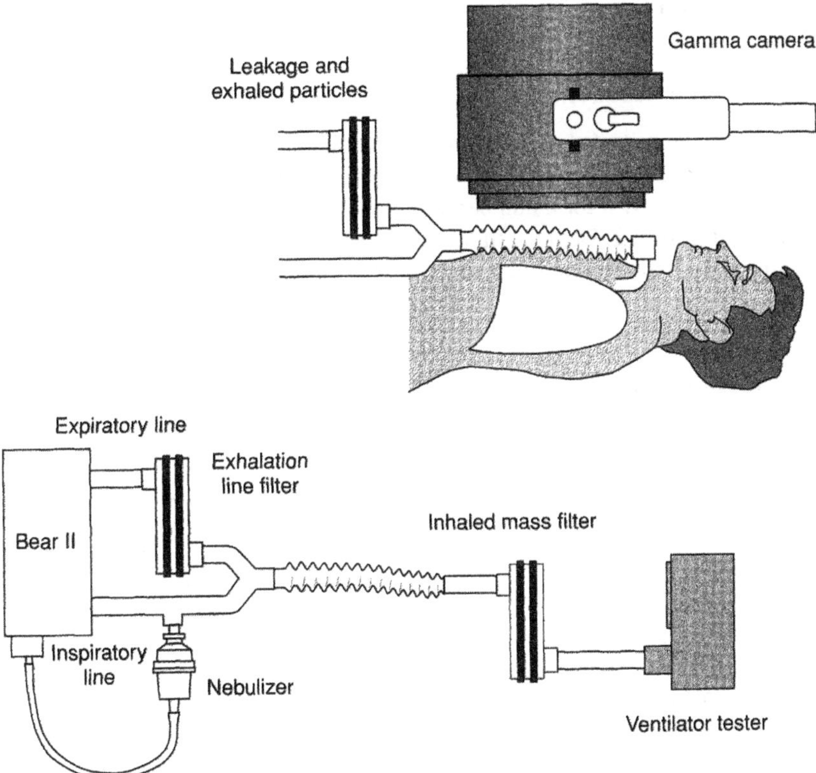

Figure 20 Sketch of ventilator circuit incorporating jet nebulization. The lower panel describes method for measuring inhaled mass *in vitro,* the upper panel, *in vivo* gamma camera scanning. (From Ref. 35.)

The filter measures inhaled mass. In the insert is a sketch of the filter configuration used to measure exhaled particles (and hence deposition) and a gamma camera for regional studies.

The ventilator itself can influence aerosol production. Figure 21 shows the inhaled mass over time generated by a typical nebulizer for four commercially available ventilators. The breathing pattern was fixed by the ventilator settings (tidal volume 1.0 L, frequency 15 breaths per minute, duty cycle 0.33). As shown in the figure, the inhaled mass for three of the ventilators ranged between 10 and 15% of the nebulizer charge in 15–20 min, while one device nebulized approximately 2.5% in 75 min (32). While all the tested ventilators performed mechanical ventilation within usual tolerances, the nebulizing system for the latter device was inadequate because the operating pressure in the nebulizer drive line was too low to drive the nebulizers tested. Manufacturers or regulatory agencies have not set standards for nebulization via mechanical ventilation.

B. The Nebulizer

Nebulizers can be tested in a given ventilator circuit and, as shown in Fig. 22, the choice of nebulizer can have a significant impact on drug delivery. Inhaled mass versus time is shown for a number of common nebulizers, including the devices first tested in Fig. 5. Devices shown to be efficient for spontaneously breathing patients are often even more efficient on the ventilator provided that the ventila-

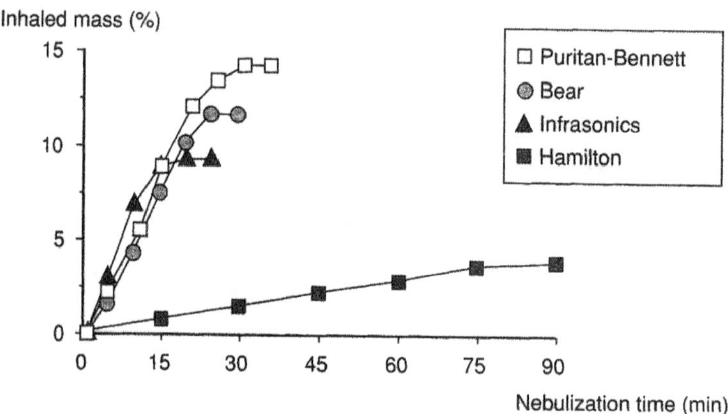

Figure 21 Influence of ventilator choice on aerosol output expressed as inhaled mass (%) versus time for four ventilators utilizing the Misty-Neb nebulizer. (Baxter Healthcare Corp., Valencia CA; from Ref. 32.)

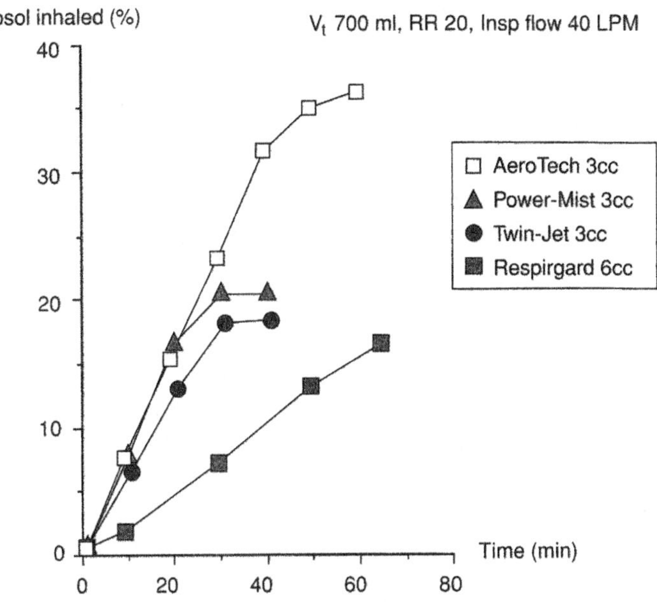

Figure 22 Importance of nebulizer choice in aerosol delivery via mechanical ventilation. The breathing pattern was fixed and inhaled mass (%) is plotted against time for four different nebulizers. (From Ref. 27.)

tor nebulizer flow system supplies adequate flow and driving pressure. The AeroTech II, for example, demonstrates an efficiency plateau of 35% for a volume fill of only 3 mL (compared to 22% for 4 mL of pentamidine in Fig. 5). The reason for this increased efficiency is the fact that when triggered by the ventilator (Bear II, Bear Medical Systems, Riverside, CA), the nebulizer is essentially a "breath actuated" device. The slope of the output curve is decreased (a treatment takes longer), but the plateau is increased (27).

C. Humidification

Ventilator circuits are often humidified and heated. Hygroscopic effects are complex in that there is considerable condensation and rainout of water in the connecting tubing between the nebulizer and the patient. This liquid is not recycled and aerosol lost is not recovered. The conditions in ventilator tubing are likely to be supersaturated and the aerosol particles serve as nuclei. Approximately 40–50% of drug can be lost when the circuit is humidified (for aerosols produced via nebulizer or MDI (27,33).

The data shown in Figs. 21 and 22 represent aerosol runs performed with the humidifier of the ventilator circuit "bypassed"; that is, the output from the humidifier is recycled directly back into it. This is equivalent to turning it off—a configuration that is useful when maximal efficiency and deposition are the goals of therapy (34). The patient still receives some humidified gases from the nebulizer itself (if the solution is aqueous), but the ventilator tubing is not supersaturated. After nebulization, the humidifier bypass is removed and full humidification restored. For "standard" aerosol treatments with bronchodilators, humidification is usually maintained during therapy.

D. The Endotracheal Tube

A low-flow cascade impactor can be inserted into the ventilator circuit between the distal tip of the endotracheal (or tracheostomy) tube and the inhaled mass filter. Impaction experiments have repeatedly shown that the aerosols leaving the tube and entering the patient are similar to those produced by small-particle nebulizers such as the AeroTech II. Often the MMADs are about 1.0 μm (27).

Deposition in the tubing can approach approximately 30% of lung deposition (27,31,35). However, recent studies in patients utilizing efficient nebulizers and optimized circuits have shown that approximately half of the deposition in the tube occurs during expiration, and therefore the tube is not a major impediment to drug delivery to the lungs (35). Finally, recent *in vivo* studies have confirmed that deposition of antibiotics in the airways of tracheostomized patients can exceed that found in spontaneously breathing patients provided that the factors known to affect drug delivery, described above, are optimized. Representative data are shown in Fig. 23, sputum levels from mechanically ventilated patients following aerosolized aminoglycoside therapy averaged 1200 μg/mL (34).

E. Considerations for Ventilated Neonates

The situation is very different for intubated neonates. A typical neonatal ventilator circuit is shown in Fig. 24. The major difference between this system and an adult ventilator circuit is the presence of a constant flow of gases through the respirator tubing. In the adult system, flow in the inspiratory line is initiated during inspiration and shuts off at the end of the breath. Therefore, all aerosol particles entering the neonatal circuit are swept away and only a few pass into the endotracheal tube. Further, flow of gas into the infant can be very small, especially for very preterm neonates. These losses, coupled with endotracheal tube losses, total over 90% (36). Because of the small size of neonates, deposition per kilogram may be adequate, but at a tremendous cost in efficiency. For inexpensive drugs, this problem may not be significant; but as the costs of drugs increase, losses will obviously become more important.

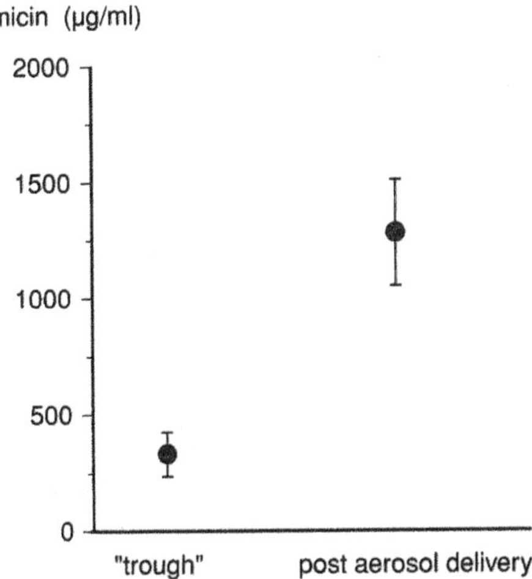

Figure 23 Sputum aminoglycoside level (µg/mL) sampled from patients maintained on mechanical ventilation. The patients were receiving gentamicin (80 mg every 8 h) and clinically were in a steady state. The "trough" level was from sputum sampled just prior to an aerosol treatment. Following aerosol therapy, average values of gentamicin exceeded 1200 µg. (From Ref. 34.)

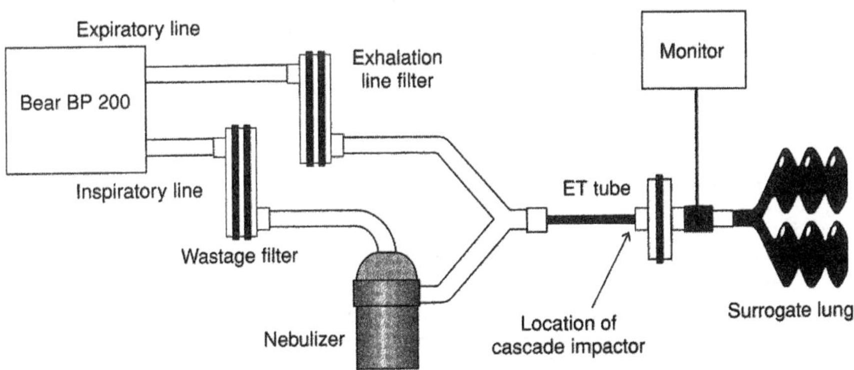

Figure 24 Diagram of neonatal ventilator circuit incorporating a nebulizer. This example illustrates an ultrasonic device. Cascade impaction can be performed at the distal tip of the endotracheal tube. (From Ref. 36.)

XIII. Summary

In summary, the ability of a nebulizer to deliver drug by aerosol to a patient is strongly dependent on a number of variables including the nebulizer itself (e.g., breath actuation, breath enhancement), the physical properties of the solution, and the patient's pattern of breathing (tidal volume, frequency, duty cycle). How can these variables be controlled to allow a reasonable estimate of dose delivery in a given clinical situation? The answer lies in preclinical bench testing. Because it is not possible to predict with certainty the function of any nebulizer from first principles, the ability of a device to deliver a reasonable amount of drug must be tested on the bench prior to any clinical trial. The experimental setup should be designed to simulate as closely as possible the actual clinical situation. The device should be tested with the actual drug to account for rheology effects of the liquid in the nebulizer. All tubing and connectors should mimic the clinical situation. In these tests, care is needed for the breathing pattern to reflect the actual clinical situation with reasonable accuracy. In adults, given the relatively small range of patient size and therefore breathing patterns, the provision of an appropriate example of an adult breathing pattern for use with the simulator should produce results that give a reliable estimate of the quantity of drug available by inhalation to a given patient population. For pediatric tests, more care is needed owing to the much greater range of inspiratory and expiratory flows in infants and children. In some instances, *in vivo* filter tests using children actually breathing on the apparatus under investigation will be needed to ensure that the *in vitro* tests are representative. Failure to perform these studies in advance of clinical trials may result in inadequate drug delivery to the respiratory tract or may increase the risk of overdosage and toxicity.

References

1. Kollef MH. The prevention of ventilator-associated pneumonia. N Engl J Med 1999; 340:627–634.
2. Smaldone GC. Determinants of dose and response to inhaled therapeutic agents in asthma. In: Schleimer R, Busse W, O'Byrne P, eds. Inhaled Glucocorticoids in Asthma—Mechanisms and Clinical Actions. New York: Marcel Dekker, 1997
3. O'Riordan TG, Smaldone GC. Aerosols. In: Adkinson NF Jr, Busse WW, Ellis EF, Middleton E Jr, Reed C, Yunginger JW, eds. Allergy, Principles and Practices, 5th ed. St. Louis: Mosby, 1998.
4. Niven RW. Atomization and nebulizers. In: Hickey AJ, ed. Inhalation Aerosols: Physical and Biological Basis for Therapy. New York: Marcel Dekker, 1996:273–312.
5. Rosenthal RR: Methodologies of aerosol delivery. In: Spector SL, ed. Provocation Testing in Clinical Practice. Vol. 5. New York: Marcel Dekker, 1995:215.

6. Loffert D, Ikle D, Nelson H. A comparison of commercial jet nebulizers. Chest 1994; 106:1788–1793.
7. Tandon R, McPeck M, Smaldone GC. Measuring nebulizer output: aerosol production vs gravimetric analysis. Chest 1997; 111:1361–1365.
8. Smaldone GC. Drug delivery via aerosol systems: concept of "aerosol inhaled." J Aerosol Med 1991; 4:229–235.
9. Smaldone GC, Fuhrer J, Steigbigel RT, McPeck M. Factors determining pulmonary deposition of aerosolized pentamidine in patients with human immunodeficiency virus infection. Amer Rev Respir Dis 1991; 143:727–737.
10. Smaldone GC, Perry RJ, Deutsch DG. Characteristics of nebulizers used in the treatment of AIDS-related *Pneumocystis carinii* pneumonia. J Aerosol Med 1988; 1:113–126.
11. Collis GG, Cole HC, Le Souef PN. Dilution of nebulised aerosols by air entrainment in children. Lancet 1990; 336:341–343.
12. Devadason SG, Everard ML, Linto JM, Le Souef PN. Comparison of drug delivery from conventional versus "Venturi" nebulisers. Eur Respir J 1997; 10:2479–2483.
13. McPeck M, Tandon R, Hughes K, Smaldone GC. Aerosol delivery during continuous nebulization Chest 1997; 111:1200–1205.
14. Nikander K, Deyner J, Smaldone GC. Effects of equipment dead space and pediatric breathing patterns on inhaled mass of nebulized budesonide. J Aerosol Med 1999; 12:67–73.
15. O'Riordan TG, Iacono A., Keenan RJ, Duncan SR, Burckart GJ, Griffith BP, Smaldone GC. Delivery and distribution of aerosolized cyclosporine in lung allograft recipients. Am J Respir Crit Care Med 1995; 151:516–521.
16. Iacono AT, Smaldone GC, Keenan RJ, Diot P, Dauber JH, Zeevi A, Burckart GJ, Griffith BP. Dose-related reversal of acute lung rejection by aerosolized cyclosporine. Am J Respir Crit Care Med 1997; 155:1690–1698.
17. Iacono AT, Keenan RJ, Duncan SR, Smaldone GC, Dauber JH, Paridis IL, Ohori NP, Grgurich WF, Burckart GJ, Zeevi A, Delgado E, O'Riordan TG, Zendarsky MM, Yousem S, Griffith BP. Aerosolized cyclosporine in lung recipients with refractory chronic rejection. Am J Respir Crit Care Med 1996; 153:1451–1455.
18. Jackson WF, ed. Nebulized Budesonide Therapy in Asthma. Oxfordshire, UK: Clinical Vision, 1995:40–41.
19. Smaldone GC, Cruz-Rivera M, Nikander K. *In vitro* determination of inhaled mass and particle distribution for budesonide nebulizing suspension. J Aerosol Med 1998; 11:113–125.
20. Smaldone GC, Dickinson G. Factors important in the deposition of aerosolized pentamidine. In: Masuda S, Takahashi K, eds. Aerosols, Science, Industry, Health and Environment. Vol 1. Oxford, England: Pergamon Press, 1990:109–112.
21. Smaldone GC, Dickinson G, Marcial E, Young E, Seymour J. Deposition of aerosolized pentamidine and failure of Pneumocystis prophylaxis. Chest 1991; 101:82–87.
22. O'Riordan TG, Baughman RP, Dohn M, Shipley R, Buchsbaum JA, Frame PT, Smaldone GC. Lobar pentamidine levels and *Pneumocystis carinii* pneumonia following aerosolized pentamidine. Chest 1994; 105:53–56.

23. Smaldone GC, Walser L, Perry RJ, Ilowite JS, Bennett WD, Greco M. Generation and administration of aerosols for medical and physiological research studies. J Aerosol Med 1989; 2:81–87.
24. O'Riordan TG, Smaldone GC. Regional deposition and regional ventilation during inhalation of pentamidine. Chest 1994; 105:396–401.
25. Finlay WH, Estimating the type of hygroscopic behavior exhibited by aqueous droplets. J Aerosol Med 1998; 11:221–229.
26. Finlay WH, Smaldone GC. Editorial: hygroscopic behavior of nebulized aerosols: not as important as we thought? J Aerosol Med 1998; 11:193–195.
27. O'Riordan TG, Greco MJ, Smaldone GC. Nebulizer function during mechanical ventilation. Am Rev Respir Dis 1992; 145:1117–1122.
28. Everard ML. Studies using radio-labelled aerosols in children. Thorax 1994; 49:1259–1266.
29. Chua HK, Collis GG, Newbury AM, Chan K, Bower G, Sly PD, Le Souef PN. The influence of age on aerosol deposition in children with cystic fibrosis. Eur Respir J 1994; 7:2185–2191.
30. Fuller HD, Dolovich MB, Posmituck G, Wong Pack W, Newhouse MT. Pressurized aerosol versus jet aerosol delivery to mechanically ventilated patients. Am Rev Respir Dis 1989; 141:440–444.
31. MacIntyre N, Silver R, Miller C, Schuler F, Coleman E. Aerosol delivery to intubated, mechanically ventilated patients. Crit Care Med 1985; 13:81–84.
32. McPeck M, O'Riordan TG, Smaldone GC. Choice of mechanical ventilator: influence on nebulizer performance. Respir Care 1993; 38:887–895.
33. Diot P, Morra L, Smaldone GC. Albuterol delivery in a model of mechanical ventilation: comparison of MDI and nebulizer efficiency. Am J Respir Crit Care Med 1995; 152:1391–1394.
34. Palmer LB, Smaldone GC, Simon SR, O'Riordan TG, Cuccia A. Aerosolized antibiotics in mechanically ventilated patients: delivery and response. Crit Care Med 1998; 26:31–39.
35. O'Riordan TG, Palmer L, Smaldone GC. Aerosol deposition in mechanically ventilated patients: optimizing nebulizer delivery. Am J Respir Crit Care Med 1994; 149:214–219.
36. O'Riordan TG, Kleinman LI, Hughes K, Smaldone GC. Predicting aerosol deposition during neonatal ventilation: feasibility of bench testing. Respir Care 1994; 39:1162–1168.

9

New Nebulizer Technology

JOHN H. DENNIS

University of Bradford
Bradford, West Yorkshire,
England

OLA NERBRINK

AstraZeneca R&D
Lund, Sweden

I. Introduction

Many different devices are available for the inhalation of drug aerosols for deposition to the respiratory tract. Based on pharmaceutical formulation, these devices fall into three categories: pressurized metered dose inhalers (pMDIs), dry-powder inhalers (DPIs), and nebulizers. pMDIs and DPIs are the most common means of drug aerosol delivery, though both fall short of the ideal delivery device due to problems in formulation, dispensing, penetration into the respiratory tract, and patient coordination and handling. The traditional view of nebulizers is that they are expensive and bulky as well as inconvenient to handle, wash, and maintain; also that they are relatively inefficient. As a consequence they are relegated to third division in the marketplace. However, perhaps as a direct consequence of a lack of pharmaceutical vested interest, nebulizers remain poorly researched and understood by many clinicians and aerosol scientists. As a result, nebulizers may hold great potential, yet to be developed. Advancement in new nebulizer and inhalation technology, together with increased understanding of the physics of nebulized drug aerosol, offers greatly increased efficiency in nebulized drug aerosol delivery. At the current time, new nebulizer technologies offer convenient alternatives to less efficient pMDIs. It is conceivable that the development of new, more efficient and convenient nebulizer systems will lead to the possibility that these systems will eventually become the drug delivery method of choice in the development of new pharmaceutical products.

II. Background

It may be useful to define terminology that is so often misused in regards to the traditional nebulizer. Many researchers refer to the nebulizer they have used in their study simply by the brand name, with little or no consideration to other crucial component parts of the nebulizer system. Among the most influential are the compressor or line feed applied to the nebulizer resulting in specific air flow rates (for jet nebulizers), mode of operation (continuous or breath-activated), residual volume, and the use of face mask or mouthpiece, the latter often being "valved" for expired air. Each of these significantly influences the total amount received by the patient during therapy, the rate of nebulized aerosol output, and the aerosol droplet size distribution. It is far more appropriate to refer to the *nebulizer system* in its entirety, in which these components play a significant role in influencing nebulized drug aerosol delivery and its characteristics. Simply identifying the brand of nebulizer used without additional information on the nebulizer system is inappropriate and confounds the interpretation of many studies. If any significant component part of a nebulizer system is replaced by another, then the nebulizer system has changed and the aerosol output characteristics will have been significantly altered.

Characteristics of traditional nebulizer design (1–2) and clinical application (3–5) are well documented in the literature. Nebulized drug solutions offer convenient formulations often unavailable in pMDI and DPI formulations. However, at the present time manufacturers of pMDIs are struggling to cope with imposed change of formulations due to environmental damage caused toy CFC propellants. DPIs are dependent on the patient's ability to perform a force-pull inhalation in order to release and disperse the powder formulation into an aerosol. This is not the case with any currently available nebulizer. Concurrently, patented DPI devices are expensive to develop and manufactures continue their struggle to optimize efficient release mechanisms and delivery of powder formulations for all patient groups. Though pMDIs and DPIs face difficult technological challenges, rapid development of nanotechnology, microelectronics, and battery power, coupled with an inherent ease of aqueous drug formulation, has provided a massive boost to the development of new and greatly improved nebulizer technology. We are currently in the middle of an exciting developmental phase in nebulizer-related technology. The aim of this chapter is to introduce this range of new and emerging nebulizer technologies and to evaluate their potential impact on drug aerosol delivery and clinical practice.

Traditional nebulizers are generally regarded as relatively inefficient drug delivery devices. The amount of drug reaching the lungs from a nebulizer is typically only 5–20% of the nominal dose placed in the nebulizer. The inefficiency of the traditional nebulizer principally results from a combination of three factors. First, a large residual volume (typically 1 mL) is usually left in the nebulizer at the end of treatment, which accounts for the largest proportion of waste—particularly as most typical nebulizer volume fills are on the order of 2–3 mL. Due to evaporation during nebulization, the remaining drug solution or suspension becomes increasingly concentrated. Thus the 1 mL remaining may contain 20–30% (6) more drug than expected, a situation enhanced in breath-enhanced jet nebulizer designs, where there is further entrainment of ambient air through the nebulizer (7). Second, a significant proportion of the aerosol generated is released during exhalation or respiratory pauses and will not be inhaled. Aerosol lost on exhalation is usually emitted into the home or hospital environment, which may create a health risk to others; though with some nebulizer designs, waste aerosol can be collected on optional filters or other scavenging systems. The third factor contributing to the inefficiency of traditional nebulizers is inappropriate droplet size. Inevitably, a proportion of inhaled aerosol will be too large to penetrate through the upper airway and will deposit in mouth, nose, or pharynx, potentially contributing to local and systemic side effects.

However, a pMDI without spacer or a DPI with a poor inhalation maneuver is an equally inefficient drug aerosol delivery device. Further, a greater proportion of drug aerosol from pMDIs and DPIs is usually deposited in the mouth, throat, and upper respiratory tract, where the drug is of no therapeutic consequence and may contribute to unwanted local or systemic side effects.

Traditional jet nebulizer devices deliver a variety of drug formulations. As such, for regulatory purposes, there is an effective separation between drug delivery device and pharmaceutical preparation. This forms a loophole in which nebulized drug delivery can bypass regulatory requirements (clinical trials) applying to pMDIs, DPIs, and other devices sold in combination with drug formulations. This has the disadvantage and risk that nebulized drug delivery is rarely supported by evidence-based medicine. When evidence from clinical trials is available, it is often confounded by a reluctance to specify operating conditions and identify all relevant components of the nebulizer system.

Without regulatory input and without a clear indication of safety and efficacy of nebulized drug delivery, patients receiving nebulized drugs are perhaps more vulnerable than those receiving drugs from more controlled delivery systems. It is conceivable and perhaps inevitable that patients receiving nebulized drugs from the new generation of nebulizer devices, with increased efficiencies, will receive greatly increased doses of drug aerosol if the same nominal dose is prescribed. Without proper understanding of the anticipated improvements in nebulized drug aerosol generation and delivery, and effective monitoring and modification of prescribing habits in clinical practice, problems will occur. However, if appropriate action is taken to review and modify prescribing habits in relation to the efficiency of new-generation nebulizers, the technology offers greater portability, ease of use, speed of drug delivery, and control of dose delivered.

III. New Nebulizer Technology

For the purposes of this chapter, new nebulizer technologies include technology developed and introduced after 1990 that further, are regarded as fundamentally different from traditional nebulizers. New nebulizer technology introduced in this chapter is presented as four classes:

1. New adaptations of existing jet nebulizer technology to produce dosimetric systems for conventional generic nebulized drug delivery—e.g., Halolite and Circulaire
2. New ultrasonic nebulizer technology for conventional generic drug delivery—e.g., AeroNeb and Omron.
3. New nebulizer delivery devices designed to deliver specific drug formulations that have undergone clinical trials to establish safety and efficacy as part of the regulatory process—e.g., Respimat and AERx.
4. New nebulizer designs that are only just emerging whose nebulized aerosol applications have not yet been fully defined—e.g., TouchSpray, Microjet, and Gañan-Calvo technology.

Classes 1 and 2 are modifications of conventional nebulizing therapy in the perspective that these have operational times lasting minutes or more. The last two classes introduce novel nebulizer technology that is fundamentally different in that delivery time for drug aerosol is very short, typically 1 or 2 s. Further, the latter two classes offer the convenience and portability more common to the DPI or pMDI than to traditional nebulizers.

New nebulizer technologies present an opportunity that should transform the stereotypical image of the traditional inefficient nebulizer. Some of these new technologies offer the convenience, portability, and ease of use of more popular pMDIs and DPIs. For some drugs, new nebulizer technology should have fewer and potentially easier technological and formulation problems to solve. Many new nebulizer technologies offer greatly improved efficiency in aerosol delivery. It remains largely up to prescribers of nebulized drugs to fully appreciate how increased efficiency will result in a corresponding increase in dose delivery with new and emerging nebulizer technologies. This understanding would be improved with more cooperation and involvement from both nebulizer and pharmaceutical companies together with participation of regulatory authorities.

IV. The Ideal Nebulizer

It may not be possible or even necessary to accommodate all the features of an "ideal" nebulizer system. Below is a "wish list" of desirable features.

1. A minimum residual volume (< 0.5 mL)
2. Aerosol delivered only during inhalation
3. No waste aerosol released to the environment
4. Aerosol delivered with a droplet size distribution suitable for pulmonary or tracheobronchial deposition
5. Small and portable: similar to the more popular pMDIs and DPIs (and ideally no more expensive)
6. Rapid treatment time, quiet and unobtrusive in use
7. Finally, perhaps also a means to monitor patient compliance

At present, there is little understanding of nebulizer performance by the typical decision makers within a hospital or community health care organization. Usually the bottom-line factor dictating which nebulizer system to purchase is cost. Consider what would result if an ideal nebulizer design, incorporating the desirable features described above, were to be made available and was proven to be both efficient and cheap. Competitive marketing of desirable features and low cost would quickly convince most decision makers and prescribers to adopt this design for use by their patients. Previous therapies given with relatively inefficient nebulizers would presumably be prescribed in the same manner—i.e., *X* mg dose in *Y* mL diluent volume. If the traits of the ideal nebulizer shown above were real, an increase in actual dose delivered to the patient would result. Half the residual volume would double the dose, and aerosol release only during inhalation would double it again. The increase in nebulized aerosol dose received by the patient may be even greater if increased compliance were taken into consideration. Adverse noticeable side effects may well provide feedback to reduce subsequent doses prescribed, though this would not apply to all nebulized drugs. It is unclear whose responsibility it is to regulate nebulized drug delivery and to ensure minimum standards of safety and efficacy. Nevertheless, if the consequences of choosing different "generic" nebulizer/drug combinations were apparent to the prescriber and the effect of improved and more accurate drug delivery obvious, resulting better therapy would decrease patient relapse involving hospitalization. A small increase in costs of purchasing new nebulizer technology would be small compared to potential savings from patient hospitalization. If true, a decrease in net cost should appeal to decision makers within hospitals and community health care organizations.

In the absence of clinical trials to establish safety and efficacy, assessment of efficiency of nebulizer systems relies largely on in vitro assessment of nebulizer performance. However, a number of factors conspire to confuse understanding of in vitro nebulizer performance. Nebulized aerosol does not behave in the same way as aerosols from pMDIs or DPIs. Extending in vitro methods of MDI assessment to nebulized aerosol is simply wrong if the objective of in vitro assessment is to reflect clinical use. The mode of drug inhalation is different between nebulizers and pMDIs and DPIs; the stability of droplet size is also different. Evaporation of the pMDI propellant is more rapid than the evaporation of water from nebulizer droplets. In vitro methods for pMDIs and DPIs using, for example, high-flow (continuous at 28.3 or 60 L/min) cascade impaction have been designed in part to reflect in vivo (variable-flow) conditions of the pMDI breath maneuver and dose delivered with it. The high airflow and evaporation effects will assess the generated droplet size distribution differently and most certainly give markedly different results for the pMDI, DPI, and nebulizer respectively. The continuous tidal breathing associated with nebulizer therapy is very different and requires different in vitro methods to assess aerosol output and size of nebulizer design performance if in vitro tests are to be predictive of in vivo performance.

A basic lack of understanding of nebulized aerosol physics, the impact of nebulizer design on aerosol generation, and the influence of patient breathing patterns on nebulizer output have given rise to a plethora of different methods of measurement. This has resulted in a wide range of different in vitro methods to assess nebulizer performance. Because in vitro assessment of nebulizer system output will continue to be an important consideration in assessing the potential benefits of most new nebulizer technologies, this chapter includes a brief introduction and description of two European initiatives. The first relates to the pending publication of a new European (Comité Europeen de Normalisation, or CEN) standard incorporating clinically reflective in vitro standard methods to assess nebulizer system performance for aerosol output and droplet size distribution. The second is an introduction to the pending publication of Clinical Nebulizer Guidelines through the European Respiratory Society, which will in part rely on the new European in vitro standard. From a clinical perspective, the development of evidence-based clinical guidelines for nebulizers should be of interest, as this presents a forum in which the development and introduction of new nebulizer technology with potentially greatly improved efficiency can be assessed and monitored to guide clinical practice. The authors are not aware of any similar developments in North America or elsewhere to assess and control nebulized drug aerosol delivery.

Nebulizers are principally used by children (<5 years) and adults (<55 years) who have difficulty coordinating the use of MDIs and DPIs, by patients with severe asthma or chronic obstructive pulmonary disease (COPD), and in the emergency room for acute episodes of bronchospasm. Today the bulk and cost of nebulizers relative to MDIs and DPIs makes them inappropriate for the majority of patients. However, pMDIs using chlorofluorocarbons (CFCs) contribute to ozone depletion (8), with subsequent environmental and public health impacts. The pending ban on CFCs for use in medical aerosols has resulted in research being directed toward providing efficient alternative methods for pulmonary delivery of drugs, particularly using alternative propellants such as hydrofluoroalkanes (HFAs) or alcohol, DPIs, and new nebulizer delivery systems. Presumed environmental problems with the HFAs may further promote development of new nebulizer technologies as well as further DPI development.

Examples of recent developments in new nebulizer technologies and significant new modifications to traditional nebulizer technologies are considered in turn below.

V. Examples of New Nebulizer Technologies

A. Traditional Nebulizer Technology Modified for Improved Generic Use (Halolite, Circulaire)

Both the Halolite and Ciculaire nebulizer systems aim to deliver a more controlled aerosol dose to the patient by different means. The Halolite emits aerosol for a fraction of each inhalation cycle before ceasing when a preset cumulative dose has been delivered. Circulaire uses a reservoir bag to conserve continuously emitted aerosol, which in principle increases the amount of aerosol available for inhalation. Both these systems rely on preexisting jet nebulizer technology designs which have then been adapted to provide dosimetric systems. In the case of Halolite, the doses delivered are relatively small, though reproducibility of dose delivery is considerably better than that from Circulaire, whose aerosol dose delivery is related to the total aerosol output of the nebulizer less deposition in the nebulizer system.

Halolite Medic-Aid

Halolite is a hand-held delivery system incorporating a jet nebulizer operated from a dedicated compressor (Fig. 1). The Halolite uses a software-driven monitoring and control system marketed as adaptive aerosol delivery (AAD). AAD monitors patient breathing parameters known to influence the aerosol delivery and respiratory tract deposition such as inhalation flow, breath frequency, and inspiratory time. This is done by monitoring the last three breaths in a continuous fashion, thereby allowing calculation of an appropriate aerosol pulse time. Aerosol is delivered within the first half of each predicted inhalation and the AAD system continues to adapt to changes in breathing pattern throughout the treatment. The system software is intended recognize when a patient has temporarily ceased breathing through the system (for example, to cough or speak), and the nebulizing process is suspended until the patient resumes treatment. This ensures that a precise preset dose is delivered to each patient, independent of his

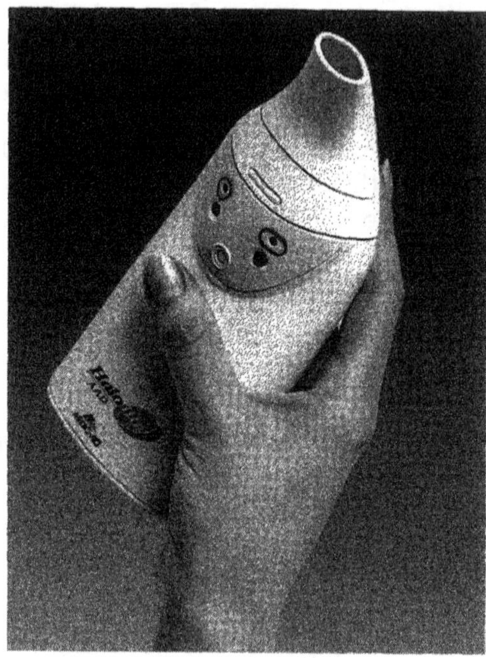

Figure 1 The Halolite nebulizer (compressor not shown).

or her breathing pattern or any interruption to the treatment (Fig. 2). The system indicates when treatment is complete after a preprogrammed total nebulization time has passed—nebulization time in this regard is linearly related to aerosol dose emitted and delivered to the patient. In a laboratory trial of 19 patients, Halolite reportedly demonstrated delivery of a preset dose with a CoV = 17% (9) and a high proportion of treatments delivered to the preset dose (10). Compared with traditional nebulizers the Halolite nebulizer system shows a significant improvement in the control of delivered doses irrespective of the patient's adherence to regimen (10).

The Halolite nebulizer system can also incorporate a patient logging system, which records the date, time, and dose received for each treatment. This allows objective measures of compliance to be made. Halolite provides a delivery system that can react to the patient's breathing pattern and target aerosol delivery to help ensure that aerosol is delivered only during the initial inspiratory phase of the patient's inhalation cycle in an effort to maximize lung deposition. The system is relatively simple to use. Once appropriately connected to the compressor and switched on, the Halolite system is fully automatic, requiring no individual adjustment, and is thought to be suitable for patients from 3 years of age. The

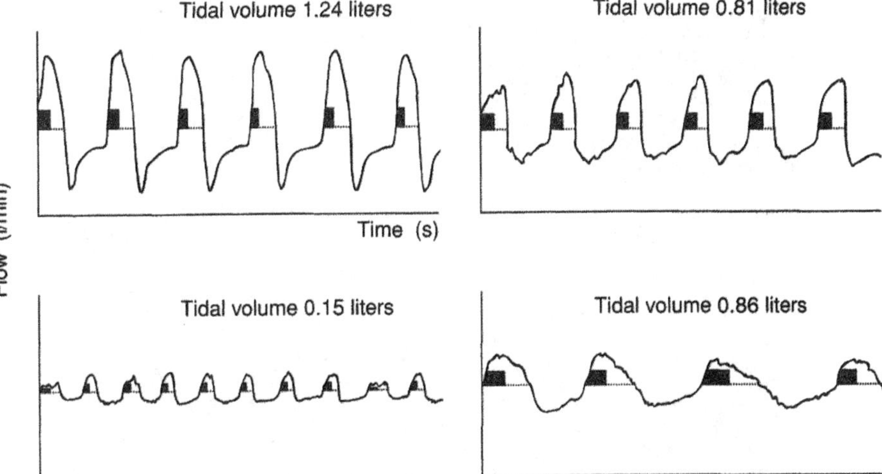

Figure 2 Schematic illustrating adaptive aerosol delivery from Halolite. Solid boxes represent periods of aerosol delivery for four different breathing patterns. Aerosol is only delivered during the first half of each inspiration. The HaloLite system indicates when the preprogrammed dose has been delivered. In each of the four examples, the dose delivered is the same but the treatment time will be different. The treatment time is dependent on the ratio of inspiratory to expiratory time and the number of breaths per minute. (From Ref. 11.)

provision of patient feedback helps promote effective and consistent delivery of the preset dose. The Halolite may be used with existing liquid drug preparations and unit-dose vials. The device is still cumbersome and requires the same rigorous cleaning regime as a reusable traditional nebulizer system.

Circulaire WestMed

Traditional nebulizers are made particularly inefficient by having a high residual volume and continuing to emit aerosol during patients' breath-holds and exhalations. The solution presented in the Circulaire nebulizer system (Fig. 3) was to add an exhalation valve and plastic reservoir bag intended to minimize waste aerosol. In theory, assuming a near balance between total nebulizer compressed airflow and overall patient inspiratory rate, no aerosol released from the nebulizer would be emitted to the environment. Any aerosol generated during patient breath-hold or expiration is stored in the flexible reservoir until the next inspiration, though it is not clear how much drug aerosol is deposited on the bag walls. Though this system does nothing to reduce the drug solution lost as residual vol-

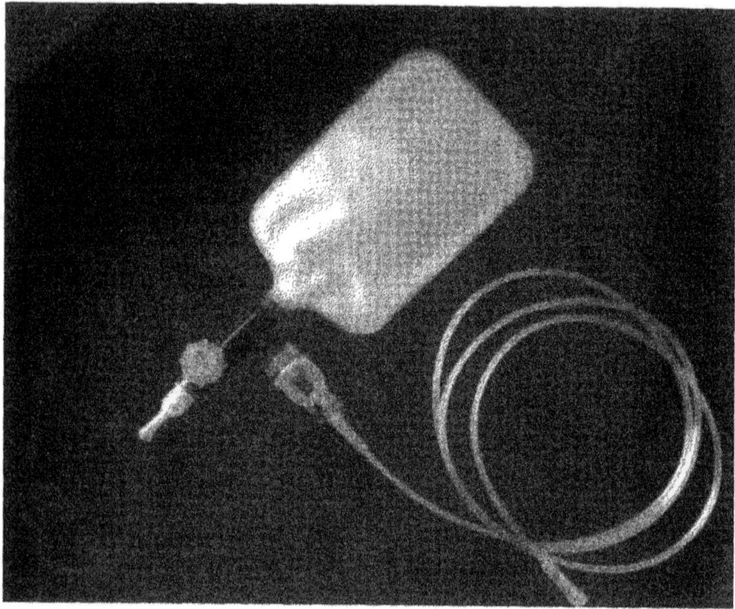

Figure 3 Circulaire nebulizer system. A traditional constant output jet nebulizer produces aerosol continuously by compressed air (compressor not shown). During patient inhalation, aerosol is drawn from the system by patient inspiration. During patient breath hold and exhalation (through one-way valve adjacent to mouthpiece) decompressed jet nebulized air containing aerosol fills an inflatable plastic bag for inhalation during subsequent breaths.

ume within the traditional nebulizer, it does potentially eliminate aerosol wasted to the environment. Instead, a proportion of this aerosol is made available for inhalation thus increasing the overall dose.

The Circulaire nebulizer system increases the rate and total aerosol dose delivered to the patient compared to the traditional constant-output nebulizer alone, and this has savings in treatment time as well as potentially reducing costs (12). Further, aerosol wasted to the environment is minimized, which, in turn, minimizes occupational exposures to drug aerosol (13,14). As with the Halolite system, the Circulaire is cumbersome and complicated to clean.

Synopsis

The Halolite uses existing drug formulations, which have been registered separately. The AAD technology allows the Halolite to deliver accurate doses to the patient with minimal wastage; the feedback to the patient might improve patient compliance. These features overcome many of the disadvantages of conventional nebulizers while using the existing drug formulations, but they do necessitate consideration of what delivered dose is required for different drugs rather than prescribing volume fill.

The reservoir incorporated within the Circulaire nebulizer system may help increase the inhaled proportion of aerosol from a given fill volume compared to the same driving nebulizer without incorporation of the valved reservoir bag system. Like the Halolite, this implies reconsideration of prescribed doses and volume fills of drug solution to avoid overdosing. The extent to which the droplet size from conventional nebulizers is affected by adaptations in Halolite and Circulaire nebulizer system is not clear. Meaning in vitro measurements (e.g., European standard) characterizing droplet size from either system is not available.

The small amounts of aerosol generated by a system such as Halolite are produced over relatively short time period (< 1 s) in a discrete bolus. This bolus is entrained with ambient air during patient inhalation and one would expect a considerable amount of mixing to occur. As ambient air has a significant capacity to absorb water vapor from nebulized aerosol (relative humidity normally <70%), evaporation of aqueous aerosol would be inevitable and rapid. The reduction in droplet size would be expected to be inconsistent, as the rate of evaporation will depend on the speed of inhalation which defines degree of dilution as well as temperature and humidity of ambient air. In contrast, aerosol-laden air inhaled from the Circulaire nebulizer system will entrain little ambient air and is therefore relatively less sensitive to any reduction in droplet size due to evaporation. To what extent evaporation reduces droplet size from Halolite is not known and deserves further investigation.

B. New Generic Nebulizer Technology: Omron and Aeroneb Ultrasonic Nebulizers

Omron Ultrasonic Nebulizer

Though ultrasonic nebulizer technology is not new in itself, an ultrasonic nebulizer that works reliably with both solutions and suspensions would be new, as many past devices have been either unreliable, have been unable to nebulize suspensions, and/or have produced droplets too large to penetrate to the lower respiratory tract.

Omron launched a battery-operated hand-held nebulizer in 1994 (in Japan, model NE-U03) (15), which has recently been updated (in Japan, model NE-U14). The Omron nebulizer employs a ceramic mesh and double-horn oscillator that combine to release a fairly fine liquid aerosol with relatively low power consumption. A unit is pictured in Fig. 4 and its operation schematically

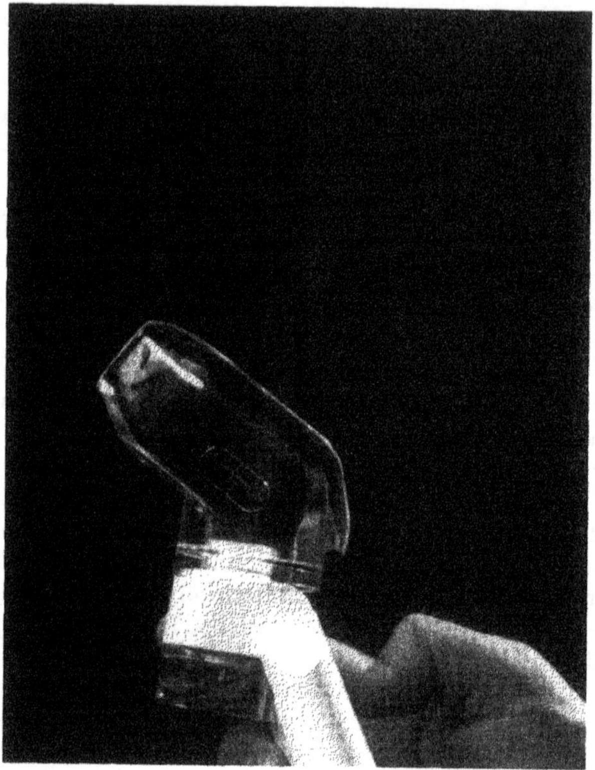

Figure 4 Omron NU-14.

represented in Fig. 5. Desirable features of the Omron ultrasonic nebulizer include portability (150 g), with power supplied by four AA batteries, there is a relatively minute residual volume (0.3 mL), and little degradation of complex drug formulations (16).

Limitations of the first Omron product include an inability to control nebulization of drugs present as suspensions due to incorporation of a small mesh hole size (between 3 and 4 μm), which could trap suspension droplets (Omron, unpublished data). The latest unit operates at 6 MHz (compared to 65 kHz for the previous unit) and is reported to generate finer aerosol droplets with a lower dependence on mesh size, which has been increased to 5 μm for the newer model (K. Kuki, personal communication 1999). Though published performance data on the unit are limited (17), manufacturer's data (unpublished) suggest that the latest unit (NE-U14) has a sufficiently large mesh hole size (5 μm) to facilitate passage and nebulization of drug suspensions, though this remains controversial. If

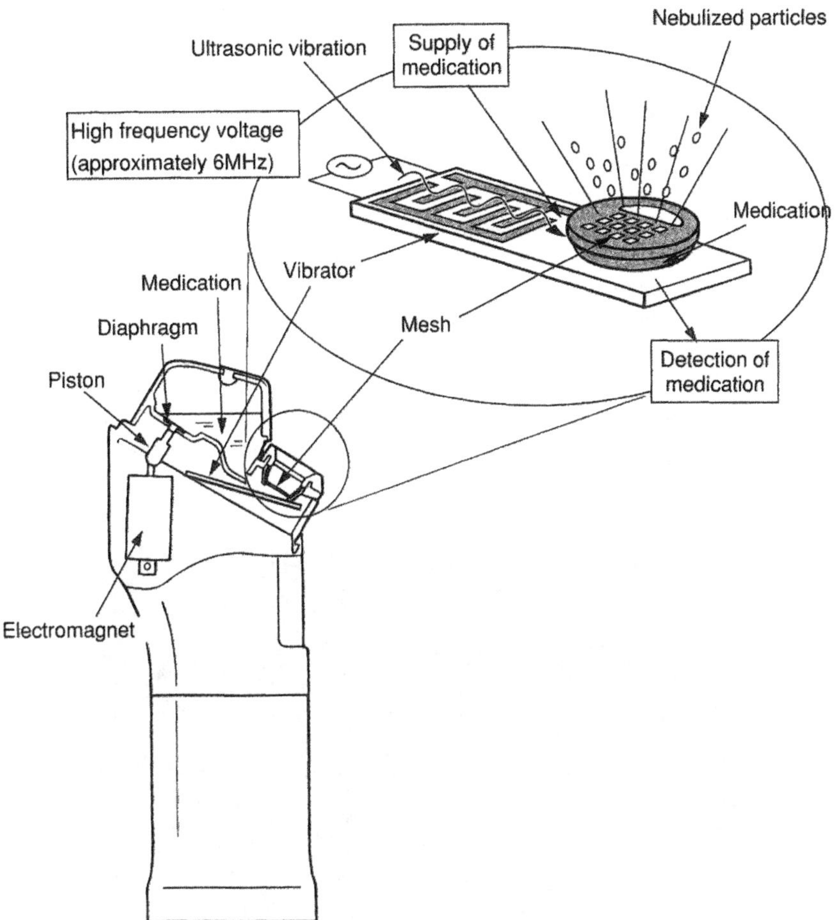

Figure 5 Schematic of Omron NE-UI4. When the power is turned on, the piston is operated by the electromagnet and pushes up the diaphragm at the bottom of the "medication bottle." Medication is then supplied to the area between the vibrator and the mesh. The ultrasonic energy generated from the vibrator is transmitted to the medication, which then is nebulized through microholes in the mesh.

true, however, practicalities of cleaning and maintenance require further investigation. A further subtle technical limitation of the early Omron nebulizer was a constant power function that did not have the ability to change with different medications, so a medication with very high viscosity or a medication with a very low surface tension could alter the rate of nebulization and also affect droplet size. However, the latest unit (NE-U14) has a power control/feedback system, which reportedly allows it to more consistently nebulize a wide range of medications (manufacturer, personal communication).

AeroNeb Aerogen

The AeroNeb is a silent, portable nebulizer system (Fig. 6) which is designed to nebulize most liquid drug formulations. In principle it is ultrasonic-like in its operation. The atomization technology eliminates the compressor required with a pneumatic nebulizer; no tubing is needed, thereby reducing costs and maintenance. The AeroNeb is low-power (1 W), and this allows it to operate from a portable battery pack using AA batteries or, alternatively, from an AC power supply or a car cigarette lighter.

AeroNeb comprises a reservoir cup for storing the liquid drug. A capillary system supplies the liquid drug to the rear surface of a shell containing an array of conical holes. A piezoelectric crystal generates a vibratory energy that bends

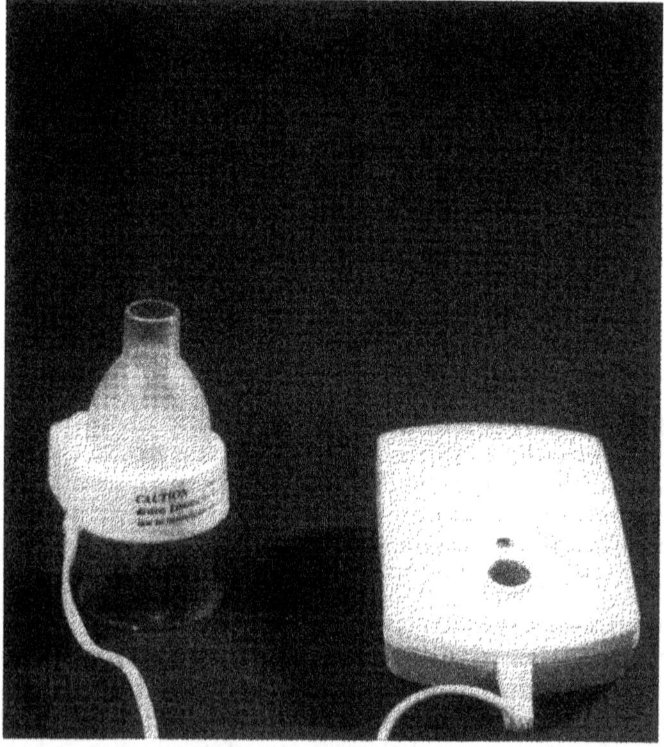

Figure 6 AeroNeb.

or oscillates the shell, which induces instability in the liquid jets emitted from the holes in the shell, causing the liquid to break up into uniform small droplets. Droplet size distribution is reported to range from 1 to 6 μm, with over 80% mass of the drug in a respirable range. The aerosol leaves the shell with little momentum and therefore has a low velocity. Current nebulizers typically require a minimum reservoir volume of 0.5–1.0 mL to be operational, so some drug remains in the system after nebulization is complete. The AeroNeb reservoir can hold up to 6 mL of liquid and nebulize virtually the entire drug solution, minimizing waste and increasing drug aerosol delivery.

In principle, both the AeroNeb and Omron nebulizer system incorporate desirable features that are absent in conventional nebulizer designs. Both systems are hand-held, portable, and reusable; both have have low running costs. However, it is worth bearing in mind that few clinicians and/or users will be aware of the higher doses of nebulized drug aerosol being delivered, given the current prescribing conventions detailing drug per volume fill as opposed to drug delivered to patient Significantly higher doses may produce unwanted clinical side effects. Given a patient coping well with a traditional nebulizer prescription, it might be prudent to consider reducing the drug prescribed in the Omron or AeroNeb systems in order to approach an equivalent delivered dose. However, as with all nebulizer systems, it has been difficult, to date, to obtain reliable and meaningful comparative figures on nebulizer performance.

Synopsis

The performance of new nebulizer technology incorporated in Aeroneb and Omron is not too dissimilar to that of traditional nebulizer technology. Both generate aerosol on a continuous basis that is not synchronized with the patient inhalation. There is a facility on the latest version of the Omron device to manually activate the nebulizer during patient inhalation only, though this requires a high degree of coordination and compliance from the patient. In any case, the development of low-power battery-operated ultrasonic nebulizer technology offers the convenience of portability. In both units, the battery power consumption is sufficiently low to facilitate use over many treatments before recharging. Efficient design of solution-holding chambers within the internal nebulizing units of each system has been developed to ensure that only a minimum reservoir volume remains in the nebulizer on cessation of nebulization. This, coupled with reasonable rates of aerosol output, should ensure that the nebulized dose delivered from both of these units will be substantially greater than nebulized drug aerosol output from traditional nebulizers, given similarly prescribed drug dose and volume. These systems are clearly more convenient and efficient than traditional technology, and this deserves consideration in their clinical application. In nebulized drug applications where side effects are not an issue and the goal is to deliver as much nebulized aerosol as possible within a time frame most acceptable to the patient, the new technology presented by both Omron and Aerogen offers superior systems compared to traditional nebulizer technology.

C. New Nebulizer Technology Developed for Specific Drug Applications: Respimat and AERx

In recent years, the advent of new methods of aerosolization of solutions without propellants and the improvement in microelectronic dosimetric systems has led to the development of more efficient designs, two of which, Respimat and AERx, combine the drug formulation and delivery system. Though these systems are in principle nebulizers, their application is more analogous to pMDIs and DPIs in terms of regulatory development, portability, and use. However, they may prove to offer significant advantages over pMDIs and DPIs in terms of drug delivery efficiency, and patient compliance.

Respimat Boehringer Ingelheim

Technically, Boehringer Ingelheim's Respimat technology does fall within the definition of a nebulizer, as Respimat transforms aqueous liquid solution to liquid aerosol droplets suitable for inhalation. In recognition that the Respimat is a new type of device, Boehringer Ingelheim has coined the phrase *soft mist inhaler* (SMI). Respimat differs in important respects from traditional nebulizer designs in that it is a single-phase pneumatic system in which the delivery device is matched to particular drug solutions. Because it is sold as a matched drug-device delivery system, it has developed under FDA regulatory control. Respimat is a propellant-free, hand-held (Fig. 7) multidose inhaler, that emits a metered dose of drug solution of 15 μL volume, with high lung deposition. The low volume delivered implies a higher concentration of the drug in the solution, which will present formulation challenges to the pharmaceutical company. It retains the convenience and ease of use of MDIs while not requiring a spacer or a battery-driven power source and can be reused by replacing the drug cartridge.

Respimat uses a new, propellant-free propulsion method schematically illustrated Fig. 8. The device is prepared for use by turning the lower half of the device through 180 degrees, thereby compressing a spring. Simultaneously, a measured amount of drug solution is drawn up from the drug cartridge into the dosing system. Actuation of the device by pressing the dose button releases the spring. This raises the pressure and forces the solution through a nozzle structure within a uniblock, which has two narrow outlet channels 8 μm in diameter, etched using microchip technology (18). The two jets of drug solution converge and the impact generates a polydisperse respirable aerosol. Respirability of nebulized droplets is determined by both droplet size and velocity of air within

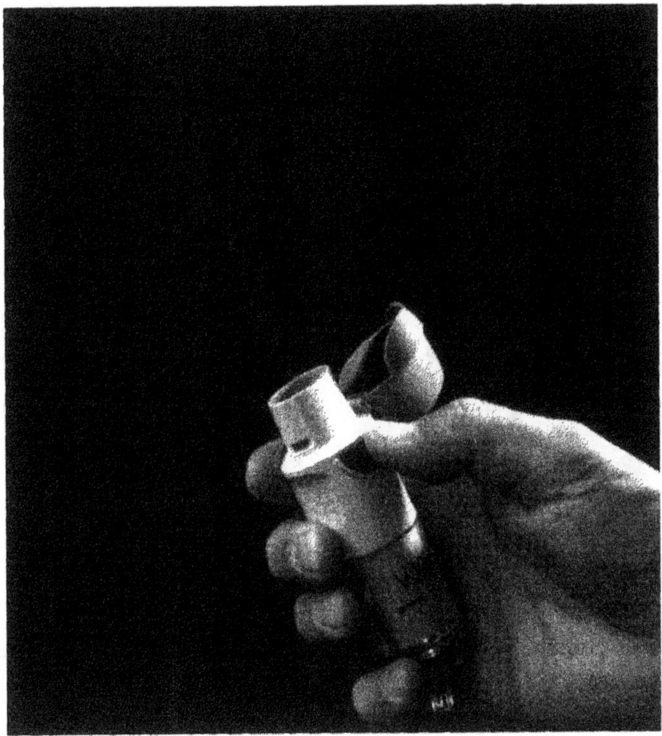

Figure 7 Respimat.

which they are inhaled (19). To avoid blocking of the nozzles, Respimat contains two prefilters within the silicon uniblock.

The aerosol fine droplet fraction from Respimat is reported to be approximately double that for a CFC-MDI (20), though the in vitro methods used to characterize droplet size of the rapidly evaporated pMDI residue aerosols cannot be meaningfully applied to characterizing largely aqueous nebulized aerosol droplets. More importantly, the aerosol emitted from Respimat is released very slowly and with a velocity approximately four times less than that from CFC MDIs. This greatly reduces the potential for drug impaction in the oropharynx (18), which remains a great limitation of pMDIs. In addition, the relatively long duration over which the dose is expelled from Respimat (about 1.2 s, compared with 0.1 s from pMDIs), would be expected to greatly reduce the need to coordinate actuation and inspiration, thus improving the potential for greater lung deposition. Improved drug delivery to the lungs has been confirmed in scintigraphic deposition studies (21), where Respimat has been shown to pro-

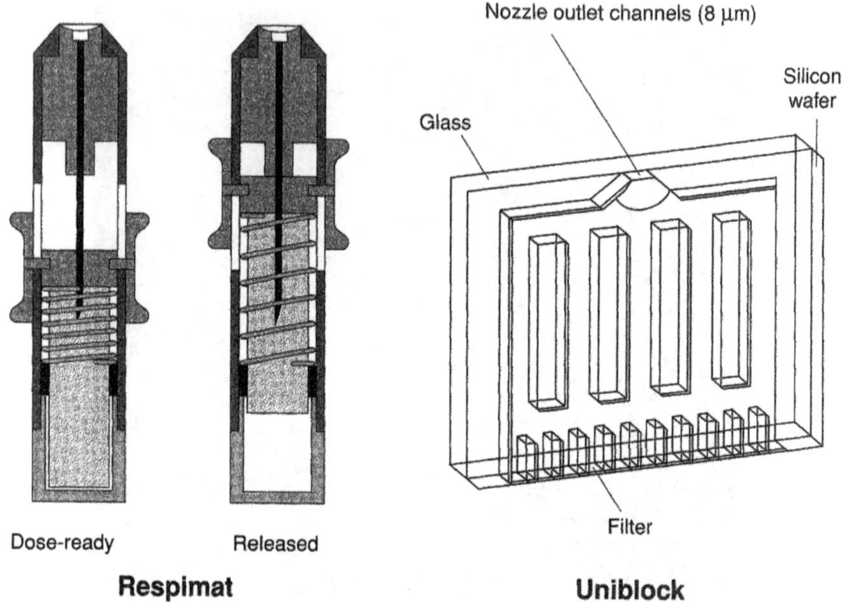

Figure 8 Schematic diagram of Respimat illustrating principle of actuation and design of the uniblock (see text for description of operation).

duce a two-to threefold increase in lung deposition of drug in comparison with a pMDI. In general the oropharyngeal deposition when drugs are inhaled from Respimat is much less than from a pMDI (22). Further, clinical studies of inhaled fenoterol alone or combined with ipatropium bromide in asthmatic patients indicated that lower doses administered by Respimat can produce a bronchodilatory effect and safety profile similar to that obtained with standard doses administered via a pMDI (23).

AERx Aradigm

Like Respimat, the AERx system is a drug- and device-specific nebulizing system. As such it can be formulated with different drug solutions that have been or currently are going through the regulatory process, and a considerable amount is becoming known concerning its clinical effectiveness. AERx is a portable handheld system (Fig. 9) consisting of a disposable dosage form containing prepacked doses as individual packets or on a blister strip enclosed in a disposable cartridge. The device contains aerosol generation hardware and electronics associated with breath actuation and compliance monitoring (24,25).

One of the design principles behind development of the AERx system is to

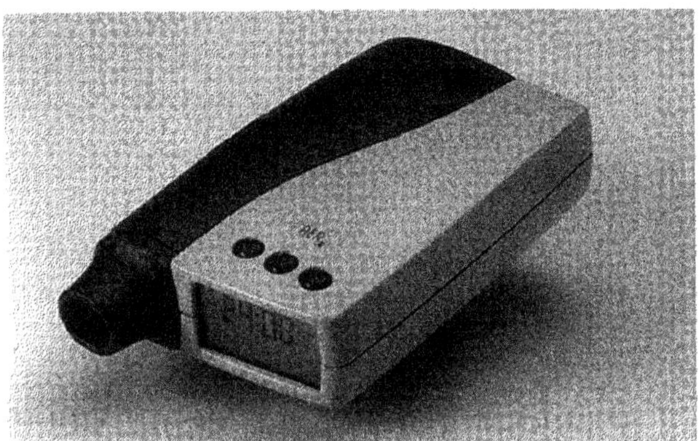

Figure 9 AERx.

reexamine and improve on deficiencies with pMDIs and DPIs in terms of the amount and consistency of delivered dose. The AERx system is designed to obviate the requirement for patients to remember and comply with instructions for use. Perhaps one of the most significant variables in drug aerosol delivery from pMDIs, DPIs, and most nebulizer systems resides in breathing patterns within and between patients. AERx technology should help reduce these variables by encouraging optimum breathing through flow-sensing technology linked to electronic feedback to the patient to optimize a full exhalation, followed by actuation of the device early in inspiration and a relatively low inspiratory flow AERx visually guides the patient to inhale in the optimum range of the inspiratory flow and delivers the aerosol pulse only at a predetermined combination of inspired volume and inspiratory flow; it provides the user with a timer to control the breath-holding maneuver. The aerosol is not emitted unless the patient is breathing at the correct flow and there is still enough inspired volume reserve to allow the drug to clear the physiological dead space of the lung. In this way, if a patient initiates the inhalation at a high velocity and subsequently corrects this guided by the appropriate LED indication, the aerosol may still not be emitted if the inspired volume is excessive (I. Gonda, personal communication, 1999).

Currently the AERx system yields an emitted dose in a range of 60–75% of the dose inserted. A schematic diagram depicting the operation of AERx is shown in Fig. 10. The formulation is contained in a predosed blister with a volume of 50 μL and beside it a multilayer lid. The lid has a micromachined array of holes that are sealed from the blister. On pressurization of the blister, the seal breaks, which forces the liquid formulation through the nozzle array into the inhalation path. In order to reduce variability due to changes in ambient conditions, a temperature-controlling module is used to warm inspired air before the generation of aerosol. The authors believe that this last innovation is an impor-

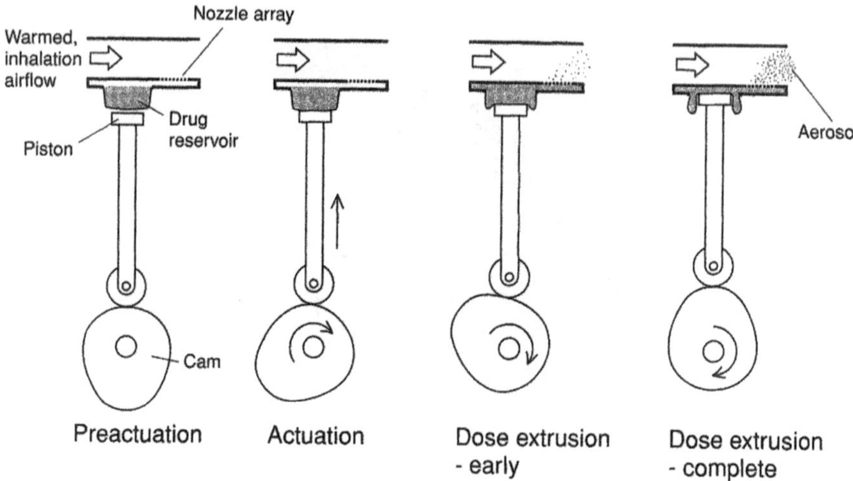

Figure 10 AERx schematic showing four stages of aerosol generation.

tant development, as no other nebulizer design even attempts to control the dynamic droplet size characteristics of liquid aerosols affected by ambient temperature and humidity conditions. A drawback is the fact that heating consumes energy that has to come from the battery source and this in turn increases the size of the device. The improved precision and reproducibility of dose delivery from AERx is reported to be substantially greater than the comparative imprecision of dose delivery from pMDIs and DPIs (I. Gonda, personal communication, 1999), though this deserves further investigation.

Technology underlying the AERx system provides a simple system for the patient to use and provides effective feedback on the efficiency of aerosol delivery. This is important for the accurate dose delivery of systemically acting drugs with a relatively narrow therapeutic index. The disposable dosage vial provides stable drug storage in a single-use aerosolization system, minimizing the risk of contamination or device malfunction. As a nebulizer system, AERx represents a great improvement over existing technology in terms of consistency, efficiency, and precision of nebulized drug delivery. The AERx system is being developed for the delivery of specific drugs requiring accurate control of dosage, including insulin (phase II); morphine (phase II); a drug to aid mucociliary clearance in COPD in collaboration with Inspire (INS 365), currently in phase I; proteins, in early phase II; recombinant human deoxyribonuclease with Genentech (phase I); and nonviral gene therapy, which is currently preclinical stage (I. Gonda, personal communication, 1999).

Synopsis

The characteristics of both Respimat and AERx clearly differentiate them from traditional nebulizers and those traditional nebulizer systems that have been modified to increase output (Circulaire) or deliver discrete doses (Halolite). Both are being developed and marketed in conjunction with specific drugs that subsequently undergo clinical trials. Both are dosimetric in operation, are reported to have very low residual volumes, have low or no electrical power requirements, and both Respimat and AERx are thought to have good dose reproducibility.

D. Emerging Nebulizer Technology: TouchSpray and Microjet

Two new nebulizer technologies have only recently been introduced in principle; their specific system design and application have not yet been publicized. Each utilizes distinctly different new nebulizer technology. Each would be expected to offer exciting new applications in nebulized aerosol therapy, though this will depend in part on how the technology is fully developed in collaboration with industrial partners.

TouchSpray TTP

TouchSpray can best be described as a vibrating-orifice ultrasonic nebulizer and was developed by the Technology Partnership (TTP), U.K. This technology has only recently been announced and little is as yet published (26). This new method for aerosol generation is compact (Fig. 11) and based on sound pressure, which forces fluids through small holes in a membrane. Unlike traditional

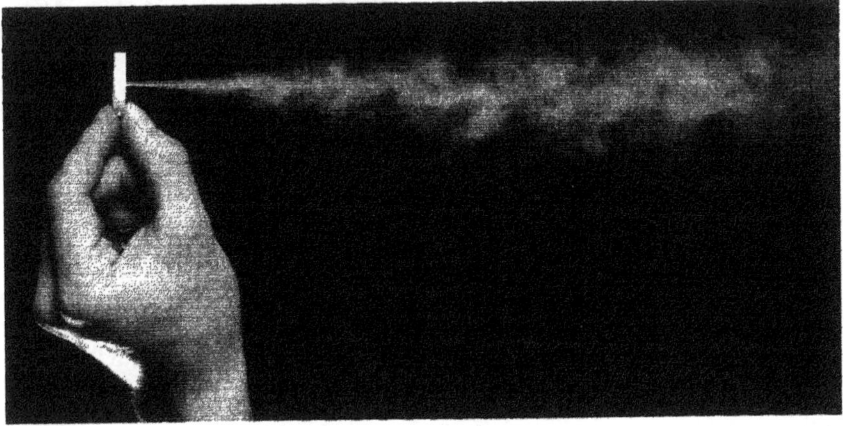

Figure 11 Prototype touchspray.

jet or ultrasonic nebulizers, the primary aerosol generated by TouchSpray is already of a sufficiently small droplet size for respirable drug aerosol delivery. Two components, a membrane and a piezoelectric element, are at the core of this nebulizer. The membrane consists of a circular, wafer-thin metal plate with small holes (Fig. 12). A ring-shaped piezoelectric actuator excites the membrane to vibrate, driven by an electronic circuit. During the vibrational motion, sound pressure is built up in the vicinity of the membrane, thus ejecting the fluid through the holes as droplets and creating the aerosol. The technology is very similar to the technology used by Aerogen in their nebulizer, the AeroNeb. This method of droplet generation is different from that of a traditional ultrasonic nebulizer, where surface acoustic waves generate the aerosol. TouchSpray technology would seem to offer the ability to circumvent difficulties in the ultrasonic nebulization of suspension, though to the authors' knowledge this has not been as yet been proven.

The power consumption of the vibrating membrane is low; allowing small batteries to power the device. Because the additional components (fluid reservoir, electronics, mouthpiece, and valves) do not require large volumes, it should be feasible to develop a small, portable nebulizer with a self-contained battery

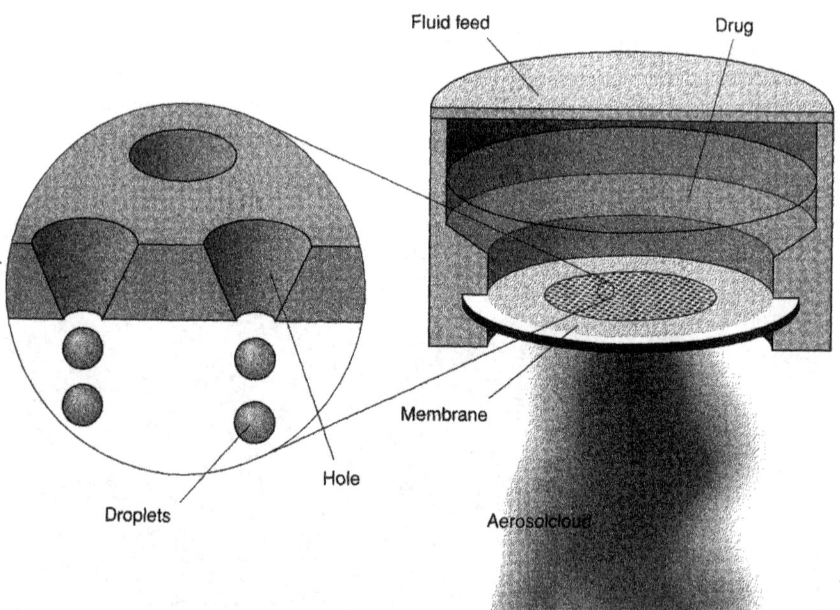

Figure 12 Touchspray schematic. Sound pressure forces fluid through small holes in a water-thin metal membrane which is vibrated by a piezoelectric actuator.

power source. The outlet velocity of the aerosol is expected to be similar to that of Aeroneb.

The proportion of respirable aerosol output from TouchSpray technology has not yet been fully evaluated. However, the manufacturer reports a high proportion of respirable aerosol due mainly to the aerosol generation process, which produces a fine primary aerosol; thus no filtering of the larger droplets using baffle structures within the nebulizer interior is required. The rate of monomodality of the aerosol produced has yet to be verified. The lack of need for a baffle system minimizes the wetted area of the nebulizer and the retention of droplet impaction on the walls. In this respect, the TouchSpray technology is similar in principle to the Omron ultrasonic generation system, which also avoids use of baffle structures. There is additional benefit from the feeding mechanism of the drug, which allows a nearly complete nebulization, thus minimizing residual volumes.

Microjet Pneumatic Nebulizer Ganan-Calvo

Ganan-Calvo and colleagues at Seville University have recently published a novel pneumatic technique to generate steady capillary microjets (27). In the near future, this technology could be applied to a number of applications including combustion, coating, microencapsulation, high-quality fiber or powder production, as well as therapeutic application in pulmonary drug delivery. The basic physical mechanism is based on the generation of a steady microscopic liquid jet by a coaxial, highly accelerated laminar gas stream. Under certain conditions, the breakup process of the jet stream is predicted by Rayleigh theory and the resulting spray approaches a monodisperse distribution. Depending on the conditions used, droplet size distributions with mass median aerodynamic diameters ranging from 0.1 to 10 μm can be realized. It was clear that a single jet nozzle producing 1-μm droplets has a very low output, though this could be increased by a nozzle array assembly that increases the output but does not alter the droplet size (27). However, to the authors' knowledge, this technology is in very early stages of development, and it is not yet clear how it will eventually appear as a means of delivering nebulized drug aerosols.

Synopsis

Commercial development of TouchSpray and Microjet technology has not yet occurred and we can only speculate on how each will be developed. TouchSpray seems to offer potential as an MDI replacement but also offers traditional nebulization applications with convenience and portability, given its small size and low power requirements. If it is manufactured in high numbers, the overall costs would be expected to be low. TouchSpray technology developed from ink-jet printing technology—the latter now a commonplace and relatively inexpensive consumer product. Microjet technology relies on a source of compressed air, and this has clearly been a barrier in the development of new nebulizer technology, in adding a large component penalty to aerosol generation and portability. It is not correct to speculate and comment further on either technology given the relatively early stage of their development.

VI. Assessment of Performance of New Nebulizer Technology

Because of regulatory loopholes (see Sec. II), most new nebulizer technologies will be made available with little or no evidence of safety and efficacy. In the absence of good in vivo data, reliance is based on laboratory studies. However, in vitro data describing aerosol output and size supplied by each manufacturer can be based on a range of methods and, further, is often not validated by independent laboratories. How then can clinicians make informed and reliable decisions on what nebulizer system is best for their patient groups? The authors believe that common misunderstanding between many scientists and research physicians is so great that a standard is required in the nebulizer field. Furthermore, the authors hold that standards should reflect as closely as practicable conditions of clinical use; this was also a unanimous decision taken during an International Society of Aerosols in Medicine Focus Symposium (28) by a significant number of aerosol scientists, pharmaceutical company scientists, and clinicians. In vitro data providing a consistent and clinically relevant estimate of aerosol output and droplet size would help clarify performance of available systems. Standard methods to estimate nebulizer output and size are being developed. If widely adopted, these should provide a consistent and meaningful comparison of nebulizer system performance to help guide clinicians in choosing the most appropriate nebulizer system for their patients. Given the present situation, a meaningful comparison is not possible.

A. British Standard on In Vitro Assessment of Nebulizer Performance

The first attempt by any nation to establish a standard method for assessing nebulizer performance was made in the U.K. in 1994. Though now outdated and technically limited (29), this published standard set a precedent and a foundation for further research and development of test methods. Much has happened to progress the understanding of nebulizer performance in recent years which has, in part, led to the development of the widely resourced European standard in assessing nebulizer performance.

B. European Standard on In Vitro Assessment of Nebulizer Performance

A draft European Nebulizer Standard (30) has been submitted for formal approval to CEN (Comité Européen de Normalisation: European Committee for Standardization). CEN is responsible for European standardization in all fields except Electrotechnical (CENELEC) and Telecommunications (ETSI). Publication of the European Nebulizer Standard is expected during 2001. Included within the European standard are detailed descriptions of two test methods for (1) assessing nebulizer aerosol output "inhaled" using breath simulation similar to that described previously and (2) assessing nebulized aerosol droplet size using "low-flow" cascade impaction. Because this standard is expected to be adopted throughout Europe (and possibly more widely), a summary of its contents may be useful to readers.

Aerosol Output Measurement Using Breath Simulation

It is well documented that much of the drug aerosol emitted from many traditional types of continuously operating nebulizers is emitted during patient exhalation and either passes into the environment or is collected on waste filters or by scavenging systems. With the exception of diagnostic applications using dosimetry, nebulizer therapy is given over a period of time during tidal breathing at rest. During this time, traditional nebulizers continue to emit and/or waste aerosol. Breath enhanced nebulizer designs increase aerosol output during inhalation by channeling inhaled air through the nebulizer which temporarily increases output. By incorporating a simulated breathing pattern (Fig. 13) similar to that described earlier (see Chap. 8), the test method becomes more

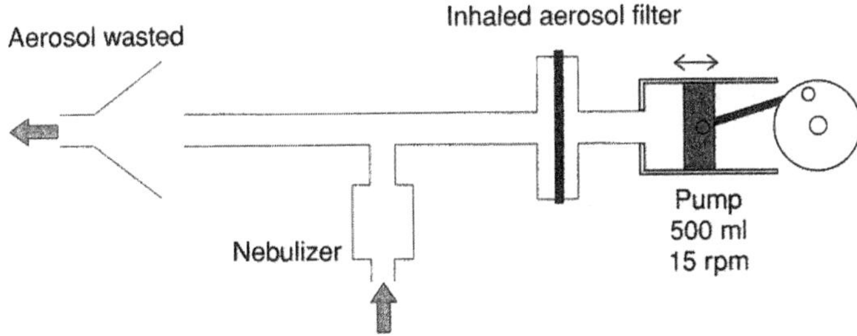

Figure 13 In vitro assessment of aerosol output in the European Standard. A simulated breathing pattern of 500 mL tidal volume and 15 breaths per minute is generated by a breathing machine in a sinus flow pattern. A low-resistance electrostatic filter at the patient interface collects all "inhaled" aerosol, which can be subsequently analyzed. Dead space in the tubing and filter is required to be <10% of tidal volume (i.e., <5 mL).

clinically representative of patient nebulizer use. Partly as a response to the need to harmonize with other European standards and partly as a practical technical issue, a sinus flow breathing simulation of 15 breaths per minute and 500 mL tidal volume has been adopted within the standard. It is well known that patients' breathing patterns are complex and varied (30) and that this influences aerosol deposition. Despite this, practical problems in limiting the number of permutations of breath simulation coupled with known difficulties of standardizing any flow regimen other than sinus flow led the European standard working group to adopt this largely artificial but fairly representative standard breathing pattern. It should be borne in mind that although the European standard will require use of this standard sinus flow pattern within its test protocols, manufacturers will be able to include additional flow patterns to emphasize specific therapeutic applications (e.g., pediatric use requiring smaller tidal volumes with greater frequency).

Aerosol Size Measurement Using Low-Flow Cascade Impaction

Since the 1970s laser sizers have offered convenient and rapid estimation of the optical size distributions of nebulized aerosol size distributions. However, just as weight loss as a measure of aerosol output is confounded by evaporation, droplet size distributions are now clearly understood also to be affected by evaporation once the aerosol cloud is mixed with drier ambient air. The methodology adopted within the European standard was inevitably a compromise but may arguably present the most representative clinical compromise.

A simulated inhalation flow fixed at 15 L/min was selected as a standard test condition. This total inhalation flow is positioned (operated by pump or vacuum line) in the patient's mouth; it is made up of both the primary flow of compressed air through the jet nebulizer (e.g., 8 L/min) the remainder (e.g., 7 L/min) drawn from the ambient environment (Fig. 14). A flow at 15 L/min was chosen for two reasons. First, 15 L/min represents the midpoint flow of the standardized breathing pattern (15 breaths per minute × 500 mL) as well as approximating the average inhalation flow of an adult during tidal breathing.

A cascade impactor operating at 15 L/min would provide an ideal instrument to employ in this standard. Unfortunately, no such device is available. Furthermore, even it were, an impactor operating at 15 L/min would not be able to cope with extension studies requiring lower airflow rates in, for example, pediatric applications. There are a limited number of devices which operate at lower flows of 1, 2, or 3 L/min; of these, the Graseby Anderson 290 series impactor was selected and, in collaboration with the manufacturer, was modified to accommodate nebulized aerosol. This low-flow impactor has additional physical features that help to produce a meaningful estimate of nebulized droplet size, including

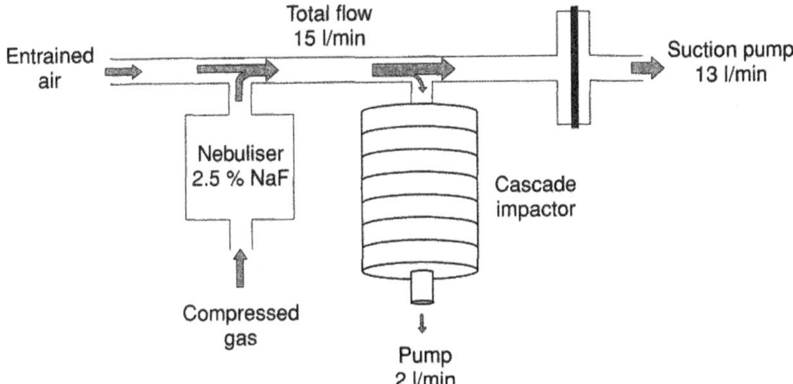

Figure 14 In vitro assessment of droplet size measurement in the European Standard. Simulated patient inhalation at 15 L/min draws air over (or through) the nebulizer where entrained ambient air mixes with nebulized aerosol. A sample of the air at 2 L/min is drawn into a Marple Series 290 cascade impactor, which sizes aerosol droplets in relation to aerodynamic diameter. Impacted aerosol solute (e.g., NaF or drug) can be subsequently desorbed and quantified from each impaction stage.

1. Relatively short residence time.
2. A low thermal capacity to warm the cooled nebulizer output air-aerosol mixture, which has been reported with other cascade impactors to further evaporate liquid aerosol and confound interpretation of droplet size measurements (32).
3. Relatively high capacity to load impaction stages when fitted with absorbent glass fiber filter substrates.

This last feature is particularly important in obtaining high-resolution droplet size distributions, as the maximum loading capacity on any particular stage determines the total amount of aerosol that can be collected. This implies that on less popular stages, the actual amount of aerosol impacted can be very small in comparison to that impacted on the most popular stage, and this has implications for analytical detection limits. Droplet bounce could confound interpretation of size distribution results and has been known to be a problem in sizing dry aerosol with this impactor (V. Marple, personal communication, 1999). However, droplet bounce has been demonstrated not to be a factor with wet Liquid droplets (unpublished data).

This low-flow cascade impaction method differs in a subtle but important manner from methods described earlier (Chap. 8, Fig. 7) in which the low-flow cascade is incorporated within a simulated breathing pattern. Here the cascade samples at a relatively low constant flow (2 L/min) within a sinus flow breathing pattern, which creates overall flows between 0 and approximately 20 L/min. During the beginning and end of the sinus flow–simulated inhalation, the low-flow cascade impactor samples aerosol whose droplet size has not been affected by any entrained ambient air. This aerosol is suspended in air that has been saturated with water vapor (100% relative humidity) from the nebulizer reservoir. Aerosol sampled during these initial and final phases is concentrated compared to aerosol sampled at the middle of the inhalation phase, which has been considerably diluted (perhaps by as much as 1:5) with ambient air. At the middle of the sinus flow, the entrained ambient air not only dilutes the aerosol-laden air but rapidly absorbs water vapor from the liquid droplets until it reaches saturation (100% RH). Thus any measure of droplet size distribution within the cascade impactor is a composite and dynamic mix of (1) concentrated unevaporated nebulized aerosol and (2) less concentrated nebulized aerosol droplets diluted by various degrees by entrained ambient air, which causes evaporation of solvent from the nebulized aerosol droplets. Preliminary calculations of the net affect of the sampling ratio within the simulated breathing pattern suggest that the resulting size distribution would be heavily biased in favor of the low-dilution aerosol and the analyzed droplet size distribution (R. Sugg, personal communication, 1999). For this reason, the CEN committee developing the European standard developed the aerosol sizing method shown in Fig. 14, which is believed to provide a clinically representative measure of nebulized aerosol size distribution.

During development of the European standard, an interlaboratory trial was organized involving six laboratories within Europe to follow a defined protocol to assess aerosol output and size from two fundamentally different nebulizer systems. Results demonstrated that the methods were repeatable within +/– 10% of mean return for both aerosol output and aerosol size (unpublished data). Results of preliminary research investigating the correlation between in vivo response and in vitro estimate of aerosol output and size show a promising correlation (33), though further work is needed in this area.

VII. Development of Clinical Nebulizer Guidelines Within the European Respiratory Society

A decision to establish an ERS Task Force to draft clinical nebulizer guidelines was made by the ERS executive in early 1998. Technical (34) and clinical workshops (35) have since helped formulate draft guidelines, which will be submitted to the ERS Executive in 2000. An important aspect of the ERS nebulizer guidelines is that they will recommend performance data obtained from European standard methodology to help guide clinicians in chosing a suitable nebulizer system.

VIII. Summary

Manufactures of pMDIs continued struggle to overcome technological problems in propellant reformulation and require a space- or breath-actuated system to achieve reasonable amounts of aerosol deposition in poor coordinators. Both pMDIs and DPIs have a potentially greater dependence on active patient cooperation and coordination than many of the new nebulizer technologies introduced above. DPIs seem to offer more efficient drug aerosol delivery compared to MDIs; but for most applications, difficulties and expense of DPI drug formulation and technical difficulties in designing effective aerosol release mechanisms prove a disadvantage compared to the apparent ease of formulation and delivery of nebulizer solutions. Over the last decade, rapid technological development in nanotechnology, microelectronics, and advanced battery technology have driven development of new nebulizer technologies, which will provide far greater efficiency of aerosol drug dose delivery than traditional nebulizers. The full impact of the new nebulizer technologies introduced and described in this chapter is not yet know but should offers realistic alternatives to the pMDI and DPI aerosol delivery systems.

The devices described above all fall into the category of new nebulizer technology. However, because they are new (some having emerged only in the past year or so), it is difficult to compare their output performance characteristics and less data exists to evaluate their clinical value. For some of the devices, a final design has not yet been fully developed. For others, where output data are available, they are obtained using a wide variety of in vitro methods, which makes meaningful comparison impossible without details of test methodology. This would be of little interest to the reader and is beyond the scope of this chapter. Despite these limitations, a summary of important design characteristics of each device compared to a typical traditional jet nebulizer is presented in Table 1. It is clear that some of the new technology should enable therapy to proceed more efficiently. Higher outputs imply faster rates of delivery, lower residual volumes imply higher dose delivery; portable and quite operation may imply better compliance, which leads again to higher dose delivery.

New devices like Respimat and AERx will undergo the same regulatory procedure as DPIs and pMDIs, as they are drug- and device-specific. The outcome will benefit the end user, as the dosing properties, accuracy, and clinical efficacy will be proven. However, many of the new technologies described above will be supplied as device only, without drug, and as such are exempt from regulatory involvement. This new nebulizer technology presents greatly improved convenience, output rates, doses, and even dose accuracy of drug aerosol delivery compared to traditional nebulizer technology. To ensure continuation of appropriate drug aerosol delivery, care must be taken in clinical practice when transferring patients from less efficient traditional nebulizers to the increasingly

Table 1 Summary of Relative Designed Aerosol Output Characteristics of New Nebulizer Technologies Compared with a Traditional Nebulizer and a Typical pMDI

	Integrated drug and device	Clinically trialed	Single/ continuous operation	Breath-activated	Delivers multiple doses before reloading is needed
Traditional nebulizer system	No	No	Cont	No	No
Typical pMDI	Yes	Yes	Single	No	Yes
Halolite	No	Partly	Cont/single	Yes	No
Circulaire	No	No	Cont	No	No
Omron	No	No	Cont	No	No
Aeroneb	No	No	Cont	No	No
Respimat	Yes	Yes	Single	No	Yes
AERx	Yes	Yes	Single	Yes	Yes
Touchspray	?	No	?	?	?
Microjet	?	No	?	?	?

more efficient new nebulizer technologies. Safety and efficacy are particularly problematic given commonly used methods of prescribing drugs for delivery by nebulizer, as the relative efficiency of the nebulizer delivery system is not taken into consideration. Given the lack of formal regulatory control over separate supply of drug and device in relation to nebulized drug delivery, it seems appropriate for respiratory societies, at both the national and international levels, to take further interest in the development and pending integration of new nebulizer technologies.

The new generation of nebulizer technology requires a more comprehensive study and dissemination of in vitro test results to characterize performance. Clinicians could then use in vitro–based assessments of output in deciding which system is most appropriate for their application.

The European Standard presents a set of in vitro methods that are expected to reflect in vivo deposition and have been shown to provide repeatable and consistent results. It is clear that some nebulizer designs cannot easily be adapted into this or any other standard and that some flexibility is required in interpreting and applying such to these systems. In particular, obtaining a realistic profile of aerosol size distribution from the small aerosol boluses mixed with entrained ambient air from the Halolite, Circulaire, and AERx is particularly problematic. However, such technical difficulties can be overcome and realistic measures of

Table 1 Continued

Requires cleaning after each dose is given	Cost	Proportion of initial charge delivered to lungs	Residual volume as proportion of initial charge	Quiet during treat-ment	Portable
Yes	Low	Low	High	No	No
No	Low	Low	Low	Yes	Yes
Yes	High	Low	High	No	No
Yes	Med	Med	High	Yes	No
Yes	High	High	Low	Yes	Yes
Yes	High	High	Low	Yes	Yes
No	Med	High	Low	Yes	Yes
No	High	High	Low	Yes	Yes
?	?	? (high)	Low	Yes	Likely
?	?	?	?	?	?

aerosol size obtained with prudent adaptation of test methods. Within the proposed ERS Clinical Nebulizer Guidelines, it is important that it is made clear what type of products the guidelines apply to. All the devices introduced above convert liquid into an aerosol using a range of different aerosol generation technologies. They include both multidose and unit dose systems. The term *nebulizer* in the clinic is typically applied to a device used to generate an aerosol from an aqueous drug solution or suspension, the drug being supplied separately to the device as a unit dose vial. It is important that clinicians and users understand how to use a device correctly, and the general classification of devices can be useful in selecting the appropriate device for a patient. However, this approach is not helpful if it leads to the wrong instructions being given. This issue is of increasing importance due to the proliferation of delivery devices on the market. In any case, clinical use of both Respimat and AERx will be outside the normal scope of nebulizer guidelines, as they have been developed and are being marketed as drug-device combinations in which patient safety and drug efficacy have been proven.

Nebulized drug delivery is possibly the most confused area of clinical practice, largely as a result of little or no regulatory control. New nebulizer technology offers greater convenience and portability and a significant increase in aerosol dose delivery. On one hand, this new, more efficient technology offers obvious benefit to patients. On the other hand, adoption of this new and improved nebulizer technology without due consideration of the consequences of increased dosing presents potential risk if drug regulatory bodies or academic societies are not willing or able to help manage the transition.

XI. Final Note

Descriptions of new nebulizer technologies included in this chapter have variable lengths. This may give the reader the false impression that some technologies were more favorably presented than others. This was not intended, as it was more the scarcity of published data relating to some new nebulizer technology that proved limiting.

Acknowledgments

The authors are grateful to manufacturers who provided information and samples of their devices, and to AstraZeneca for sponsoring meetings during preparation of this chapter.

References

1. Nikander K. Some technical, physicochemical and physiological aspects of nebulization of drugs. Eur Respir J 1997; 7(44): 168–172.
2. Dennis JH, Hendrick DJ. Design characteristics for drug nebulizers. J Med Eng Technol 1992; 16(2):63–68.
3. Smye SW. The physics of corticosteroid nebulization. Eur Respir J 1997; 7(44):184–188.
4. Geddes DM. Nebulized therapy and cystic fibrosis. Eur Respir J 1997; 7(44):173–176.
5. Muers MF. The rational use of nebulizers in clinical practice. Eur Respir J 1997; 7(44):189–197. 1997.
6. Dennis JH, Stenton SC, Beach JR, Avery AJ, Walters EH, Hendrick DJ. Jet and ultrasonic nebulizer output: use of a new method to measure aerosol output directly. Thorax 1990; 45:728–732.
7. Dennis JH. Drug nebulizer design and performance: breath-enhanced jet vs constant output jet vs ultrasonic. J Aerosol Med 1995; 8(3):277–280.
8. Pavia D, McLeod L. The environmental impact of inhaled aerosols. Eur Respir Rev 1994; 4(suppl 18):75–77.
9. Denyer J, Dyche A, Nikander K, Newman S, Richards J, Dean A. HaloLite A novel liquid drug aerosol delivery system. Thorax 1997; 52(6):A83.
10. Denyer J, Dyche A. Patient compliance with inhaled treatment using a novel aerosol delivery system. Eur Respir J 1998; 12(S28):P0647.

11. HaloLite: A novel liquid drug aerosol delivery system. J. Denyer, K. Nikander. RDD VI May 1998.
12. Miller WC, Mason JW. Abbreviated aerosol therapy for improved efficiency. J Aerosol Med 1998; 11(3):127–131.
13. Stenton SC, Dennis JH, Hendrick DJ. Occupational asthma due to ceftazidime. Eur J Respir Dis 1995; 8:1421–1423.
14. Alberts WM. Occupational asthma in the respiratory care workers. Respir Care 1993; 38(9):977–1004.
15. Noone PG, Regnis JA, Liu X, Brouwer KL, Robinson M, Edwards L, Knowles MR. Airway deposition and clearance and systemic pharmacokinetics of amiloride following aerosolization with an ultrasonic nebulizer to normal airways. Chest 1997; 112(5):1283–1290.
16. Ito K, Kikuchi S, Yamada M, Torii S, Yoshida M. Time course of drug concentrations in nebulizers and nebulized solutions. Arerugi 1992; 41(7):772–777 (in Japanese)
17. Takano H, Nakazawa M, Asai K, Itoh M. Performances of a new clinical nebulizer for drug administration based on the mesh-type ultrasonic atomization by elastic surface waves. J Aerosol Med 1999; 12(2):98.
18. Zierenberg B, Eicher J, Dunne S, Freund B. Boehringer Ingelheim Nebulizer BINEB, a new approach to inhalation therapy. In Respiratory Drug Delivery V. Buffalo Grove, IL: Interpharm Press, 1996:187–193.
19. Pavia D, Thomson ML, Clarke SW, Shannon HS. Effect of lung function and mode of inhalation on penetration of aerosol into the human lung. Thorax 1977; 32:194–197.
20. Whelan AM, Hahn NW. Optimizing drug delivery from metered-dose inhalers. DICP Ann Pharmacother 1991; 25:638–645.
21. Newman SP, Brown J, Steed KP, Reader SJ, Kladders H. Lung deposition of fenoterol and flunisolide using a novel device for inhaled medicines: comparison of RESPIMAT with conventional metered-dose inhalers with and without spacer devices. Chest 1998; 113:957–963.
22. Newman SP, Steed KP, Reader SJ, Hooper G, Zierenberg B. Efficient delivery to the lungs of flunisolide aerosol from a new portable hand-held multidose nebulizer. J Pharm Sci 1996; 85:960–964.
23. Kunkel G, Magnussen H, Bergmann K-C, Juergens U, De May C, Freund E, Hinzmann R, Jahnel B. Cumulative dose response study comparing a new soft mist inhaler with a conventional MDI for delivery of fenoterol/ipratropium bromide combination in patients with asthma. Eur Respir J 1997; 10(suppl 25):104s.
24. Schuster G, Rubsamen R, Lloyd P, Lloyd G. The AERx aerosol delivery system. Pharm Res 1997; 14:354–357.
25. Schuster G, Farr S, Chipolla D, Wilbanks T, Rosell J, Lloyd P, Gonda I. Design and performance validation of highly efficient and reproducible compact aerosol delivery system AER_x Respiratory Drug Delivery VI. Buffalo Grove, IL: Interpharm Press, 1998:83–90.
26. Stangl R, Lauangkhot N, Liening-Ewert R, Jahn D Characterising the functional model of a vibrating membrane nebulizer. Paper presented at the Aerosol Society, Dublin, 1999.

27. Ganan-Calvo AM, Barrero A. A Novel pneumatic technique to generate steady capillary microjets. J Aerosol Sci 1999; 30(1):117–125.
28. Clark AR, Gonda I, Newhouse MT. Towards meaningful laboratory tests for evaluation of pharmaceutical aerosols. J Aerosol Med 1998; 11(suppl 1):S1–S7.
29. Dennis JH, Pierron CA, Nerbrink O. Standards in assessing in vitro nebulizer performance. Eur Respir J. In press.
30. Draft European Nebuliser Standard. prEN13544 13544-1. Respiratory Therapy Equipment Part 1: Nebulizing Systems (available through all national European Standards bodies, e.g., in UK available through BSI ref BS 99/5662734DC).
31. Denyer J. Breathing patterns in adult patients. J Aerosol Med 1997; 10(1):99.
32. Stapleton KW, Finlay WH. Errors in characterizing nebulized particle size Distributions with cascade impactors. J Aerosol Med 1998; 11(Suppl 1):80–83.
33. Silkstone VL, Dennis JH, Chrystyn H. In-vivo/in-vitro correlation for nebulizers. In: Drug Delivery to the Lungs X. London:1999.
34. Boe J, Dennis JH. European Respiratory Society nebulizer guidelines: technical aspects. Eur Respir Rev 2000; 73:
35. Boe J, O'Driscoll R, Dennis JH. European Respiratory Society Nebulizer Guidelines: clinical aspects. Eur Respir Rev. In press.

10

The Metered-Dose Inhaler

CHRIS O'CALLAGHAN

University of Leicester
Leicester, England

PAUL WRIGHT

Astra Zeneca R&D
Charnwood, Loughborough, England

I. Introduction

Many drugs have been formulated for use with pressurized metered-dose inhalers (pMDIs) (Table 1). The main market for these devices is in the treatment of asthma, allergic diseases, and chronic obstructive pulmonary disease (COPD), for which approximately 500 million pMDIs are produced each year. Their major selling points are that they are cheap and portable. Despite their huge sales, there is increasing concern that the dose of drug patients with asthma receive will vary considerably due to their inhalational technique and to a lesser extent to the variability of dose delivery from the pMDI. It is likely, however, that the popularity of pMDIs will continue due to various modifications and additions that are aimed to help with inhalational technique and improve drug delivery. Examples of these include breath-actuated devices, discussed in this chapter, and spacer devices discussed in a subsequent chapter.

The initial part of this review focuses on the traditional chlorinated fluorocarbon (CFC) pMDIs that are still by far the most common formulations available at present. Developments in pMDI technology relating to the ongoing switch to non-CFC pMDIs (hydrofluoroalkanes, or HFAs) are highlighted toward the end of this chapter.

Table 1 Drugs Formulated for Administration via pMDIs

$Beta_2$ agonists
Ipratropium bromide
Isoprenaline
Epinephrine
Sodium cromoglycate
Steroids
Ergotamine

II. What Is a Pressurized Metered-Dose Inhaler (pMDI)?

The pMDI (Fig. 1) delivers a metered dose of a CFC or HFA drug suspension or solution. It consists of three major components:

1. A reservoir, containing drug suspended or dissolved in liquefied gas propellant
2. A metering valve, which when depressed delivers a known volume
3. A spray actuator, which, combined with the stem of the metering valve, comprises a twin orifice expansion chamber and spray nozzle

A. Formulation

A typical pMDI contains:

Drug substance
Up to three different propellants
One or more surfactants or lubricants

Most current CFC-containing pMDIs are formulated using micronized or spray-dried drug particles held in suspension. Surfactants are used to disperse drug particles in suspension and for valve lubrication. Surfactant molecules interact with each other, with drug particles, and with the propellant, to stabilize drug particles in a predominantly nonpolar propellant environment (1). Oleic acid, sorbitan mono-oleate(Span80), sorbitan tri-oleate (Span85) and phosphatidyl lecithin choline are the commonly used surfactants in CFC containing pMDIs in concentrations typically around 0.1% w/w but sometimes as high as 2%w/w. High concentrations of nonvolatile surfactants increase emitted droplet size, as they do not evaporate from the surface of drug particles and may slow down evaporation of volatile propellants.

At low drug concentration, emitted droplets will contain a single drug

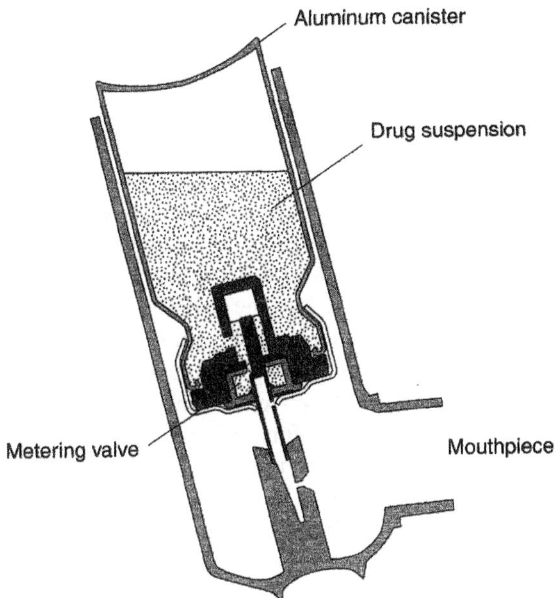

Figure 1 A schematic section through a typical pressurized metered dose inhaler (pMDI).

particle and approximate to the original micronized size (2). However, at higher drug concentrations, droplets containing multiple drug particles will be produced, leading to an increase in droplet size and reducing drug delivery to the lungs.

The final particle size of solution formulations, in contrast, will depend on the initial droplet size, the concentration of nonvolatile components in the droplet, and the ambient conditions. It is possible to use the drug concentration to alter the final particle size. In practice, it is often difficult to dissolve drug in CFC propellants, and drug may be lost to the elastomers in the MDI valve (3). As will be discussed later, the problems of solution aerosols of steroids using HFA propellants have recently been overcome. Dissolved mint extracts and micronized saccharin have been added to formulations in an attempt to improve patient acceptability.

B. Metering Valves

The main function of the metering valve is to deliver a reproducible amount of the liquid phase of the formulation in which the medication is either dissolved or dispersed. Each valve consists of several components made of inert materials. The metering tank contains a single dose of drug, usually in the range of 25–100 μL (Fig. 2). Some valves such as the 3M Neotechnic are surrounded by a larger reservoir known as the retaining cup, which contains the next few doses of drug. When the valve is actuated by depressing the valve stem, the communication between the metering tank and the retaining cup is closed, and the metering tank empties through the opening of the valve stem. The metered dose is ejected from the metering chamber under the pressure of the boiling liquid propellant. The vapor/liquid drug mixture then flows through the valve stem orifice into the valve stem. When in the valve stem, it expands by further vapor formation before discharge through the spray orifice. The atomization process at the final spray orifice is a two-phase gas/liquid air blast (4). However, after droplet formation has taken place, the droplets of the emerging cloud quickly evaporate and lose their forward velocity (5). It is the CFC's capacity to both generate sufficient vapor to produce sufficient two-phase atomization without the need for an external power source and to evaporate quickly after droplet generation has taken place that makes the pMDI such a successful inhalational delivery system. After actuation, the spring returns the valve to the resting position and the metering tank refills from the retaining cup. The retaining cup may hold as many as four or more doses depending on the pMDI. The retaining cup is refilled from the main reservoir through the opening in its base. The concentration of suspension mixture available at the inlet between

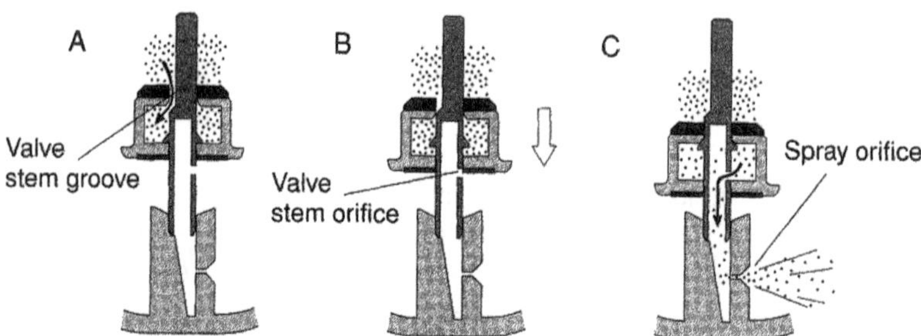

Figure 2 The metering valve of one variety of pMDI. The metering chamber holds the next dose. In the resting state, it communicates with the contents of the larger retaining cup (tank) holding further doses. This, in turn, communicates with the main reservoir. The retaining cup allows the inhaler to be used until it is virtually empty. When the inhaler is activated by compressing the valve stem, the communication between the metering tank and the retaining cup is closed and the metering tank empties through the opening in the valve stem. After actuation, the spring returns the valve stem to the resting position and the metering tank refills from the retaining cup. The retaining cup is refilled from the main reservoir through an opening in its base. (From Ref. 5.)

the main reservoir and the retaining cup is therefore very important in metering subsequent doses. If the concentration of drug is low at the inlet, a low drug dose concentration will appear in the retaining cup and the metering tank and the patient will inhale a low dose. Variation in drug delivery due to this problem is discussed later in this chapter.

C. Aerosol Containers

Both aluminum and glass aerosol containers are available. Aluminum aerosol canisters are light, impervious to light, robust, and cheap to make. Glass containers are now very rare. Typically they are laminated or plastic-coated so they can withstand pressures of up to 150 psig. Occasionally the inert nature of glass containers makes them a more suitable choice for some solution formulations.

D. Mouthpiece Design

Mouthpieces are usually made of polypropylene or polyethylene materials. The stem of the MDI fits into the actuator part of the mouthpiece, against which the valve of the MDI is pressed. Depression of the valve allows discharge of the aerosol through the small jet orifice of the mouthpiece. The aerosol cloud generated after depression of the valve stem is dependent on the geometric size of the active drug particles (in the case of suspension), the volume of the metering chamber, the vapor pressure of the propellant formulation, and the diameter of the jet orifice in the mouthpiece. The diameter of this orifice controls the rate of spray of the formulation (6) and has a critical effect on the aerosol particle size produced. To make sure that this orifice does not become blocked during repeated use with medications with a high drug load, such as sodium cromoglycate 5-mg pMDIs, regular removal and washing of the mouthpiece is recommended. Drying is essential prior to further use.

III. pMDI Technique

Surprisingly the optimal method of pMDI use is still debated. Newman et al. (7,8) demonstrated maximal bronchodilatation and lung deposition with the MDI in the mouth (the closed-mouth technique), (Table 2) slow (about 30 L/min), deep inhalation, and a 10-s breath-hold. Faster inhalation was less effective, with more aerosol impacting on the oropharynx, while a shorter period of breath-holding allows insufficient time for sedimentation of particles in the airways. Extending the breath-holding pause to 20 s has not been shown to enhance bronchodilatation (9). Others have found a greater bronchodilator response at an inhalation rate of 64 L/min compared to a very high inhalation rate of 192 L/min (10).

Table 2 Correct Metered-Dose Inhaler Technique[a]

1. Remove the cap and shake the canister thoroughly.
2. Hold the canister upright and breathe out fully.
3. Place the mouthpiece between the lips, or 3–4 cm in front of the open mouth.
4. Fire the inhaler while inhaling slowly and deeply.
5. Hold the breath for 10 s, or for as long as possible.
6. Wait approximately 1 min before taking a second dose.

[a] In very severe airways obstruction more than one actuation may be necessary.

Hindle and colleagues (11), using urinary salbutamol excretion, have assessed the closed-mouth technique in detail. A greater relative lung bioavailability of the drug was observed with inhalation to residual volume, slow inhalation with MDI actuation, and a 10-s breath-hold following inhalation. In contrast, Dolovich (12) obtained the greatest delivery of radiolabeled aerosol to the lungs and Thomas (13) the greatest degree of bronchodilatation using the open mouth technique with the pMDI held 4 cm from the wide open mouth. Others have not found this method beneficial (14–16).

There is even disagreement as to the lung volume at which the aerosol should be inhaled. Newman and colleagues (7,8) found that actuation at 20% of vital capacity gave greater or similar bronchodilatation and lung deposition than that achieved following actuation at 80% of vital capacity. Riley et al. (17,18) found that isoprenaline was more effective when actuated at a vital capacity of 80% as compared with a vital capacity of 20%. Although patients are usually told to inhale maximally, beginning at residual volume, inhalation of a fenoterol aerosol starting at functional residual capacity has been shown to be equally effective (19).

The time interval between successive doses of bronchodilator has been debated. Although manufacturers often recommend a 1- to 2-min interval between successive actuations, a longer time interval of 10–20 min has been suggested. This has the theoretical advantage of allowing the second dose to penetrate further into the airways (20). Other factors influencing dose delivery from pMDIs are discussed below (Table 3).

A. Shaking the pMDI and Low First-Spray Drug Contents from pMDIs

Patients are always instructed to shake their pMDI prior to inhalation because of the potential problem of separation of drug particles from the suspension (21). Berg (22) visually demonstrated the importance of shaking a MDI prior to inhalation. She was able to transfer budesonide suspension from a pMDI to a pMDI with a glass canister that allowed the behavior of the micronized drug sus-

Table 3 Factors Influencing Dose Delivery from pMDI

Coordination requirements
pMDI design
Reformulation from CFC to HFA propellants
Distance from actuation orifice
Temperature
Separation of drug and solvent

pension to be observed (Fig. 3). As the drug particles in the suspension were less dense than the propellants, drug gradually separated from the formulation, forming a cream-like layer at the top of the propellant/surfactant mixture. Thus, the concentration of drug substance in the lower, metering valve end of the pMDI decreases. If the drug particles were denser than the propellant, however, they would settle in the reservoir of the pMDI, thus increasing the drug concentration near the metering valve. Whether drugs either cream or settle depends upon the difference in densities between the drug substance and the propellant mixture.

Berg (22) made a theoretical calculation of the effects of occasional failure to shake the pMDI on the dose of drug released following actuation. The marked variation in the dose of drug delivered is shown in Fig. 4. This work was based on a sequence of 10 consecutive doses with shaking prior to actua-

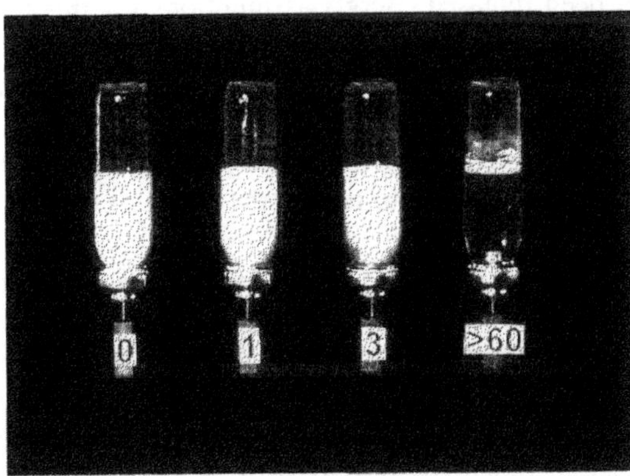

Figure 3 The behavior of the contents of a pMDI in glass-walled containers. The pMDI contains a suspension of micronized budesonide identical to that used in the production pMDIs. It was shaken immediately before time zero. Separation of the contents begins as soon as the pMDI is left in an undisturbed state. Complete separation of the contents has occurred within 60 min of shaking. (From Ref. 22.)

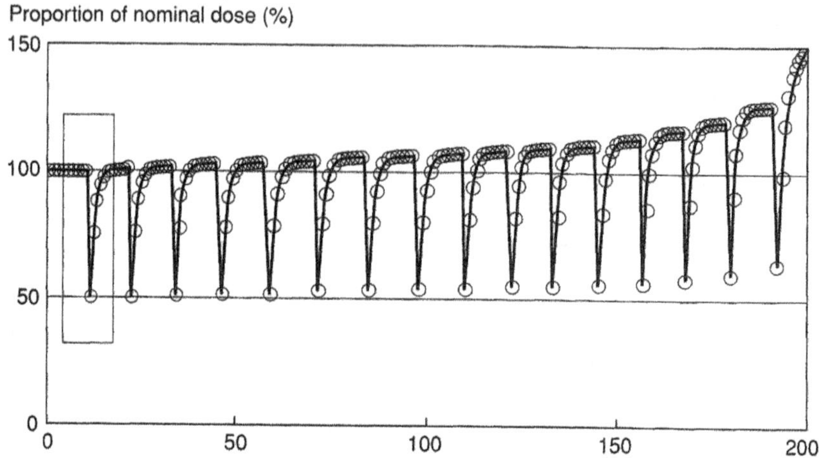

Figure 4 Theoretical calculation of the effects of occasional failure to shake a pMDI on the dose released. The tank retaining cup holds two doses, and the calculation has been based upon the sequence of each 10 consecutive doses with shaking followed by one dose without shaking. It is assumed that the drug floats ("creams") and that complete separation from the liquid propellant/surfactant has occurred before the unshaken dose is administered. (From Ref. 22.)

tion followed by one dose without shaking. This sequence was repeated until 200 doses had been released. Berg's assumptions for this were that the drug creams without shaking, the retaining cup contains two doses, more than 1 h has elapsed since shaking for the unshaken dose, and complete mixing has occurred in the retaining cup. The next dose to be delivered enters the metering valve when the last shot has been fired, thus shaking of the pMDI should occur immediately prior to actuation to reduce the effect of creaming or sedimentation of a drug in suspension.

In laboratory trials of pMDIs, the inhalers are usually primed by actuating on several occasions before testing to encourage reproducible performance. However, patients do not routinely prime their pMDI by firing shots to waste before actuating and inhaling. Cyr and colleagues (23) showed that this might result in considerable variation in the amount of drug they receive. They studied the output of salbutamol from pMDIs of three different manufacturers. Each pMDI was primed and then stored valve-down for 3 h. The pMDIs were then shaken for 5 s and actuated. This was repeated on three occasions and the salbutamol content of each puff measured. Five groups of three actuations were collected from each pMDI, beginning at actuation 10, 50, 100, 150, 198. The intervening actuations were discharged to waste. The drug content in the first spray was found to be very erratic and was usually substantially less than the 100 μg claimed on the label. However, occasional first sprays contained very high levels of drug, up to 208 μg, for a label claim of 100 μg. The mean drug contents of the second and third sprays were much closer to the label claim and less variable (Fig. 5).

Byron (24) also investigated the dose of salbutamol released from salbutamol inhalers under various conditions and found that when the pMDI was primed, shaken, and immediately fired, the average dose per spray was close to the "label claim," with a low variability. When a 30-s delay was introduced between shaking and firing, the first dose per actuation was a mean of 87.5% of the label claim. Subsequent doses were close to the label claim. Storage valve down for 24 h after shaking gave a first dose per actuation of 49.5% of the label claim. The second dose after shaking was 63% of label claim and the third and fourth were close to label claim. If the inhaler was shaken before the first dose after a 24-h delay in the valve-down position, the first dose was a mean of 81.3% of the label claim and subsequent doses were close to 100%. If the inhaler was shaken before the first dose after a 24-h delay in the valve-up position, the doses were very close to the label claim. In the more likely clinical scenario of the inhaler being shaken before the first dose, after a 24 h delay with the inhaler stored on its side, the first and subsequent actuations were very close to the label claim. Everard et al. (25) found that not shaking a salbutamol pMDI before use reduced the total and "respirable dose" by 25 and 35%, respectively. They also found that very rapid actuations could reduce the dose delivered per actuation, but that a

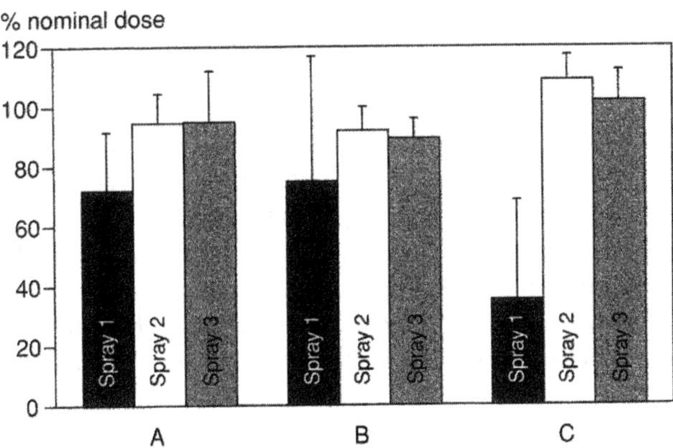

Figure 5 Salbutamol content of the first, second, and third actuations from pMDIs produced by three different manufacturers. The pMDIs were primed and left in a valve-down position for 3 h before testing. There is a marked variation in the dose emitted. (From Ref. 23.)

salbutamol pMDI can be actuated immediately after a 10-s breath-holding pause without affecting the dose delivered.

To overcome the need for repriming, Schultz and colleagues (26) developed a design where the fixed metering tank is eliminated and each dose is drawn directly from the main reservoir. A more consistent dose is delivered even after 24 h of storage in the valve-down position. Valois has an ACT valve, aimed at solutions, where the fixed metering chamber is eliminated. Information released from manufacturers regarding the new valves designed for use with the new HFA metered-dose inhalers show very little variation in dose output compared to the CFC inhalers. This is discussed later in the chapter.

B. When Is a pMDI Empty?

To obtain regulatory approval, manufacturers must demonstrate consistent and accurate medication concentration for actuation up to a specified number of actuations per canister (27). Beyond this specified number of actuations, some drug may still be expelled from the canister. Pharmaceutical companies now have to provide data in their registration dossiers to show an acceptably fast tail-off. It has been suggested that using MDIs beyond the maximum number of specified actuations may possibly be a contributing factor for the rise in asthma morbidity and even mortality (28). Ogren and colleagues (29) found that 54% of the patients they surveyed were unaware of the specified maximum number of actuations listed by the manufacturer for the inhalers they were using, and only 8% counted the number of actuations they were using. The group looked at the most commonly taught method of assessing whether a replacement MDI was required—that is, the flotation technique. It has been claimed that pMDIs float in water when they have delivered their licensed number of doses and suggested that they should be replaced at this time (30). As can be seen from Fig. 6A, a full MDI should lie on the bottom of a container of water, whereas an empty canister floats on top. Ogren (29) clearly demonstrated that this is a very inappropriate technique, as there was no universal flotation status when the inhalers had reached their respective specified maximum number of actuations (Fig. 6B). Concern also exists that immersing the pMDI in water may cause the valve stem to become clogged with a thick drug paste.

Dose counters are already available for dry-powder inhalers (DPIs), and there is little doubt that they will also become a feature of pMDIs.

IV. Airway Deposition and the Effects of Anti-Asthma Drugs Delivered from MDIs

There are three main components to inhalation therapy. The first is the dose delivered from the inhaler, the second the pulmonary deposition of some of the de-

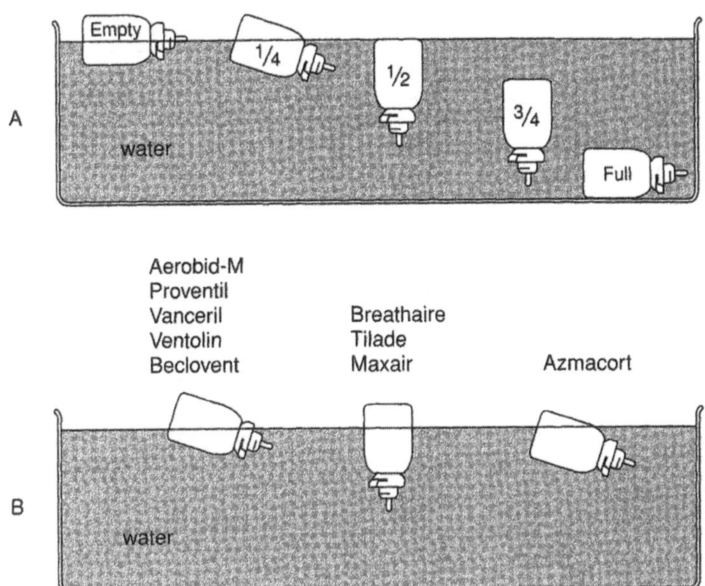

Figure 6 The commonly used flotation diagram is shown in A. The actual flotation status of MDIs at manufacturer's recommended number of actuations to denote replacement status of the canister is shown below, in B. This highlights the problems with using the flotation technique to determine the contents of a pMDI. (From Ref. 29.)

livered dose, and third the functional response to the deposited dose. The first two steps are covered in this chapter. The third step involves the nature of the drug, such as its potency, full or partial and agonist activity, and whether the inhaler constituents can induce irritation or even bronchoconstriction.

Initial deposition studies were performed in healthy volunteers by Davies (31), who found lung deposition to be less than 10%. The approximate lung dose was calculated from a difference in isoprenaline metabolism when the drug was administered via the intravenous and inhaled routes. Radiolabeling of inhaled drugs was first used in the early 1980s to study lung deposition of aerosolised drugs (12,32,33). Pauwels et al. (34) have recently reviewed the airway deposition and airways effects of antiasthma drugs delivered from pMDIs. Table 4 shows the lung deposition after inhalation of different substances via pMDIs. When available, data on inhalational flow or other inhalational parameters are given. Unfortunately, in many reports these parameters have not been documented. Pauwels and colleagues (34) concluded that in general there is a good relationship between pulmonary deposition and pulmonary effects for both bronchodilators and steroids. The information is still rather limited for inhaled

Table 4 Lung Deposition After Inhalation of Different Substances via pMDI

Inhaler	Substance	V'_I L-min[1]	Lung dose	Ref.	Comments
pMDI	Isoprenaline	—	<10	31	HV
	Ipratropium	—	–16	33	HV(n=4)
	Teflon	20	13	32	20% VC, Pts. (n=10)
	particles	120	5		
	Terbutaline	—	2.9	90	Pts, range 0.8–10.0%
	Teflon	30	14.3	77	20% VC, BHT=10 s Pts. (n=10)
	particles		14.3		50% VC
			13.8		80% VC
			11.8		20% VC, BHT = 4s
			6.5		50% VC
			6.8		80% VC
	Teflon	30	12.8	8	20% VC, BHT=4 s, Pts. (n=8)
	particles		7.5		50% VC
			7.2		80% VC
			8.4		20% VC
			7.0		50% VC
			6.0		80% VC
	Terbutaline	86	8.2	91	HV (n=11)
	DSCG	—	9.2	92	HV (n=7)
	Rudesonde	40	15	93	HV (n=24)
	DSCG	30	8.8	100	HV (n=10), 5-mg dose
	Salbutamol	—	21.6	94	HV (n=10)
			18.2		Pts (n=19)
	Salbutamol	—	24.1	95	HV (n=6)
	Terbutaline	34	16.7	96	HV (n=8)
	Terbutaline	37	10.7	97	HV (n=8)
		151			
pMDI	Salbutamol	—	18.6	69	Pts. good coordination, (n=10)
BA pMDI			11.2[a]		
pMDI			10.4		Pts. bad coordination, (n=8)
BA pMDI			7.2[a]		
SmartMist/	Salbutamol	30	14.1	98	HV (n=9)
pMDI		90	18.6		
		270	7.6[b]		
Gentlehaler	Salbutamol	—	18.8	99	pMDI, Pts. (n=10)
			19.6		Gentlehaler

Key: pMDI, pressurized metered-dose inhaler; VC, vital capacity; BHT, breath holding time; BA, breath-actuated measured by scintigraphy.
[a] Measured by charcoal-block method.
[b] Late actuation.
Source: Ref. 34

steroids; this may be explained by the difficulty in obtaining a dose-response relationship for their clinical effects. Pauwels et al. also point out that the development of an increasing number of inhalational devices will result in increasing demand for studies comparing the efficacy of the different devices. The need for comparative clinical studies using these different devices will obviously remain. However, methods for estimating pulmonary deposition by in vitro, pharmacokinetic, or radioisotope studies could help in optimizing inhalation therapy with regard to both inhalation technique and inhalation device.

C. Incorrect pMDI Technique

As far back as 1965, Saunders (35) found that 14 out of 46 patients studied were not using their inhalers correctly, and 11 of these were not achieving maximum therapeutic effect. It is now accepted that many adults and most children use their pMDIs incorrectly (35–41), and most health care workers are also uncertain about their correct use (42–47). It is estimated that between 25 and 38% of patients who use a pMDI have never received verbal instructions on how to use their device from a health care professional (37,48) and many patients do not receive follow-up assessment and retraining (48,39).

The most common errors are the inability to coordinate inhalation with MDI actuation, to inhale too quickly, and to exhale without a breath-hold (12,49,50). Crompton (49) identified 215 patients with inadequate inhaler technique. Of these, 50% failed to synchronize aerosol release with inhalation and 36% stopped inhaling when the propellant spray hit the back of the throat. Patients may stop breathing in when propellants impact on the back of the throat and rapidly evaporate, causing almost instantaneous cooling in that area. This is known as the "cold freon" effect (51). It is difficult to argue with the advice that old patients, young patients, and anyone else should be assumed to be unable to use pMDIs properly unless proved otherwise (49). Nasal inhalation is also a common error among children (51).

V. Use of pMDIs in the Very Young and in the Elderly

It is now widely accepted that pMDIs should not be used alone by children 6 years of age or less. Even children older than this should probably avoid using a pMDI unless in the form of a breath-actuated inhaler or via a spacer device.

Older adults may be at an increased risk of incorrect pMDI use because of associated disease or physical and cognitive decline (52,48). Increased risk for incorrect pMDI technique is greater in those with reduced cognitive status (53,52). A low score on a mental state questionnaire is associated with both incorrect pMDI technique and inability to learn correct pMDI technique despite retraining (52). The fact that pMDI performance is influenced by cognitive status may explain the conflicting results on the influence of age on inhaler technique. Gray and colleagues (53) did not find age to be a predictor of incorrect inhaler technique in patients ranging from 50 to 87 years, which is consistent with previous reports that have included all age groups (37,39). Others have reported significantly lower rates of correct use in many older patients and the inability of many older patients to learn correct techniques despite retraining (48,54). This variation in findings may be due to the failure to assess cognitive function among subjects or to control for it. As impaired cognitive status is more common in the elderly, poor pMDI technique may be related more to cognition than to age. Cognitive status should be controlled for in any subsequent studies on inhaler technique.

Gray and colleagues (53) recently investigated whether hand strength and various demographic variables were predictive of correct use of pMDIs in older subjects. They found hand strength to be an independent predictor of correct pMDI technique, even though subjects had enough hand strength to depress their canister. This suggests that adequate hand strength beyond the minimum required to depress the pMDI canister is important. Potentially, decreased hand strength may interfere with coordination of inhalation with actuation. From a practice point of view, it is recommended that patients demonstrate their ability to depress the canister to their health care professional. This is now considered essential, as Armitage and Williams (48) found that one-third of the older patients they tested did not have adequate strength to generate the minimum force required to actuate their inhalers.

It is uncertain whether the use of breath-actuated inhalers offer an advantage over the pMDI for patients with neurological deficits or other conditions that cause decreased hand strength. However, Chapman et al. (55) found that pMDI-familiar and pMDI-naive elderly subjects preferred a breath-actuated device over the pMDI.

VI. Safety of pMDIs

Patients and physicians need to be aware that although antiasthma drugs inhaled from pMDIs do not usually produce adverse effects, they can make symptoms worse. Paradoxical bronchospasm has been associated with the use of beta$_2$ agonists and corticosteroids inhaled from MDIs (56–58). Decreases in FEV$_1$, of more than 10% have been reported to occur in as many as 4.4% of subjects (59). Nicklas (58) reviewed adverse reaction reports submitted to the Center for Drug Evaluation and Research of the FDA between 1974 and 1988; of these, 126 reports associated with the use of these drugs by MDI, which were consistent with the diagnosis of paradoxical bronchospasm, were observed. More recently, Wilkinson et al. (60) reported paradoxical bronchoconstriction in asthmatic patients after inhaling salmeterol by a pMDI but not via a DPI.

The additives in the pMDI are probably causative agents of adverse effects of paradoxical bronchoconstriction linked to pMDI use, as similar bronchoconstriction occurs after inhalation from a placebo pMDI, but not when $beta_2$ agonist is inhaled from a DPI or nebulizer (60–62). It is still unknown whether new HFA pMDIs will perform better in this respect. In clinical practice, the bronchodilator drugs administered often mask bronchoconstriction of this kind. Alcohol present in inhalers might also produce bronchospasm (63).

Safety concerns have been raised with regard to the large amount of oropharyngeal deposition of drug combined with a relatively unpredictable dose to the lungs when pMDIs are used. Oropharyngeal deposition is some 50–80% of the nominal dose (8,64,65), while the lung dose is variable. Lipworth (101) has shown that the vast majority of systemic activity of inhaled steroids is due to the dose of drug reaching the lungs. With some inhaled steroids, a small but still significant contribution to the systematic availability of the steroid is due to gastrointestinal absorption. This is especially true for beclomethasone dipropionate. Oropharyngeal deposition and related systemic absorption may be very greatly reduced by use of a spacer device.

VII. Breath-Actuated MDIs

Although it is likely that breath-actuated MDIs will be more popular than the standard MDI in many countries, the clinical data available on these devices is surprisingly limited. Crompton (66) first described a breath-actuated inhaler, designed by Charlie Theil of 3M, in 1971. This early model, containing isoprenaline, was unsuccessful for several reasons. It was bulky, some patients had difficulty in generating a sufficient flow to trigger the valve mechanism, and its operation was somewhat noisy and violent. The Autohaler replaced this device.

A. The Autohaler

This is a compact device (Fig. 7); it is quiet in operation and functions at a low inhaled flow rate that is easily achieved by patients with obstructive airways disease (67).

The features that distinguish it from a standard inhaler are that:

The aerosol canister is completely enclosed within the body of the device.
There is a latching lever at the top of the inhaler, which the patient lifts to prime the device prior to inhalation.

To operate the device, the patient:

Removes the mouthpiece cover.
Lifts the priming lever.
Inhales through the mouthpiece.

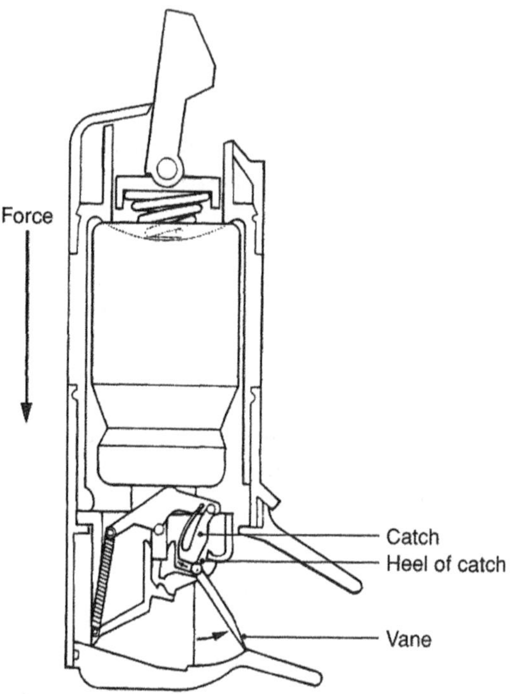

Figure 7 The Aerolin Autohaler. Arrows indicate the direction of movement of the catch and vane. The lever at the top of the device has been pushed into an upright position, thus compressing the spring. When the patient inhales, the vane moves, allowing the compressed spring to force the MDI downward and the valve to actuate. (From Ref. 69.)

The act of inhalation actuates the metering valve and allows a dose of drug to be released, eliminating the need for coordination.

Elevation of the priming lever compresses a spring above the base of the MDI. A mechanical obstruction prevents movement of the aerosol canister within the plastic moulding until the patient inhales. Inhalation rotates a small vane within the mouthpiece, removing the obstacle and allowing the aerosol canister to move down sufficiently to actuate the MDI. Unscrewing the removable sleeve can open the Autohaler. This allows the MDI to be removed and the mouthpiece adapter to be washed (68).

Newman and colleagues (69) studied the radioaerosol deposition and bronchodilator response to 100 μg salbutamol administered from a conventional MDI and from the Autohaler in 18 asthmatic patients. In the 10 patients who could coordinate actuation and inhalation of their own MDIs, deposition of aerosol in the lungs and bronchodilator response were equivalent. In contrast, for the 8 patients who could not coordinate, the mean (SEM) percentage of the dose deposited in the lungs with their own inhaler technique was lower [7.2% (3.4%)] than when they were taught to use their MDI correctly [23% (2.5%)] or when an Autohaler was used [20.8%(1.7%)]. The increase in FEV_1 was significantly greater in the group taught to use their MDIs correctly and in the Autohaler group than in those who used the device incorrectly. The Autohaler will not, however, help patients who stop inhaling at the moment of actuation (70) (Fig. 8).

The data on drug delivery to children via the Authohaler are limited. Ruggins and colleagues (71) compared the effect of giving salbutamol via the Rotahaler (400 μg) and the Autohaler (200 μg) in 51 children aged from 4–13. They found no significant difference in peak expiratory flow rate between the two devices. Only 11 children less than 6 years were studied, of whom one 4-year-old

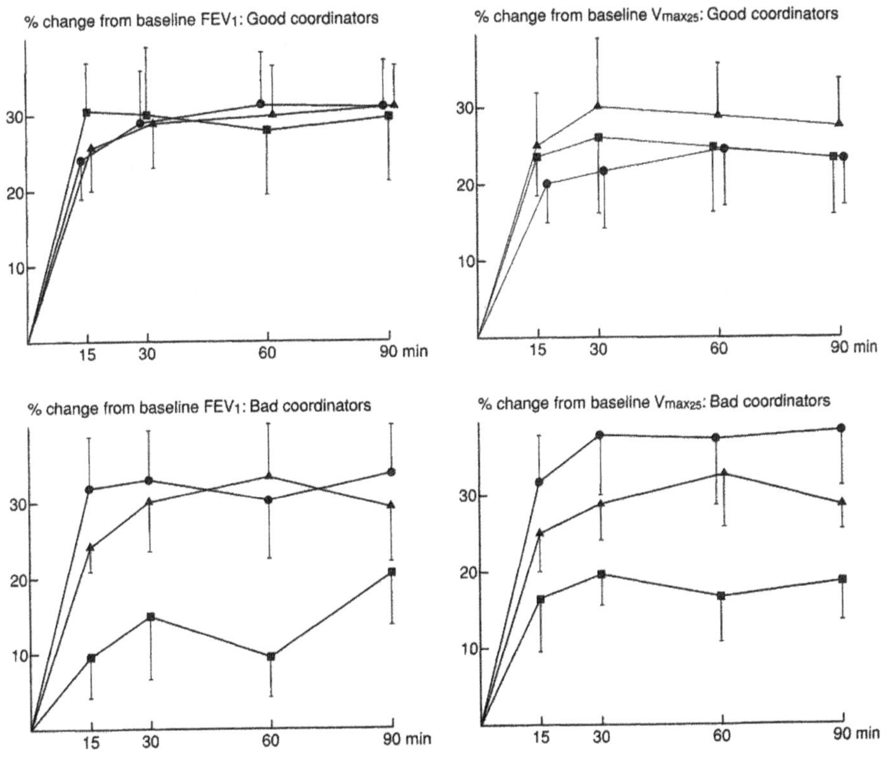

Figure 8 Mean percentage changes in FEV_1 (with standard errors) and maximal expiratory flow at 75% of forced vital capacity ($V_{max}25$) in 10 good coordinators (upper figures) and in 8 bad coordinators (lower figures) for studies with their own pMDI technique (■), the taught MDI technique (♦), and the Autohaler (▲). (From Ref. 69.)

was unable to trigger the Autohaler. Of the other 10 children, only 50% showed some improvement in peak expiratory flow rate. None of the children of 6 years or less were able to clear the Rotahaler of salbutamol. Caution is required in the interpretation of these results, as the inclusion criteria were biased in that the children needed to be able to perform the measurements of peak inspiratory and peak expiratory flow rates. From these data it is clear that breath-actuated devices should not be the device of first choice in children aged 5 or less.

B. The Easi-Breathe Inhaler

The Easi-Breathe is a breath-actuated metered-dose aerosol inhaler developed by Norton Healthcare. The device is primed when the mouthpiece is opened. When the patient breathes in, the mechanism is triggered and a dose is automatically released into the airstream. The inhaler works on a pneumatic principle. An internal vacuum restrains an operating spring. A valve that is operated in response to the patient's inhalation that allows the spring to fire the canister releases the vacuum. It can be actuated at a very low flow of approximately 20 L/min (72). Not surprisingly the device scored better than a pMDI on a number of features, including ease of use and having an attached mouthpiece cover. Practice nurses found it easier to teach and patients easier to learn to use than a conventional pMDI (73).

The Optimiser is a small-volume open-tube spacer device that was developed for use with the Easi-Breathe beclomethasone dipropionate inhalers. It is a plastic 10-cm tube with a volume of 50 mL that can be slotted onto the end of the Easi-Breathe device. Hardy and colleagues (72) compared drug delivery from Becotide 100 Easi-Breathe alone and with the Optimiser, Becotide 100 with a Volumatic, and Baker Norton's standard 100-μg MDI with and without training. Eight volunteers inhaled radiolabeled beclomethasone dipropionate (100 μg) from each of the inhalers on two separate occasions. The Easi-Breathe and Optimiser combination produced significantly better lung deposition than the other devices. Oropharyngeal deposition was markedly reduced using the Easi-Breathe and Optimiser combination, with 55% of the dose remaining in the Optimiser.

Again, the clinical data on using these devices are limited. There are no direct clinical trials comparing the efficacy of beclomethasone dipropionate delivered via the Easi-Breathe with that of BDP delivered via the pMDI.

C. The Easidose

The Easidose (74) is best characterized as a breath coordinated device as opposed to a breath-activated system. At rest no (or minimal) airflow can be achieved through the device. The stem of the valve is linked to a spring-biased vane, incorporating lost motion. When the patient fires the MDI unit, the vane moves open allowing airflow before the valve fires the dose. So as the patients begin to inhale from the device, they cannot do so. However, when they press the inhaler down, a valve opens, resulting in airflow through the device. Thus, the patient is inhaling when actuation of the inhaler occurs.

D. Microprocessor-Controlled MDIs

Optimizing the lung deposition, regional distribution and reproducibility of an inhaled drug could improve its therapeutic efficacy. Optimized delivery will be essential if the inhaled route is to provide a viable method for delivering systemically active drugs that are poorly absorbed from other sites of administration. For example, differences in regional distribution profoundly affect the bioavailability of macromolecular drugs such as insulin following delivery to the lung (75).

The SmartMist (Aradigm Corporation, Hayward, CA) is a hand-held breath-actuated microprocessor-controlled accessory for use with MDIs. The device is shown in Fig. 9. It can be loaded with some of the standard pMDI canisters. It con-

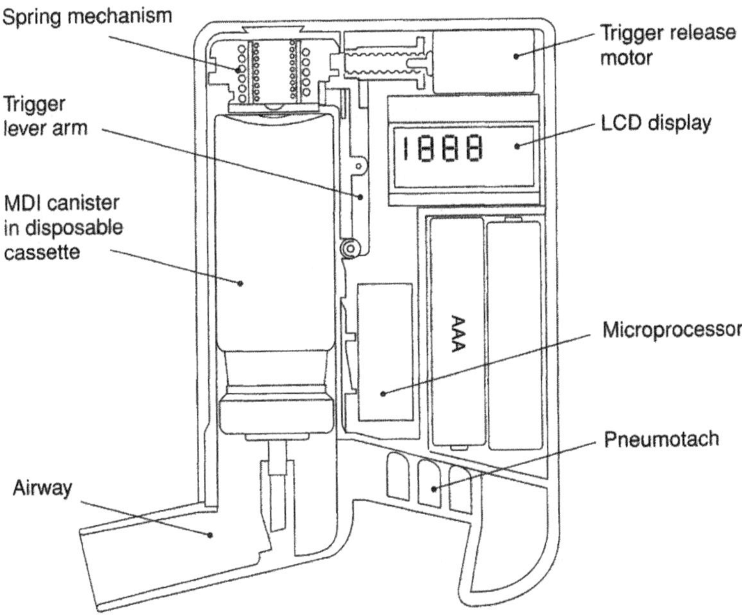

Figure 9 Cutaway view of the Smart Mist device loaded with a pMDI. The Smart Mist device allows reproducible actuation of a pMDI at a preprogrammed point during inhalation. This system analyzes the inspiratory flow profile and automatically actuates the MDI when the predefined conditions of flow and cumulative inspired volume coincide. (From Ref. 76.)

tains a microprocessor that analyzes an inspiratory flow profile and automatically actuates the pMDI when predefined conditions of flow rate and cumulative inspired volume coincide. Inhalation flow is measured before, during and after drug administration and may be recorded in solid-state memory for computer download.

Farr and colleagues (76) used gamma scintigraphy to determine the lung dose of salbutamol delivered, using the SmartMist, to a group of healthy volunteers using various inspiratory flows (30 L/min, slow; 90 L/min, medium; 270 L/min, fast) combined with different cumulative inspired volumes (early, 300 mL; late, 3000 mL). The SmartMist firing at medium flow and early in the cumulative inspired volume resulted in the highest lung deposition [18.6(1.42)%]. The slow early setting gave the second highest deposition [14.1 (2)%]. The peripheral lung deposition was similar between the medium/early [9.1(0.9)% and slow/early (7.5(1)%] settings. Improved lung deposition with this system at a flow of 90 L/min is different to earlier lung deposition studies, mentioned above, where the optimum inhalation rate was approximately 30 L/min. In these studies inspiratory flows approaching 100 L/min were considered too fast (77). The reason for these conflicting data is not entirely clear.

VIII. The Synchroner

The Synchroner is a standard metered-dose inhaler with a convenient integral open-tube spacer that adds little to the size of the MDI. When not in use, the spacer is folded against the main body of the canister holder and is held in place by the dust cap. When the inhaler is used, the dust cap is removed and the spacer with mouthpiece is moved until it is at right angles to the inhaler. The device provides a 10-cm gap between the aerosol canister and the patient's mouth, which slows the aerosol down after it comes out of the MDI.

The Synchroner is also designed to help patients coordinate actuation of the aerosol canister and inspiration. If the inhalation and actuation are mistimed when using the Synchroner, the aerosol cloud escapes from the open tube. This may be seen by the patient and give instant feedback of their poor technique. If patients inhale correctly no cloud appears.

Newman and colleagues (78), found lung deposition was improved over the metered-dose inhaler alone at both slow (25 L/min) and fast (100 L/min) inhalation rates, with the slower inhalation rate achieving the highest total and peripheral lung delivery. Oropharyngeal deposition was halved.

IX. The Spacehaler

The Spacehaler (Fig. 10) is a relatively new actuator/mouthpiece designed to be used in conjunction with a pressurized metered-dose canister. The mouthpiece is

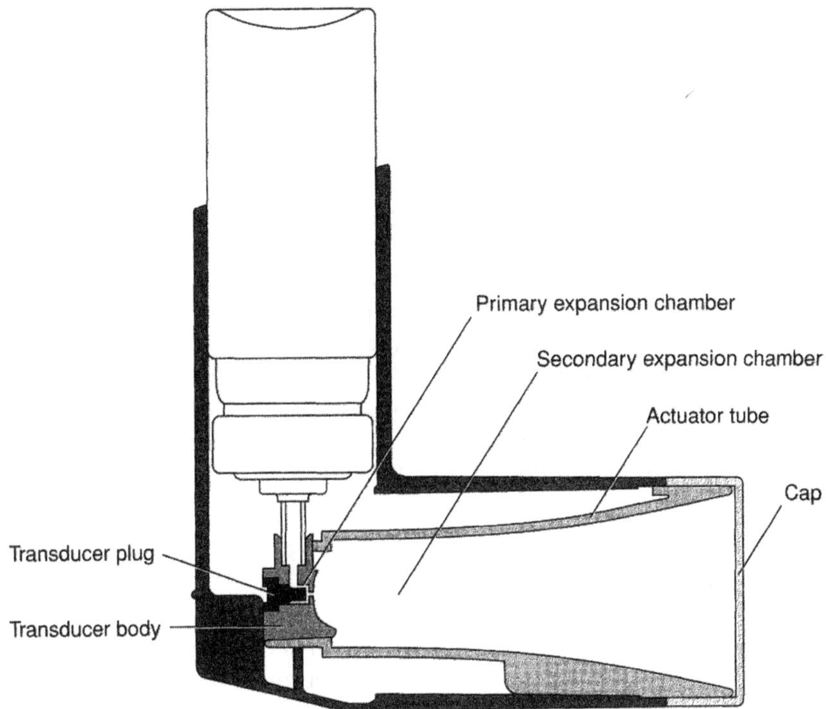

Figure 10 A cross-sectional view of the Spacehaler. The design slows the aerosol plume prior to inhalation.

slightly extended compared with the standard actuator. The purported benefits of this device are that the velocity of the emitted dose is reduced to approximately 2 m/s compared with the 30 m/s commonly seen with a standard actuator.

From depression of the drug canister, material is forcibly expelled and passes into the transducer inlet at very high speed. It travels along the inlet passage and into the first expansion chamber, where it encounters a "bluff body." This gives rise to a number of standing shock waves and the generation of a large number of vortices in the immediate vicinity of the bluff body. These vortices have axes parallel to the bluff body and, owing to the pressure gradient throughout the expansion chamber, the vortices are compressed and forced toward the outlet orifice. On passing through the outlet orifice into the secondary expansion chamber, some expansion into a single large vortex takes place. At this stage the emitted cloud is a rapidly spinning vortex and large particles within the cloud collide with the side of the actuator tube and some deposition of the large particles occurs. This has the effect of removing the majority of nonrespirable drug particles and theoretically increasing the proportion of respirable particles within the emitted cloud. Published data on the use of the Spacehaler are limited, particularly its use in childhood.

X. Generic pMDIs—Salbutamol and Steroids

There has been considerable debate on the issue of generic and innovator salbutamol and steroid pMDIs (79,80). In contrast to the procedure for oral medications, the Medicines Control Agency only required in vitro testing for inhaled forms of generic salbutamol before licensing. With salbutamol there is some variation between generic and innovator products in terms of the total dose available per actuation. However, Clark et al. (81) found no difference in terms of two generic and innovator formulations of salbutamol MDIs in terms of bioavailability. Newman (82) found minor differences in the fine particle mass of an innovator and two generic beclomethasone dipropionate pMDIs. The clinical relevance of these slight differences is unclear.

XI. CFC-Free MDIs

Over the last 40 years, pMDIs have contained chlorofluorocarbons (CFCs) as propellants. Although safe for human use when given in the recommended dosage, chlorine atoms in CFCs have been shown to deplete the earth's stratospheric ozone layer, which filters out harmful ultraviolet rays from the sun. As described in the chapter on propellants, the use of CFCs in pMDIs has continued under temporary exemptions that were included in the Montreal protocol for "essential users." This exemption was granted to pharmaceutical companies, giving them the time to complete thorough safety testing on appropriate alternative propellants. In response to the Montreal protocol, two propellants were identified as replacements for chlorofluorocarbons (CFCs). One such compound was the hydrofluoroalkane (HFA), 1,1,1,2-tetrafluoroethane (HFA 134a). HFA 134a contains only carbon, hydrogen, and fluorine, replacing the chlorine of the CFCs. It is used in the HFA pMDIs released to date. The other propellant—1,1,1,2,3,3,3-heptafluoropropane (HFC-227)—is under active investigation.

Major physicochemical characteristics of HFA 134a had to be overcome for formulation and manufacture. HFA 134a has a low boiling point (-27°C). The CFC contained in MDIs currently available—for example, those produced by 3M—contains CFC11 and 12 that have boiling points of +24°C and -30°C respectively. CFC11 has a high boiling point, so that, at room temperature, it is a liquid in which the drug can be dissolved or dispersed. This mixture is then metered into a canister, the valve crimped into place, and CFC12, which provides the driving force for atomization of the drug, can be pressure-filled through the valve. HFA 134a is equivalent to CFC12 in that it provides the propelling force, but a replacement for CFC11 has not been identified. Thus a new manufacturing process was developed. However, ethanol is used as a cosolvent and this can take the place of CFC11.

The surfactants commonly used in CFC pMDIs, such as oleic acid and lecithin, are insoluble in HFA134a. Possible solutions to this problem involved the removal of the surfactant, the use of an HFA-soluble surfactant, or the addition of ethanol to aid the dissolution of the surfactant. The Ventolin Evohaler, for example, contains drug and HFA 134a propellant only, as does the CFC-free fluticasone propionate. The surfactant has been eliminated. To prevent drug from being deposited on the inhaler walls, the internal surface of the ventolin Evohaler is coated with a Teflon-like fluoropolymer with a low surface energy, preventing drug from being attracted to it. Rubber seals have also been changed within the valve system.

The Ventolin (salbutamol) Evohaler from GlaxoSmith Kline comprises a suspension of micronized salbutamol sulfate in liquefied CFC-free propellant (HFA 134a) contained in an aluminum alloy canister. The canister is sealed with a metering valve that contains a peroxide-cured nitrile rubber seal. The actuators are identical to those used for the ventolin inhaler. Advantages of the new valve system with the ventolin Evohaler are that drug delivery has been shown to be reproducible regardless of storage orientation of the inhaler between actuations. The dose delivered is also consistent throughout the intended life span of the device (83). The fine particle mass of the ventolin Evohaler has also been shown to be comparable to that of the conventional ventolin inhaler, allowing a direct exchange of the product.

Ross and Gabrio (84) compared various aspects of the function of a new CFC-free MDI containing salbutamol sulfate (Airomir, 3M) with traditional CFC-containing salbutamol pMDIs. In addition to the new formulation of HFA 134a propellant drug, a new inhaler was developed incorporating a new metering valve with seals made of elastomers compatible with the HFA propellant. A smaller valve size of 25 μL and a smaller actuator spray exit orifice diameter were also incorporated into the product. The new actuator features are a reshaped round mouthpiece that is intended to open the patient's mouth wider. The following performance aspects of the new salbutamol inhalers were studied:

Consistent dosing through to the end of canister life: The valves currently used on salbutamol CFC pMDIs do not uniformly deliver drug when the canister is nearly empty because of inconsistency of filling up the metering tank. This is referred to as tail-off. If the canister is used beyond the label number of doses, the delivered dose may become unpredictable and subject to wide variation (85). The tail-off pattern of the new CFC-free salbutamol inhaler (Airomir) shows that once valve delivery dropped below 85% of the baseline value, very little drug was delivered. The authors consider that this would present a clear indication to the patient that the inhaler was empty. In contrast, the CFC salbutamol product they studied had an erratic dose pattern at the end of the canister life, fluctuating between normal and low doses before consistently falling below 85% of the baseline drug delivery. The authors suggest this may make it difficult for the patient to determine if the canister is nearly empty (Fig. 11).

Storage orientation effects: Studies on the CFC-free MDIs stored either valve up or valve down without disturbance for up to 14 days demonstrated that the first dose actuated consistently delivered the drug label claim (86) (Fig. 12). This is a clear advantage over the CFC-containing salbutamol MDIs and the findings of Cyr et al. (23)

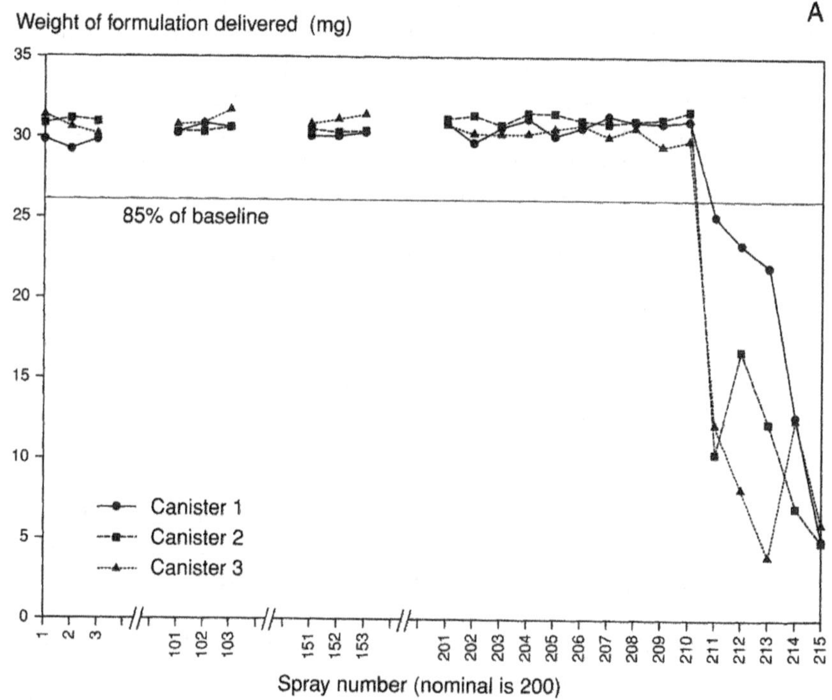

Figure 11 Tail-off of delivery of salbutamol from CFC and CFC-free pMDIs. A. CFC-free salbutamol MDI showing relatively quick tail-off after the 200th actuation is reached. B. CFC salbutamol tail-off showing very variable tail-off once the 200th dose has been passed. (From Ref. 85.)

Effect of storage temperature: CFC-free salbutamol was shown to deliver a more consistent dose and a more consistent fine particle mass over a range of temperatures from –20 to 20°C. Only at temperatures less than –10°C did the fine particle mass as a percentage of the initial dose, decrease, and then only to approximately 65%.

Spray plume temperature: Proventor HFA (Schering-Plough, Madison, NJ) produced a significantly softer and warmer aerosol spray than other products tested. Plume temperatures for various CFC and CFC-free salbutamol pMDIs are shown in Fig. 13.

XII. CFC-Free Steroids Delivered by pMDI

In contrast to CFC-based formulations, the new beclomethasone dipropionate available in a CFC-free pMDI is in solution. The solution contains hydrofluoroalkane-134a (HFA-134a) and ethanol. There is no added surfactant in this preparation.

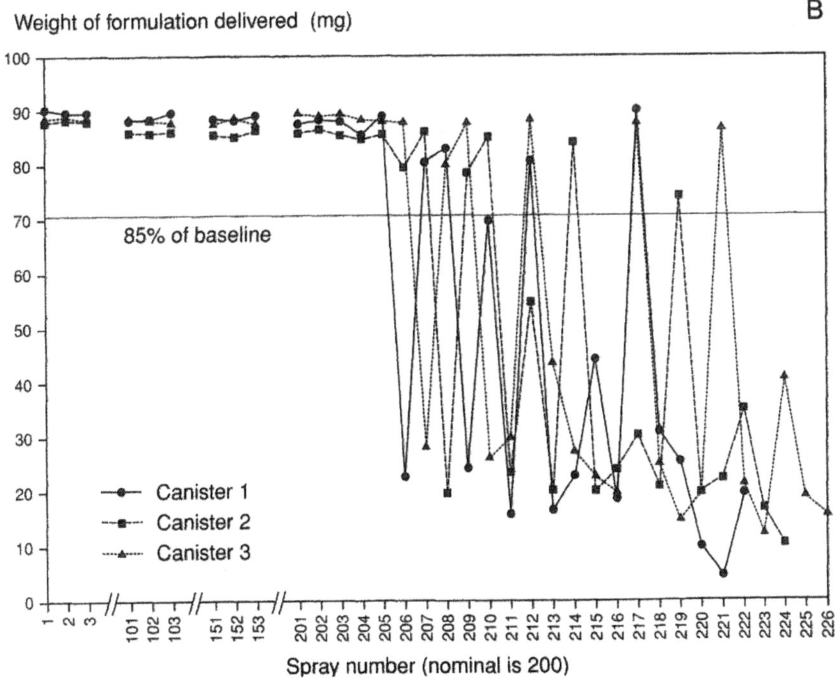

Figure 11 Continued.

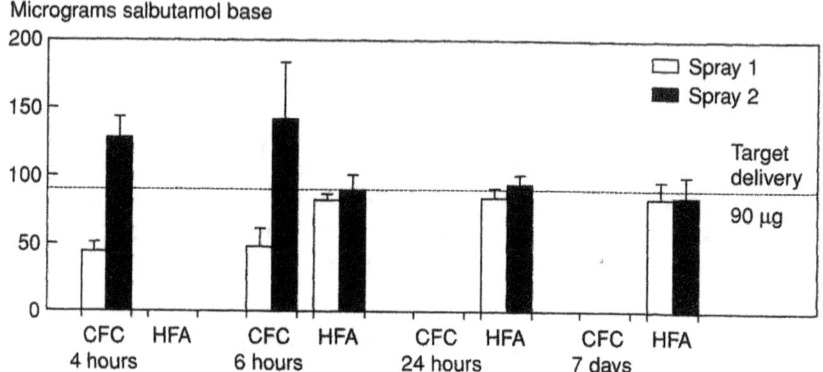

Figure 12 The effect of storage orientation on the output of CFC-free salbutamol pMDIs. There is a very consistent dose output with the HFA inhalers over the study period when stored in the inverted position. Horizontal and upright storage also showed consistent drug output from the HFA inhalers over a period of up to 7 days. (From Ref. 85.)

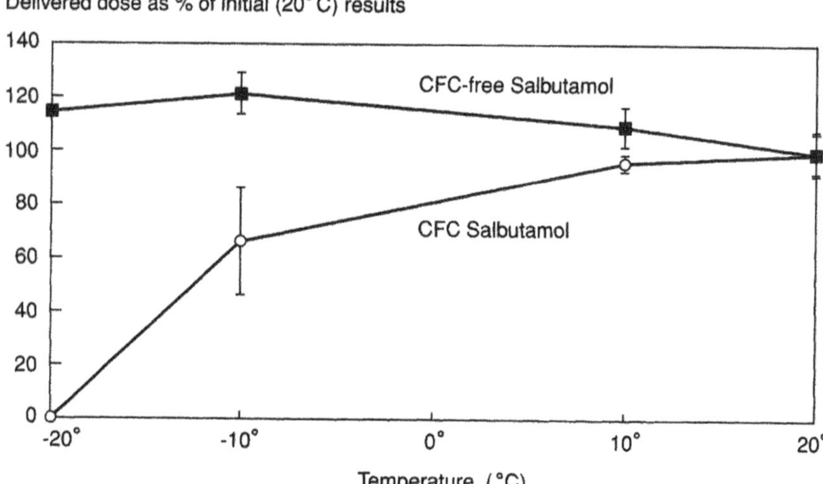

Figure 13 Plume temperature of CFC and CFC-free salbutamol MDIs. (From Ref. 85.)

The solution aerosol has the effect of markedly reducing the particle size of the drug aerosol. When actuated, 60% of the particles are in the respirable range and they have an average size three times smaller than with the CFC-BDP (1.1 versus 3.4–4 μm) (87). Using radiolabeled techniques, the percentage deposition in the lungs is considerably greater with solution BDP than with the CFC-BDP, while the oropharyngeal deposition is reduced. The actual values when six normal volunteers were studied are shown in Table 5 (88). Plasma profiles following delivery of CFC-BDP or solution HFA-BDP reflect the relative delivery of drugs to the airways. In patients, it takes twice as much CFC-BDP to achieve similar total plasma levels as solution HFA-BDP. Inhaled BDP is rapidly metabolized in the lung to the active metabolite 17-BMP and absorbed into the systemic circulation. CFC-BDP plasma levels reach a peak within 2 h and within 30 min with solution HFA-BDP. Across a dose range for 100–800 μg/day, it has been shown that a 2.6 times higher dose of CFC-BDP is required to achieve the same level of efficacy (FEV_1 response) as solution HFA-BDP. These studies were in adults and it is suggested that the dose delivery of the HFA-BDP solution should be half that of the conventional CFC-BDP.

Baker Norton has launched another solution HFA-134a BDP preparation in certain countries, which is recommended as a direct microgram-for-microgram replacement for CFC-BDP (89). This is surprising, as the particle size and dose delivered from this preparation is similar to that of the 3M HFA preparation described above. Serum cortisol levels taken at 9 A.M. were compared following very large doses of BDP-CFC or BDP-HFA 500 μg for 12 weeks. No statistical difference was found. It is likely that prescribing different doses of what appear to be similar HFA-BDP solutions will cause confusion.

XIII. Compliance Monitors

Most compliance monitors will only tell if the pMDI has been actuated, not whether the patient has taken the dose. For example, actuating the pMDI when

Table 5 Deposition of a HFA Beclomethasone Dipropionate Solution pMDI Compared to a CFC Preparation, Expressed as a Percentage of Ex-Actuator Dose (mean ± SE)

	n	Oropharynx	Lungs	Abdomen	Exhaled
HFA BDP Solution 100 μg	3	27±11	60±8	2±1	11±2
CFC-BDP 250 μg	4	84±7	7±1	6±5	2±1

the mouthpiece cap is in place will not be recognized, nor will actuation during exhalation. A second potential drawback of some devices is that the pMDI can and valve in question is fitted into the monitoring devices body where the monitoring actuator stem and mouthpiece may be different, leading to a modified aerosol cloud.

There are also two ways to look at compliance monitors, whether they are to help the patient to follow his or her dosing regime or whether they are for the physician to check if the patient is following this regime. In the simplest case, numerical dose counters now being fitted to breath-activated inhalers enable a patient—or perhaps more importantly a child's parent—to check if the dose has been taken. This assumes the discipline of keeping track of the previous dose number.

However, more sophisticated monitors require a power source, usually batteries, so that more complex information can be recorded and transcribed. This also requires the use of electronics that are becoming more common; but a mass-produced electronic chip will be necessary for low cost. Hence a number of compliance monitors at present have been developed within companies for internal use, including clinical trials, but are relatively crude prototype devices.

Medtrac Technologies (102,103) have the MDI Chronolog, which holds the canister, and the unit can record the date and time of actuations. This information can then be downloaded to a computer for analysis. Other studies (104) have attached a nebulizer chronology from Forefront Technologies to a MDI, again to determine the patterns of actuations.

More sophisticated systems have been reported, such as those from Miras Medical Corporation (105), whose device presents overuse for pain relief programs with an inhaler. Medtrac Technologies (106) have a patent for an electronic device that not only measures and records the dosing parameters but also can control the timing of the dose. Aradigm as well as their standard unit for recording data reference have a patent (107) for control of actuation.

XIV. Future Research

The pMDI will continue to be one of the most popular drug delivery devices for inhaled antiasthma drugs. The increasing number of modifications to the standard inhaler should improve drug delivery.

Future research is required in three main areas: first, to reduce the marked variability in deposition of drug in the lower airway; second, to reduce the upper air way deposition of inhaled drug; and third, to include compliance monitors in the delivery device.

Acknowledgments

We would like to thank Judy White, Judith Jackson, John Chege, Elna Berg, and Peter Barry for their helpful and constructive comments on this chapter.

References

1. Bower C. Washington C, Purewal TS. Characterisation of surfactant effect on aggregates in model aerosol propellant suspensions. J Pharm Pharmacol 1996; 48:337–341.
2. Gonda I. Development of a systematic theory of suspension inhalation aerosols: I. A framework to study the effects of aggregation on the aerodynamic behaviour of drug particles. Int J Pharm 1985; 27:99–116.
3. Atkins PJ. The development of new solution metered dose inhaler delivery systems. Proceedings of the Second Conference on Respiratory Drug Delivery. Lexington, KY: University of Kentucky, 1991: 416–445.
4. Clark AR. PhD thesis. Loughborough University of Technology, 1991.
5. Clark AR. Medical aerosol inhalers: past, Present, and future. Aerosol Sci Technol 1995, 22:374–391.
6. Byron PR. Aerosol formulation, generation, and delivery using metered systems. In: Byron PR, ed. Respiratory Drug Delivery. Boca Raton, FL: CRC Press, 1990: 171–174.
7. Newman S, Pavia D, Clarke S. Improving the bronchial deposition of pressurised aerosols. Chest 1981; 80:909–911.
8. Newman S, Pavia D, Garland N, Clarke S. Effects of various inhalation modes on the deposition of radioactive pressurised aerosols. Eur J Respir Dis 1982; 63:57–65.
9. Newman SP, Bateman JRN, Pavia D, Clarke SW. In: Baron D, ed. Recent Advances in Aerosol Therapy. Brussels: UCB Pharmaceuticals, 1979:117–122.
10. Lawford P, MacKenzie D. Does inspiratory flow rate affect broncodilator response to an aerosol beta-2 agonist? Thorax 1981; 36:714.
11. Hindle M, Newton DA, Chrystyn H. Investigations of an optimal inhaler technique with the use of urinary salbutamol excretion as a measure of relative bioavailability to the lung. Thorax 1993; 48:607–610.
12. Dolovich M, Ruffin RA, Roberts R, Newhouse MT. Optimal delivery of aerosol through metered dose inhalers. Chest 1981; 80:911–915.
13. Thomas P, Williams T, Riley PA, Bradley D. Modifying delivery technique of fenoterol from a metered dose inhaler. Ann Allergy 1984; 52:279–281.
14. Newman SP, Pavia D, Clarke SW. How should a pressurised beta adrenergic bronchodilator be inhaled? Eur J Respir Dis 1981; 62:3–21.
15. Lawford P, MacKenzie F. Pressurised bronchodilator aerosol technique: influence of breath holding, time and relationship of inhaler to the mouth. Br J Dis Chest 1982; 76:229–233.
16. Chhabra SK. A comparison of closed and open mouthed techniques of inhalation of salbutamol metered dose inhaler. J Asthma 1994; 31:123–125.

17. Riley DJ, Liu RT, Edelman NH. Enhanced responses to aerosolised bronchodilator therapy in asthma using respiratory manoeuvres. Chest 1979; 76:501–507.
18. Riley DJ, Weitz BW, Edelman NH. The responses of asthmatic subjects to isoproterenol inhaled at differing lung volumes. Am Rev Respir Dis 1976; 114:509–515.
19. Lawford P, MacKenzie D. Pressurised aerosol technique. Lancet 1981; 1:1003–1004.
20. Heimer D, Shim C, Williams MH. The effect of sequential inhalations of metaproterenol aerosol in asthma. J Allergy Clin Immunol 1980; 66:75–77.
21. Moran F. Aerosol dosage forms and formulations. In: Moran F, Dolovitch MB, Newhouse MT, Newman SP, eds. Aerosols in Medicine, Principles, Diagnosis and Therapy, 2d ed. Amsterdam: Elsevier Science, 1993: 321–350.
22. Berg E. In vitro properties of pressurised metered done inhalers with and without spacer devices J Aerosol Med 1995; 8:S3–S11.
23. Cyr TD, Graham SJ, Lee KYR, Lovering E.G. Low first-spray drug content in albuterol metered dose inhalers. Pharm Res 1991; 8:658–660.
24. Byron PR. Dosing reproducibility from experimental albuterol suspension metered dose inhalers. Pharm Res 1994; 11:580–584.
25. Everard MT., Devadason SG, Summers QA, Le Souef PN. Factors affecting total and respirable "dose" delivered by a salbutamol metered dose inhaler. Thorax 1995; 50:746–749.
26. Schulze MD, Riebe MT, Martin NB, Ryder SM, Shurkus DD, Ashurst IC. Development and performance of a new HFA-based metered dose inhaler (MDI) system for salbutamol sulphate. Eur Respir J 1997; 10(suppl 25): 38S.
27. Weiss W, Bodenheimer S, Bergner A, et al. Metered dose inhalers: drug delivery over the life of a canister. JAMA 1993; 270:2050–2051.
28. Bergner A, Griesner WA, Bergner RK. Metered dose inhalers: the specified number of sprays. JAMA 1993; 269:1506.
29. Ogren RA, Baldwin JL, Simon RA. How patients determine when to replace their metered dose inhalers. Ann Allergy Asthma Immunol 1995; 75:485–489.
30. Williams DJ, Williams AC, Kruchek DG. Problems in assessing contents of metered dose inhalers. Br Med J 1993; 307:771–772.
31. Davies D. Pharmacokinetics of inhaled substances. Postgrad Med J 1975; 51:69–75.
32. Newman SP, Pavia D, Morean F, Sheahan NF, Clarke SW. Deposition of presssurised aerosols in the human respiratory tract. Thorax 1981; 36:52–55.
33. Short M, Singh C, Few J, Studdy P, Heaf P, Spiro S. The labelling and monitoring of lung deposition of an inhaled synthetic anticholinergic bronchodilating agent. Chest 1981; 80:918–921.
34. Pauwels R, Newman S, Borgstrom L. Airways deposition and airway effects of anti-asthma drugs delivered from metered dose inhalers. Eur Respir J 1997; 10:2127–2138.
35. Saunders KB. Misuse of inhaled bronchodilating agents. Br Med J 1965; 1:1037–1038.
36. Patterson IC, Crompton GK. Use of pressurised aerosols by asthmatic patients. Br Med J 1976; 1:76–77.
37. Epstein SW, Manning CPR, Ashley MJ, Corey PN. Survey of the clinical use of pressurised aerosol inhalers. Can Med Assoc J 1979; 120:813–816.

38. Pedersen S, Frost L, Arnfred T. Errors in inhalation technique and efficiency in inhaler use in asthmatic children. Allergy 1986; 41:118–124.
39. De Blaquiere P Christensen DB, Carter WB, Martin TR. Use and misuse of metered dose inhalers by patients with chronic lung disease. Am Rev Respir Dis 1989; 140:910–916.
40. Larsen JS, Hahn M, Ekholm B, Wick KA. Evaluation of conventional press and breathe metered dose inhaler technique in 501 patients. J Asthma 1994; 31:193–199.
41. Van Beerendonk I, Mesters I, Mudde AN, Tan TD. Assessment of the inhalation technique in outpatients with chronic obstructive pulmonary disease using a metered dose inhaler or dry powder device. J Asthma 1998; 35:273–279.
42. Kelling JS, Strohl KP, Smith RL, Altose MD. Physician knowledge of the use of canister nebulisers. Chest 1983; 83:612–614.
43. Guidry GG, Brown WD, Stogner SW, George RB. Incorrect use of metered dose inhalers by medical personnel. Chest 1992; 101:31–33.
44. Kesten S, Zive K, Chapman KR. Pharmacists' knowledge and ability of use inhaled medication delivery systems. Chest 1993; 104:1737–1742.
45. Hanania NA, Wittman R, Kesten S, Chapman KR. Medical personnel's knowledge of and ability to use inhaling devices: metered dose inhalers, spacer chambers, and breath actuated dry powder inhalers. Chest 1994; 105:111–116.
46. Amiravi I, Goren A, Pawlowski NA. What do paediatricians in training know about the correct use of inhalers and spacer devices? J Allergy Clin Immunol 1994; 99:669–675.
47. Amirav I, Goran A, Kravitz RM, Pawlowski NA. Physician targeted programme on inhaled therapy for childhood asthma. J Allergy Clin Immunol 1995; 95:818–823.
48. Armitage JM, Williams SJ. Inhaler technique in the elderly. Age Ageing 1988; 17:275–278.
49. Crompton GK. Problems patients have using pressurised aerosol inhalers. Eur J Respir Dis 1982; 19(Suppl):101–104.
50. Newman SP Aerosol deposition considerations in inhalation therapy. Chest 1985; 88:142S–160S.
51. Pedersen S, Ostergaard PA. Nasal inhalation as cause of inefficient pulmonary aerosol technique in children. Allergy 1983; 38:191–194.
52. Allen SC, Prior A. What determines whether an elderly patient can use a metered dose aerosol correctly? Br J Dis Chest 1986; 80:45–49.
53. Gray SL, Williams DM, Pullan CC, Sirgo MA, Bishop AL, Donohue JF. Characteristics predicting incorrect metered dose inhaler technique in older subjects. Arch Intern Med 1996; 156:984–988.
54. Horsley MG, Baille GR. Risk factors for inadequate use of pressurised aerosol inhalers. J Clin Pharm Ther 1988; 13:139–143.
55. Chapman KR, Love L, Brubaker H. A comparison of breath-actuated and conventional metered-dose inhalation techniques in elderly subjects. Chest 1993: 104:1332–1337.
56. Bryant DH, Pepys J. Bronchial reactions to aerosol inhalant vehicle. Br Med J 1976; 1:1319–1320.

57. Reisman RE. Asthma induced by adrenergic aerosols. J Allergy 1970; 46:162.
58. Nicklas RA. Paradoxical bronchospasm associated with the use of inhaled beta agonists. J Allergy Clin Immunol 1990; 85:959–964.
59. Yarborough J, Mansfield L, Ting S. Metered dose inhaler induced bronchospasm in asthmatic patients. Ann Allergy 1985; 55:25–27.
60. Wilkinson JRW, Roberts JA, Brading P, Holgate ST, Howarth PH. Paradoxical restriction in asthmatic patients after salmeterol by metered dose inhaler. Br Med J 1992; 305:931–932.
61. Jackson L, Stahl E, Holgate ST. Terbutaline via a pressurised metered dose inhaler (pMDI) and Turbuhaler in highly reactive asthmatic patients. Eur Respir J 1994; 7:1598–1601.
62. Selroos O, Lofroos AB, Pietinalho A, Riska H. Comparison of terbutaline and placebo from a pressurised metered dose inhaler and a dry powder inhaler in a subgroup of patients with asthma. Thorax 1994; 49:1228–1230.
63. Gong HR, Taskin DP, Calvarese BM. Alcohol induced bronchospasm in an asthmatic patient: pharmacologic evaluation of the mechanism. Chest 1981; 80:167–173.
64. Borgstrom L, Newman S. Total and regional lung deposition of terbutaline sulphate inhaled via a pressurised MDI or Turbuhaler. Int J Pharm 1993; 97:47–53.
65. Newman SP. Deposition and effects of inhalation aerosols. Thesis, Rahms Tryckeri, Lund, Sweden, 1983.
66. Crompton GK. Breath-activated aerosol. Br Med J 1971; 2:652–653.
67. Wallace WAH, Lenny J, Cooksey E, Greening AP, Crompton GK. Ability of patients with severe air flow limitation to trigger a new breath actuated inhaler. Thorax 1989; 44:318.
68. Baum EA, Design, development and testing of a new breath actuated inhaler. Inspiration, development in inhalational therapy; meeting proceedings. Medicine Publishing Foundation, 1988:20–30.
69. Newman S, Weisz A, Talace N, Clarke S. Improvement of drug delivery with a breath-actuated pressurised aerosol for patients with poor inhalation technique. Thorax 1991; 46:712–716.
69. Pederson S, Mortensen S. Use of different inhalational devices in children. Lung 1990; 168 (suppl):653–657.
71. Ruggins, NR, Milner AD, Swarbrick A. An assessment of a new breath actuated inhaler device in acutely wheezy children. Arch Dis Child 1993; 68:477–480.
72. Hardy J, Jasuja A, Frier M, Perkins A. A small volume spacer for use with a breath-operated pressurised metered dose inhaler. Int J Pharm 1996; 142:129–133.
73. Price DB, Pearce L, Powell SR, Shirley J, Sayers MK. Handling and acceptiability of the Easi-Breathe device compared with a conventional metered dose inhaler by patients and practice nurses. Int J Clin Pract 1999; 53:31–36.
74. Howlett D. Determination and improvement of patients' co-ordination with pMDIs: Drug delivery to the lungs IX. Aerosol Soc 1998; 184–187.
75. Colthorpe P, Farr SJ, Taylor G, Smith IJ, Wyatt, D. The pharmacokinetics of pulmonary delivered insulin: a comparison of intratracheal and aerosol administration to the rabbit. Pharm Res 1992; 9:764–768.

76. Farr SJ, Rowe AM, Rubsamen R, Taylor G. Aerosol deposition in the human lung following administration from a microprocessor controlled metered dose inhaler. Thorax 1995; 50:639–644.
77. Newman SP, Pavia D, Garland N, Clarke SW. Effects of various inhalation modes on the deposition of radio active pressurised aerosols. Eur J Respir Dis 1982; 119 (suppl):57–65.
78. Newman SP, Clark AR, Talaee N, Clarke SW. Pressurised aerosol deposition in the human lung with and without an "open" spacer device. Thorax 1989; 44:706–710.
79. Pearson M, Lewis R, Watson J, Ayres J, Ibbotson G, Ryan D. Generic inhalers for asthma. Br Med J 1994; 309:1440.
80. Struke G. Generic inhalers for asthma: patients titrate dose against response. Br Med J 1995;310:602.
81. Clarke DJ, Gordon-Smith J, McPhate G, Clark G, Lipworth BJ. Lung bioavailability of generic and innovator salbutamol metered dose inhalers. Thorax 1996; 51:325–326.
82. Kenyon CJ, Dewsbury NJ, Newman SP. Differences in aerodynamic particle size distributions of innovator and generic beclomethasone dipropionate aerosols used with and without a large-volume spacer. Thorax 1995; 50:846–850.
83. Schultz RK, Dupont RL, Ledoux KA. Issues surrounding metered dose valve technology: past, present and future perspectives. In: Respiratory Drug Delivery IV. Buffalo Grove, IL: Interpharm Press, 1994:211–219.
84. Ross D, Carlson S, June D. Comparison of a new HFA albuterol metered dose inhaler (MDI) to a marketed CFC albuterol MDI—effect of storage orientation, end of canister life and temperature on dosing consistency. Am J Respir Crit Care Med 1996; 153:A62.
85. Ross DL, Gabrio BJ. Advances in metered dose inhaler technology with the development of a chlorofluorocarbon-free drug delivery system. J Aerosol Med 1999; 12:151–160.
86. Tansey I. Technological development of Airomir (salbutamol sulphate in CFC-free system) MDI. Br J Clin Pract 1995; (suppl 79):13–15.
87. Leach C. Improved delivery of inhaled steroids to enlarge small airways. Respir Med 1998; 92(suppl A):3–8.
88. Harrison L, Leach C, Seale P. Improvement in topical lung vs systemic availability of bectomethasone dipropionate from an extra-fine aerosol formulation. Eur Respir J 1997; 10(suppl 25):349s.
89. Milanowski J, Qualtrough J, Perrin VL. Inhaled beclomethasone (BDP) with non-CFC propellant (HFA 134a) is equivalent to BDP-CFC for the treatment of asthma. Respir Med 1999; 93:245–251.
90. Davies D. Pharmacokinetic studies with inhaled drugs. Eur J Respir Dis 1982; 63:67–72.
91. Borgstrom L, Nilsson M. A method for determination of the absolute pulmonary bioavailability of inhaled drugs: terbutaline. Pharm Res 1990; 7:1068–1070.
92. Vidgren M, Karkaainen A, Akarjalainen P, Nuutinen J, Paronen P. In vitro and in vivo deposition of drug particles inhaled from pressurized aerosol and dry powder inhaler. Drug Dev Ind Pharm 1988; 14:2649–2665.

93. Thorsson L, Edsbacker S, Conradson T-B. Lung deposition of budesonide from Turbohaler is twice that from a pressurised metered dose inhaler (pMDI). Eur Respir J 1994; 7:1839–1844.
94. Melchor R, Biddiscombe M, Mak V, Short M, Spiro S. Lung deposition patterns of directly labelled salbutamol in normal subjects and in patients with reversible airflow obstruction. Thorax 1993; 48:506–511.
95. Biddiscombe M, Melchor R, Mak V, et al. The lung deposition of salbutamol, directly labelled with technetium-99m, delivered by pressurised metered dose and dry powder inhalers. Int J Pharm 1993; 91:111–121.
96. Borgstrom L. Methodological studies on lung deposition. Evalutation of inhalational devices and absorption mechanisms. Comprehensive summaries of Uppsala disserations from the Faculty Pharmacy 105. Acta Univ Uppsala 1993; 1–51.
97. Newman S, Steed K, Hooper G, Kallen A, Borgstrom L. Comparison of gamma scintigraphy and pharmacokinetic technique for assessing pulmonary deposition of terbutaline sulphate delivered by pressurised metered dose inhaler. Pharm Res 1995; 12:231–236.
98. Farr S, Rowe A, Rubsamen R, Taylor G. Optimisation of aerosol inhalation from metered dose inhalers by use of a novel microprocessor controlled device. Pharm Res 1994; 11–158.
99. Newman S, Clarke S. Bronchodilator delivery from Gentlehaler, a new low-velocity pressurised aerosol inhaler. Chest 1993; 103:1442–1446.
100. Newman S, Clark A, Talace N, Clarke S. Lung deposition of 5 mg of Intal from a pressurised metered dose inhaler assessed by radiotracer technique. Int J Pharm 1991; 74:203–208.
101. Lipworth BJ. New perspectives on inhaled drug delivery and systemic bioactivity. Thorax 1995; 50:105–110.
102. Cramer JA. Microelectronic systems for monitoring and enhancing patient compliance with medication regimens. Drugs 1995; 49:321–327.
103. Milgrom H. Bender B. Ackerson L. Bowry P. Smith B. Rand C. Noncompliance and treatment failure in children with asthma. J Allergy Clin Immunol 1996; 98(6/1):1051–1057.
104. Simmons M, Nides MA, Rand CS, Wise RA, Tashkin DP. Trends in compliance with bronchodilator inhaler use between follow up visits in a clinical trial. Chest 1996; 109(4):963–968.
105. Rubsman R. Intrapulmonary delivery of narcotics. Patent: WO 94/16755, 1994.
106. Wolf J. Electronic medication Chronolog device. Patent: WO 97/13553, 1997.
107. Rubasmen R. Intrapulmonary delivery of hematopoietic drug. Patent: WO 96/30068, 1996.

11

Propellants

MARTYN R. PARTRIDGE

Whipps Cross University Hospital
London, England

ASHLEY A. WOODCOCK

Wythenshawe Hospital
Manchester, England

I. Introduction

The pressurized metered dose inhaler (pMDI) is a pocket sized, hand-held drug delivery system designed to deliver consistent small doses of medicines directly to the patient's lungs. The essential constituents are the medicine, the propellant, and a storage canister, a metering valve, and an actuator. This chapter is concerned with the propellants. It addresses

Current propellants and why they are being changed
The new propellants and new pMDIs
The process of transition from new to old
Issues for the next 3–5 years
What may happen to propellants and pMDIs over the next 5–20 years

II. The Background

Existing pMDIs contain chlorofluorocarbon (CFCs) propellants. These are a class of organic chemicals containing chlorine, fluorine, and carbon. The main

CFCs are CFC-11, CFC-12, CFC-113, CFC-114, and CFC-115. CFCs were originally developed in the 1930s and, while originally used as refrigerants, they have been used for a variety of purposes over the last 30 years. Uses have included air conditioning systems, as cleaning solvents, in foam blowing in the manufacture of insulation materials, and as propellants in aerosol sprays containing everything from deodorant to insect killers, furniture polish to pMDIs. The structure of the CFCs used in the production of pMDIs and as propellants in pMDIs is shown in Fig. 1 and compared with the main replacement propellant HFC 134a.

In June 1974, in an important paper published in *Nature,* Molina and Rowland raised the possibility that CFCs could lead to depletion of the ozone layer (1). They pointed out the increasing use of these chemicals—and that although they are inert at ground level, they have such long natural lives that they eventually migrate to the stratosphere where, over time, the sun initiates the process of their decompensation. CFC 11, for example, has a lifetime of 65 years; CFC 12, 120 years; and CFC 114, a lifetime of 200 years.

CFCs are released into the atmosphere when aerosol sprays are activated, when there are leaks from air conditioning systems in cars or buildings, and when refrigerators are broken up. These CFCs pass through the lower atmosphere unchanged; but in the stratosphere, around 25 km above the earth's surface, the effect of pronounced solar radiation breaks them up to release reactive chlorine fragments (Cl and ClO). Molina and Rowland suggested that these fragments could then initiate an extensive catalytic chain reaction leading to the net destruction of O_3 and O in the stratosphere:

$$Cl + O_3 \rightarrow ClO + O_2$$

$$ClO + O \rightarrow Cl + O_2$$

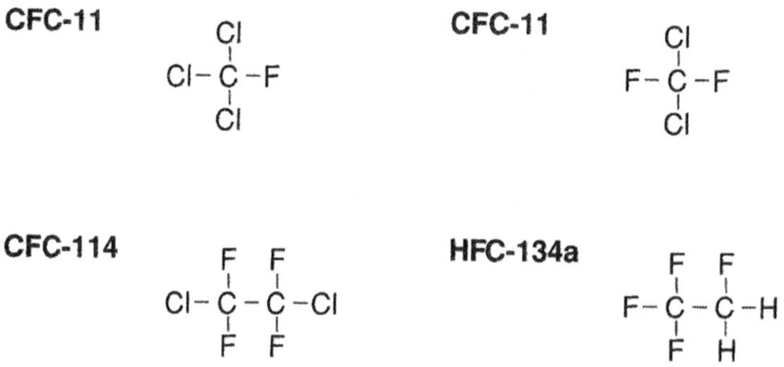

CFC-11

```
    Cl
    |
Cl- C -F
    |
    Cl
```

CFC-11

```
   Cl
   |
F- C -F
   |
   Cl
```

CFC-114

```
    F   F
    |   |
Cl- C - C -Cl
    |   |
    F   F
```

HFC-134a

```
   F   F
   |   |
F- C - C -H
   |   |
   F   H
```

Figure 1 The chemical structure of commonly used propellants.

It was initially felt that the threat, while real, would be small; but in 1985 the British Antarctic Survey scientists reported thinning of the ozone layer over the Antarctic (2). Subsequent surveys, satellite studies, and aeroplane sampling studies have confirmed the accuracy of the predictions of Molina and Rowland, suggesting a faster onset of likely problems than had been originally realized (Fig. 2, see color plate).

Reduction in thickness of the ozone layer permits increased levels of damaging ultraviolet B radiation to reach the earth's surface. The potential medical consequences of this are shown in Table 1 and have been comprehensively reviewed elsewhere (3–5).

III. Government Response

Studies performed after Molina and Rowland's original hypothesis suggested that their predictions were likely to come true; but even before 1985, when the British Antarctic Survey scientists were able to demonstrate an accelerated decline in the ozone layer, multinational government action was initiated to address the problem. In 1981, the United Nations Environment Programme (UNEP) began negotiations to develop protection of the ozone layer from damage caused by CFCs, halons, and other ozone-damaging substances. Their actions resulted in the Vienna Convention for the Protection of the Ozone layer in March 1985. This initial international government action was concerned with data collection, exchange of information, and monitoring; as a result of these processes the Montreal Protocol was signed by 24 nations in September 1987. (By 1994 a total of 128 nations covering 100% of the world's production of ozone-damaging substances and up to 96% of global consumption had signed the protocol.) The original Montreal Protocol limited production of each CFC as shown in Table 2. However, it was soon clear that the potential rate of damage to the ozone layer was such that these rates of reduction in CFC production were going to be too low. In June 1990, governments meeting in London accelerated the targets for reducing CFC production and ratified a total phase-out by the year 2000—the London Agreement (Table 3). Scientific study even then showed that the unexpected accelerated decline in the ozone layer would mean that such action would

Table 1 Possible Effects of Enhanced Levels of UVB Radiation

Increase the prevalence of nonmelanoma skin cancers
Increase the incidence of other keratoses, skin aging and sunburn
Possibly affect the incidence of melanomas
Damage the eye (corneal photokeratitis, cataracts, pterygium, retinal damage)
Suppress the immune system
Affect plant life and the food cycle

Table 2 Modifications to the Montreal Protocol

The original Montreal Protocol signed in September 1987 came into force on January 1, 1989. The production limits for CFCs, relative to 1986 levels, were:	
Action 1	Production levels frozen at 1986 levels by 1989
Action 2	Production levels to be reduced by 10% by July 1, 1993
Action 3	Production levels to be reduced by a further 30% by July 1, 1998

not reverse the damage for decades; the Copenhagen amendment to the protocol was therefore ratified in 1992 (Table 3). That this was necessary was shown by the fact that ozone thinning over Antarctica continued to get worse. Measurements made in 1992 to 1993 were the most severe on record (6). The necessity for this action is underlined by the long latent period between reduction in production and regeneration of the zone layer (Fig. 3).

As a result of the Montreal Protocol, almost imperceptibly, aerosol deodorants, furniture polishes, and hair sprays were reformulated with alternative, often inflammable propellants, and CFCs were phased out as refrigerants. Such replacement propellants were not suitable for use in pMDIs for reasons of flammability and toxicity, and the Montreal Protocol recognized that some temporary exemption from the protocol may be necessary to allow identification of alternative propellants. It provided for this eventuality by means of an "essential-use exemption" clause. "Essentiality" exists when:

1. There are no technically feasible alternatives to the use of a CFC in the product.
2. The product provides a substantial health environmental or other public benefit that would not be obtainable without the use of the CFC.
3. The use does not involve a significant release of CFCs into the atmosphere or, if it does, the release is warranted by the consequences if the use were not permitted.

Table 3 Amendments to the Montreal Protocol

Amendments to the Montreal Protocol accelerated the production phase out of CFCs 11, 12, 13, 114, and 115. Figures shown represent reduction compared to the 1986 production levels.

	London Amendment, 1990	Copenhagen Amendment, 1992
Action 1	Reduce by 50% by 1995	Reduce by 75% by 1994
Action 2	Reduce by 85% by 1997	Total phase out by 1996
Action 3	Total phase out by 2000	

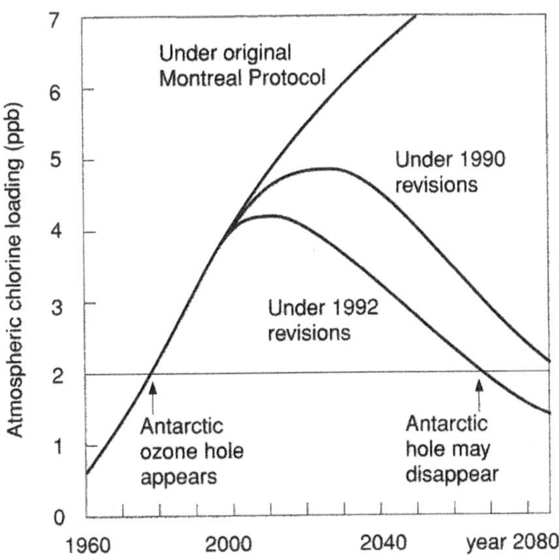

Figure 3 The World Meteorological Organization have shown graphically how action now only leads to satisfactory regeneration of the ozone layer years later because of the longevity of CFCs in the stratosphere.

Essentiality is reexamined on an annual basis and the signatories to the Montreal Protocol are advised by a preparatory meeting of a body known as the Open Ended Working Group (OEWG). The OEWG is advised by three advisory panels, one of which is the Technical and Economic Assessment Panel (TEAP), which coordinates the work of seven Technical Options Committees (TOCs), one of which looks specifically and in depth at aerosol use. This TOC contains a mixture of technical experts, manufacturers, environmentalists, and clinicians who do not make policy but make assessments, identify alternatives, highlights their advantages and disadvantages, answer queries and make recommendations to the TEAP. With regard to classification of pMDIs as an essential use, the TOC recognized a number of points before making a recommendation. The most obvious was that pMDIs represent the bulk of the respiratory therapy worldwide, accounting for three-quarters of all inhaled therapy (dry-powder devices accounted for most of the rest). The TOC recognized that theoretically there were some currently available alternatives to pMDIs, such as:

1. Dry-powder inhalers (single-or multidose)
2. Nebulizers
3. Orally administered drugs (tablets, liquids, syrups)
4. Injectable drugs

Alternatives in the future might also include:

1. pMDIs with new propellants
2. New nebulizers (either handheld and mechanical or electric)
3. New forms of dry-powder inhalers
4. New (more effective) tablet therapies
5. New modalities of treatment

Recognizing the fact that pMDIs were the most widely used form of inhaled therapy and available in all markets for all types of inhaled respiratory medicine, it was felt that their use did justify an essential use exemption from the Montreal Protocol. Dry-powder devices were recognized as an alternative for many, but they were not available in all countries for all medicines and were not always suitable for the young and those with low inspiratory flow rates; also, they may not be suitable in certain humid climates. In some markets their extra cost would also deprive many of necessary treatment.

Designation of the pMDI as an essential use of CFCs did not cover its use for all medications. The commonly used treatments for asthma and COPD, delivered via the pMDI, were classified as essential. pMDIs used to deliver intranasal steroids were not defined as essential (because mechanical propulsion of solutions was equally effective), nor was the use of a pMDI to deliver epinephrine to the upper airways in cases of laryngeal edema and anaphylaxis (alternative methods of administration of the drug were regarded as acceptable).

IV. New Propellants for pMDIs

In response to the Montreal Protocol, pharmaceutical users of CFCs had to look for alternative propellants or alternative methods of delivering medicine to the 600 million people worldwide with airway diseases. While new modalities of treatment and new forms of inhaler devices were possible for the more distant future, initial solutions were to lie with the substitution of non-CFC for CFC propellants. Designation of CFC use as essential gave some breathing space, but it was clear that with pMDIs being the only remaining user of CFCs, their production was likely to become unattractive both financially and environmentally, and they may no longer be available long term irrespective of the Montreal Protocol. Stockpiling of large quantities of CFCs was considered but felt to be inappropriate because accidental loss could suddenly jeopardize pMDI users and lead to an environmental catastrophe. Recycling of CFCs previously used as refrigerants was not an option because the CFCs were not of pharmaceutical quality. The search for new propellants therefore began, and the length of the process likely to be involved was predicted as being up to 10 years even at the outset (Fig. 4).

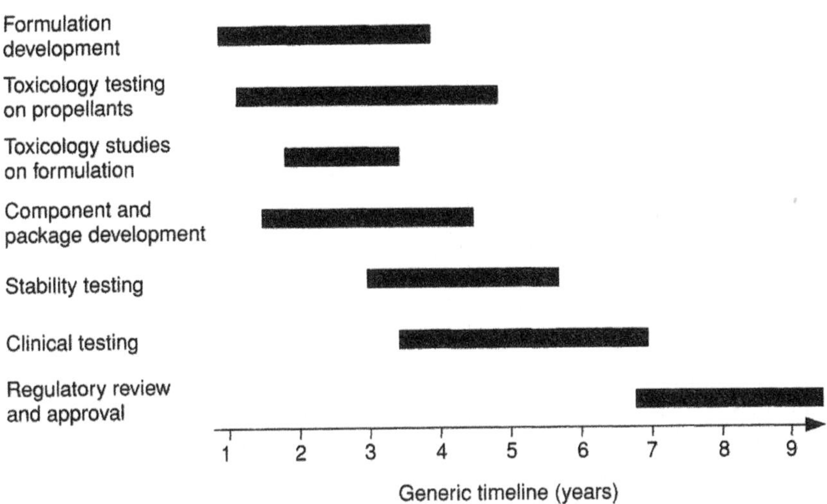

Figure 4 Replacement of CFC propellants with non-CFC propellants within an MDI is far from a simple matter of direct substitution. For use in humans, toxicity testing is clearly essential, and use of new propellants necessitates redesign of aerosols to accommodate the propellants' differing physicochemical characteristics, followed by extensive testing when reformulation with each of the medicines involved has been done. The time scale of this process is shown here. (Redrawn from material originally supplied by the International Pharmaceutical Aerosols Consortium.)

The criteria for a propellant for possible use in a pMDI is shown in Table 4. Possible alternatives theoretically included:

Compressed gases
Hydrocarbons
Hydrochlorofluororocarbons (HCFCs)
Hydrodrofluorocarbons (HFCs)

Nonliquefied compressed gases are of no use for pMDIs because "liquid" is needed for suspension of the drug and the addition of water makes propulsion of the aerosol in an appropriate manner technically impossible. Hydrocarbons in general have the wrong density for use as propellants in pMDIs. While suitable as propellants for some nonmedicinal household purposes, they are difficult to use in a situation where dose reproducibility is essential, and most are of course flammable and thus inappropriate for inhalation. The HCFCs are ozone-damaging and additionally have adverse toxicological effects on the heart and some biochemical hepatic functions.

Table 4 Criteria for an MDI propellant

An MDI propellant must:
Be nonflammable
Have negligible toxicity
Be a liquefied gas
Be stable chemically
Have appropriate solvency characteristics
Be acceptable to patients (i.e., smell, taste)
Be of appropriate density

Most attention for alternative propellants therefore focused upon new hydrofluorocarbons. Working in a collaborative way to save time, consortia of pharmaceutical companies combined efforts in the identification of propellants, toxicology testing, and physicochemical evaluation and identified HFC 134a as being likely to be very suitable for their use in pMDIs. (Groups of chemical manufacturers had also identified this product as being a suitable replacement for CFC 12 for refrigeration purposes.) Subsequently HFC 227 was also identified as being safe when inhaled, and subsequent development has therefore concentrated on these two chemicals.

A summary of the differing environmental effects of the old and new propellants is shown in Table 5.

Reformulation of existing medicines with the new propellants was soon realized to involve far more than simply a matter of direct substitution for CFCs. Existing inhalers contain medicine, propellant, and surfactant—the latter being necessary to suspend the drug and lubricate the valve. Conventional surfactants such as oleic acid, sorbitan trioleate, and lecithin were found to be insoluble in

Table 5 Environmental Effects of New and Old pMDI Propellants, CFCs, and HFCs

Propellant	ODP[a]	Duration	GWP[b]
CFC 11	1	60 years	3800
CFC 12	1	125 years	8100
CFC 114	0.7	200 years	9300
HFC 134a	0	16 years	1300
HFC 227	0	33 years	2900

[a]ODP = ozone-damaging potential.
[b]GWP = global warming potential.
Source: Data from the U.N.E.P Aerosol Technical Options Committee report, 1994.

HFC 134a. Use of HFC 134a also necessitated change of the rubber component of the valve. When all these new components were combined, it was discovered that in some cases the aerosol spray had quite different characteristics from its predecessor, necessitating change in the actuator to produce a spray with the desired particle size (and subsequent respirable mass).

Clinical and regulatory authorities then required adequate clinical studies for the replacement products, such as

- Initial safety, efficacy, and dose-ranging studies
- Acute dosing studies to determine the efficacy of short-acting drugs such as bronchodilators
- Chronic dosing studies and/or bronchial challenge studies for anti-inflammatory medicines
- Safety data—both short-term (acute toxicity) and long-term clinical experience (and postmarketing surveillance)
- Separate studies for adults and children

These studies clearly have to be of sufficient size to avoid type II (statistical) errors and confirm that the two products are truly clinically equivalent.

Clearly the solutions to some of the reformulation problems have varied from product to product and between manufacturers; some problems have been solved, with the new product already in the marketplace, while other medicines may be some years off reformulation if indeed reformulation proves possible. Not all of the process, however, has been one of redevelopment merely to "stand still" with an identical product. The reformulation process has in many ways provided us with more information about our inhaled medication than was previously known. The process has led to improvements in inhaler design such that there is greater consistency of dosing from first dose to last with the new inhaler and fewer problems related to whether the inhaler is stored on its side or upside down as compared with the older inhalers. For most of the newly reformulated products, it will now also be more obvious to users when the pMDI is empty.

A. Clinical Trials Using Non-CFC-Propellant pMDIs

Studies on bronchodilators include single-dose and 3-month efficacy and safety studies. There are satisfactory data on equivalence for two HFC MDIs for salbutamol, and both are launched in much of Europe. In addition more than 2 million patient-years of experience has now been accumulated with Airomir (3M), and no unpredicted adverse events have occurred in postmarketing surveillance.

Studies on inhaled steroids are more difficult to design and carry out because of the insensitivity of markers of efficacy and the difficulty in interpreting data on systemic effects. In particular there is a flat dose-response curve for any effects on lung function, which means that studies must be large to be of adequate power. Generally, studies must be carried out in patients who are capable of responding to inhaled steroids (nonresponders are likely to show equivalence), with a minimum of 100 patients per group. Inadequate statistical power has been a historical problem in comparative studies of inhaled steroids and is a common cause of misinterpretation of clinical equivalence by both authors and pharmaceutical companies. For example, this is true for almost all trials investigating inhaled steroids in Rotahaler and Turbuhaler devices. More recently introduced DPIs—e.g., the Diskhaler—generally have adequate studies to show clinical equivalence to MDIs as part of the regulatory application. These studies show equivalence for fluticasone (7) at the same dose and for beclomethasone (8) at twice the dose from a Diskhaler compared to a CFC MDI.

Differences in the formulation for HFC MDIs can lead to differences in the amount of drug deposited in the lung and also where it is deposited. Pharmaceutical data may not predict with precision the relative potency or the therapeutic ratio in patients. For example, Qvar (3M), the only formulated HFC beclomethasone with published information, has a smaller particle size, and radiolabeling data show that up to eight times the dose is delivered to the lungs, while three times less is delivered to the oropharynx (9). Clinical studies have shown that Qvar is equivalent to twice the dose of CFC beclomethasone (10,11)—i.e., the dose will need to be halved when transition occurs. In contrast, HFC fluticasone (Glaxo Wellcome) more closely resembles the CFC version, and studies have shown clinical equivalence at the same dose (12,13).

The size of the problem of reformulation of medicines contained within pMDIs with new propellants should not be underestimated and is summarized in Table 6. Over 10 pharmaceutical companies have been involved, with work being done in 22 laboratories involving an estimated 1400 scientists, and nearly £1 billion have been invested in research and development of the new inhalers and their production.

From the patients' point of view, the whole process has been designed to ensure continuous availability of trusted and effective medication. Nevertheless, changes in aerosol design necessitated by reformulation with new propellants have led to some discernible changes in some of the end products. For those prod-

Table 6 What Has Been Involved in Replacing CFCs in pMDIs?[a]

Identification of alternative propellants likely to be free of ozone-damaging potential and global warming effects
Extensive toxicological testing of the new propellants
Redesign of the MDIs to cope with the new propellants
Testing the safety and interaction of the drug/propellant mixture
Clinical trials of efficacy and equivalence

[a]Many drugs, many manufacturers, many countries!

ucts about which information is currently available, it is clear that reformulation can result in change to the shape and feel of the inhaler, change in oropharyngeal deposition of aerosol, changes in taste, and—in some circumstances—changes in pulmonary deposition of the aerosolized drug, which may necessitate dose changes (14).

V. Implementing the Montreal Protocol

A. A Transition to New Non-CFC pMDIs

With the process of transition to new propellants now well under way, all involved wish it to be completed as speedily and safely as possible. However the rate of transition depends on the rate of reformulation of the products, the overcoming of technical problems, clinical testing, and regulatory approval. Marketing of the new products is then necessary, and health professionals must be informed of the need to change prescriptions; in turn, users of the products must be prepared for the change.

Driving the whole process as the environmental controller is the Montreal Protocol. Ultimately, complete transition to new inhalers will take place only when the final essential use exemption is withdrawn. At present, each signatory government to the protocol that manufactures CFC-containing pMDIs makes an application, usually 2 years ahead, for a certain tonnage of CFCs, which they anticipate they will require. This application must include information about planned usage in the year for which application is made compared to historical usage, justification for essential use, and information about the proportion of pMDIs for use within that country and the amount going for export. Some stockpiling of CFCs to allow for transportation difficulties or other impediments to manufacture is allowed, but the size of stockpiles is carefully monitored. Each year applications for future uses of CFCs are carefully scrutinised by the TOC, which gives advice to the TEAP which makes recommendations to the OEWG. This process of implementation of the Montreal Protocol is clearly the ultimate control process overseeing phase-out, with the mechanism by which this happens being the withdrawal of essential use exemptions and thus the withdrawal of CFCs. It is an ultimate guillotine rather than a finely tuned process, and the signatories to the Montreal Protocol, in conjunction with the United Nations Environmental Programme, have recommended that each country should develop a national strategy for the smooth and planned changeover from CFC to non-CFC propellant pMDIs.

B. Transition Strategies

Most countries, in preparing transition strategies, have recognized that many different drugs are involved (see Table 7) and that more than one phase-out strategy can operate in parallel. "Brand-by-brand" transition is without the Montreal Pro-

Table 7 The Categories of Drugs Involved in pMDI Transition

A. Short-acting beta-agonist bronchodilators—e.g., salbutamol (albuterol in the United States), terbutaline, fenoterol
B. Inhaled steroids—e.g., beclomethasone, budesonide, flunisolide, fluticasone, triamcinolone
C. Nonsteroidal anti-inflammatory agents—e.g., cromoglycate, nedocromil
D. Anticholinergic bronchodilators—e.g., ipratropium
E. Long-acting beta-agonist bronchodilators—e.g., salmeterol, formoterol
F. Combinations of the above—e.g., ipratropium and fenoterol, salmeterol and fluticasone

tocol, and the term merely describes a situation whereby as a particular pharmaceutical company reformulates a branded product with non-CFC propellants, they withdraw the older CFC-containing product over a period consistent with constraints of production, supply, and postmarketing surveillance.

The other two modalities of transition are under the control of the Montreal Protocol, involving individual producer countries not applying for essential use exemption for CFCs in pMDIs once sufficient alternative products are available. Category-by-category transition considers each of the categories listed in Table 7 in turn. Thus, in considering steroid inhalers, for example, one nation's transition strategy might decree that once two beclomethasone pMDIs and one budesonide and one fluticasone pMDI (for example) were reformulated with non-CFC propellants, that country would no longer regard CFCs as essential. They would no longer apply for any of those propellants for use with inhaled steroids, the effect being that those manufacturers who had not reformulated their products would be "starved" of supplies. In drug-by-drug transition, it could be deemed that once a certain drug is available in a reformulated form and has undergone a reasonable period of postmarketing surveillance, then, irrespective of manufacturer, all other CFC-containing versions of that drug would be withdrawn by removing their source of CFCs. This type of transition could be varied to permit more than one (two or three) companies to reformulate before phase-out, and the period of phase-out could also vary.

National strategies will have to vary between countries to reflect national interests and preferences for different medications and to accommodate differing regulatory processes. In some countries, licenses to manufacture a particular medicine can be withdrawn by government order, which could then expedite transition. In other countries there is no legal mechanism to withdraw a production license for a product that is medically safe; therefore withdrawal can only occur by cutting CFC supply. Whatever the form of a national strategy in any country, the paramount consideration will be that of patient safety.

C. Special Issues for Developing Countries

Developing countries and countries with economies in transition have a 10-year grace period before they are required to cease use of CFCs in pMDIs. Some of these countries currently import finished products from multinational companies based elsewhere; others have production facilities belonging to multinational firms based within their countries, while yet others have their own national industry which, in some countries, involves quite small firms manufacturing CFC-containing medical aerosol products for local use. As with all environmental change, the financial burden of transition in these countries may be considerable; unless effectively undertaken, it will lead to unnecessary suffering where essential medicines are available to a smaller proportion of those who need them than had been the case previously. Resolution of these inequities will involve either medicines being sold more cheaply in those countries, establishment of local factories by multinational companies, joint ventures, technology transfer, and/or international World Bank–type subsidy of local manufacturers with subsidy for reestablishment of production lines for non-CFC-containing pMDIs. How this problem will be solved is still not clear, and the 10-year grace period may well be unrealistic if CFCs become unavailable before that time. WHO backed World Asthma Day in May 2000 focused in a major way on effective medicines being available for all.

D. Implementation of National Transition Strategies: The National-to-District Step

Different countries have implemented their national strategies in different manners and within different time frames; some of their experiences will be of interest to those in Article 5 countries who are yet to change. While brand by brand transition is largely within the control of the individual pharmaceutical companies, some form of coordinated transition planning group has been recommended to oversee the rest of the national-to-district process (15). An appropriate cascade of information and advice involves guidance being made available by governments and health departments and the use of journals and symposia to inform health professionals of the reasons behind the changeover and the logistics to be addressed.

In some countries this process began with priming editorials in journals as much as 6 years before transition really began (16,17), and stakeholders such as government departments and organizations representing pharmacists, doctors, nurses, and patients as well as the pharmaceutical industry met in a collaborative way to identify potential problems and aid in the dissemination of information. At local levels, some countries have then found it helpful to have district planning teams to oversee and advise on transition, with these involving primary and secondary care physicians, nurses, allergists, pediatricians, community pharmacists, and local health managers. The advantages of planning transition at a district level are shown in Table 8.

E. What Does Transition Mean for Patients and Health Professionals?

The changeover from CFC-containing pMDIs to CFC-free pMDIs has involved more patients than any other changeover of medicines throughout history. Health professionals have needed to understand the reasons behind the change and what the change involves; because of the numbers involved, the changeover has necessitated a teamwork approach, for extra doctor/patient consultations with all users of pMDIs is logistically difficult. The actual changeover at a practice/local level has involved all or some of the processes shown in Table 9. Whichever method is used, it is important to remember that 50% of all that is said during a consultation will be forgotten within 5 min. The spoken word therefore needs to be reinforced with the written word. In the U.K., the National Asthma Campaign produced fact sheets on transition and the government's Department of Health,

Table 8 Advantages of District Transition Policies

Coordinated district, hospital, or clinic switch strategies have the advantage of:
Coordination of common messages between community pharmacists, doctors, and nurses
Reducing primary and secondary care interface problems
Utilizing local media to inform patients of transition
Reduction in problems associated with dual availability (unused stock, shortage of new products, mistakes, inadvertent switching back, shelf-space problems, etc.)

Table 9 Methods Used to Aid in the Transition of Patients from Use of CFC pMDIs to non-CFC pMDIs at a Practice/Clinic/Local Level

Informing patients of imminent transition by means of local newspaper articles, posters in clinics and pharmacies, letters given at time of previous prescription
Use of diagnostic registers to identify patients needing a letter to inform them of transition, and then planned changeover
Opportunist transition during routine review in asthma clinics or during routine doctor/nurse consultations
Automatic substitution of old inhaler by a choice of new on computerized prescribing systems
Brand-by-brand substitution at a community pharmacy level where transition involves transition to an "identical" product
Reinforcement of spoken messages with written materials, leaflets, use of videotapes, etc.

in conjunction with the National Asthma Campaign and British Lung Foundation, produced a leaflet available free for distribution in primary and secondary care and in community pharmacies.

The key points that need emphasizing to patients are that:

The process affects only pMDIs (not dry-powder devices).

The new inhalers contain exactly the same medicines as previously and have been fully tested and shown to be as safe and effective as their predecessors. However, a dose change may be necessary with some products.

The previous inhalers were environmentally damaging but in no way damaging to the individual.

The new inhalers may look, feel, and taste different.

F. How Is the Transition Going So Far?

The rate of changeover to new pMDIs has varied from country to country as a result of different timings for launch of new products, waits for regulatory approval, health professional practice, and differences within national strategies. In some countries previous use of dry-powder inhalers (DPIs) represented 60–80% of inhaler usage, and the proportion of inhaler users needing to undergo transition was clearly less. In other countries, dry-powder inhaler usage represents 20% or less, and transition in those countries will involve change from CFC-containing pMDIs to either CFC free pMDIs or dry-powder devices. In some countries few dry-powder devices have historically been available. In others, where they are available, the cost of dry-powder inhalers has been higher than that of MDIs, and where that has been the case, it may have acted as a barrier to change from CFC pMDIs to DPIs. Health professionals therefore must be made aware of all of the alternatives to CFC pMDIs, so that the best choice may be made for the individual patient. Even when new CFC-free pMDIs reach the marketplace their use may initially be low. Early experience suggests that voluntary changeover occurs most readily with brand-by-brand substitution driven by individual pharmaceutical companies, and this happens to the greater degree when the companies impose a voluntary withdrawal of the CFC-containing product after a certain time interval. Mere launch of a new reformulated product will not necessarily be followed by use; for example, in one country it is estimated that many months after launch of a CFC-free inhaled steroid, less than 10,000 of 1,150,000 current users had been changed to the new formulation. Such slow transition may reflect lack of marketing pressure, reluctance of health professionals to change, lack of clear government or health department advice, or fear of incurring extra costs. This last is often not, in fact, a genuine concern, with new products often being introduced at the same price as the old. Where sizable numbers have changed over to the new inhalers, experience shows that this has been far less problematic than many had anticipated. In the U.K., a National Telephone Helpline run by the National Asthma Campaign was extended to cope with an anticipated increase in callers concerned by the CFC transition issue, but in the event calls regarding this issue represented less than 2% of the total.

VI. The Kyoto and the Montreal Protocol

The next major environmental challenge will be that of global warming. At the third conference of parties to the Framework Convention of Climate Change, the Kyoto Protocol, which was concluded in 1997, controlled a basket of greenhouse gases including carbon dioxide, methane, nitrous oxide, HFCs, PFCs, and sulfur hexafluoride. HFC use has increased rapidly since 1990, when they were introduced widely as substitutes for ozone-damaging substances (ODS). Although they have about one-sixth of the global warming potential of CFCs [and zero ozone-damaging potential (ODP)] it is, nevertheless estimated that they will constitute approximately 5% of European Union (EU) greenhouse gas emissions by the year 2005. This must be taken in the context of global emissions for all greenhouse gases in 2005 (approximately 52.5 billion tons of CO_2 equivalent), of which HFCs in MDIs constitute about 0.07%.

Under the Kyoto protocol, there has been an overall agreement to reduce greenhouse gases by 5.2% below 1990 levels between 2008 and 2012, although some parties have agreed to go further than this (e.g., European Union, 8% reduction; United States, 7% reduction). Initially this will be achieved mainly by attempting to reduce energy demand via energy taxes and reducing car emissions (even in the face of increasing numbers of motor vehicles). However, since HFCs have a relatively high global warming potential (GWP) compared to CO_2, they are likely to be an early target for control. They are likely to be replaced in nonmedical aerosols by hydrocarbons. HFC self-chilling cans are now banned in the United States and their inventor has agreed to discourage their use. There are alternatives in some areas, but they are less than satisfactory (e.g., portable compressed-gas dusters, used in using compressed-air computer cleaners, have fewer blasts per can. Signaling horns on boats could use hydrocarbons, but these may be hazardous in case of fire).

It is therefore likely that, over the next 10 to 20 years, the use of HFCs as MDI propellants is likely to come under environmental pressure; as a consequence, a search for new alternatives will continue. Experience shows that it will have taken almost two decades to phase CFCs from MDIs by the time transition is completed, and it is likely to be another 20 years before HFCs are entirely phased out from MDIs. Even the alternatives of aqueous sprays and DPIs are not environmentally neutral, since their manufacture requires energy. At the present time, we can speculate that HFCs for MDIs could receive some sort of temporary exemption/protection under the Kyoto Protocol, just as CFC MDIs were deemed essential for patient health and received temporary exemption under the Montreal Protocol.

VII. MDI Propellants: Where Will We Be in 2015?

The last few years of the old millennium and the first of the new have seen environmentalists, governments, the pharmaceutical industry, health professionals, and patients involved in the major exercise of changeover from CFC-containing to non-CFC pMDIs. The cost of this exercise to all concerned has been phenomenal. As a result of the transition, ozone-damaging substances have been largely eliminated. The new propellants do have some global warming effect, but at a practical level it can be argued that the effect resulting from use of HFAs in pMDIs is likely to be very small. No one can anticipate that the industry and others would wish to now embark on another major transition to non-global-warming propellants, even if they could be identified. However, we need to recognize that the effect of environmental action on these substances is going to be an ongoing pressure to reduce their use. As a result, scientific and industrial energy is more likely to be channeled into new methods of delivering aerosolized medications to the airways than into a search for new chemical propellants. These new methods are likely to involve newer handheld mechanical or electrical nebulizers and increasing moves toward use of breath-actuated devices and dry-powder devices. As a result, pMDI usage is likely to decline significantly over the next decade or so, but we need to monitor this situation to ensure that it in no way disadvantages those in developing countries. In parallel with a change in method of delivering medicines to the lung may come a decline in the prevalence of the airway disorders they are used to treat. After a period of rapidly increased suffering due to asthma, there now comes the possibility that we will shortly be able to offer advice and interventions that may reduce the likelihood that those with an inherited tendency will develop the condition. If this were to be paralleled by firm international government action to control the problem of tobacco use (perhaps a Montreal Protocol on the phase-out of tobaco substances), then the number of people suffering from smoking-induced airway diseases worldwide may also decline, and with it the need for inhaled therapy.

> We must ensure that today's patients with asthma and chronic obstructive pulmonary disease are comfortable with their new inhalers, and that the world is a safer place for their grandchildren (17).

References

1. Molina MJ, Rowland FS. Stratospheric sink for chlorofluoromethanes: chlorine atom—catalysed destruction of ozone. Nature 1974; 249:810–814.

2. Farman JC, Gardiner BG, Shanklin JD. Large losses of total ozone in Antarctica reveal seasonal C10x/Nox/C interaction. Nature 1985; 315:207–210.
3. Lloyd SA. Stratospheric ozone depletion Lancet 1993; 342:1156–1158.
4. Jeevan A, Kripke ML. Ozone depletion and the immune system. Lancet 1993; 342:1159–1160.
5. Young AR. The biological effects of ozone depletion. Br J Clin Pract (Suppl) 1997; 89:10–15.
6. World Meteorological Organisation. Scientific assessment of ozone depletion: 1994. World Meteorological Organisation Global Ozone Research and Monitoring Project Report 37. Geneva: WMO, 1995.
7. Lundbeck B, Dahl R, De Jonghe M, Ilyldebrandt N, Valta R, Payne SL. A comparison of fluticasone propionate when delivered by either the metered dose inhaler or the Diskhaler in the treatment of mild-to-moderate asthma. Eur J Respir 1994; 5:11–19.
8. Drepaul BA, Paylor D, Qualtrough JE, Perry IJ, Reeve FBA, Charlton SC. Becotide or Becodisks? A controlled trial in general practice. Clin Trials J 1989; 26:335–344.
9. Leach CI. Improved delivery of inhaled steroids to the large and small airways. Respir Med 1998; 92(suppl A):3–8.
10. Cohen RM. Assessment of switching patients taking CFC-BDP to Qvar at approximately half the dose. Am J Respir Crit Care Med 1998; 157:A405.
11. Busse W, Colice G, Donnell D, Hannon S. A dose response comparison of HFA BDP and CFC BDP based on FEV1 and FEF 25–75%. Am J Respir Crit Care Med 1998; 157:A405.
12. Perruchoud AP, Jones AL. A 12-month multi-national study comparing the efficacy and safety of fluticasone propionate propelled by CFCs 11 and 12 or an alternative propellant GR 106642X in adults. Am J Respir Crit Care Med 1996; 153:A338.
13. Ayres J, Millar A, Williams E. A 12 week multicentre study comparing the efficacy and tolerability of fluticasone propionate "mg daily propelled by CFCs 11 and 12 or an alternative propellant, GR 106642X in adults with severe asthma. Eur Respir J 1995; 8:157s.
14. Thompson PJ, Davies RJ, Young WF, Grossman AB, Donnell D. Safety of hydrofluoroalkane-134a beclomethasone dipropionate extra fine aerosol. Respir Med (1998); 92(suppl A):33–39.
15. Partridge MR. Managing the change issues for healthcare professionals, physicians and patients. Eur Respir Rev 1997; 41:40–41.
16. Partridge MR. Metered dose inhalers and CFCs; what respiratory physicians need to know. Respir Med 1994; 88:645–647.
17. Partridge M, Woodcock A. Metered dose inhalers free of chlorofluorocarbons. Br Med J 1995; 310:684–685.

12

Spacer Devices

HANS BISGAARD and JACOB ANHØJ

Copenhagen University Hospital
Rigshospitalet
Copenhagen, Denmark

JOHANNES H. WILDHABER

University Children's Hospital
Zurich, Switzerland

I. Introduction

The aerosol cloud from a pressurized metered dose inhaler (pMDI) leaves the canister at a very high speed after actuation. As a result, coordination of actuation and inhalation can be very difficult, resulting in a high aerosol deposition in the oropharynx and variation in the lung dose. Spacers and holding chambers have been developed in an attempt to overcome this problem. In principle, spacers are extensions of the pMDI canister, allowing deceleration and maturation of aerosol, while holding chambers are valved spacers allowing breathing from a standing cloud of aerosol. In clinical practice, the term *spacer* is used to denote either of such inhalation aids, and this term is used in the present review.

Franklin (1958) developed a spacer to aid delivery of hydrocortisone to the lungs via pMDI. He used a 14-in. plastic tube, noting that approximately 50% of the steroid delivered was deposited on the wall of the tube, and that "the use of the plastic tube unquestionably decreased the dose of steroid administered, but had the desirable effect of increasing the proportion entering the airway as compared with that retained in the mouth" (1).

Two decades later, various designs—including large-volume spacers, small-volume spacers, and tube-extensions—had been developed for general clinical use (2–4), and the spacer concept was subsequently extended to young children and infants (5–7). The clinical effects of bronchodilators (ipratropium bromide, salbutamol) (6–11), and inhaled steroids (8) delivered by pMDI and spacer for young children were documented.

The requirements for optimal drug delivery from spacers are most critical in young children with irregular and shallow breathing; although similar principles apply to all patients, this difficult group makes the greatest demands on a spacer. The recent interest in spacers for this group of patients has led to increased understanding of the technical requirements for a spacer. Therefore, this chapter discusses critical aspects of spacer construction in general and with an emphasis on young children.

II. The Objectives of a Spacer Device

The primary objective of a spacer is to minimize the need for coordination between actuation of the pMDI and inhalation. In addition, the spacer should ensure that the aerosol particles trail the inspiratory flow of the patient, reduce the proportion of the dose contained in large particles, and increase the proportion contained in small particles (12). The need for coordination between actuation and inhalation is reduced by presenting the aerosol to the patient as a standing cloud of particles, which decreases oropharyngeal deposition. Oropharyngeal deposition with the actuator alone ranges from 30 to 70%, compared with 5–10% with spacer devices (13,14).

The aerosol cloud should be available over a prolonged period to minimize still further the need for coordination between actuation and inhalation. This is particularly important in young children with poor compliance, and shallow and irregular breathing patterns (Fig. 1). If inspiratory flow and tidal volume are low, several breaths may be required to obtain the whole volume of aerosol retained in the spacer. These factors may also be important in older children and adults with faulty coordination between inhalation and actuation, in whom emptying of a large volume spacer may be delayed.

When a drug is inhaled from a spacer, the aerosol particles will trail the inspiratory flow of the patient. This improves drug targeting to the lungs compared with an aerosol with an inherent flow, such as that generated by a nebulizer or pMDI alone, where the flow of aerosol may be misdirected and hence depositing on the skin or in the oropharynx.

Large particles tend to deposit in the upper airways and, depending on the drug, this may add to the risk of both local side effects and systemic absorption. Fine particles add to the desired clinical effect and, by increasing the ratio between fine and large particles, the therapeutic index of the treatment is improved

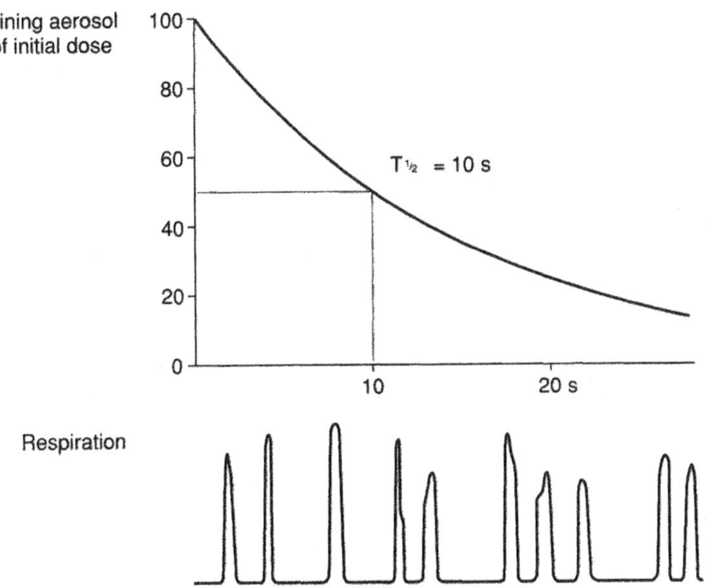

Figure 1 The effect of aerosol fallout on dose delivery. The irregular breathing pattern in a 2-year-old child is compared with the exponential passive fallout of aerosol to illustrate the importance of a stable aerosol for optimal drug delivery to young children.

and the cost decreased (15). Obviously such improved therapeutic index and cost of treatment assumes that the clinician takes advantage of the improved drug delivery and reduces the prescribed dose.

The spacer improves the particle profile by two mechanisms. First, the spacer acts as a settling bag, allowing large particles to impact or sediment. Second, the micronized drug particles from a pMDI are wet particles enveloped in propellant, which evaporates within the spacer and thus reduces the particle size; only a minor proportion of the propellant flashes immediately into vapor as the propellants leave the pMDI. Further evaporation of the liquid droplets occurs during passage through the air. Thus, the size of the drug-containing droplets depends on the time available for evaporation of the propellants and the distance from the actuator orifice.

Key Points:

- Spacers reduce the need for coordination between actuation and inhalation.
- Spacers may improve the therapeutic index of inhaled therapy.
- Spacers may reduce cost of treatment from improved drug delivery.

III. When Should a Spacer Be Used?

Determining the suitability of various devices for different patients will improve the response to drug therapy and thus ultimately improve the treatment of asthma.

Figure 2 presents a suggestion for the choice of device in various age groups. In brief, nebulizers are rarely indicated for maintenance treatment. pMDI and spacer with face mask or mouthpiece is the preferred device for maintenance treatment until the child is sufficiently mature to reliably use a dry-powder inhaler (DPI) or breath-operated pMDI (12).

The use of a spacer improves the predictability of drug delivery from a pMDI in patients with a potential coordination difficulty. The clinical benefit of administering bronchodilators from pMDIs with spacers has been proven for patients with faulty inhalation techniques but not those who can correctly use a pMDI alone (16–18). Children often have difficulty coordinating actuation of the pMDI with inhalation of the aerosol, which leads to inadequate delivery of drug to the lungs and a diminished therapeutic effect (19). In particular, coordination is not reliable in young children. In children, therefore, pMDIs should seldom be used without a spacer. Even adults, however, often use pMDIs ineffectively and incorrectly; handicapped and aged patients often have considerable difficulty using pMDIs and indeed may be unable to use these devices.

The use of a spacer improves the safety of treatment with a pMDI com-

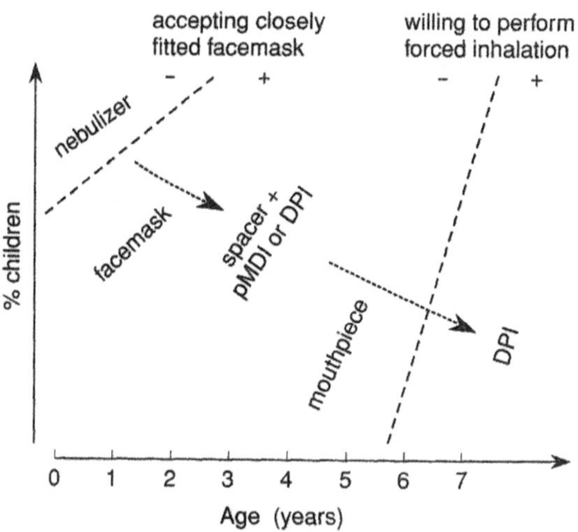

Figure 2 Choice of delivery device in children of different ages. (From Ref. 12.)

pared to other devices because of the improved particle size profile. In particular, patients on high-dose topical steroid therapy will benefit from the reduced oral deposition, as oral deposition presents a risk of local side effects, such as candidiasis and hoarseness (20) and may add to the systemic load of drug.

Nebulizers, which may represent the alternative to pMDIs for most young children and other patients with coordination difficulties, deliver a constant flow of aerosol during both inspiration and expiration, which may result in excessive exposure of the patient's skin and eyes to the drug. Drug loss to the environment may also result in unwanted exposure of caregivers to a nebulized aerosol. By contrast, aerosol from spacers reaches the lungs with little loss in the upper airways and minimal exposure of face and eyes to drug, since the aerosol passively follows the patient's inspiration with no inherent flow. Dosimetric nebulizers are being developed where the aerosol is delivered on demand only during the inspiratory phase. Still, they are expensive, bulky, and technically complicated devices.

pMDIs with spacers are more portable than nebulizers, though the size of most spacers is inconvenient to older children and adults, for whom more portable alternatives such as DPIs are available. The time needed for drug administration with spacers is much shorter than with nebulizers, which aids compliance. In addition, spacers are less expensive, and intuitively simpler to use than nebulizers.

For these reasons, a pMDI with spacer should be preferred to a nebulizer for maintenance treatment; moreover, pMDIs appear to be as effective as nebulizers in patients with acute asthma (21,22). pMDIs with spacers are therefore convenient for use as first-line treatment of acute severe asthma in primary care (23). However, it is a common clinical observation (though certainly not evidence-based) that nebulizer treatment is more efficient than treatment with a pMDI and spacer in young children with acute severe asthma. If this is not merely a personal bias, it may be explained by the longer aerosol availability provided by the nebulizer. Furthermore, additives in pMDIs can cause airway irritation, which is exaggerated during acute severe asthma. In hospital settings, nebulizers are often the preferred mode of treating acute asthma in children.

Face masks should be used with spacers unless it is certain that the patient will not entrain though the nose or around the mouthpiece. This is often difficult to confirm in young children, who should therefore use face masks in most cases until about the age of 4 years, after which a mouthpiece should be used. The age at which devices such as DPIs, requiring active cooperation, may be used depends on the individual patient. It should be emphasized that the choice of device should not be based on the physical ability to achieve certain inhalation flows but rather on the maturity and willingness of the patient to comply under all conditions. Young children can often use more demanding devices correctly under optimal conditions but may not do so at all times, particularly during respiratory distress. From the age of 7 years, however, most children will cooperate reliably and can be switched to a DPI.

Key Points:

- pMDIs should always be used with spacers in children.
- Nebulizers should not be used for maintenance treatment but may be useful in children with acute severe asthma.
- Spacers should be used with facemasks in young children until they can be trusted to inhale from a mouthpiece, usually from around age 4.
- DPIs or breath-operated pMDIs are recommended for patients who can reliably be expected to cooperate in all circumstances.

IV. Specifications of Spacer Devices

A. Approval

At present, spacers are not considered to be medical products and can therefore be marketed without any documentation. The performance characteristics of pMDIs are required to be strictly documented before approval by drug regulatory authorities; considering the significant influence of spacers on pMDI performance, it would seem logical to require similar documentation of the pMDI-spacer combination before approval and marketing. Spacers should not be considered generic devices that can be used with any pMDI. In the future, spacers should be tested for their effect on aerosol delivery with specified pMDIs and marketed only for use with these pMDIs.

Key Point:

- Spacers should be considered to be medical products, and formal documentation and approval should be required in the future.

B. In Vitro Measurement of Delivered Doses from Spacers

The delivered dose from spacers is sometimes reported as the dose at the time of pMDI actuation—i.e., the dose is measured in vitro by emptying the spacer immediately upon pMDI actuation. This, however, does not take account of the delayed emptying by children with variable and shallow breathing maneuvers. The aerosol is lost passively during such a period between actuation of the pMDI and in vivo emptying of the spacer (Fig. 1). Since the aim of a spacer is to provide a stable aerosol to avoid the need for coordination between actuation and inhalation, dose measurement concomitant with actuation of the pMDI seems irrelevant. The dose from the spacer should be defined after a period of 10 or 20 s, which would be a more realistic reflection of the situation in clinical use. The passive loss of aerosol is monoexponential and can be described by its half-life (24).

Although the initial dose at the time of actuation may be satisfactory, it is of little use if the half-life is short, since the patient may not be able to empty the aerosol before a considerable and variable fraction is lost within the spacer. Young children often breathe irregularly, with periods of breath-holding and shallow breathing, when presented with a face mask (Fig. 1); thus a stable aerosol with a long half-life would be advantageous. The longer the aerosol is available after actuation, the less coordination is required between actuation and inspiration. A long half-life is important to ensure adequate delivery of aerosol to young children; an aerosol with a short half-life within the spacer increases the need for coordination between actuation and inhalation and will not deliver a full and predictable dose. Conversely, a long aerosol half-life improves the predictability of dosing.

Key Point:

- Measurement of drug delivery from spacers should consider the time-dependent passive loss of aerosol and assess the delayed dose delivered and aerosol half-life.

V. Sources of Aerosol Loss Within Spacers

One of the aims of spacer devices is the removal of large aerosol particles. However, the loss of fine particles reduces the cost-effectiveness of treatment (15). Furthermore, such losses may be variable, leading to unpredictable dosing and disease control.

The major causes of aerosol loss from a pMDI delivered into a spacer are illustrated in Fig. 3. The larger particles impact on the spacer wall due to the inertia in the jet of particles from the pMDI. Particles sediment due to the progressively reduced velocity of the aerosol. In addition, particles can be adsorbed to the spacer wall if this carries electrostatic charges. Aerosol loss is partly instanta-

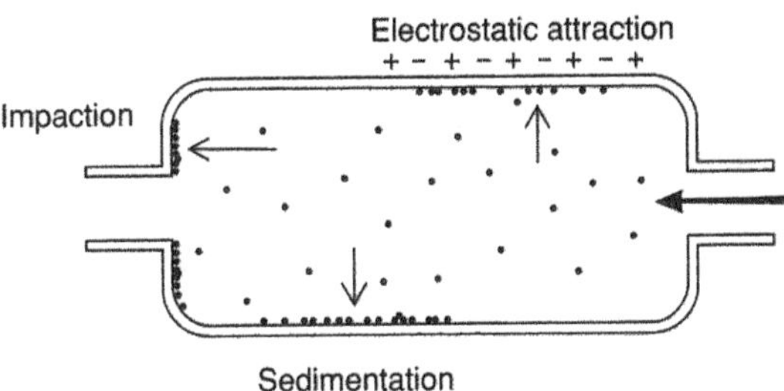

Figure 3 Mechanisms of loss of aerosol in a spacer. (1) impaction due to inertia of the particle jet; (2) sedimentation; (3) attraction of drug particles to the spacer wall due to electrostatic charges.

neous due to impaction after actuation of the spray into the spacer, while additional loss due to the sedimentation and electrostatic attraction is time-dependent.

Aerosol can also be lost in any dead space common to the inspiratory and expiratory lines in a device; a certain amount of dead space cannot be avoided in a face mask. Finally, aerosol may be lost because of valve insufficiency and other leaks.

A mathematical model incorporating impaction, aerosol half-life, spacer volume, dead space, and leakage was recently developed and validated (25). This model correctly predicted the aerosol delivery from common spacers.

A. Impaction

pMDIs produce a jet of particles at very high speed (up to 50 m/s). These particles have to be decelerated within the spacer in order to remain airborne as an aerosol. The large "ballistic" droplets have the greatest inertia and will impact on the spacer wall. The impaction of aerosol is critically dependent on the relationship between the speed of the jet and the size and shape of the spacer. Loss due to impaction occurs before the other factors influencing aerosol loss have had significant effects. In addition, part of the aerosol jet may escape backward around the aerosol canister. Such losses account for the major loss of aerosol; therefore spacer volume and shape are critical to the dose delivered from a particular pMDI.

The volume of the spacer is critical; the larger the spacer, the greater the amount of drug that will remain airborne and eventually be delivered (26). The available fraction of aerosol immediately after actuation of a budesonide pMDI into the 145-mL AeroChamber spacer was 27%, compared with 63% from the 750 mL-Nebuhaler spacer (25). Similarly, the fine-particle fraction (mass median aerodynamic diameter, or MMAD, < 5 μm) of salbutamol CFC pMDI from the 750-mL Volumatic spacer was almost three times that from Aerochamber (27). In vivo, the lung dose from Nebuhaler with hydrofluoroalkane (HFA) pMDI was 1.6-fold higher than that from AeroChamber (28).

The vapor pressure and the design of the canister nozzle determine the aerosol jet and eventually impaction. Low vapor pressure increases drug delivery from a particular spacer due to a reduced jet and therefore reduced impaction. Airomir salbutamol pMDI containing HFA propellant delivered less drug as fine particles (MMAD < 5 μm) compared with the Ventolin salbutamol pMDI containing chlorofluorocarbon (CFC) propellant but a higher output from a spacer, probably due to a lower jet velocity (29).

This interaction between spacer volume and pMDI vapor pressure can cause a twofold change in the fine-particle output from different pMDI and spacer combinations (14).

The shape of the spacer may also affect the degree of impaction within the spacer to some extent. The volume and shape of spacers have seemingly often been designed with reference to the visible plume of the aerosol (2). High-speed video studies have shown that this plume consists of an initial jet phase traversing 5–10 cm, followed by dispersion into a cone-shaped cloud (30). However, the visible plume consists mainly of propellants and additives and does not correspond to the distribution of drug particles. Thus, cone-shaped spacers may not be ideal. A spherical spacer apparently causes the aerosol jet to vortex within the spacer, thereby reducing impaction and increasing dose output (31).

Impaction accounts for most of the large particle trap effect of the spacer. This is illustrated in Fig. 4, which shows the fine and coarse particle doses obtained from a budesonide pMDI (Pulmicort, AstraZeneca, Sweden) actuated into a metal spacer. The spacer was initially 23 cm long, and subsequent reduction in the length of the spacer caused a reduction in both the coarse- and eventually also the fine-particle doses. Even the initial shortening of the spacer reduced the coarse particle dose, whereas the fine-particle dose was unaffected; thus, the total particle dose was reduced, but the ratio between fine and coarse particles was improved by shortening the spacer. Thus, the spacer length is critical for the fine-particle dose and the ratio of fine to coarse particles. Different pMDIs have different vapor pressures and therefore different aerosol velocities and volumes; as a result, the optimal spacer length is specific to a particular pMDI. Moreover, the spacer should be adapted to the particular aerosol jet. For this reason, the op-

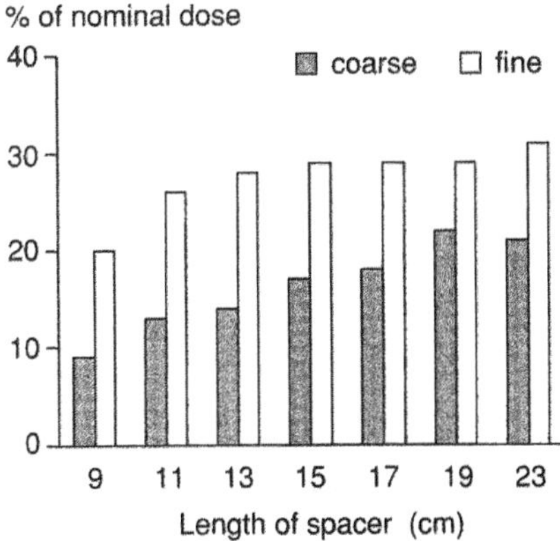

Figure 4 The effect of spacer length on dose delivery. Fine (< 4.7-μm) and coarse (> 4.7-μm) budesonide particles delivered from a pMDI with a metal spacer of different lengths. The aerosol was analyzed by an Anderson impactor (U.S. throat) 2 s after actuation (28 L/min). The optimal ratio between fine and coarse particles was obtained with a spacer of 13 cm for this particular pMDI. Other pMDIs will have different optimum spacer sizes, depending on vapor pressure.

timal shape and size of a spacer for use with one pMDI cannot be extrapolated to other pMDIs.

It is inappropriate to use any pMDI with any spacer without considering the aerosol characteristics, even if the pMDI adaptor fits. The use of a universal spacer common to all pMDIs will result in unpredictable dosing.

Key Points:

- Impaction is the single most important factor affecting drug output and the ratio between large and fine particles.
- Drug output increases with spacer volume.
- The ratio of fine to coarse particles is dependent on spacer volume, spacer shape, and pMDI vapor pressure.
- Spacer-pMDI combinations should be considered individual entities and the use of a "universal" spacer for different pMDIs should be avoided.

B. Sedimentation of the Aerosol

Sedimentation of drug particles in the aerosol is another factor that reduces the available aerosol and shortens the time available for inhalation after actuation. The velocity of sedimentation is proportional to the aerodynamic diameter of the particles. In a narrow spacer, the sedimentation distance is short and therefore the loss of aerosol is faster in small-volume tube spacers than in large-volume spacers. This principle is taken to its extreme in a vertical spacer, compared with the traditional horizontal spacer.

The effect of sedimentation was illustrated in an in vitro study in which a budesonide pMDI was delivered through two different spacers, Nebuhaler (Astra Zeneca, Sweden) and Babyhaler (GlaxoWellcome, UK) (Fig. 5). Both spacers are of similar length (200 mm) but have different diameters (80 versus 50 mm); both were primed before use to prevent electrostatic charge effects (see below). The total dose was increased in the wider spacer, mainly due to an increased coarse particle dose, and the half-life of the fine particle fraction was longer (33 versus 23 s).

Key Point:

- Increased sedimentation distance within the spacer increases the total dose and prolongs the half-life of fine particles at the cost of a higher coarse-particle fraction.

C. Electrostatic Attraction

Aerosolization induces a static electric charge by triboelectrification of aerosol particles or droplets, including particles from pMDIs, DPIs and nebulizers. In addition, all plastic devices, including plastic spacers, carry random electrostatic

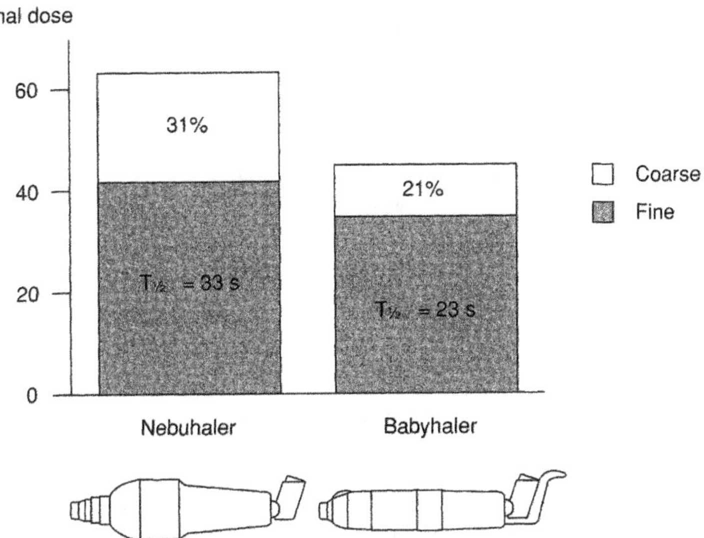

Figure 5 The effect of spacer volume on dose delivery. The aerosol from a budesonide pMDI was analyzed by the Anderson impactor (U.S. throat) 2 s after actuation (28 L/min) through Nebuhaler and Babyhaler, both of which had been primed to prevent electrostatic effects. Both spacers are of similar length but have different diameters (80 versus 50 mm). The aerosol was airborne for a longer time in the spacer with the larger diameter; correspondingly, the total dose was larger, mainly due to an increased coarse particle dose.

charges. The net effect of these electrostatic charges is attraction of aerosol particles onto plastic surfaces. This will significantly reduce the drug aerosol available for inhalation from plastic spacers; the electrostatic activity of plastic spacers reduces the initial dose available for inhalation and reduce the aerosol half-life of aerosol in the spacer, thus reducing the time available for inhalation.

In vitro studies have shown that drug delivery is enhanced by the use of an antistatic lining on a plastic spacer (32), and that a steel spacer (inherently nonelectrostatic) produces a significantly higher dose compared with a plastic spacer (24,33,34). The dramatic effect of the electrostatic charge on the delivered dose is illustrated in Fig. 6, together with data on the increased drug delivery resulting from priming by repeated use of pMDI. Such a priming effect during repeated use was also seen in a field study of drug delivery to young children from the Babyhaler plastic spacer; drug delivery measured at home showed a 0.8% increase per day (35). In another study, the fine-particle fraction of salbutamol delivered from a plastic spacer handled by several different techniques showed an inverse correlation with the static voltage on the spacer device (36,37).

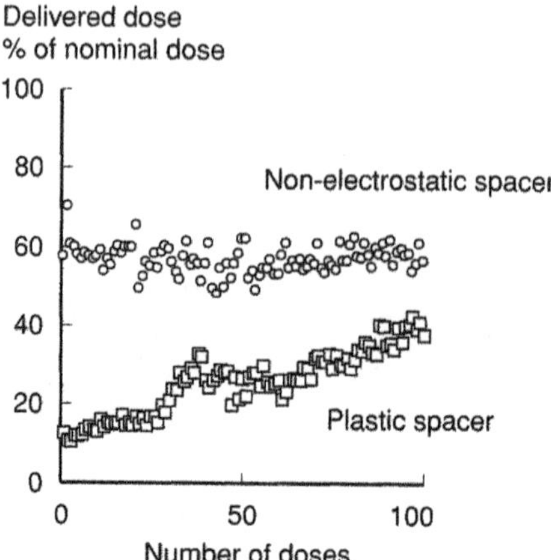

Figure 6 The effect of an electrostatics on dose delivery. Dose delivered to filter during 100 consecutive actuations of budesonide pMDI via a metal (nonelectrostatic) spacer (Nebuchamber) (o) and fluticasone propionate pMDI via a plastic (electrostatic) spacer (Babyhaler) (□). (From Ref. 38.)

Electrostatic attraction causes a continuous and rapid disappearance of the aerosol; in plastic spacers, the aerosol half-life is typically 10 s, compared with 30 s if the static charge is abolished (24,37,38). Because of this short residence time in plastic spacers, the inhalation must be coordinated with actuation of the pMDI to obtain an optimal dose. This obviously negates one of the major advantages of spacers.

The effect of electrostatic charge has also been shown in in vivo measurements. The lung dose of salbutamol in children, estimated by a pharmacokinetic method, was halved when an ordinary plastic spacer was used compared with the same spacer after antistatic priming (39). In a similar study in adults, however, this effect was not apparent (40); this may have been because adults can empty the spacer in one or two breaths coordinated with actuation, which would reduce the importance of the electrostatic charge. Two further studies have used scintigraphic estimates of lung dose after administration of radiolabeled drug to investigate the effect of electrostatic charge (41,42). In one study, the lung dose improved 1.5-fold, while in the other study, the lung dose increased fourfold; the latter study reported an unusually high lung dose of 46% from coated spacers. Such differing results may partly be ascribed to poor standardization of the scintigraphic method, and they should be interpreted cautiously. However, the overall conclusion from in vivo studies seems to be that electrostatic charges significantly affect the dose delivered to the lungs from plastic spacers.

The electrostatic charge of plastic spacers may be reduced in various ways. Priming should coat the inner surface of the spacer with a conducting layer, thereby reducing electrostatic charge;

1. Antistatic paints have been used successfully (32,43).
2. Immersion in household detergents is also effective, ionic detergents being more efficient than nonionic detergents (42,44). This effect may last for several weeks (42), though the data are inconsistent (44). If detergent is used, it is very important not to rinse the spacer in water or to dry the plastic with a cloth, since this immediately recharges the spacer; and the spacer should be stored unwrapped (44).
3. Benzalkonium chloride is effective in neutralizing the electrostatic charge of plastic spacers (38).
4. Repeated use of the pMDI itself primes the plastic to some extent (38). This priming effect is time-dependent; the effect is not immediate but builds up over days (38). As with other priming procedures, the effect is reversible with ordinary washing.

The various priming options should be compared with respect to the stability of the effect during routine use. Potential toxicity from inhaled residues of the chemical used for priming must also be studied. The risk of contact dermatitis from use of various coating including detergents should be evaluated. Possible interactions between priming chemicals and the aerosolized drug should be tested, and patient compliance with priming procedures should be considered.

Washing the plastic spacer may remove any priming layer, resulting in the spacer reverting to its original charged state. The spacer could then go through cycles of high and low drug delivery, as the priming layer builds up on the walls with use, and is removed during washing. The delivered dose may be low immediately after washing, gradually increasing with use until the spacer is washed again. This leads to both intersubject and intrasubject variations in dosage, since patients will clean their spacers in different ways.

It seems obvious that manufacturers of spacer devices should use only nonelectrostatic materials in the future. Certainly, it is not satisfactory to require the patient to remember a certain priming procedure, which is likely to jeopardize compliance. Metal is an obvious, robust, and safe choice for a nonelectrostatic spacer (24,34), since it carries no charge no matter how it is handled and requires no chemical treatment. Alternatively a nonelectrostatic plastic material (carbon black) has been produced by mixing a conductive material into the plastic during the moulding procedure; other nonelectrostatic materials may be developed in the future.

Key Points:

- Electrostatic charges in plastic spacers cause a clinically significant reduction of lung dose.
- Possible priming procedures for available plastic spacers should be studied with respect to stability, toxicity, drug interactions, and impact on patient compliance.
- Only nonelectrostatic devices should be used in the future.

D. Valves

The valves controlling inhalation of aerosol from the spacer and exhalation from the face mask must operate effectively over the entire range of pressures from those encountered in the shallow breathing of a sleeping child (pressure changes $< \pm 0.01$ kPa) to those in a crying baby (pressure changes > 0.5 kPa) (25). Leakage through an inefficient inspiratory valve blows aerosol out of the spacer during expiration. An inefficient expiratory valve dilutes the inspiration with air from outside the spacer, resulting in delayed aerosol delivery and increased loss due to passive fallout of aerosol in the spacer. These factors can significantly impair drug delivery.

Some spacer adaptations lack a valve at the expiratory outlet. This may not be essential in older children and adults, since the volume shift during inspiration is sufficient despite the open expiratory outlet. In young children with shallow breathing, however, an open outlet will allow significant air entrainment during inspiration, attenuating the inspiratory volume shift from the spacer and thus delaying emptying of the spacer. During this delay, fallout of the aerosol within the spacer will reduce dose availability (24).

In an in vitro study, the pressure change at the valves varied from between -0.2 kPa and +0.7 kPa with the high-resistance NebuChamber to between -0.02 and +0.01 kPa with the low-resistance Babyhaler during simulated regular breathing of toddlers. During tidal breathing, the typical flow varied from 8 to 16 L/min (25). A low-pressure swing at low-resistance valves may not always assure efficient opening and closure of the valves; thus, leakage through the valves was more common in the low-resistance valves than the high-resistance valves (25). High-pressure swings present no difficulty to young children or infants (for comparison, applied positive expiratory pressure in infants with respiratory distress uses pressures of 0.5–0.8 kPa) and assure more reliable opening and closure of valves.

Key Points:

- Inlets should have valves; for use in children, outlets should also have valves.
- Leakage though valves reduces drug delivery. Leakage is more common through low-resistance valves.

E. Dead Space

Any volume common to the inspiratory and expiratory lines in a device is dead space, which means that drug in this volume will not contribute to the lung dose but will be lost in each breath. A certain amount of dead space cannot be avoided in a face mask but should be minimized by reducing the volume of the mask.

The effect of dead space on drug delivery from spacers was illustrated in a study in which the fine particle dose obtained by evacuating the spacer with a ventilator mimicking the breathing of a young child (tidal volume 195 mL; respiratory frequency 20; inspiratory:expiratory ratio 1:2) was expressed as a percentage of the dose obtained by evacuating the spacer by a constant flow (38). The effect of leaky valves may have added to the loss during breathing. When breathing from a spacer with high-resistance valves with no dead space, 95% of the dose was recovered, while only approximately 60% was obtained by breathing from a spacer with low-resistance valves and a 40-mL dead space.

Key Point:

- Drug delivery is reduced by the proportion of dead space to tidal volume.

VI. Effect of Spacer Construction on Dose Delivery

Drug delivery from a spacer is critically dependent on the factors outlined above, including the volume and shape of the spacer, valves, and spacer material. The influence of these factors can be illustrated with reference to three of the more commonly used spacers.

NebuChamber is a 250-mL metal spacer with high-resistance valves and no dead space between the valves.

Babyhaler is a 350-mL plastic spacer with low-resistance valves and a 40-mL dead space between inlet and outlet valves.

AeroChamber is a 145-mL plastic spacer with low-resistance valves and no dead space between the valves.

The comparative efficiency of these spacers has been documented in vitro (38) and in vivo (24,34,35) by collecting the dose delivered to a filter in front of the spacers. The in vitro measurements were performed with a ventilator mimicking the breathing of a toddler, while the in vivo measurements were performed by sampling aerosol in front of the face mask of young children. The doses measured were adjusted for the fraction of small droplets (< 4.7 μm) in the aerosol and calculated as percentages of the nominal dose. The delivered doses were 35% from NebuChamber (budesonide pMDI), 22% from Babyhaler (fluticasone pMDI), and 13% from AeroChamber (budesonide pMDI) (38). The relative efficiency of the devices to deliver fine particles could thus be determined by relating the output from Babyhaler to the output from NebuChamber (0.22/0.35 = 63%) and the output from AeroChamber to the output from NebuChamber (0.13/0.35 = 37%). From such in vitro estimates, the relative efficiencies of these three devices for the delivery of fine particles appear to be 10:6:4. This indicates that the nominal dose used in an AeroChamber should be increased by a factor of 2.5 compared with NebuChamber to obtain a defined clinical effect in the lungs of a young child. Suboptimal spacer performance was ascribed to inefficient valve control, dead space in the inspiratory line, loss of aerosol by residual electrostatic attraction in the primed plastic spacers, and inappropriate spacer volumes.

Similar differences have been described among other spacers. The fine particle dose varied by twofold between commonly used "universal" plastic spacers (45).

Such differences in dose delivery highlight the significance of the choice of device in relation to dose recommendations and cost-effectiveness of treatment (15).

Key Points:

- Differences in spacer construction may change drug delivery by several-fold.
- Predictable dosing assumes a fixed combination of pMDI and spacer

VII. The Optimal Spacer for Young Children

The optimal spacer for young children would show the following features:

1. A volume of intermediate size, permitting the chamber to be emptied in a few breaths, but not so small that the bulk of the delivered dose from the pMDI impacts on the walls at the moment of actuation
2. Nonelectrostatic material
3. An efficient one-way inspiratory and expiratory valve system to assure opening and closing even during the shallow breathing of a young baby
4. Minimal dead space in the valve and face mask
5. A long half-life for the aerosol in the chamber
6. A tight-fitting face mask.

Such an optimal spacer is not yet available.

VIII. Choice of Spacer Depends on Choice of Drug

The drug to be delivered determines the choice of spacer. The requirements for the delivery of bronchodilators and inhaled steroids are so different that different devices should be recommended.

A. Bronchodilators

The metered doses of salbutamol and fenoterol in commercially available pMDIs are several-fold higher than those that produce maximal effects on the airways (46,47). Therefore, it may be possible to lose a large proportion of drug through poor inhalation technique, while still obtaining maximal bronchodilatation. Indeed, in one study, no change in bronchodilator response was seen when actuation of a pMDI was deliberately desynchronized from inhalation (48,49). In contrast, the metered dose of commercially available terbutaline pMDI appears to be less than the dose required for maximal bronchodilatation (50), and changes in the efficiency of the delivery device significantly affect the lung dose and the clinical response (51).

Bronchodilators have a high therapeutic index and are comparatively inexpensive. Thus inefficient or unpredictable drug delivery can be compensated for by increasing the prescribed dose at little cost, and with low risk of incurring side effects.

Bronchodilators are used on an "as-required" basis. Therefore, spacers for bronchodilators should be conveniently portable.

B. Inhaled Steroids

Inhaled steroids have a narrow therapeutic index and therefore it is essential that the particle profile is optimal, with a high proportion of fine particles and a low proportion of large particles. Moreover, inhaled steroids are relatively costly and thus the fraction of the nominal (labeled) dose delivered should be optimized. Inhaled steroids are normally given once or twice daily, and therefore portability is less of an issue than with bronchodilators.

Price often determines the choice of spacers. However, the price of wasted drug also contributes to the cost-effectiveness of treatment (15). Optimally designed spacers may be relatively expensive but, in the case of inhaled steroids, loss of drug from inefficient spacers is probably more costly in the long term than even the most expensive spacer, since inefficient spacers require higher prescribed doses (15). Such estimates of cost-effectiveness may be less clear for bronchodilators.

The single most important factor determining drug delivery is the size of the spacer; large-volume spacers deliver more drug than small-volume spacers. The optimal size depends on the pMDI, and therefore dedicated spacers should be preferred to universal spacers. Small-volume spacers such as AeroChamber were designed to overcome problems of coordination, rather than to optimize lung dose (3,52). Accordingly, they provide significantly reduced drug delivery compared with intermediate- or large-volume spacers (13,24,27,38,39,52–54).

Simple containers may provide suitable aerosols even for infants. Saline containers (55) and coffee cups (56,57) have been shown to provide clinically effective bronchodilator aerosol delivery. Undoubtedly, even the simplest of containers aids coordination between pMDI actuation and inhalation. However, the loss of drug is likely to be considerable and such containers probably do not improve on the particle profile. Such delivery may suffice for bronchodilators but not for inhaled steroids.

In large parts of the world, socioeconomic conditions often preclude the use of more advanced spacers as patients are unable to afford imported devices. Local production should be encouraged to reduce costs. In fact, simple and efficient spacers that conform to the requirements described above have been produced for the delivery of bronchodilators (58,59).

Key Points:

- The choice of spacer depends on the drug to be delivered. The requirements for delivery of bronchodilators and steroids differ, and different devices may be required.
- Inexpensive but ineffective spacers may cause expensive loss of drug.
- Spacers developed and documented for particular pMDIs should be preferred over universal spacers.
- Simple containers or small-volume spacers may be used for bronchodilators.
- Optimized spacers are essential for delivery of inhaled steroids.

IX. Use of Spacers

A number of recommendations can be made for the optimal use of spacers. Slow inhalation is preferable since the impaction of particles is proportional to velocity and particle size. A slow flow reduces the risk of impaction on valves and anatomic structures such as the pharynx or vocal cords. In addition, high flow rates enhance central airway deposition caused by inertial impaction and therefore reduce deposition in peripheral airways.

It is essential that a pMDI is shaken before every use (see Chap. 10), since failure to do this will dramatically reduce drug delivery (60,61). The spacer should be positioned before actuating the pMDI because the fallout of aerosol reduces the available dose over time. Movement of the spacer should be avoided, as this will reduce the drug available for inhalation due to impaction on the sides of the spacer wall (62).

If multiple doses are prescribed, they should be given separately, since simultaneous administration causes a significant reduction in the recovered dose (44,63,64). This may be less of a concern with nonelectrostatic spacers.

The number of breaths required to empty a spacer obviously depends on the size of the patient and the spacer. The aerosol empties from a spacer in an exponential manner, since inhaled aerosol is replaced by air thus diluting the remaining aerosol. Adults may empty a spacer in one to two inhalations, whereas in laboratory studies in which ventilators were used to mimick the breathing of toddlers, commonly used spacers for young children were emptied in two to four breaths (25). A safe recommendation would be to suggest 10 breaths in infants, 5 breaths in toddlers and 2 slow deep inhalations in older children and adults.

In a previous study, crying did not have an important impact on drug delivery to the patient (65), but lung deposition has been shown to be much lower in a screaming child than in quietly and tidally breathing children (66,67). Tidal volume and inspiratory flows are increased during crying, whereas breathing frequency and the inspiration/expiration ratio are decreased. Such changes in breathing patterns may greatly influence drug distribution in the patient and thus lung deposition.

Key Points:

- Slow inhalation is optimal.
- Multiple doses should be given as separate inhalations.
- The spacer should be positioned before actuation.
- Ten breaths in infants, 5 breaths, in toddlers and 2 breaths in older children and adults.

X. Use of Facemasks with Spacers

The pressure measured within the facemask is often much lower than that observed in an in vitro situation, which suggests that leakage between the mask and the face is a common problem (25). Similarly, the recovered dose is lower and more variable in vivo (24,34) than in vitro (25). This also suggests problems with the fit of the mask. This leakage is probably an important factor contributing to variable drug delivery. In addition, the use of a facemask adds to the dead space, and optimization of facemask design is necessary.

The nose efficiently filters particles from the inhaled air and thus can potentially reduce the amount of drug inhaled. One study reported that lung dose was reduced by half in schoolchildren inhaling through the nose as compared with mouth inhalation (68). This filter effect appears to be inversely related to age, and the lower airways seem to be less well protected in younger children (69). Interestingly, a recent study reported no difference between lung deposition after inhalation via facemask or mouthpiece in forty 3- to 7-year-old children (70). The efficiency of nasal filtration is unknown in very young children. Even though the available evidence is conflicting, it is likely that lung dose is reduced with nasal inhalation in infants as it is in older children. Such a filter effect in the nose is unfortunate for at least three reasons. First, the nasal mucosa readily absorbs most drugs, which thereby bypass first-pass metabolism in the liver; thus nasal inhalation adds significantly to the systemic bioavailability of inhaled drugs. Second, nasal breathing reduces the lung dose, which hampers clinical control and the cost-effectiveness and safety of treatment. Finally, changing between nasal and mouth breathing will increase variability of dosing. Inhalation of aerosolized drug for the lower airways should therefore be via the mouth only.

We recently developed a facemask which allows only mouth breathing (Fig. 7). A septum separates the nose from the mouth within the facemask, thereby preventing nasal breathing. Since young children are habitual nose breathers, this may be less acceptable to them at first, but initial experience has shown that acceptance is soon obtained. In preliminary tests, this facemask successfully prevented air leakage from the nose in a group of 0.5- to 4-year-old children. The facemask is designed to have minimal dead space and the inlet and outlet valves are integrated into the mask, which avoids any dead space in the inhalation and exhalation lines. These features can be expected to improve delivery of aerosol to the lungs.

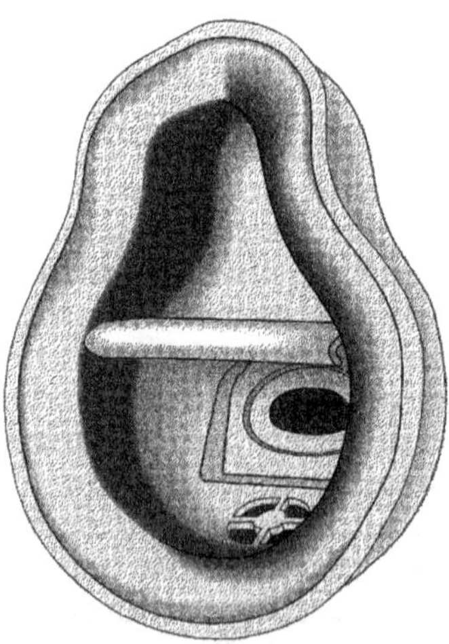

Figure 7 Prototype facemask occluding the nose. This ensures mouth breathing, thereby avoiding nasal drug deposition.

Key Points:

- Leakage around the facemask and nasal breathing from within a facemask are critical factors in drug delivery from pMDIs with spacers and facemasks.
- A facemask to prevent nasal breathing is suggested.

XI. Use of Spacers in Neonates and Infants

In recent years, bronchodilator aerosol therapy with pMDIs and spacers has been shown to be effective not only in mechanically ventilated but also in spontaneously breathing preterm and term neonates as well as in infants (71,72). Delivery of bronchodilators and inhaled steroids by pMDI and spacer has been shown to have a clinical benefit even in the youngest age group (73,74). Breathing patterns during spontaneous respiration during the neonatal period and infancy differ from those of older children. Breathing often is irregular and tidal volumes and inspiratory flows are low and vary greatly (75). The tidal volume is proportionate to the weight. These factors are very likely to have an important impact on aerosol delivery. In addition, breathing patterns may be altered in respiratory illnesses and may thus influence drug delivery (76,77). Parameters discussed previously—such as spacer volume, electrostatic charge, valve systems and dead volume—greatly influence the efficiency of drug delivery. Especially at the low tidal volumes characteristic for neonates and infants, the clearance of aerosol is more efficient in small-compared to large-volume spacers (27). Instrumental dead space is known to alter breathing patterns and pulmonary mechanics (78). The spacer for neonates should therefore have a small volume, a low-resistance inspiratory and expiratory valve system, and a reduced dead volume between the device and the patient (including the facemask); it should be made of nonelectrostatic material.

Delivery of bronchodilators to spontaneously breathing neonates from a pMDI through a nonelectrostatic spacer is more efficient than delivery from a nebulizer (65,79).

Key Points:

- Delivery of bronchodilators through spacers is clinically effective in spontaneously breathing neonates and infants.

XII. Use of Spacers in Ventilated Patients

In-line spacers have been developed to enhance lung deposition of aerosols from pMDIs into the ventilator setting. The advantage of a spacer inserted in the ventilator circuit is that the actuated aerosol cloud is retained within the chamber and hence, impaction of the drug within the ventilator circuit is reduced. Spacers have been shown to be superior to nonchamber devices (80). The factors influencing delivery to spontaneously breathing patients do generally also apply to ventilated patients. Large-volume spacers would be expected to be more efficient than small-volume spacers due to decreased loss of aerosol in the spacer. However, when a large in-line spacer without a valve system is inserted in the ventilator circuit next to the tracheal tube, it might not be totally cleared in inspiration and hence will be cleared in subsequent expiration, wasting drug during the expiratory phase. In-line spacers are efficiently cleared only in inspiration, when the tidal volume exceeds the volume of the in-line holding chamber (81). Alternatively, a large-volume spacer may be inserted in the inspiratory limb of the ventilator circuit, which will overcome the problem of aerosol wasting during expiration. Small-volume nebulizers can also effectively deliver aerosols in a ventilator model (82–84), but in vitro and in vivo studies suggest that pMDIs are more efficient in aerosol delivery than small-volume nebulizers (71,85–88). Bronchodilator delivery by pMDI and spacer has also been shown to be superior to delivery by nebulizer in ventilated infants (89). Respiratory system compliance improved more after pMDI and spacer than after nebulizer treatment. In addition to known factors (such as pMDI dose, design of spacer, and its position in the ventilator setting) specific ventilator parameters (such as ventilator mode, inspiratory flow pattern, humidity, and spontaneous respiratory effort) can greatly influence bronchodilator delivery (84). Delivery shows a linear correlation with both inspiratory time and duty cycle. A change in the compliance of the lung model while maintaining the same ventilator settings did not alter drug delivery. Delivery of bronchodilators is greater under dry than under humidified conditions (82). Humidification may lead to hygroscopic growth of the aerosols and increased impaction of aerosols on the chamber surface and hence decreased delivery.

Key Point:

- Spacers are more efficient than nebulizers for aerosol delivery to a ventilated patient.

XIII. Influence of Spacers on Lung Dose

In adults, the lung dose achieved with intermediate- and large-volume spacers is about twice that obtained with the corresponding pMDI alone (i.e., 20–35% of the metered dose) (28,61,90–92). In one study, lung doses from pMDIs with and without a large-volume spacer were similar (93), which may be explained by a lack of priming of the plastic spacer. The small-volume spacer AeroChamber delivers a lung dose similar to that of the corresponding pMDI (28). In one study on pMDI dose delivery to young children (3 months to 6 years of age) of salbutamol labeled with technetium 99m (^{99m}Tc) and inhaled via a small-volume plastic spacer (AeroChamber), a lung dose of 2% of the delivered dose was obtained (66). However, these data are difficult to interpret, since codeposition of drug and isotope was not confirmed. Clinical reports confirm the improved efficacy achieved with a spacer device in adults (94–96), and children (16,97), although not with the small-volume AeroChamber (52,98).

In addition to the total lung dose, the distribution of aerosol within the lungs may affect the clinical response. The aerosol characteristics are changed in a spacer, resulting in smaller particles that are likely to penetrate into smaller airways. However, little is known about the exact anatomic targets of various drugs within the airways.

A. Lung Dose and Age

Dose correction is normally based on body size. This may not be appropriate, however, as airway geometry may reduce lung dose in proportion to body size. In a pharmacokinetic study of a fixed dose of budesonide inhaled via Nebuchamber spacer, area under plasma concentration versus time curve (AUC) was similar in young children and adults (99). As AUC reflects the systemic *concentration* of drug, systemic *dose* reflecting lung dose must have been reduced in the children compared to the adults. This represents a highly important topic for future research, and if this observation is confirmed, it may lead to revision of current guidelines.

Key Point:

- Lung deposition from spacers depends on device characteristics and age-specific breathing patterns and airway morphology.

XIV. A Spacer for a Dry-Powder Inhaler

The combination of a spacer and face mask with a pMDI was the breakthrough that allowed the benefits of inhaled therapy to be offered to the large number of young patients with wheezing. However, pMDIs have significant disadvantages, including the irritant effect of additives, problems of dose consistency (see Chap. 10), and environmental concerns over both CFC and HFA propellants (see Chap. 11).

Because of these disadvantages, it has been suggested that a DPI could be used with a spacer device in young children (100), DPIs lack propellants, lubricants, surfactants, and other potentially harmful additives; thus this concept maintains the advantages of a pMDI plus spacer without the disadvantages associated with pMDIs.

The working principle of this device is a mechanical "inhalation" from the DPI into a spacer (Fig. 8). This inhalation is caused by the release of a spring-loaded piston underneath the spacer chamber. The inhalation draws the metered dose as an aerosol from the DPI into the spacer. After inhalation, the piston is compressed upon the spring and locks in place, ready for the next use. As a consequence of the standardized nature of the mechanical actuation, there is no requirement for forced inspiration, and repeatability of dosing is high. The use of a vertical spacer position opposed to the traditional horizontal position increases the sedimentation distance, which prolongs the half-life of the aerosol and thus increases the time available for inhalation.

In vitro tests with the prototype have shown that it produces a remarkably stable fine-particle aerosol with a MMAD of 2.8 μm. The half-life of the fine-particle aerosol in the spacer is approximately 1.5 min. Even in the case of a non-compliant toddler, who may breath-hold or perform periods of shallow breathing, passive fallout of aerosol will have little effect on the dose obtained.

In summary, the mechanical actuation of a DPI into a spacer provides a new option for aerosol treatment. In addition to the general advantages offered by a spacer, this device provides the advantage of a drug aerosol delivered without use of potentially harmful additives and propellants. The mechanical actuation ensures a high repeatability of drug delivery. Finally, the tower-shaped spacer and its nonelectrostatic properties ensure a stable aerosol, which remains airborne for a prolonged period. This makes coordination and forced inspiration unnecessary and should permit effective inhalation, even by children who have previously been unable to use spacer devices effectively.

In conclusion, this device utilizes the new understanding of the essential aspects of spacer function that has been obtained in recent years. Such developments should improve our ability to treat young children with inhaled drug aerosols.

Key Points:

- The use of a DPI plus a spacer avoids the problems of propellants and irritants inherent to all pMDIs.
- Mechanical actuation of a DPI into a spacer avoids the requirements of coordination and forced inhalation.

XV. Conclusion

Spacers reduce the need for coordination, improve the therapeutic index of aerosol treatment, and reduce the cost of treatment. In children, pMDIs should not be used without spacers, but pMDIs with spacers are the devices of choice

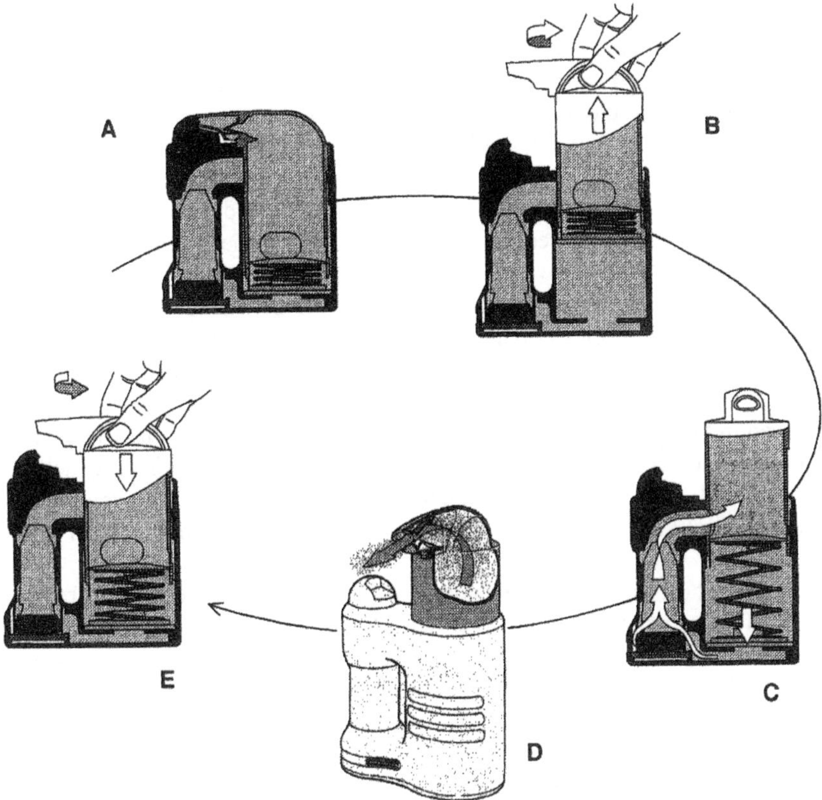

Figure 8 DPI with spacer. (A) A section through the device in the resting state. The drug is dispensed from a standard dry-powder inhaler (Turbuhaler). The spacer chamber to the right is closed. Beneath the spacer a compressed spring is under tension. (B) The device is activated by lifting the spacer chamber. The compressed spring is locked between the bottom of the spacer and a piston. (C) Actuation of the device is accomplished by twisting the spacer chamber through degrees. This action primes the inhaler via a gearing system and also releases the spring. Release and expansion of the spring creates a partial vacuum, thus drawing air through the inhaler, dispersing the aerosol, and drawing it into the spacer. (D) The aerosol is available for inhalation. Due to the vertical position of the spacer and the nonelectrostatic material used in its construction, the aerosol is stable with a half-life of approximately 1.5 min. A face mask may be fitted for use by younger children. (E) After inhalation, the spacer chamber is rotated back 90 degrees to its original position. The spacer chamber is pushed firmly down, compressing the spring and storing the energy for the next actuation.

for maintenance treatment in patients who cannot reliably use DPIs or breath-actuated pMDIs. Spacers should be used with a face masks in patients who cannot reliably be expected not to entrain through their nose and mouth, and a mouthpiece should be used until the child can reliably be expected to cooperate under all circumstances with the inhalation maneuvers required for the use of a DPI or breath-actuated pMDI.

Measurements of drug delivery from spacers should consider the fallout of aerosol and provide delayed dose measurements and measurements of aerosol half-life.

The drug output increases with spacer volume, while the ratio between fine and coarse particles is dependent on the balance between spacer volume and pMDI vapor pressure. Electrostatic charges in plastic spacers cause a clinically significant reduction of lung dose; thus, nonelectrostatic devices should be used in the future. Drug delivery is reduced by the proportion dead space to tidal volume. Differences in spacer construction may change drug delivery several-fold. Therefore each pMDI-spacer combination should be considered a separate entity and the use of a "universal" spacer for different pMDIs should be avoided.

The choice of spacer depends on the drug to be delivered. The requirements for delivery of bronchodilators and steroids differ, and different devices may be advisable. Simple containers or small-volume spacers may be used for bronchodilators, whereas optimized spacers are essential for delivery of inhaled steroids. Inexpensive but ineffective spacers may cause expensive loss of drug.

Aerosol should be inhaled from a spacer by slow inhalation, and multiple doses should be given as separate inhalations. The spacer should be positioned before actuation. Infants should empty the spacer by 10 breaths, toddlers by 5 breaths, and older children and adults by 2 breaths.

Leakage around the face mask and nasal breathing from within a face mask are critical factors affecting drug delivery from a pMDI with spacer and facemask. A facemask with a septum separating the nasal cavity from the mouth to prevent nasal breathing is suggested.

Little is known of how to adjust the dose in different age groups; this needs to be elucidated in future studies. Lung deposition from spacers depends on device characteristics and age-specific breathing patterns and airway morphology.

The use of a DPI with spacer avoids the problems of propellants and irritants inherent to all pMDIs. Mechanical actuation of a DPI into a spacer avoids the requirements of coordination and forced inhalation.

Increased understanding of the factors affecting aerosol drug delivery has provided better spacer devices. The next major step forward depends on the willingness of all involved parties to standardize recommendations based on this knowledge. This will ultimately improve the treatment of asthma.

References

1. Franklin W, Lowell F, Michelson AL, Schiller I. Aerosolized steroids in bronchial asthma. J Allergy 1958; 29:214–221.
2. Moren F. Drug deposition of pressurized inhalation aerosols: influence of actuator tube design. Int J Pharm 1978; 1:205–212.
3. Corr D, Dolovich M, McCormack D, Ruffin R, Obminski G, Newhouse M. Design and characteristics of a protable breath actuated, particle size selective medical aerosol inhaler. J Aerosol Sci 1982; 13:1–7.
4. Bloomfield P, Crompton GK, Winsey NJP. A tube spacer to improve inhalation of drugs from pressurised aerosols. Br Med J 1979; 2:1479.
5. Bisgaard H, Olsson S. PEP-spacer: an adaptation for administration of metered-dose inhalers to infants. Allergy 1989; 44:363–364.
6. O'Callaghan C, Milner AD, Swarbrick A. Spacer device with face mask attachment for giving bronchodilators to infants with asthma. Br Med J 1989; 298:160–161.
7. Conner WT, Dolovich MB, Frame RA, Newhouse MT. Reliable salbutamol administration in 6- to 36-month-old children by means of a metered dose inhaler and Aerochamber with mask. Pediatr Pulmonol 1989; 6:263–267.
8. Bisgaard H, Munck SL, Nielsen JP, Petersen W, Ohlsson SV. Inhaled budesonide for treatment of recurrent wheezing in early childhood. Lancet 1990; 336:649–651.
9. Kraemer R, Frey U, Sommer W, Russi E. Short-term effect of albuterol, delivered via a new auxiliary device in wheezy infants. Am Rev Respir Dis 1991; 144:347–351.
10. Kraemer R, Birrer P, Modelska K, Casaulta Aebischer C, Schöni MH. A new baby-spacer device for aerosolized bronchodilator administration in infants with bronchopulmonary disease. Eur J Pediatr 1992; 151:57–60.
11. Clarke JR, Aston H, Silverman M. Delivery of salbutamol by metered dose inhaler and valved spacer to wheezy infants: effect on bronchial responsiveness. Arch Dis Child 1993;69:125–129.
12. Bisgaard H. Delivery of inhaled medication to children. J Asthma 1997; 34:443–468.
13. Kim CS, Eldridge A, Sackner MA. Oropharyngeal deposition and delivery aspects of metered-dose inhaler aerosols. Am Rev Respir Dis 1987; 135:157–164.
14. Ahrens R, Lux C, Bahl T, Han S-H. Choosing the metered-dose inhaler spacer or holding chamber that matches the patient's need: evidence that the specific drug being delivered is an important consideration. J Allergy Clin Immunol 1995; 96:288–294.
15. Bisgaard H. Drug delivery from inhaler devices (Editorial). Br Med J 1996; 313:895–896.
16. Pedersen S. Aerosol treatment of bronchoconstriction in children with or without a tube spacer. N Engl J Med 1983; 308:1328–1330.
17. Lee H, Evans HE. Evaluation of inhalation aids of metered dose inhalers in asthmatic children. Chest 1987; 91:366–369.

18. König P. Spacer devices used with metered-dose inhalers—breakthrough or gimmick? Chest 1985; 88:276–284.
19. Pedersen S. Inhaler use in children with asthma. Danish Med Bull 1987; 34:234–249.
20. Salzman GA, Pyszczynski DR. Oropharyngeal candidiasis in patients treated with beclomethasone dipropionate delivered by metered-dose inhaler alone and with AeroChamber. J Allergy Clin Immunol 1988; 81:424–428.
21. Morgan M, Singh B, Frame M, Williams S. Terbutaline aerosol given through a pear spacer in acute severe asthma. Br Med J 1982; 285:849–850.
22. Fuglsang G, Pedersen S. Comparison of Nebuhaler and nebuliser treatment of acute severe asthma in children. Eur J Respir Dis 1986; 69:109–113.
23. Keeley D. Large volume plastic spacers in asthma (commentary). Br Med J 1992; 305:598–599.
24. Bisgaard H, Anhøj J, Klug B, Berg E. A non-electrostatic spacer for aerosol delivery. Arch Dis Child 1995; 73:226–230.
25. Zak M, Madsen J, Berg E, Bülow J, Bisgaard H. A mathematical model of aerosol holding chambers. J Aerosol Med 1999; 12: 187–196.
26. Levison H, Reilly PA, Worsley GH. Spacing devices and metered-dose inhalers in childhood asthma. J Pediatr 1985; 107:662–668.
27. Barry PW, O'Callaghan C. Inhalational drug delivery from seven different spacer devices. Thorax 1996; 51:835–840.
28. Lipworth BJ, Clark DJ. Early lung absorption profile of non-CFC salbutamol via small and large volume spacer devices. Br J Clin Pharmacol 1998; 46:45–48.
29. Barry PW, O'Callaghan C. In vitro comparison of the amount of salbutamol available for inhalation from different formulations used with different spacer devices. Eur Respir J 1997; 10:1345–1348.
30. Dhand R, Malik K, Balakrishnan M, Verma SR. High speed photographic analysis of aerosols produced by metered dose inhalers. J Pharm Pharmacol 1988; 40:429–480.
31. Laschka B, PernPeintner A. Strömungsverhalten bei "Rondo"—Ringwirbelvernebelung zur optimierten Dosier-Aerosol-Inhalation. Atemz Lungenkrkh 1990; 16:S40–S44.
32. O'Callaghan C, Lynch J, Cant M, Robertson C. Improvement in sodium cromoglycate delivery from a spacer device used of antistatic lining, immediate inhalation, and avoiding multiple actuations of drug. Thorax 1993; 48:603–606.
33. Bisgaard H. Dose of aerosol inhaled in young children from a small-volume spacer. Eur J Respir Dis 1993; 6:352.
34. Bisgaard H. A metal aerosol holding chamber devised for young children with asthma. Eur Respir J 1995; 8:856–860.
35. Janssens HM, Devadason SG, Hop WCJ, LeSouëf PN, De Jongste JC, Tiddens HAWM. Variability of aerosol delivery via spacer devices in young asthmatic children in daily life. Eur Respir J 1999; 13:787–791.
36. Dewsbury NJ, Kenyon CJ, Newman SP. The effect of handling techniques on electrostatic charge on spacer devices: a correlation with in vitro particle size analysis. Int J Pharm 1996; 137:261–264.

37. Wildhaber JH, Devadason SG, Hayden MJ, James R, Dufty AP, Fox RA, Summers QA, LeSouëf PN. Electrostatic charge on a plastic spacer device influences the delivery of salbutamol. Eur Respir J 1996; 9:1943–1946.
38. Berg E, Madsen, J, Bisgaard H. In vitro performance of three combinations of spacers and pressurized metered dose inhalers for treatment of children. Eur Respir J 1998; 12:472–476.
39. Anhøj J, Bisgaard H, Lipworth BJ. Effect of electrostatic charge in plastic spacers on the lung delivery of HFA-salbutamol in children. Br J Clin Pharmacol 1999; 47:333–336.
40. Clark DJ, Lipworth BJ. Effect of multiple actuations, delayed inhalation and antistatic treatment on the lung bioavailability of salbutamol via a spacer device. Thorax 1996;51:981–984.
41. Kenyon CJ, Thorsson L, Borgström L, Newman SP. The effects of static charge in spacer devices on glucocorticosteroid aerosol deposition in asthmatic patients. Eur Respir J 1998; 11:606–610.
42. Piérart F, Wildhaber JH, Vrancken I, Devadason SG, Le Souëf PN. Washing plastic spacers in household detergent reduces electrostatic charge and greatly improves delivery. Eur Respir J 1999; 13:673–678.
43. Barry PW, O'Callaghan C. The effect of delay, multiple actuations and spacer static charge on the in vitro delivery of budesonide from the Nebuhaler. Br J Clin Pharmacol 1995; 40:76–78.
44. Wildhaber JH, Devadason SG, Eber E, Hayden MJ, Everard ML, Summers QA, LeSoüef PN. Effect of electrostatic charge, flow, delay and multiple actuations on the in vitro delivery of salbutamol from different small volume spacers for infants. Thorax 1996; 51:985–988.
45. Finlay WH, Zuberbuhler P. In vitro comparison of beclomethasone and salbutamol metered-dose inhaler aerosols inhaled during pediatric tidal breathing from four valved holding chambers. Chest 1998; 114:1676–1680.
46. Reilly PA, Yahav J, Mindorff C et al. Dose-response characteristics of nebulized fenoterol in asthmatic children. J Pediatr 1983; 103:121–126.
47. Harvey JE, Tattersfield AE. Airway response to salbutamol: effect of regular salbutamol inhalations in normal atopic and asthmatic subjects. Thorax 1982; 37:280–287.
48. Rivlin J, Mindorff C, Levison H, et al. Effect of administration technique on bronchodilator response to fenoterol in a metered dose inhaler. J Pediatr 1983; 102:470–472.
49. Shore SC, Weinberg EG. Administration of bronchodilator to young children. Br Med J 1973; 2:350.
50. Cushley MJ, Lewis RA, Tattersfield AE. Comparison of three techniques of inhalation on the airway response to terbutaline. Thorax 1983; 38:908–913.
51. Borgström L, Derom E, Ståhl E, Wåhlin-Boll E, Pauwels R. The inhalation device influences lung deposition and bronchodilating effect of terbutaline. Am J Respir Crit Care Med 1996; 153:1636–1640.
52. Dolovich M, Ruffin R, Corr D et al. Clinical evaluation of a simple demand inhalation MDI aerosol delivery device. Chest 1983; 84:36–41.

53. Ashurt IC, Ambrose CV, Russel DJ. Pharmaceutical evaluation of a new spacer device for delivery of metered-dose inhalers to infants and young children. J Aerosol Sci 1992; 23:S499–S502.
54. Agertoft L, Pedersen S. Influence of spacer device on drug delivery to young children with asthma. Arch Dis Child 1994; 71:217–220.
55. Mallol J, Barrueto L, Girardi G, Toro O. Bronchodilator effect of fenoterol and ipratropium bromide in infants with acute wheezing: use of pMDI with a spacer device. Pediatr Pulmonol 1987; 3:352–356.
56. Henry RL, Milner AD, Davies JG. Simple drug delivery system for use by young asthmatics. Br Med J 1983; 286:2021.
57. Yuksel B, Greenough A, Maconochie I. Effective bronchodilator treatment by a simple spacer device for wheezy premature infants. Arch Dis Child 1990; 65:782–785.
58. Sritara P, Janvitayanuchit S. Improvement of inhaler efficacy by home-made spacer. J Med Assoc Thai 1993; 76(12):693–697.
59. Zar HJ, Liebenberg M, Weinberg EG, Binns HJ, Mann MD. The efficacy of alternative spacer devices for delivery of aerosol therapy to children with asthma. Ann Trop Paediatr 1998; 18(2):75–79.
60. Berg E. In vitro properties of pressurized metered dose inhalers with and without spacer devices. J Aerosol Med 1995; 8(suppl 3):3–11.
61. Thorsson L, Edsbäcker S. Lung deposition of budesonide from a pressurized metered-dose inhaler attached to a spacer. Eur Respir J 1998; 12:1340–1345.
62. Everard ML, Clark AR, Milner AD. Drug delivery from holding chambers with attached facemask. Arch Dis Child 1992; 67:580–585.
63. Barry PW, O'Callaghan C. Multiple actuations of salbutamol MDI into a spacer device reduce the amount of drug recovered in the respirable range. Eur Respir J 1994; 7:1707–1709.
64. Rau JL, Restrepo RD, Deshpande V. Inhalation of single vs multiple metered-dose bronchodilator actuations from reservoir devices. Chest 1996; 109;109:969–974.
65. Uhlig T, Eber E, Devadason SG, Pemberton P, Badawi N, LeSouëf PN, Wildhaber JH. Aerosol delivery to spontaneously breathing neonates: spacer or nebulizer? Pediatr Asthma Allergy Immunol 1997; 11:111–117.
66. Tal A, Golan H, Grauer N, Aviram M, Albin D, Quastel MR. Deposition pattern of radiolabeled salbutamol inhaled from a metered-dose inhaler by means of a spacer with mask in young children with airway obstruction. J Pediatr 1996; 128:479–484.
67. Wildhaber JH, Dore ND, Wilson JM, Devadason SG, LeSouëf PN. Inhalation therapy in asthma: nebulizer or pressurized metered-dose inhaler with holding chamber? In vivo comparison of lung deposition in children. J Pediatr 1999; 135:28–33.
68. Chua HL, Collis GG, Newbury AM, Chan K, Bower GD, Sly PD, Le Souëf PN. The influence of age on aerosol deposition in children with cystic fibrosis. Eur Respir J 1994; 7:2185–2191.
69. Becquemin MH, Swift DL, Bouchikhi A, Roy M, Teillac A. Particle deposition and resistance in the nose of adults and children. Eur Respir J 1991; 4:694–702.

70. Zar HJ, Weinberg EG, Binns HJ, Gallie F, Mann MD. Lung deposition of aerosol—a comparison of different spacers. Arch Dis Child 2000; 82(6):495–498.
71. Wilkie RA, Bryan MH. Effect of bronchodilators on airway resistance in ventilator-dependent neonates with chronic lung disease. J Pediatr 1987; 111:278–282.
72. Lee H, Arnon S, Silverman M. Bronchodilator aerosol administered by metered dose inhaler and spacer in subacute neonatal respiratory distress syndrome. Arch Dis Child 1994; 70:F218–F222.
73. Gappa M, Gartner M, Poets CF, von der Hardt H. Effects of salbutamol delivery from a metered dose inhaler versus jet nebulizer on dynamic lung mechanics in very preterm infants with chronic lung disease. Pediatr Pulmonol 1997; 23:442–448.
74. Yuksel B, Greenough A. Randomised trial of inhaled steroids in preterm infants with respiratory symptoms at follow up. Thorax 1992; 47:910–913.
75. Fisher JT, Mortola JP, Smith JB, Fox GS, Weeks S. Respiration in newborns: development of the control of breathing. Am Rev Respir Dis 1982; 125:650–657.
76. Benito-Zaballos MP, Pedraz Garcia C, Salazar A, Villalobos V. Pulmonary function in preterm and full term infants during the neonatal period: 1. Respiratory pattern. Ann Esp Ped 1991; 35:243–247.
77. Riedler J, Robertson CF. Effect of tidal volume on the output and particle size distribution of hypertonic saline from an ultrasonic nebulizer. Eur Resp J 1994; 7:998–1002.
78. Marsh MJ, Ingram D, Milner AD. The effect of instrumental dead space on measurement of breathing pattern and pulmonary mechanics in the newborn. Pediatr Pulmonol 1993; 16:316–322.
79. Fok TF, Monkman S, Dolovich M, Gray S, Coates G, Paes B, Rashid F, Newhouse M, Kirpalani H, Efficiency of aerosol medication delivery from a metered dose inhaler versus jet nebulizer in infants with bronchopulmonary dysplasia. Pediatr Pulmonol 1996; 21:301–309.
80. Rau JL, Harwood RJ, Groff JL. Evaluation of a reservoir device for metered-dose bronchodilator delivery to intubated adults: an in vitro study. Chest 1992; 102:924–930.
81. Wildhaber JH, Hayden MJ, Dore ND, Devadason SG, LeSouëf PN. Salbutamol delivery from a HFA pMDI in paediatric ventilator circuits. An in vitro study. Chest 1998; 113:186–191.
82. Diot P, Morra L, Smaldone GC. Albuterol delivery in a model of mechanical ventilation: comparison of metered-dose inhaler and nebulizer efficiency. Am J Respir Crit Care Med 1995; 152:1391–1394.
83. Everard ML, Stammers J, Hardy JG, Milner AD. New aerosol delivery system for neonatal ventilator circuits. Arch Dis Child 1992; 67:826–830.
84. Fink JB, Dhand R, Duarte AGJenne JW, Tobin MJ. Aerosol delivery from a metered-dose inhaler during mechanical ventilation: an in vitro model. Am J Respir Crit Care Med 1996; 154:382–387.
85. Fuller HD, Dolovich MB, Chambers C, Newhouse MT. Aerosol delivery during mechanical ventilation: a predictive in-vitro lung model. J Aerosol Med 1992; 5:251–259.

86. Arnon S, Grigg J, Nikander K, Silverman M. Delivery of micronized budesonide suspension by metered dose inhaler and jet nebulizer into a neonatal ventilator circuit. Pediatr Pulmonol 1992; 13:172–175.
87. Gay PC, Patel HG, Nelson SB, Gilles B, Hubmayr RD. Metered dose inhalers for bronchodilator delivery in intubated, mechanically ventilated patients. Chest 1991; 99:66–71.
88. Fuller HD, Dolovich MB, Posmituck G, Pack WW, Newhouse MT. Pressurised aerosol versus jet aerosol delivery to mechanically ventilated patients. Am Rev Respir Dis 1990; 141:440–444.
89. Sivakumar D, Bosque E, Goldman SL. Bronchodilator delivered by metered dose inhaler and spacer improves respiratory system compliance more than nebulizer-delivered bronchodilator in ventilated premature infants. Pediatr Pulmonol 1999; 27:208–212.
90. Newman SP, Steed K, Hooper G, Källén A, Borgström L. Comparison of gamma scintigraphy and a pharmacokinetic technique for assessing pulmonary deposition of terbutaline sulphate delivered by pressurized metered dose inhaler. Pharm Res 1995; 12:231–236.
91. Vidgren P, Vidgren M, Paronen P, Vainio P, Nuutinen J. Effects of inspirease holding chamber on the deposition of metered dose inhalation aerosols. Eur J Drug Metab Pharmacokinet 1991; 3:419–425.
92. Thorsson L, Kenyon C, Newman SP, Borgström L. Lung deposition of budesonide in asthmatics: a comparison of different formulations. Int J Pharm 1998: 119–127.
93. Melchor R, Biddiscombe MF, Mak VHF, Short MD, Spiro SG. Lung deposition patterns of directly labelled salbutamol in normal subjects and in patients with reversible airflow obstruction. Thorax 1993; 48:506–511.
94. Tobin MT, Jenouri G, Danta I, Kim CS, Watson H, Sackner MA. Response to bronchodilator drug administration by a new reservoir aerosol delivery system and a review of other auxiliary systems. Am Rev Respir Dis 1982; 126:670–675.
95. Morris J, Milledge JS, Moszoro H, Higgins A. The efficacy of drug delivery by a pear-shaped spacer and metered dose inhaler. Br J Dis Chest 1984; 78:383–389.
96. Hindle M, Chrystyn H. Nebuhaler and volumatic improve pulmonary delivery. Arch Dis Child 1992;67:580–585.
97. Fuglsang G, Pedersen S. Cumulative dose response relationship of terbutaline delivered by three different inhalers. Allergy 1988;43:348–352.
98. Gurwitz D, Levison H, Mindorff C, Reilly P, Worsley G. Assessment of a new device (Aerochamber) for use with aerosol drugs in asthmatic children. Ann Allergy 1983; 50:166–170.
99. Anhøj J, Thorsson L, Bisgaard H. Lung deposition of inhaled drugs increases with age. Am J Respir Crit Care Med 2000.
100. Bisgaard H. Automatic actuation of a dry powder inhaler into a nonelectrostatic spacer. Am J Respir Crit Care Med 1998; 157:518–521.

13

Dry-Powder Inhalers

LARS BORGSTRÖM

AstraZeneca R&D
Lund
Uppsala University
Uppsala, Sweden

HANS BISGAARD

Copenhagen University Hospital
Rigshospitalet
Copenhagen, Denmark

CHRIS O'CALLAGHAN

University of Leicester
Leicester, England

SØREN PEDERSEN

University of Southern Denmark
Odense, Denmark
McMaster University
Hamilton, Ontario, Canada

I. Introduction

The first commercially successful dry-powder inhaler (DPI) was Spinhaler, introduced by Fisons 30 years ago for the delivery of disodium cromoglycate (DSCG) (1). A number of DPIs using different dosing principles have since then reached the market. Rotahaler (GlaxoSmithKline, UK) (2) and Cyclohaler/Aerolizer (ISF, Italy; Novartis, Switzerland) use single prefilled capsules, while Diskhaler (GlaxoSmithKline, UK) (3) is a multidose system using disks with four or eight doses. The first modern DPI, Turbuhaler (AstraZeneca, Sweden), is a multidose reservoir-type of inhaler using a dosing disk to meter the dose (4). Diskus/Accuhaler (GlaxoSmithKline, UK) (5) was launched in the mid-1990s and has an internal system reminiscent of that used in an old-fashioned cap gun. This involves a blister strip of double foil, with each of the 60 blisters containing a set dose of powder. The simplicity and the ability of the new DPIs to deliver multiple doses of the drug over a prolonged period of time, together with an indicator/warning system allowing the patient to know when devices were running out, has established dry-powder devices as a major competitor to the pressurized metered-dose inhaler (pMDI).

The popularity of DPIs received a major boost following the implementation of the 1989 Montreal Protocol, which aims to phase out the use of chlorofluorocarbons (CFCs) due to their potential to breakdown of the earth's protective ozone layer. Since this time, DPIs have appeared to many as an obvious replacement for the delivery of drugs via pMDIs using CFC propellants. A change of pMDI propellant from CFCs to hydrofluoroalkanes (HFAs) is ongoing, but concerns have been expressed about the global warming potential of HFAs. A major practical advantage with DPIs as compared with pMDIs is that there is no need to coordinate actuation and inhalation, since the dose will follow the inhaled air into the lungs (6). In addition, some patients using a pMDI stop inhaling when they feel the aerosol cloud in their mouths. Multidose DPIs are as simple to operate as the pMDIs and their size and compact design make them equally convenient.

The chapter starts with a brief overview of different principles for dry powder formulation and continues with how the particles are generated at inhalation. Then the importance—for both children and adults—of the intrinsic resistance of an inhaler for the clinical outcome is discussed. Before enumerating the marketed and also some investigational inhalers, a quick word on the importance of humidity for their performances is given. Finally, lung deposition and its variability is dealt with before the chapter is rounded off by some safety aspects of DPIs.

II. Dry-Powder Formulations

An inhaled formulation—be it a pMDI, nebulized, or dry-powder formulation—is made up of two components: the device and the pharmaceutical formulation (see Fig. 1). The device determines the aerodynamic and flow properties and the

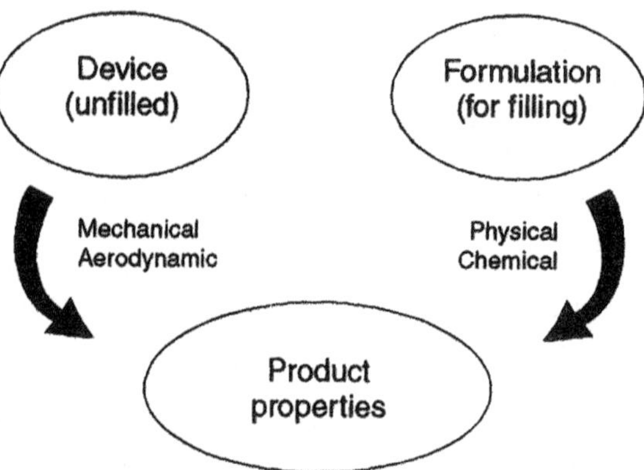

Figure 1 An inhaled formulation is composed of the unfilled device and the pharmaceutical formulation.

pharmaceutical formulation sets the physical and chemical properties of the resulting formulation. Differences in the aerodynamic and mechanical properties of the inhaler thus will affect the quality of the resulting aerosol. Each combination of device and pharmaceutical formulation has to be judged on its own merits. Thus, we should not, for instance, take a gelatin capsule for Aerolizer and use it in Rotahaler to gain information on how the Aerolizer caspule or Rotahaler device performs. Of special interest for DPIs is the intrinsic inhalation resistance of a device. All currently marketed DPIs rely on the inspiratory effort of the patient to lift the powder from the drug reservoir, the dosing disk, the blister, the capsule, etc. The same effort also deaggregates the powder into particles small enough to have a fair chance to reach the patient's lungs. A more forceful inhalation through an inspiratory flow driven inhaler will result in better deaggregation, more fine particles, and a higher amount of drug reaching the lungs (7).

With regard to the pharmaceutical formulation the size of the substance crystals, or particles, after manufacturing is much too large to allow the particles to reach the airways at inhalation. The particles in the generated aerosol cloud should have an aerodynamic diameter of about 2–4 μm (8) or smaller (9) to have a good chance of reaching the lower airways during inhalation. In addition, it has been shown that the fine-particle dose, defined as the dose of drug in particles <5 μm, is linearly correlated to the degree of lung deposition for a range of DPIs (10). Thus, the manufactured large particles must be made smaller, and it is common to mill or micronize the crystals/particles down to the more optimal particle size, in most cases around 2–4 μm. An alternative to milling for the production of the fine powder is spray drying, which allows more control of particle shape, surface properties, and size (11). For example, it has been shown that a spray-dried powder formulation of DSCG can produce more drug in fine particles than when the drug is micronized (12). Milling, or spray drying however, generates another problem. The resulting small particles cannot be handled in the pharmaceutical production or in an inhaler, as the particles will adhere to most surfaces due to Van der Waals and electrostatic forces. The particles must be made larger again! This problem has been solved in two distinctly different ways. The one way is to use large, about 30- to 300-μm (most often 50- to 150-μm) carrier particles, such as lactose or glucose, which are blended with the smaller drug particles. The surface of the carrier particles has energy-rich sites and the small drug particles adhere to these sites on the carrier particles at blending (13,14). First, the most energy-rich sites are covered with drug particles and eventually also the less energy-rich sites. The properties of the resulting, ordered mixture pharmaceutical formulation, means that the powder now can be handled in the production process, in the inhaler, and at inhalation (Fig. 2). The adhesion of the small particles to the carrier must not be too strong as they should detach during inhalation. The roughness of the carrier and the time and speed of mixing may have a significant effect on the adhesion of the small particles to the carrier particle. Lactose

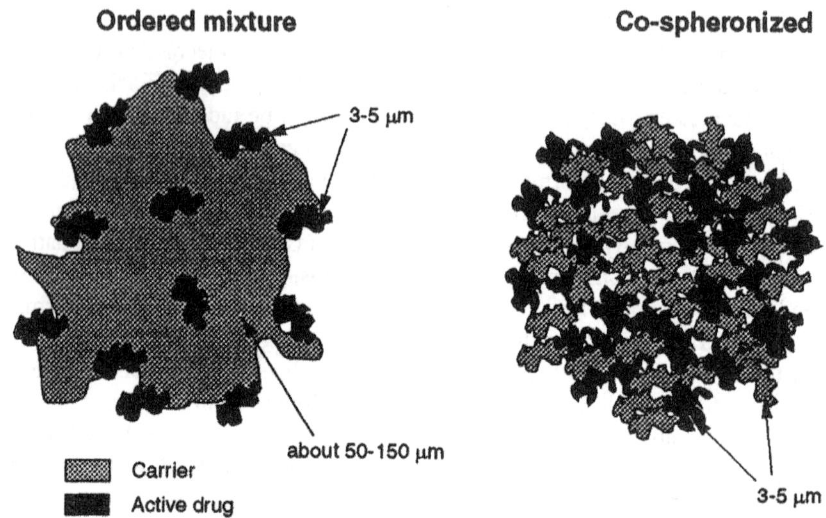

Figure 2 An ordered mixture and a co-spheronized formulation. The active drug particles are of the same size, while the lactose components are of very different size in the two formulations.

with a smooth surface has been shown to deliver a significantly higher fine-particle fraction than lactose particles with a rougher surface (15,16). For practical reasons, the different dose strengths of the same formulation use the same amount of carrier and thus, for the higher doses, each carrier particle carries more drug. For the higher doses, where also the less energy-rich sites are covered with drug particles, the mean strength of the drug–carrier binding becomes weaker [e.g., the 500-μg fluticasone Diskus will deliver about 120 μg (24% of the nominal dose) as fine particles, while the 50-μg fluticasone Diskus will deliver only about 7 μg (14% of the nominal dose) as fine particles—a 20- instead of the expected 10-fold difference (17). Optimization of the drug/carrier ratio as well as reduction in carrier particle size has been shown to increase the fine-particle fraction of drug in the aerosol. Additional formulation components such as L-leucine or magnesium stearate will change the binding forces between drug and carrier and can increase the fine-particle fraction.

The other way to solve the problem with the small particles and the Van der Waals and electrostatic forces is to tumble the 2- to 4-μm particles to form larger spheres. The resulting spheres have free-flowing properties, meaning that they can be handled in the pharmaceutical production and in the inhaler. This method has been used for the Turbuhaler formulations. The method is the same whether the pharmaceutical formulation contains only pure drug, as is the case for Pulmicort (budesonide) Turbuhaler, or when a mixture of pure drug(s) and micronized lactose is used, as is the case for Oxis (formoterol and lactose) and Symbicort (budesonide, formoterol, and lactose) Turbuhaler. This pharmaceutical principle will not give rise to any nonlinearity when different strengths of the same substance are formulated, as the resulting pharmaceutical formulation is a homogeneous mixture of the micronized components (17).

A third way to formulate a dry powder is to take advantage of the difference between geometric and aerodynamic diameter. The aerodynamic diameter of a particle is equivalent to the diameter of a unit-density sphere that has the same terminal settling velocity in still air, and is the best parameter for defining the dimension of aerosol particles. It has been suggested that administering particles with a large geometric diameter to the lungs may increase bioavailability by reducing phagocytosis (18). Porous particles, also known as large fluffy particles, have been designed to reach the lower airways. They have a large geometric but a "normal" aerodynamic diameter. Their actual geometric dimensions can be greater than 30 μm, but as they have a low density, their aerodynamic diameter can still be less than 5 μm, small enough to deposit in the lungs (19).

III. Dispersion of Powders in a DPI

There are a number of forces that influence the dispersion of the dry-powder particles into an aerosolized cloud suitable for inhalation. These include Van der Waals, electrostatic, capillary, and friction forces. Attraction of like materials—that is, drug particle to drug particle—are called *cohesive forces* and attraction of materials that are unlike each other—for example, the carrier particle to the drug particle or the drug particle to the delivery device surface—are called *adhesive forces*. Within a dry powder, Van der Waals forces are dominant. However, under special conditions, capillary forces can be very much higher than both Van der Waals and electrostatic forces. Fortunately, capillary forces are produced only at humidities that tend to rise to greater than 65%. They are formed by the condensation of water that may form high tensile liquid bridges. The observed electrostatic charge is generated from particles that are separated from the bulk material or where there is contact to other surfaces. Mechanical interlocking and friction may be significant between irregular, large carrier particles and small drug particles. For example, small drug particles may enter into cavities within the carrier particle, from which it may be difficult for them to escape.

IV. Aerosol Generation from a DPI

When the inhalation starts, the powder is contained in the dosing disk, the capsule, or the blister. The inhalation initiates the dispersion of particles when enough space is created between the particles for them to pass around and over each other in the direction of the flow. The flow of the particles is not predictable due to the nonuniform shape of dry powders and the various adhesive and cohesive forces. When more air is drawn through the powder, it starts to fluidize. Fluidization is defined as the mobilization of a bulk powder by air. In gas-assisted fluidization, gas (air) is actually forced through the powder and fluidization occurs when a low-pressure field is established close to the powder. A pressure difference between the air contained in the powder and the motion of air passing over the powder is developed and the powder is fluidized. Shear force fluidization occurs when a gas stream is passed over a powder source and the particles on the surface experience reduced interparticulate forces. Collisions with other particles may occur and the particles bounce, resulting in incipient fluidization. Vibrational fluidization occurs, for example, when the powder is shaken and falls through the air by gravitational forces.

Aggregates of carriers and drug particles, or drug clusters, are dispersed into primary particles in a process known as *deaggregation* (see Fig. 3). Adhesive and cohesive forces between small particles need to be overcome for deaggregation to occur. The principal force leading to deaggregation is thought to be turbulence. But also shear stress, electrostatics, collision, and relative motion are involved. In the overall process a portion of the metered dry-powder dose is turned into an aerosol cloud to be inhaled by the patient. Even for an efficient inhaler, not more than around 50% of the metered dose is turned into fine particles that have a good chance of reaching the lungs. The remaining portion leaves the inhaler as aggregates or is retained in the device. For a general discussion of in vitro delivery from DPIs see the articles by de Boer (20–22).

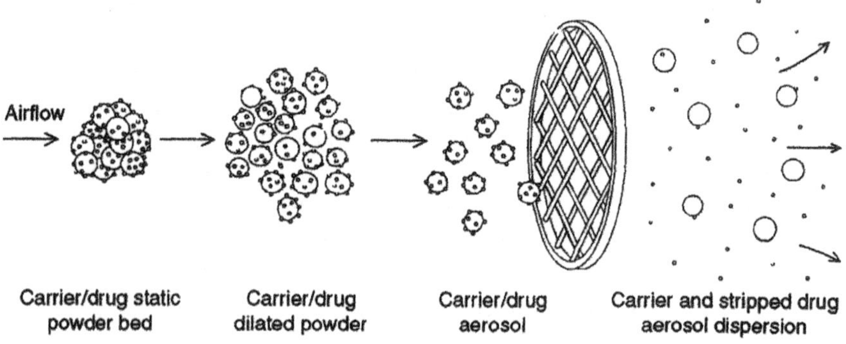

Figure 3 A schematic diagram of the deaggregation of an ordered mixture formula.

V. Particle Size Determination from DPIs

Determination of the aerosol particle size is currently performed using a variety of impactor systems, including the twin, Andersen, and multistage liquid impingers (see Chap. 4, "Predictability of in Vitro Measurements for Lung Deposition"). The traditional methods of sizing particles in an aerosol are designed to study aerosols already generated and presented as a standing cloud of particles at a defined constant flow. The aerosol passes through the device and is fractionated with progressively smaller and smaller particles being collected on the distal stages. A standardized constant flow is a prerequisite for the assumption of a defined particle size at a defined stage of the impactor device. The use of this equipment for studying dry-powder inhalers presents two fundamental problems.

A. Flow

The energy input dispersing the aerosol is related to the flow through and the resistance of the device. Therefore, DPIs of different resistances cannot be compared at similar flows. Rather the devices should be compared at a similar inspiratory effort which is reflected in the European Pharmacopoiea recommendation to test DPIs at the same 4-kPa pressure drop (23). The ability to inhale and generate this effort could be dependent on age, patient group, etc., and this information should be obtained for the different DPIs—e.g., by measuring flow through various resistances or inhalers by patients belonging to different groups. The use of effort instead of flow as comparator has improved the relevance of comparison between DPIs (24).

B. Flow Profile

Particle size impactors operate at constant flows. The aerosol output from DPIs has often been studied by abruptly increasing the flow through the DPI in a stepwise fashion. That is, the rise time from zero to desired flow is extremely short and does not necessarily mimic patient inhalation. Flow acceleration at the start of inhalation is probably more important in terms of aerosol dispersion than the actual flow achieved (see below) (25).

A new development in methodology, the electronic lung, has tried to address this problem. The patient's inhalation profile, pressure versus time, through a device is recorded and subsequently replayed in the laboratory. This allows aerosol output to be evaluated from each individual patient's performance in a laboratory setting with a given device. The recorded inhalation profiles are replayed and used to control a piston creating a true image of the patient's inhalation maneuver: The simulated inhalation actuates the DPI into a large metal holding chamber where the aerosol is available as a standing cloud ready to be analyzed by a routine impactor method. Bisgaard and colleagues recently used this system to study the performance of the Diskus and Turbuhaler DPIs in two groups of children aged 4 (n=18) and 8 years (n=18), respectively (25). The children had been trained intensively in a clinic and by their parents. Initial results demonstrated a very highly variable inhalation performance both between and within the children. Second, it became apparent that the peak inspiratory flow (PIF) was often reached long after the aerosol had been emitted from the DPI. The initial acceleration of flow seemed a more relevant determinant of the aerosol characteristics. For a normal inhalation PIF can be seen as a surrogate parameter for the flow at dose release. A higher PIF will mean that the dose has been released at a higher flow and a steeper flow acceleration than a lower PIF.

The fine-particle dose in this in vitro setup was significantly increased in the 8-year-old children as compared with the 4-year-old children for both devices. The relative difference was larger for Turbuhaler. The fine-particle dose for Turbuhaler in the 8-year-old children was approximately twice that of Diskus. The coefficient of variation (CV) for the interindividual scatter around the mean was approximately 28% in the 8-year-olds using Turbuhaler but 10% from Diskus. The CV was even higher from Turbuhaler in 4-year-olds, while the CV in 4- and 8-years-olds using Diskus was the same. The results suggested that the Diskus inhaler might be expected to provide the same dose reproducibility in children aged 4 and 8. For a discussion on the relevance of in vitro variability for the in vivo variability see below, under "Variability in Lung Deposition."

VI. Inhalation Resistance of DPIs

In an acute asthma exacerbation, a constrained situation, it is a common misconception that the inspiratory flow is heavily reduced. This is not the case! In the constricted lung, airway resistance increases at expiration due to the increased pressure on the airways. Expiration becomes slow and difficult resulting in a heavily reduced maximal expiratory flow. At inhalation, the lung volume increases, pressure on the airways lessens and is reversed, and maximal inspiratory flow is thus less affected by the asthmatic bronchial narrowing than is maximal expiratory flow (26,27). Specifically it has been shown that expiratory flow decreased from 320 L/min at a low degree of dyspnea to 45 L/min in heavily dyspneic subjects (27). Inspiratory flow decreased much less, from 269 to 188 L/min over the same range of dyspnea; the ratio of mean expiratory versus mean inspiratory flow decreased from 1.20 to 0.23. In other words, the asthmatic patient, even in an acute situation, can generate a high inhalation flow through a DPI, but for a much shorter time due to the low inhaled volume. What is more, a DPI will probably perform better than a pMDI in acute asthma, as it is not the inhalation force that is reduced but rather the inhaled volume. When a pMDI is used in an acute situation, the coordination of actuation and inhalation becomes more critical.

Different DPIs have different intrinsic inhalation resistances which govern the resulting peak inhalation flow generated by the patient at inhalation (24,28–30). All inhalers need a certain effort to lift the dry powder from the dose-metering unit and to disperse the powder into a dry-powder aerosol. Assuming the same inhalation effort, a high-resistance inhaler will perform adequately at a lower inhalation flow than a low-resistance inhaler (Fig. 4). At inhalation, the lung and the inhaler are in series and the total pressure drop (R_{tot}) is the sum of the pressure drop over the inhaler (R_{inh}) and the airways (R_{airw}); this equals the total pressure drop that is developed by the chest muscles: $R_{tot}=R_{inh} + R_{airw}$. The smallest cross-sectional area determines the resistance. For high-resistance inhalers, it is the inhaler that determines the resistance: $R_{inh}>>R_{airw}$. For low-resistance inhalers, both the inhaler and the lung influence the overall resistance: $R_{inh}\approx R_{airw}$. This means that the performance of a low-resistance inhaler will be more sensitive to the patient's degree of bronchoconstriction than the performance of a high-resistance inhaler. With a low-resistance inhaler, the patient will not be able to generate the same peak inspiratory flow during a severe bronchoconstriction compared to when they are well, as the constriction in the lung now limits the inhalation flow. Turbuhaler has a higher resistance than Rotahaler, and the flow needed to get a good bronchodilating effect is lower (about 30 L/min) than for Rotahaler (about 70 L/min) (31,32). For the low-resistance Rotahaler, especially during an exacerbation, the resistance of the airways will proba-

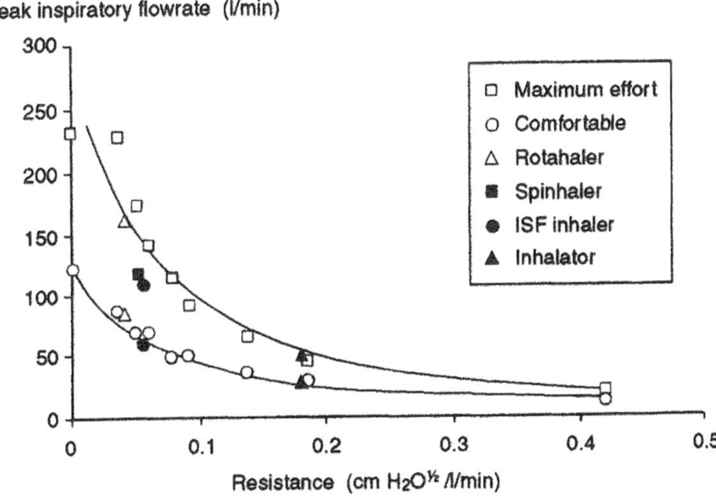

Figure 4 The relationship between the inhaler resistance and peak inhalation flow rate for healthy volunteers. The two curves indicate a maximum effort and a comfortable effort at inhalation. (From Ref. 28.)

bly influence the resulting PIF. For Turbuhaler, with its higher intrinsic resistance, the inhaler is the restrictive part while the resistance in the airways has negligible influence on the resulting PIF. Results in accordance with this theoretical discussion have been presented in two different studies from the same group. In the first study, using the low-resistance Rotahaler (32), the difference in PIF through Rotahaler at acute wheeze and when the patient's pulmonary function had improved was significant. In the second study, the PIF through Turbuhaler seemed to be less sensitive to the degree of lung restriction (31).

The difference in inhalation flow can also influence the degree of oropharyngeal deposition as has been shown for pMDIs (33). When a high inhalation flow is being used, more of the drug will deposit in the oropharynx as compared with a low inhalation flow, which is more optimal with regard to this parameter.

VII. The Clinical Importance of the Resistance of a DPI

As touched upon earlier, a more forceful inhalation through an inspiratory-flow-driven DPI will result in better deaggregation, more fine particles, and a higher amount of drug reaching the lungs (7) until a plateau level of fine-particle dose and lung deposition is reached. After the plateau has been reached, an even more forceful inhalation will decrease the amount of the inhaled drug that will impact on the back of the oral cavity during inhalation. This is due to the inertia of the particles. A higher degree of impaction will result in a lower amount of drug reaching the lungs. Theoretically, one could thus imagine a situation where the balance between deaggregation and impaction for a specific inhaler would tip over, so that a more forceful inhalation would decrease the amount of drug reaching the lungs. All DPIs on the market are driven by inspiratory flow and available information indicates that for these inhalers the flow at which this balance is reached is probably higher than the upper flow limit that the patient can achieve. Thus, to achieve a high lung deposition with a DPI, a forceful inhalation resulting in a high inhalation flow should be aimed at.

On the other hand, for a DPI that does not rely on the patient's inhalation effort to deaggregate the powder formulation, we can expect to see the reverse: a high flow will result in a decrease in the amount of drug reaching the lungs, as compared with a low flow. This has also been shown to be the case for one inhaler, Spiros (Dura Pharmaceuticals, USA), which uses an electrically driven impeller to deaggregate the powder (34,35). The situation is analogous to the one for pMDIs, where the aerosol cloud is generated by the canister pressure. For pMDIs, it has been shown that a high inhalation flow will result in a lower lung deposition and a lower effect than a low inhalation flow (36).

Thus, inhalation flow is of importance for both DPIs and pMDIs, and it is important to evaluate each DPI, and pMDI on its own merits.

It is a common misunderstanding that a DPI with a low intrinsic resistance is a better inhaler than one with a high intrinsic resistance. An interesting example of the opposite is given in a study where the same aerosol cloud was inhaled against a resistance, similar to that in the Turbuhaler inhaler, on one study day and against no resistance at another study day (37). A marked increase in lung deposition and a reduced variability in lung dose were seen when the patients inhaled against the resistance. Inhaling against a resistance probably opens up the oral cavity and thus reduces the interaction between the inhaled aerosol cloud and the cavity surfaces.

A. Asthmatic Children

Asthmatic children are often thought to have problems in generating an inhalation flow through a DPI high enough to obtain the full effect of the inhaled drug, even if the inhaler has been shown to function well in adults. The major difference between a child and an adult lies not so much in their ability to generate a good inhalation flow as in the inhaled volume and, for young children, also their ability to do a reproducible, forceful inspiratory effort. The child's smaller inhaled volume is of minor importance when using a DPI, as the dose leaves the DPI with the first few hundred milliliters of inhaled air (25). With a child's smaller inhaled volume, the inhalation time becomes shorter. This could be a problem for a child when using a pMDI, as coordination of actuation and inhalation is a major obstacle to a well-performed inhalation with a pMDI (6,38,39). The actually achieved inhalation flow does not seem to differ between children and adults when the children have been well trained in the inhalation technique. In a training study, it was shown that 3-year-old children did not improve their DPI inhalation technique at training, while 4- and 5-year-old children achieved relevant PIFs after training even if their initial PIFs were low and similar to those of the 3-year-old children (40).

The effect of using different inhalation flows on clinical performance in children has been investigated for a few inhalers. Inhalator Ingelheim (Boehringer Ingelheim, Germany) is a high-resistance inhaler, and the normal PIF through the inhaler ranges between 14 and 45 L/min in children (41). In a clinical trial of an 0.2-mg inhalation of fenoterol, a slow (17 L/min) PIF resulted in a lower increase in FEV_1 than a fast inhalation (37 L/min).

The effect in asthmatic children (7 to 14 years) of salbutamol Rotahaler when used at different peak inhalation flows has been investigated at 30–50 (slow), 60–80 (medium), and 90–120 (fast) L/min (32). The improvement in FEV_1, after inhaling 0.2 mg salbutamol after the two fastest inhalations was significantly greater than after the slow inhalation. Aerolizer has been used to deliver formoterol to children at two different PIFs (42). In the first part of the study, it was found that 60–120 L/min was the typical PIF range for children aged 3–10 years. In the subsequent clinical part of the investigation, including children aged 8–15 years (n=16), inhalation of 12 μg formoterol at the low inhalation flow did not provide a significant bronchodilatation after 4 h or bronchoprotection at 12 h, while the high-flow inhalation did so. Thus, there was a tendency to a better effect at 12 h after the high inhalation flow.

A typical PIF through Turbuhaler for 3- to 6-year-old asthmatic children was 59 L/min, while children aged 7–10 years achieved a mean PIF of 70 L/min (43). In another study, PIF through Turbuhaler for 265 healthy children, aged 3.5–15 years, was found to correlate to age and typically ranged between 30 and 90 L/min (31). The importance of different PIFs for the clinical outcome was evaluated after inhaling the β_2 agonist terbutaline through Turbuhaler. Fourteen children aged 7 to 15 years inhaled a low dose of terbutaline, 0.25 mg, through Turbuhaler at four different inhalation flows, covering a wide range of PIFs. The study was randomized and crossover and performed on four different study days. Even a PIF of 13 L/min gave an increase in FEV_1; a PIF of 22 L/min, and even more so 31 L/min, further increased the FEV_1. An increase in PIF to 60 L/min, however, did not further increase the FEV_1 in this group of asthmatic children. To assure that the observed effects were not on the top of the dose-response curve, a further 1 mg of terbutaline was given at the end of each effect-measurement period and a significant further increase was then observed at each study day. The observed lack of difference in effect between 30 and 60 L/min thus is probably not due the fact that the two different inhalations were on the top of the dose-response curve.

Diskus PIF has also been evaluated in asthmatic children (44). Children (n=129) aged 3–10 years were included and an almost linear relationship between age and PIF was found between 3 and 8 years. At the age of 8, PIF reached a plateau. As almost all children could generate a flow of at least 30 L/min, this was considered to be a relevant lower-target flow in a later part of the investigation, where protection by the β_2 agonist salmeterol against exercise-induced bronchoconstriction was investigated in a clinical trial. Twenty-six percent of the children attained 90 L/min, which was therefore considered to be a relevant upper-target flow for children using Diskus. In the clinical trial, 50 μg of salmeterol (Serevent) was given to 18 children (aged 8–15 years) with exercise-induced asthma, and at two different PIFs, 30 and 90 L/min. Exercise challenge was carried out at 1 and 12 h after the dosing, using the fall in FEV_1 as the primary parameter. There was no difference in protection at 12 h between the low- and high-flow days.

B. Asthmatic Adults

In adults, some situations are looked upon as critical in the use of an inhaler. During an asthma exacerbation the expiratory constraints, showing up as a low

FEV_1, do not, however, seem to affect the ability to generate a good inhalation flow through a DPI. This was shown in a study in acute asthma, where the PIF for Turbuhaler ranged between 30 and 90 L/min, with a mean value of around 60 L/min (45). In another study on acute asthmatic subjects (n=86), the mean PIF through Turbuhaler on reporting at the emergency ward was 49 L/min, with a range from 26–68 L/min (46). In the latter study, the clinical outcome of salbutamol given via a pMDI plus a spacer or via Turbuhaler was also evaluated. Salbutamol Turbuhaler was given in half the dose as compared with the pMDI regimen, but no difference in clinical outcome after the two regimens was observed. The results are in accord with the results from a dose-response study in stable asthmatics, where it was shown that a given dose of salbutamol administered via Turbuhaler elicited the same effect as twice the dose given via pMDI (47).

The salbutamol results are supported by the finding that when terbutaline was given to patients with acute obstructive lung disease either via Turbuhaler or via pMDI plus a spacer at the same nominal dose, the Turbuhaler treatment resulted in a significantly better effect as measured by FEV_1 (48).

An additional factor to consider in interpreting comparisons between DPIs and pMDIs in acute asthma is the potential of pMDIs to cause a transient paradoxical bronchoconstriction on inhalation (49,50). The constriction is probably caused by the nondrug components in the pMDI formulation.

Spirometry after inhaling terbutaline sulfate via Turbuhaler at 30 and 60 L/min showed that changes in FEF_{50} and FEF_{75} were significantly higher after inhalation at 60 L/min while changes in FEV_1 were similar (51). This is in contrast to the results from a study by Engel and coworkers (52). The elicited effects measured by spirometry after different inhalation modes were investigated, and comparable bronchodilation was achieved when the PIF through Turbuhaler varied between 34 and 88 L/min. The low inhalation flow (34 L/min) tended, however, to result in a slightly reduced bronchodilatation compared with the three high-inhalation flow modes. In another study, the FEV_1 response was higher, but not significantly so, after the inhalation of 0.5 mg of terbutaline via Turbuhaler at 60 L/min versus inhalation at 30 L/min (53). The increases in FEV_1 were 0.6 and 0.4 L, respectively.

Another DPI, Pulvinal (Chiesi, Italy), has been investigated in severe asthmatics and at two different inhalation flows (54). No correlation between PIF and efficacy or PIF and severity of asthma could be shown. Neither could it be shown that efficacy depended on the generated PIF. The 20% difference in lung deposition seen after a low and a high Pulvinal inhalation flow, in another study, was obviously too small to show up as a change in effect (55).

Inhalator Ingelheim with fenoterol has been evaluated in adults, and a difference, although not significant, in elicited effect was observed when the inhalation flow was 15 and 40 L/min, respectively (56).

Finally, the amount of DSCG reaching the lungs after inhaling via Spinhaler was investigated in 10 healthy volunteers inhaling at different inhalation flows (57). PIF for Spinhaler using a standard inhalation maneuver is 120 L/min; this flow and a flow of 60 L/min were tested. Lung deposition was 13.1% at the high and 5.5% at the low flow. In a study on asthmatic subjects, the protective effect against adenosine monophosphate provocation after inhaling DSCG via Spinhaler at three different flows was investigated (58). A correlation between PIF and protection and level of DSCG plasma concentration was observed. The observed differences were assigned to differences in dispersion of the powder aggregates, resulting in different fine particle doses reaching the lungs at the different inhalation flows.

Available information on the use of DPIs in asthmatic situations clearly indicates that they perform well both in the acute and the stable asthmatic situation. Inhalation flow can affect the clinical outcome, but for both Turbuhaler and Diskus no significant differences were observed between a low and a typical or high inhalation flow. For Turbuhaler, extremely low inhalation flows resulted in a significantly lower effect, but the decline was gradual. Based on this, we do not expect to see any sharp drop in drug delivery to the lungs or clinical effect when lower than normal inhalation flows are used.

VIII. Humidity

A potential problem with inhaled formulations is that the surrounding environment can affect their performance. For a pMDI, the surrounding temperature affects the canister pressure and thus the quality of the generated aerosol, while for DPIs, humidity can be a problem. Humidity at storage and humidity at inhalation are two different aspects and can influence the performance of DPI formulations in different ways. Dry-powder formulations, which contain lactose or a hygroscopic active drug, will eventually be degraded at storage if the protective cap, etc., is not put on after use. This is analogous to the situation when the lid on a tablet container is not replaced properly after use; after a while the tablets will degrade. A difference is that inhaled formulations are more sensitive than tablets, as the quality of the generated aerosol is heavily dependent on the particle properties, while a tablet can be taken and can exert the same effect even if it is affected by humidity. For formulations that are protected by a cap when not in use, humidity at storage before being used by the patient or when in use is no problem, as was shown in a study where formoterol Turbuhaler was stored at 40°C/75% for 6 months without any sign of decline in fine particle dose (59). Furthermore, exposure of Turbuhaler to a routine wash-dry cycle in a domestic washing machine (60°C) did not affect the delivered or fine particle dose. For formulations that do not come with a protective cap, storage in a humid environment can be a problem. Thus, it has been shown that storage of Diskus at, 40°C/75% relative humidity for about 2–3 months will reduce the fine particle dose to about half (60). This problem can be overcome at least partly by using a protective foil in which to package the inhaler before it is used by the patient, as is the case for the Diskus formulation when marketed in the United States. To minimize the effect of humidity on the dry powder in the inhaler, both at storage before use ad in use, some inhalers include a desiccant in the inhaler body to keep the internal milieu at a low relative humidity when the cap is on.

Another aspect is the humidity of the air at inhalation. Humidity at inhalation may lead to an increase in the adhesion between the dry-powder particles. In general it can be stated that inhalation at a very high relative humidity will tend to decrease the fine particle dose from a DPI (61,62), although there was no difference in clinical effect between a salbutamol DPI (Turbuhaler) and pMDI in hot, humid regions (63).

IX. Dry-Powder Inhalers

A. Aerolizer

Aerolizer (Novartis, Switzerland) is a single-capsule inhaler and is marketed for the inhalation of formoterol and budesonide. The same inhaler has also been marketed with salbutamol, beclomethasone, and budesonide under the Cyclohaler name. A gelatin capsule is inserted into the inhaler and pierced from the ends. At inhalation, the capsule is lifted into a chamber and rotated by the inhaled air, at the same time delivering its contents through the capsule ends.

B. Clickhaler

Clickhaler (ML Laboratories PLC, UK) is a multidose dry-powder inhaler containing up to 200 doses and is available for the delivery of salbutamol and beclomethasone dipropionate. The feel of the device is similar to that of a pMDI. A cone that sits below the drug reservoir has a series of metering cups, which are filled by gravity as they rotate and carry the dose of drug into the inhalation passage. There is minimal resistance to airflow through the device. Powder is fluidized and also impinges on the internal surfaces of the mouthpiece, providing further dispersion of agglomerated particles.

C. Diskhaler

Diskhaler (GlaxoSmithKline, UK) is a 4- or 8-dose inhaler based on a disk with aluminum foil blisters. Before inhalation, a blister is pierced and the ordered mixture formulation is inhaled.

D. Diskus/Accuhaler

Diskus/Accuhaler (GlaxoSmithKline, UK) is a multidose inhaler with 60 doses; the drug is contained in blisters on a foil strip and is blended with lactose as carrier. As a blister moves toward the mouthpiece, the covering foil is pulled off it prior to inhalation. Air is sucked through the inhaler and the powder is aerosolized by shear-force fluidization. Extra air drawn through the two holes in the mouthpiece helps with particle deaggregation by providing turbulence.

E. Easyhaler

Easyhaler (Orion Farmos, Finland) is an inhaler with 200 doses in a drug/lactose mixture. There is a gravitational flow of powder from the drug reservoir into the metering cylinder cavity. Depression of the cap places pressure on the metering cylinder, causing it to rotate, and a single dose of powder is transported to the mouthpiece. As the patient inhales, the aerosol is formed, assisted by turbulent flow along the narrow mouthpiece of the inhaler.

F. Inhalator Ingelheim

Inhalator Ingelheim (Boehringer Ingelheim, Germany) is a single-capsule device, and the formulation contains glucose as a carrier. After insertion of the gelatin capsule, it is pierced at both ends; at inhalation, air is drawn through the bottom of the inhaler, through the holes in the capsule, and out through the mouthpiece. The capsule's emptying is also supported by its vibration in the air stream.

G. Inhale Inhaler

The Inhale inhaler (Inhale Therapeutic Systems, USA) for dry-powder delivery aerosolizes the dry powder by the assistance of compressed gas. The Inhale system is being used to deliver insulin mixed with lactose. Powder ranging from 1 to 3 μm is packaged in unit-dose aluminum blisters. The inhaler is armed by the patient, resulting in a smaller amount of air being compressed. After the blister is inserted, it is punctured, and when the device is activated, compressed air is released through the powder at a very high velocity. The aerosol is thus generated in a gas-assisted fluidization process. The aerosol is suspended within the spacer device, from which it is then inhaled.

H. Novolizer

Novolizer (Asta Medica, Germany) is a reusable device. The disposable reservoir cartridges contain 200 doses of drug lactose mixture. When actuated, a slide moves at the bottom of the cartridge and a new dose is gravimetrically metered to the air channel.

Table 1 Lung Deposition After Inhalation of Different Substances via Different Dry-Powder Inhalers[a]

Inhaler	Substance	Inhalation flow (L/min)	Lung deposition (%)	Reference	Comments
Aerolizer	Formoterol	Normal	27	66	HV (n=12)
Clickhaler	BDP	35–63	31	67	HV (n=10)
Cyclohaler	Salbutamol	55	7.0	10	HV (n=11)
		107	10.7		
	DSCG	55–70	16.4	68	HV (n=7)
Diskus	Fluticasone	-	16.6	69	HV (n=12)
	Fluticasone	Normal	12.6	70	HV (n=13)
Diskhaler	Salbutamol	-	12.4	71	HV (n=10)
			11.4		Pat (n=19)
		-	11.3	72	HV (n=6)
	Fluticasone	-	11.9	69	HV (n=12)
Easyhaler	Salbutamol	58	28.9	73	HV (n=8)
		-	23.7	74	Pat (n=12)
Inhalator Ingelheim	DSCG	55–70	16.4	68	HV (n=7)
		Normal	20.9	75	HV (n=8)
Novolizer	Budesonide	54	20	76	HV (n=13)
		65	25		
		99	32		
Pulvinal	Salbutamol	28	11.7	55	HV (n=10)
		46	14.1		
Rotahaler	DSCG	55–70	6.2	68	HV (n=7)
	Salbutamol	77	3.4	10	HV (n=11)
		144	7.0		
Spinhaler	DSCG	55–70	11.5	68	HV (n=7)
		60	5.5	57	HV (n=10)
Spiros (Dryhaler)	BDP	15	40.5	35	HV (n=15); delivered dose
		30	37.5		
		60	30.4		
	Salbutamol	17.3	21.0	34	HV (n=5)
		56.5	16.1		
Taifun	Budesonide	Low	29.6	77	Pat (n=10)
		Fast	34.3		
Turbuhaler	Terbutaline	55	26.9[b]	78	HV (n=6)
			21.1[c]		
	Terbutaline	58	21	79	HV (n=8)
	Budesonide	36	15	7	HV (n=10)
		58	28		
	Budesonide	52	32	80	HV (n=24)

Table 1 Continued

Inhaler	Substance	Inhalation flow (L/min)	Lung deposition (%)	Reference	Comments
	Budesonide	67	26	81	Pat (n=8)
	Budesonide	Normal	34.1	70	HV (n=13)
	Budesonide	58	21.4	76	HV (n=13)
	Formoterol	Normal	50	66	HV (n=12); delivered dose
	Salbutamol	30 60	13.9 23.2	10	HV (n=11)

[a]Inhalation flows are given with values or estimates when available (HV=healthy volunteer; pat=patient; values are given in % of metered dose unless noted).
[b]By scintigraphy.
[c]By charcoal block.

I. Pulvinal

Pulvinal (Chiesi, Italy) is a multidose reservoir inhaler containing 100 doses of powder mixture. A protecting cap provides a moistureproof barrier. On rotation of the mouthpiece, a dose is metered volumetrically into a cavity and then transferred into an aerosolizing chamber. Upon inhalation, air is drawn through the aerosolizing chamber and the aerosol is transported out through the mouthpiece.

J. Rotahaler

Rotahaler (GlaxoSmithKline, UK) is a single-dose device using powder drugs such as beclomethasone dipropionate and salbutamol combined with a lactose carrier and contained in gelatin capsules. A capsule is inserted into the inhaler and broken; fluidization is then induced at inhalation. Particle deaggregation is mainly caused by turbulence promoted by the grid through which the drug passes before entering the mouthpiece.

K. Spinhaler

Spinhaler (Aventis, UK) is one of the first mass-produced dry-powder inhalers and used for the delivery of DSCG. A single gelatin capsule containing 20 mg of micronized drug without a carrier is mounted onto an impeller in the inhaler. A piercing mechanism punctures the capsule and inhaled air causes the impeller and capsule to rotate at a speed dependent on the airflow generated through the device by the patient. At high flows, the capsule vibrates, leading to mechanical fluidization (64). This action is supported by capillary fluidization due to the pressure drop across the capsule. The drug powder is then conveyed toward the perforations, where it is discharged into the airstream. Shear force and relative motion are the predominant mechanisms of powder deaggregation (65).

L. Spiros

Spiros (Dura Pharmaceuticals) is a reusable device containing either a disposable, prefilled plastic cassette with 30 doses or an aluminum blister disk with 16 doses. The device is breath-actuated and the inhalation flow activates a battery-driven motor, which spins an impeller that disperses the drug blend.

M. Taifun

Taifun (Leiras, Finland) is a reservoir inhaler containing 200 doses of drug mixture. One dose is gravimetrically metered when the mouthpiece is turned one full turn. The dose is then transferred from the drug reservoir into the vortex chamber. Upon inhalation, air passes through the vortex chamber, creating a grinding action that deaggregates the powder.

N. Turbuhaler

Turbuhaler (AstraZeneca, Sweden) contains up to 200 doses of drug stored in a reservoir. Initially, the micronized drug in Turbuhaler did not contain carrier particles, but in later formulations the active drug is cospheronized with lactose particles of the same size. The small pellets of powder disintegrate into their primary particles during the metering and inhalation process (4). Turning the bottom of the inhaler rotates the dosing unit. Drug is then scraped into holes within the dosing unit. As the patient inhales, air passes through the dosing unit, across the powder bed, which is fluidized by shear force. Capillary fluidization also occurs. Particle deagglomeration is caused by turbulence in the narrow inhalation channel, impaction on the bottom of the mouthpiece, and the high shear stress generated within the mouthpiece.

X. Lung Deposition via DPIs

Lung deposition of inhaled drug can be determined by both scintigraphic and pharmacokinetic methods.

A collection of relevant data is given in Table 1.

As expected, there is a large range in the degree of lung deposition from different DPIs. Values range from 5% to more than 30% of the metered dose. Thus, results from one DPI cannot be extrapolated to another DPI. It should also be observed that for the DPIs that have been investigated at different inhalation flows, there was a difference in the degree of lung deposition. In investigating lung deposition of DPIs, it is thus recommended that the subjects be asked to inhale in a clinically relevant way and that the inhalation flow be recorded.

Diskhaler and Diskus, as well as Rotahaler, use the same pharmaceutical principle, ordered mixture, and degree of lung deposition: 10–12% for Diskhaler and Diskus, with Rotahaler giving lower values about 5% (10,68,70–72). The different values indicate that both formulation and device properties are of importance for the resulting lung deposition outcome.

An interesting observation is that, for Spiros, the flow dependency is reversed, as was commented upon earlier. A higher inhalation flow will give a lower lung deposition. Turbuhaler, finally, has been thoroughly investigated with respect to lung deposition, and the general picture is that about 20–30% of the dose reaches the lung, in healthy volunteers and in patients at a typical inhalation flow, about 60 L/min (7,68,78,80,82–84).

The values given in Table 1 are from healthy volunteers and patients, and it should be observed that even if the subject has constricted lungs, as in asthma, this does not influence the total degree of lung deposition as shown in a study comparing a group of patients and a group of healthy volunteers using the same inhalation technique (71). This is what can be expected, as it is the inhalation flow that determines how much of the nominal dose will reach the lung. The regional distribution is, however, more central in the presence of airway narrowing (85,86). Very little information on the degree of lung deposition in children has been presented. In a recent study in children with cystic fibrosis (n=21) aged 4–16 years, actual lung dose was measured after inhaling from a budesonide Turbuhaler (87). The mean dose in percent of total body dose ranged between 10 and 40% and was clearly related to the age of child. The age-dependent lung dose may reflect a flow-dependent dose from the Turbuhaler or more likely the effect of the diameter and anatomy of the oropharynx on delivery in the younger children. In another Turbuhaler study in asthmatic children aged 6 to 16 years (n=23), lung deposition ranged between 16 and 47% of the metered dose (88). Degree of deposition was correlated with age, height, and PIF, with correlation coefficients of around 0.5 for all three parameters. PIF ranged between 45 and 76 L/min.

The importance of the degree of lung deposition for the elicited clinical effect is discussed in Chap. 5, but generally it can be stated that the amount of drug reaching the lungs will determine the elicited effect, as the systemic portion of total lung concentration is of minor importance for inhaled drugs. It should, however, be observed that many of the published studies comparing different inhalers and substances are done at doses that give a response that is already on the plateau of the dose-response curve; and thus cautious interpretation of comparative studies is recommended (89).

XI. Variability in Lung Deposition

The amount of drug reaching the effector site, in this context the lungs, determines the elicited effect (84,89). Thus, for inhaled drugs, it is of interest to evaluate not only the amount of drug reaching the lungs but also its variability, as a large variability in lung deposition could cause a variability in the exerted effects.

The overall delivery of inhaled drugs to the effector site can be described by a number of steps. The variability in lung deposition thus depends on a large number of in vitro and in vivo factors—e.g., device performance, handling of the device, coordination of actuation and inhalation, inhalation flow, patient anatomy, etc. Variability in the different steps will add up to an overall variability in the amount of drug reaching the lungs.

In vitro analyses are done to ascertain a good quality of the manufactured product and the analyses are done under strictly standardized conditions. The absolute amount of drug leaving the inhaler and its variability are typical in vitro parameters. The in vivo analyses include lung deposition, but also the clinical outcome. The measured in vitro variability may account for only a small portion of the overall in vivo variability observed in the clinical situation.

The variability in amount of drug reaching the lungs has specifically been determined in two studies one in healthy volunteers and one in asthmatic patients (90,91). In the two studies, both *intra-* and *inter*variability in amount of drug reaching the lungs when inhaling via a pMDI and a DPI, Turbuhaler, were determined. It was shown that the DPI, Turbuhaler, delivered a more reproducible dose to the lungs than the corresponding pMDI.

In the healthy volunteers study, the Turbuhaler and pMDI inhalers were also analyzed in vitro. Intradevice variability, expressed as a coefficient of variation (CV), was 6.4% for pMDI and 18.2% for Turbuhaler, a significant ($p<0.001$) difference. Also the *inter*device variability was significantly higher for Turbuhaler than for pMDI; the ratio of CVs was 2.0 ($p=0.023$).

The observed difference in variability in lung deposition between Tur-

Table 2 Inter- and Intravariability in Lung Deposition of Terbutaline Inhaled via pMDI or Turbuhaler[a]

	Patients		Healthy volunteers	
Device	Inter-	Intra-	Inter-	Intra-
Turbuhaler	8.17	39.3	18.5	47.1
pMDI	61.2	39.1	46.7	73.0

[a]Values are expressed as coefficients of variation (%). Values are from Beckman (90) and Borgström (91).

buhaler and pMDI probably represents a class difference between DPIs and pMDIs. This is because the generation of aerosol and inhalation is a continuous process with DPIs, in contrast to pMDIs, where aerosol generation and inhalation of the generated aerosol are two distinct processes that need to be coordinated by the inhaling subject. This difference can explain the results obtained.

XII. Safety of DPIs

Use of pMDIs plus spacer results in less oropharyngeal deposition of inhaled drugs compared to delivering the same dose via a pMDI or a DPI. This may reduce the risk of local and systemic side effects, but it must be appreciated that this can vary considerably for the inhaler and drug used. For inhaled steroids and β_2 agonists, it has become clear that the doses deposited in the lungs are the greatest contributor to the systemic effect, because steroids and β_2 agonists are absorbed directly from the lungs into the systemic circulation. Therefore the ratio between lung dose and extrapulmonary dose (L/T ratio) should be considered when comparing different treatmens like pMDI, pMDI plus spacer, and DPI (92). Not only the choice of device but also the degree of first-pass metabolism of the drug under study will influence the L/T ratio.

For DPIs that produce a very high lung dose or a drug with a high first-pass metabolism, the problem should not be as great, as both factors will improve the L/T ratio. Consequently, a high lung dose delivered from a given DPI should allow the nominal dose to be reduced, thus improving safety.

Dry-powder impaction in the oropharynx with local side effects should also be considered when DPIs are used, compared to pMDIs plus spacers.

Apart from lactose as carrier or filler, DPIs do not have to incorporate the lubricants and cosolvents needed in propellant driven pMDIs. These additives may be the cause of commonly observed cough (93) and bronchoconstriction when a patient is inhaling from a pMDI (50), though the latter is often masked by the drug effect. As mentioned earlier, the CFC propellant of the pMDI has been withdrawn due to the detrimental effect of CFCs on the ozone layer. CFCs have now been replaced by HFA propellants, which should have no effect on the ozone layer. They are, however, considered as "greenhouse" gases. In fact, they are several thousand times more potent than carbon dioxide.

XIII. Concluding Remarks

We have discussed the different principles for dry powder formulation and their potential implications for the quality of the generated aerosol and continued with how the particles were generated at inhalation. The importance of the intrinsic resistance of an inhaler for the clinical outcome was considered, and it was suggested that a high-resistance inhaler would perform in a more reproducible way. It was then shown that both children and adults can use a DPI, also when constricted. Lung deposition for a range of DPIs was given and the two aspects of humidity were discussed. The variability between DPIs and pMDIs was compared, and finally some words on the safety on DPIs were given.

Acknowledgments

It is a pleasure to acknowledge Lars Asking, Gerreke Biewenga, Eva Bondesson, Lars Thorsson, and Eva Trofast for their valuable comments and suggestions during the preparation of this manuscript.

References

1. Bell J, Hartley P, Cox J. Dry powder aerosols I: A new powder inhalation device. J Pharm Sci 1971; 60:1559–1564.
2. Hetzel M, Clark T. Comparison of salbutamol Rotahaler with conventional pressurized aerosol. Clin Allergy 1977; 7:563–568.
3. Pover G, Langdon C, Jones S, Fidler C. Evaluation of a breath operated powder inhaler. J Int Med Res 1988; 16:201–203.
4. Wetterlin K. Turbuhaler: A new powder inhaler for administration of drugs to the airways. Pharm Res 1988; 5:506–508.
5. Brindley A, Sumby B, Smith I, Prime D, Haywood P, Grant A. Design, manufacture and dose consistency of the Serevent Diskus. Pharm Technol Eur 1995; 7:16–17, 20–22.
6. Crompton G. Problems patients have using pressurized aerosol inhalers. Eur J Respir Dis 1982; 63:101–104.
7. Borgström L, Bondesson E, Morén F, Trofast E, Newman S. Lung deposition of budesonide inhaled via Turbuhaler: a comparison with terbutaline sulphate in normal subjects. Eur Respir J 1994; 7:69–73.
8. Zanen P, Go L, Lammers J-W. Optimal particle size for β_2-agonist and anticholinergic aerosols in patients with severe airflow obstruction. Thorax 1996; 51:977–980.
9. Leach C. Enhanced drug delivery through reformulating MDIs with HFA propellants-drug deposition and its effect on preclinical and clinical programs. Respiratory Drug Delivery V. Buffalo Grove, IL: Interpharm Press, 1996:133–144.
10. Olsson B, Borgström L, Asking L, Bondesson E. Effect of inlet throat on the correlation between measured fine particle dose and lung deposition. In: Dalby R, Byron P, Farr S, eds. Respiratory Drug Delivery V. Buffalo Grove, IL: Interpharm Press, 1996:273–281.
11. Sacohetti M, van Ort M. Spray-drying and supercritical fluid particle generation technique. In: Hickey AJ, ed. Inhalation Aerosols: Physical and Biological Basis for Therapy. Vol. 94. New York: Marcel Dekker, 1996:337–384.
12. Vidgren M, Vidgren P, Paronen T. Comparison of physical and inhalation properties

of spray-dried and mechanically micronized disodium cromoglycate. Int J Pharm 1987; 35:139–144.

13. Staniforth J, Rees J, Lai F, Hersey J. Interparticle forces in binary and ternary ordered powder mixes. J Pharm Pharmacol 1982; 34:141–145.
14. Hersey J. Ordered mixing: A new concept in powder mixing practice. Powder Technol 1975; 11:41–44.
15. Kassem N, Ganderton D. The influence of carrier surface on the characteristics of inspirable powder aerosols. J Pharm Pharmacol 1990; 42:11P.
16. Zeng X, Martin G, Marriott C, Pritchard J. Effects of surface smoothness of lactose on the delivery of salbutamol sulphate from dry powder inhalers. Pharm Res 1997; 14:s136.
17. Asking L, Lööf T, Pettersson G. Flutide Diskus less consistent than Pulmicort Turbuhaler with respect to in vitro fine particle dose proportionality. Am J Respir Crit Care Med 2001: Accepted.
18. Rudt S, Müller R. In vitro phagocytosis assay of nano- and microparticles by chemiluminescence: I. Effect of analytical parameters, particle size and particle concentration. J Contr Rel 1992; 22:263–272.
19. Edwards D, Hanes J, Caponetti G, et al. Large porous particles for pulmonary drug delivery. Science 1997; 276:1868.
20. de Boer AH, Winter HMI, Lerk CF. Inhalation characteristics and their effects on in vitro drug delivery from dry powder inhalers: Part I. Inhalation characteristics, work of breathing and volunteers' preference in dependence of the inhaler resistance. Int J Pharm 1996; 130:231–244.
21. de Boer A, Gjaltema D, Hagedoorn P. Inhalation characteristics and their effects on in vitro drug delivery from dry powder inhalers: Part 2. Effect of peak flow rate (PIFR) and inspiration time on the in vitro drug release from three different types of commercial dry powder inhalers. Int J Pharm 1996; 138:45–56.
22. de Boer A, Bolhuis G, Gjaltema D, Hagedoorn P. Inhalation characteristics and their effects on in vitro drug delivery from dry powder inhalers Part 3: The effect of flow increase rate (FIR) on the in vitro drug release from the Pulmicort 200 Turbuhaler. Int J Pharm 1997; 153:67–77.
23. European Pharmacopoeia, Inhalanda. Vol. 2. Strasbourg: European Pharmacopoeia Secretariat, 1999:988.
24. Olsson B, Asking L. Critical aspects of the function of inspiratory flow driven inhalers. J Aerosol Med 1994; 7(suppl 1): S43–S47.
25. Bisgaard H, Klug B, Sumby B, Burnell P. Fine particle mass from the Diskus inhaler and Turbuhaler inhaler in children with asthma. Eur Respir J 1998; 11:1111–1115.
26. Heinbecker P. A method for the demonstration of calibre changes in the bronchi in normal respiration. J Clin Invest 1927; 4:459–469.
27. McNeill R, Malcom G, Rhind Brown W. A comparison of expiratory and inspiratory flow rates in health and in chronic pulmonary disease. Thorax 1959; 14:225–231.
28. Clark A, Hollingworth A. The relationship between powder inhaler resistance and peak inspiratory conditions in healthy volunteers—implications for in vitro testing. J Aerosol Med 1993; 6:99–110.
29. Clark A. Effect of powder inhaler resistance upon inspiratory profiles in health and

disease. In: Dalby R, Byron P, Farr S, eds. Respiratory Drug Delivery IV. Buffalo Grove, IL: Interpharm Press, 1994:117–123.

30. Assi K, Chrystyn H. The device resistance of recently introduced dry-powder inhalers. J Pharm Pharmacol 2000; 52:58.
31. Pedersen S, Hansen O, Fuglsang G. Influence of inspiratory flow rate upon the effect of a Turbuhaler. Arch Dis Child 1990; 65:308–310.
32. Pedersen S. How to use a Rotahaler. Arch Dis Child 1986; 61:11–14.
33. Newman S, Pavia D, Garland N, Clarke S. Effects of various inhalation modes on the deposition of radiactive pressurized aerosols. Eur J Respir Dis 1982; 63:57–65.
34. Dolovich M, Rhem R, Rashid F, Bowen B, Coates G, Hill M. Lung deposition of albuterol sulphate from the Dura Dryhaler in normal adults. Am J Respir Crit Care Med 1996; 153:A62.
35. Warren S, Taylor G, Godfrey C, Coté G, Hill M. Gamma scintigraphic evaluation of beclomethasone dipropionate (BDP) from the Spiros dry powder inhaler. J Aerosol Med 1999; 12:117.
36. Newman S, Pavia D, Clarke S. How should a pressurized beta-adrenergic bronchodilator be inhaled? Eur J Respir Dis 1981; 62:3–21.
37. Svartengren K, Lindestad P-Å, Svartengren M, Philipsson K, Bylin G, Camner P. Added external resistance reduces oropharyngeal deposition and increases lung deposition of aerosol particles in asthmatics. Am J Respir Crit Care Med 1995; 152:32–37.
38. Pedersen S, Frost L, Arnfred T. Errors in inhalation technique and efficiency in inhaler use in asthmatic children. Allergy 1986; 41:118–124.
39. Liard R, Zurek M, Aubier M, Korobaeff M, Henry C, Neukirch F. Misuse of pressurized metered dose inhalers by asthmatic patients treated in French private practice. Rev Epidém et Santé1995; 43:242–249.
40. Agertoft L, Pedersen S. Importance of training for correct Tubuhaler use in preschool children. Acta Paediatr 1998; 87:842–847.
41. Pedersen S, Stefensen G. Fenoterol powder inhaler technique in children: Influence of inspiratory flow rate and breath-holding. Eur Respir Dis 1986; 68:207–214.
42. Nielsen K, Skov M, Klug B, Ifversen M, Bisgaard H. Flow-dependent effect of formoterol dry-powder inhaled from the Aerolizer. Eur Respir J 1997; 10:2105–2109.
43. Ståhl E, Ribeiro L, Sandahl G. Dose response to inhaled terbutaline powder and peak inspiratory flow through Turbuhaler in children with mild to moderate asthma. Pediatr Pulmonol 1996; 22:106–110.
44. Nielsen K, Auk I, Bojsen K, Ifversen M, Klug B, Bisgaard H. Clinical effect of Diskus dry-powder inhaler at low and high inspiratory flow rates in asthmatic children. Eur Respir J 1998; 11:350–354.
45. Brown P, Ning A, Greening A, McLean A, Crompton G. Peak inspiratory flow through Turbuhaler in acute asthma. Eur Respir J 1995; 8:1940–1941.
46. Nana A, Youngchaiyud P, Maranetra N, et al. β_2-agonists administered by a dry powder inhaler can be used in acute asthma. Respir Med 1998; 92:167–172.
47. Löfdahl C, Andersson L, Bondesson E, et al. Differences in bronchodilating potency of salbutamol in Turbuhaler as compared with a pressurized metered-dose inhaler

formulation in patients with reversible airway obstruction. Eur Respir J 1997; 10:2474–2478.

48. Tönnesen F, Laursen L, Evald T, Ståhl E, Ibsen T. Bronchodilating effect of terbutaline powder in acute severe bronchial obstruction. Chest 1994; 105:697–700.
49. Jackson L, Ståhl E, Holgate S. Terbutaline via pressurised metered dose inhaler (P-MDI) and turbuhaler in highly reactive asthmatic patients. Eur Respir J 1994; 7:1598–1601.
50. Selroos O, Löfroos A-B, Pietinalho A, Riska H. Comparison of terbutaline and placebo from a pressurised metered dose inhaler and a dry powder inhaler in a subgroup of patients with asthma. Thorax 1994; 49:1228–1230.
51. Dolovich M, Vanziegelheim M, Hidinger K. Influence of inspiratory flow rate on the response to terbutaline sulphate inhaled via the Turbuhaler. Am Rev Respir Dis 1988; 137:433.
52. Engel T, Scharling B, Skovstedt B, Heining J. Effects, side effects and plasma concentrations of terbutaline in adult asthmatics after inhaling from a dry powder inhaler device at different inhalation flows and volumes. Br J Clin Pharmacol 1992; 33:439–444.
53. Newman S, Morén F, Trofast E, Talaee N, Clarke S. Terbutaline sulphate Turbuhaler: effect of inhaled flow rate on drug deposition and efficacy. Int J Pharm 1991; 74:209–213.
54. Dal Negro R, Pomari C, Micheletto C, Cantini L. Peak inspiratory flow rate as measured through a new powder inhaler, does not correlate with asthma severity or influence effect of inhaled salbutamol. Adv Ther 1997; 14:181–191.
55. Pitcaim G, Lunghetti G, Ventura P, Newman S. A comparison of the lung deposition of salbutamol inhaled from a new dry powder inhaler, at two inhaled flow rates. Int J Pharm 1994; 102:11–18.
56. Groth S, Dirksen H. Optimal inhalation procedure for the fenoterol powder inhaler. Eur J Respir Dis 1983; 64:17–24.
57. Newman SP, Hollingworth A, Clark AR. Effect of different modes of inhalation on drug delivery from a dry powder inhaler. Int J Pharm 1994; 102:127–132.
58. Richards R, Simpson S, Renwick A, Holgate S. Inhalation rate of sodium cromoglycate determines plasma pharmacokinetics and protection against AMP-induced bronchoconstriction in asthma. Eur Respir J 1988; 1:896–901.
59. Shaw M. Effective and reliable drug delivery. In: Jackson W, ed. Turbuhaler. Oxford, UK: Clinical Vision, 1999.
60. Asking L, Axelsson M, Lindberg J. Aluminium blisters may fail to protect against humidity. Drug Delivery to the Lungs IX. London: The Aerosol Society, 1998:84–87.
61. Dickens C, McAughey J, Knight D, Baker S. Factors affecting in vitro testing of inhalers. J Aerosol Med 1994; 7:193–196.
62. Jashnani R, Byron P, Dalby R. Testing of dry powder aerosol formulations in different environmental conditions. Int J Pharm 1995; 113:123–130.
63. Lindsay D, Russell N, Thompson J, Warnock T, Shellshear I, Buchanan P. A multicentre comparison of the efficacy of terbutaline Turbuhaler and salbutamol pressurized metered dose inhaler in hot, humid regions. Eur Respir J 1994; 7:342–345.

64. Bell J, Hartley P, Cox J. Dry powder aerosols: I. A new powder inhalation device. J Pharm Sci 1971; 60:1559–1564.
65. Steckel H, Müller B. In vitro evaluation of dry powder inhalers: II. influence of carrier particle size and concentration on in vitro deposition. Int J Pharm 1997; 154:31–37.
66. Rosenborg J, Larsson P, Luts A, et al. Lung deposition of formoterol was greater after inhalation via the dry powder inhaler (DPI) Turbuhaler than via the DPI Aerolizer. Eur Respir J 1999; 14:62s.
67. Warren S, Taylor G. Effect of inhalation flow profiles on the deposition of radiolabelled BDP from a novel dry powder inhaler (DPI, Clickhaler), a conventional metered dose inhaler (MDI) and MDI plus spacer. In: Dalby R, Byron P, Farr S, eds. Respiratory Drug Delivery VI. Buffalo Grove, IL: Interpharm Press, 1998:453–455.
68. Vidgren M, Kärkkäinen A, Karjalainen P, Paronen P, Nuutinen J. Effect of powder inhaler design on drug deposition in the respiratory tract. Int J Pharm 1988; 42:211–216.
69. Johnson M. Fluticasone propionate: pharmacokinetic and pharmacodynamic implications of different aerosol delivery systems. In: Dalby R, Byron P, Farr S, eds. Respiratory Drug Delivery VI. Buffalo Grove, IL: Interpharm Press, 1998:61–70.
70. Thorsson L, Edsbäcker S. Lung deposition of budesonide via Turbuhaler was greater than that of fluticasone propionate via Diskus or pMDI. Am J Respir Crit Care Med 1999; 159:A118.
71. Melchor R, Biddiscombe M, Mak V, Short M, Spiro S. Lung deposition patterns of directly labelled salbutamol in normal subjects and in patients with reversible airflow obstruction. Thorax 1993; 48:506–511.
72. Biddiscombe M, Melchor R, Mak V, et al. The lung deposition of salbutamol, directly labelled with technetium-99m, delivered by pressurised metered dose and dry powder inhalers. Int J Pharm 1993; 91:111–121.
73. Vidgren M, Arppe J, Vidgren P, Vainio P, Silvasti M, Tukiainen H. Pulmonary deposition of 99mTc-labelled salbutamol particles in healthy volunteers after inhalation from a metered-dose inhaler and from a novel multiple-dose inhaler. STP Pharma Sci 1994; 4(1):29–32.
74. Vidgren M, Vidgren P, Hyvärinen L, Silvasti M, Tukiainen H. Deposition and clinical response of 99m Tc–labelled salbutamol inhaled from a novel multiple dose powder inhaler. Am Rev Respir Dis 1993; 147(suppl):A58.
75. Vidgren M, Paronen P, Vidgren P, Vaino P, Nuutinen J. Radiotracer evaluation of the deposition of drug particles inhaled from a new powder inhaler. Int J Pharm 1990; 64:1–6.
76. Newman S, Pitcairn G, Hirst P, et al. Scintigraphic comparison of budesonide deposition from two dry powder inhalers. Eur Respir J 2000; 16:178–183.
77. Pitcairn G, Lankinen T, Seppäla O-P, Newman S. Pulmonary drug delivery from the Taifun dry powder inhaler is relatively independent of the patient's inspiratory effort. J Aerosol Med 2000; 13:97–104.
78. Borgström L, Newman S, Weisz A, Morén F. Pulmonary deposition of inhaled terbutaline: comparison of scanning gamma camera and urinary excretion methods. J Pharm Sci 1992; 81:753–755.

79. Borgström L, Newman S. Total and regional lung deposition of terbutaline sulphate inhaled via a pressurised MDI or Turbuhaler. Int J Pharm 1993; 97:47–53.
80. Thorsson L, Edsbäcker S, Conradson T-B. Lung deposition of budesonide from Turbuhaler is twice that from a pressurized metered-dose inhaler P-MDI. Eur Respir J 1994; 7:1839–1844.
81. Thorsson L, Kenyon C, Newman S, Borgström L. Lung deposition of budesonide in asthmatics: a comparison of different formulations. Int J Pharm 1998; 168:119–127.
82. Newman S, Morén F, Trofast E, Talaee N, Clarke S. Terbutaline sulphate Turbuhaler: effect of inhaled flow rate on drug deposition and efficacy. Int J Pharm 1991; 74:209–213.
83. Meijer R, van der Mark T, Aalders B, Postma D, Koëter G. Home assessment of peak inspiratory flow through the Turbuhaler in asthmatic patients. Thorax 1996; 51:433–434.
84. Borgström L, Derom E, Ståhl E, Wåhlin-Boll E, Pauwels R. The inhalation device influences lung deposition and bronchodilating effect of terbutaline. Am J Respir Crit Care Med 1996; 153:1636–1640.
85. Santolicandro A, Di Mauro M, Storti S, et al. Lung deposition of budesonide inhaled through Turbuhaler in asthmatic patients before and after bronchodilatation. Am J Respir Crit Care Med 1994; 149(suppl):A220.
86. Harrison KS, Laube BL. Bronchodilator pretreatment improves aerosol deposition uniformity in HIV-positive patients who cough while inhaling aerosolized pentamidine. Chest 1994; 106:421–426.
87. Everard M, Devadason S, Macerlean C, et al. Drug delivery from Turbuhaler to children with CF. Am J Respir Crit Care Med 1996; 153:A70.
88. Wildhaber J, Devadason S, Wilson J, et al. Lung deposition of budesonide from Turbuhaler in asthmatic children. Eur J Pediatr 1998; 157:1017–1022.
89. Pauwels R, Newman S, Borgström L. Airway deposition and airway effects of antiasthma drugs delivered from metered-dose inhalers. Eur Respir J 1997; 10:2127–2138.
90. Beckman O, Bondesson E, Asking L, Källén A, Borgström L. Intra- and interindividual variations in pulmonary deposition via Turbuhaler and a pMDI. J Aerosol Med 1996; 9:449.
91. Borgström L, Bengtsson T, Derom E, Pauwels R. Variability in lung deposition of inhaled drug, within and between asthmatic patients, with a pMDI and a dry powder inhaler, Turbuhaler. Int J Pharm 2000; 193:227–230.
92. Borgström L. Local versus total systemic bioavailability as a means to compare different inhaled formulations of the same substance. J Aerosol Med 1998; 11:55–63.
93. Engel T. Patient-related side effects of CFC-propellants. J Aerosol Med 1991; 4:163–167.

14

Compliance with Asthma Medicine

MICHAEL E. HYLAND

University of Plymouth
Plymouth, England

CYNTHIA S. RAND

The Johns Hopkins School of Medicine
Baltimore, Maryland

"It is so hard that one cannot really have confidence in doctors and yet cannot do without them." Johann Wolfgang von Goethe, 1749–1832.

I. What Is Compliance?

A. Definitions and Interpretations of Compliance, Adherence, and Concordance

Noncompliance is defined as any behavior of the patient that is inconsistent with the instructions given by the doctor or health professional. Compliance is behavior consistent with those instructions. Although it seems self-evident that compliance is desirable, it is by no means universally accepted that compliance defined in this way is "good" and noncompliance is "bad." There are several reasons for dissatisfaction with the simplistic interpretation of compliance described above.

B. The Meaning of Noncompliance in Asthma

The relationship between doctor and patient is unequal in terms of power and control (1), and the term *compliance* implies a passive patient who slavishly follows what the doctor says. The acceptance of passivity on the part of the patient and omniscience on the part of the doctor may be good for neither party. The term *adherence* (2) has been suggested as a way of avoiding the inherent passivity implied in *compliance.* Alternatively, terms such as *concordance* (3), *therapeutic alliance* (2), or *therapeutic contract* have been proposed as a way of showing that the self-management plan followed by the patient is in some way negotiated between the doctor and the patient and that the doctor is therefore not omniscient. In addition, the term *intelligent noncompliance* has been suggested (4), or *rational noncompliance* (5), where the patient's noncompliance is a reasoned decision (6). This reasoned noncompliance may, in fact, prove a better alternative to that recommended by the physician. For example, patients may discover by experimentation that regimen modifications may result in improved asthma control. At other times, however, "rational nonadherence" may be dangerous and inappropriate, as when patients discontinue prophylactic therapy because they no longer have symptoms and consider the regimen burdensome. Thus, the term *compliance* has to be viewed within a modern culture where patients are not denied the freedom of choice and where the patient's own desired outcome and quality of life is important.

Rather than focus on the difference between instruction and behavior and its consequences, an alternative perspective on noncompliance—the word *compliance* seems to persist despite its critics—is that noncompliance represents a breakdown in communication and in the relationship between the health professional and the patient. Thus, it is not so much that the patient "is doing the wrong thing" but the pattern of relationship between the doctor and the patient is one that is not optimum for health care. Several different patterns may emerge where the relationship deteriorates between the physician and patient (1). The patient may feel coerced to comply against the his or her own wishes by the "powerful" doctor, leading to dissatisfaction and the risk of future noncompliance. The patient may indicate dissatisfaction with the doctor's recommendations and maintain that disagreement, leading to dissatisfaction and disapproval on the part of the doctor. The patient may outwardly agree with the doctor's recommendations but do something different, leading to a relationship that is partially dishonest. Thus, even if noncompliance does not lead to poor control of disease it is undesirable because of the strains it can place on the doctor-patient relationship.

C. Ethical Issues in Noncompliance

It is common for health care providers to talk about "good patients" and "bad patients" based on the degree to which they comply with prescribed therapy (7). As Holm has observed, "Every doctor can tell stories about the diabetic who 'cheats,' the epileptic who, without consulting the doctor, stops taking his medication, or the patient who 'misuses' her steroid cream" (8). However, this language of judgment and critical perspective ignores a core tenet of ethical medical care, that is, the patient's right to autonomy. As Coy has described, "other things being equal, competent adult patients *always* have the right to decide what ought or ought not to be done to them (provided that exercising that right does not infringe on the comparable rights of others)" (9). Clinicians who believe that compliance with therapy is in the patient's best interest may violate a patient's autonomy by pressing, coercing, or forcing compliance. This tension can create ethical dilemmas when considering compliance in clinical decision-making (10).

The term *medical paternalism* (9) is used when a health care provider, believing it to be in the best interest of the patient, challenges a patient's informed, autonomous decision to be noncompliant. While such concerns about the patient's well-being are understandable, medical paternalism is never justifiable for informed, competent adults. This means that a patient's decision to be noncompliant must be acknowledged and respected by the ethical physician. In the case of children, noncompliance may be a parental decision, and the ethical physician should respect the important relationship between child and parent. Parents react negatively to the suggestion or implication that they are poor parents, and an antagonistic relationship between clinician and parent is seldom helpful.

Despite the frustration that may be experienced when patients are noncompliant, it should not lead to the assumption that the patient is rejecting treatment and that the physician is thus absolved from ethical responsibility. On the contrary, noncompliant patients want treatment, and will often attend the clinic regularly, but they are dissatisfied with the treatment which is being given. Blaming the patient is neither productive nor is it considered ethically justified (11). Improved communication and tailored regimens are ultimately more effective and rewarding than blame. The quotation at the beginning of this chapter illustrates the kind of dilemma sometimes experienced by patients, that they are searching for the "best" form of treatment (12).

D. The Forms of Noncompliance in Asthma and Doctor Guilt

Although noncompliance is common in almost all treatments, the issue of noncompliance in respiratory disease is particularly complex. First, treatment for respiratory disease involves inhalers, and problems with technique lead to unintentional noncompliance which may not occur in other diseases. Intentional and unintentional noncompliance therefore need to be contrasted. Second, recommendations for care can vary between prescribing physicians. Not only are variations possible within the guidelines, but also the way the doctor communicates and advises patients is very much open to the doctor's own judgment and style. In particular the degree to which the patient is empowered to self-manage may vary between physicians. A patient who is noncompliant with one set of instructions may be compliant with another. Third, in the case of asthma in particular, compliance involves a repertoire of different behaviors some of which are needed depending on circumstance—e.g., regular dosing, increasing dose, peak flow monitoring, calling for assistance, etc. Thus, there are several different aspects of care with which a patient can be noncompliant.

A major disadvantage of the word *noncompliance* is that it can be interpreted as implying that there is a single behavior that can be characterized as noncompliance. The reality is that there are different behaviors and they occur for different reasons; it is only by understanding these differences that noncompliance can be managed effectively. Understanding the reason for noncompliance in an individual case is essential for management and forms a central part of this chapter.

The very fact that managing noncompliance is a responsibility of the physician, coupled with the ethical issues referred to in the previous section, can lead to feelings of guilt or inadequacy on the part of the physician when things "go wrong." There are few physicians who, knowing of one of their patients was dying from asthma, will fail to have doubts about their provision of care. Guilt can alter the physician's behavior, leading in some instances to overprescription. However, the corollary of rejecting medical paternalism (9) is that patients have free choice. The physician can educate and encourage to the best of his or her ability; however, the choice of behavior is that of the patient. If patients have free choice, then they cannot be made to behave in ideal way. Guilt should only occur if paternalism is an accepted part of the doctor-patient rela-

'Frankly, I wouldn't bother mate - try my apple and you won't want anything else.'
'Furthermore, Adam, I give you free choice whether or not to take your inhaler according to my Holy Law'.

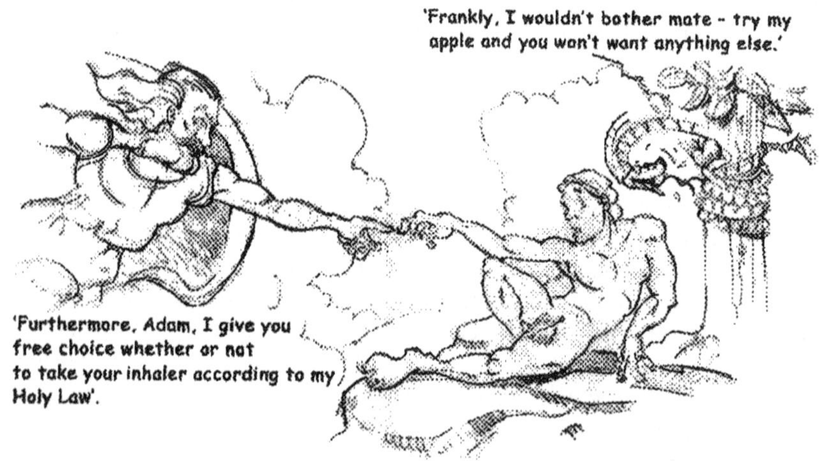

Figure 1

tionship. A similar argument occurs in religious philosophy, where an omnipotent God is said to experience regret but not guilt about the sins of sinners because of the existence of free choice. The clinician's aim should always be to provide the patient with best possible care, taking into account the sometimes suboptimal choices of patients. Finding out about those suboptimal choices is therefore essential for quality care.

- Patients have free choice and will exercise that choice.
- Patients can fail to comply for a variety of reasons.
- The clinician should aim to provide the best possible management of asthma, accommodating the suboptimal choices of some patients.

II. Measurement of Noncompliance and Prevalence

A. Patient Report

Most physicians rely on patient report when investigating noncompliance. Patients or parents of asthmatic children can be questioned either by the prescribing physician or a professional not involved in the care of the patient, the latter possibly being more reliable as patients may feel that admitting noncompliance may compromise care. In addition, admitting to noncompliance may be culture-specific. A Japanese physician wrote to the author indicating that noncompliance is seldom raised as an issue with patients, because admitting noncompliance will lead to loss of face for both patient and physician.

Studies where patients are interviewed about compliance show, however, that intentional noncompliance is common. In one study (13), 46% of patients indicated that they complied, 11% that they overused their prophylactic medicine, 28% reported underuse, and 15% reported cyclical use—i.e.,variable over- and underuse. These figures are similar to those obtained from electronic monitoring. In a study where adolescents were asked about medication, the majority reported not taking their prophylactic medicine regularly and delayed taking their bronchodilator (14). Others show that it is regular use rather than increases in use during exacerbations which is disliked by patients (15). Despite the value of these patient reports, there are two reasons why patient report might be considered unreliable. First, studies in both clinical and research settings (16–18) have found that some patients may deliberately mislead when they report on their use of inhalers. Second, patients forget and therefore give an inaccurate report unintentionally. Disparities between records from electronic inhalers (19) and diary records of inhaler use suggest that some inaccuracy in reporting may simply be due to incompetence on the part of the patient. Patients cannot be relied on to remember what they have done (20), or record accurately what they do in diary cards. To err is human.

Despite these disadvantages patient reports have certain advantages compared with more objective measures of adherence, such as biochemical measures and electronic monitors. For example, patient report provides information about how patients respond to worsening asthma. One of the assumptions of electronic monitoring is that patients should be taking a constant dose. However, some adult self-management plans include an increase in dose when asthma exacerbates (e.g., a drop in peak expiratory flow). It may be that a failure to increase when exacerbating has a more serious consequence to outcome than simply not taking the required dose regularly. Finally, patient report provides reasons why noncompliance occurs. Not only do some patients admit that they intentionally fail to comply, but they will also give clearly articulated reasons why they do so.

B. Prescription Monitoring

As computerization of pharmacy data has become more prevalent, it has become increasingly feasible to monitor patients' medication compliance by examining these records. Within an office a physician can track patient's requests for refills of asthma medications. Within a pharmacy such databases can provide information on the amount of medication dispensed, and the timing of refills. This data can be used to roughly calculate the average dose per day. In some health care data management systems prescriptions that are written but never filled can also be monitored. Pharmacy data review can reveal refill-based adherence patterns for different classes of medication or dosing regimens. For example, Kelloway et al. (21) examined pharmacy claims data within a health maintenance organization and found that asthmatic patients were significantly more adherent to prescribed tablet medication (theophylline) than with two commonly prescribed inhaled anti-inflammatory medications (inhaled corticosteroid and inhaled cromolyn). Pharmacy review to identify noncompliance has several limitations. Even when pharmacy data can determine the filling of a prescription, however, they provide no confirmation of consumption, or appropriate consumption patterns. In addition, pharmacy review cannot determine if medications sit unused; are hoarded for future use; shared or given to family and friends; or taken inappropriately. Nevertheless, as more and more pharmacy data go on line, this compliance measuring strategy has great potential (22).

C. Electronic Monitors

Over the past 10 years, electronic inhaler monitoring devices have been developed which record the date and time of actuations and can then be downloaded onto a computer. A record can then be printed which reflects a patient's pattern of inhaler use over a period of time. Electronic peak flow meters are also available which record and store peak flow values, along with date and time information. While these devices have generally been utilized exclusively for research, improved technologies are increasingly making their clinical application feasible.

Research with electronic inhalers has examined both prophylactic and bronchodilator use. In one study of prophylactic medicine use (23), only 50% of patients complied as defined by within 10% of recommended twice daily dosing, 50% underused and 10% overused. Electronic monitoring of inhaler use has documented widespread underuse of anti-inflammatory medications in both children and adults. Mawhinney et al. reported that patients used their medication as prescribed on average for 37% of the days in the 3 to 4 weeks monitoring period (24). Underuse was observed for over 38% of the monitored days. Coutts et al. monitored school-age children and observed underuse of the inhaled steroids was observed on 55% of the study days (16). Similar results on the underuse of anti-inflammatory medications have been reported elsewhere (25–27).

Nonadherence with asthma therapy can involve not only underuse of preventive medications but may also overuse or inappropriate use of rescue medications. A number of researchers have speculated that overreliance on inhaled bronchodilators may contribute to patient delays in seeking medical care for acute asthma, or that overuse of beta agonists may pose direct health risks to the asthmatic patient (28,29). As with inhaled anti-inflammatory therapy, patients may not be accurate reporters of their level of adherence with this treatment. For example, when Yeung et al. examined adherence with beta-agonist therapy using electronic monitors, they found that, in contrast to anti-inflammatory therapies, patients tended to underreport beta-agonist use (19).

Electronic devices have been used to monitor peak flow measurement, though the use of regular peak flow monitoring is not always recommended (30). In a study where patients were unaware of such electronic monitoring and were asked to monitor daily and keep a written record, 15% of days were missing from the written peak flow record after 3 weeks but 52% of days were missing from the electronic records (31). Thus, if patients are advised to monitor peak flow in order to guide therapeutic change, one should not assume that patients do as advised.

Although electronic monitoring devices can provide important insights into patients' patterns of inhaler and peak flow monitor use, this measurement strategy has some limitations. For example, electronic inhaler monitors do not show whether the patient is firing the inhaler into the air or into the mouth, and repeated actuations may be because the patient is "testing" the inhaler in the air; but nevertheless, these data overall paint a poor picture of noncompliance. Electronic records of inhaler use do not show if a patient is failing to increase medication in the event of worsening symptoms. Most importantly, such records do not show *why* the patient is engaging in noncompliant behavior.

- Noncompliance can be measured by patient reporting, prescription monitoring, and electronic inhalers. Each method has advantages and disadvantages.

- About 50% of patients fail to comply with twice daily prophylactic medication.
- Noncompliance takes a variety of different forms.
- Many patients underuse, some overuse, and some sometimes over and sometimes underuse.

The next two sections examine the several reasons for noncompliance. They draw partly on patient report but also on the more general literature and theory in psychology concerning the determinants of health-related behavior. Patients are not always able to articulate a reason for their noncompliance, so the reasons for noncompliance cannot rely only on patients. Because it is common to distinguish intentional from unintentional noncompliance, the next two sections are organised on that basis. These sections describe *reasons* for noncompliance, the *behaviors* associated with that noncompliance, and *management strategies* for dealing with that particular kind of noncompliance.

There are two types of reason for noncompliance:

- Unintentional noncompliance
- Intentional noncompliance

III. Reasons for Unintentional Noncompliance

A. Forgetting: Instructional Problems

Studies that have examined patients' recall of physicians' instructions report that patients' recall is generally poor (32). Regimens for asthma care can be particularly complex, with multiple inhalers and dosing schedules. Because there are two kinds of inhaler, a prophylactic and a bronchodilator, patients can forget which inhaler is which, though there are no clear data on the numbers who forget in this way. Patients are often taught the terms preventer and reliever, but their meaning is not always clear to patients. For some patients, the color coding of blue and brown is the easier memory cue, but the introduction of new inhalers with other color codings requires extra caution. A simple question such as "How do you use your inhalers?" can be a useful check, particularly in the case of patients whose cognitive ability may be poor.

Apart from forgetting the function of the two (or more) inhalers, patients will also forget to take their inhaler on occasion. In a study of parents of asthmatic children (33), 60% said they sometimes forget to give their child's medicine. Indeed, it seems a normal human characteristic to forget to take medicine on occasion. It will only be the exceptional patient who takes medicine exactly as instructed every day without fail. An absence of clear instructions in the self-management plan about what to do when a dose is forgotten is an important omission.

The physiological effect of forgetting to take a dose will vary with the patient. For patients whose inflammation is barely controlled by the regular dose, lack of one dose may lead to increased inflammation and a drop in peak flow. Such patients may be advised to double their dose when they realize they have forgotten. For other patients, sufficient anti-inflammatory control is achieved despite the occasional missed dose. Self-management plans should include clear instructions as to what to do when patients forget to take their prophylactic inhaler, as they inevitably will from time to time. Clinical approaches to help patients who have difficulty remembering to take their inhaler should center on strategies that cue or prompt inhaler use. Positioning the inhaler near the patient's toothbrush or kettle, reminder notes on the refrigerator, or even medication alarms can be helpful for some patients.

B. Device and Technique Problems

Correct use of a meter-dose inhaler (MDI) requires a variety of actions to be completed, including shaking the inhaler, complete exhalation, slow inhalation, coordination of actuation with inhalation, and breath-holding. Research shows that technique is poor in one or more of these actions. For example DeBlaquiere found that although all patients in a sample had received initial instruction in inhaler use, only 38% demonstrated proper technique when measured (34). However, the original training of patients may be responsible for some error (35) as evaluations of prescribing physicians have also been found to be poor (36,37). Chapman et al. suggest that physician ignorance on inhaler use arises because such skills are looked on as prosaic and of little interest to medicine (38). The use of nurses and physiotherapists in training patients may have advantages. In addition to incorrect voluntary actions by the patient, patients may also demonstrate an involuntary constriction of the throat, the "cold freon effect," which even with training may be difficult to eliminate.

Difficulties in the way patients use MDIs has been one factor in the development of other forms of inhaler, in particular dry-powder inhalers (DPIs) and breath-actuated MDIs. These newer devices produce better compliance in terms of technique (whether they affect other reasons for noncompliance is less clear), but even here, some are better than others. One study of dry-powder inhaler technique found that that 5% had good technique, 5% were adequate, and 27% were insufficient (39). For example, in the case of DPI, it is necessary to inhale reasonably fast, though the extent to which the rate of inhalation affects deposition varies between inhalers. Some DPIs show less variation and are tolerant of lower inhalation rates compared with others. The wide range of inhalers now available varies on a number of different criteria, and some inhalers will be more suited to some patients than others. Devices may not be equally suited to children, young adults, or the elderly.

Checking of technique can take place in the clinic and normally provides a reasonably accurate estimate of the patient's technique when at home. Because inhaler technique tends to deteriorate over a period of time, review of technique should be a regular component of follow-up care.

For patients whose poor inhaler technique cannot be modified, alternatives include the use of a spacer or switching to an inhaler device or alternative therapy (e.g., oral) with which the patient is more comfortable and competent. A sensible recommendation is that patients should play an active role in choosing the device which suits them best—for example, they are given a choice from a limited selection previously decided by the physician. Providing patients with choice may lead to greater perceived control and hence better compliance.

In some health care systems, the selection of an appropriate device for the patient is affected by cost. It is important to recognize, however, that although an MDI with spacer may be the most economic way of drug delivery, providing patients with a device which is poorly accepted can lead to poor compliance and may therefore lead to increased health care costs overall. Hence, cost should never be the only factor taken into account when selecting between devices.

C. Respiratory Insensitivity

The relationship between peak expiratory flow (PEF) and symptoms is good for some patients, but for others the relationship is very poor (40). Patients with chronically poor symptom perception may consider their asthma "under control" and as a result fail to comply with prophylactic therapy. Some patients are unaware of worsening asthma, in particular slow declines in PEF. Such patients will not take appropriate action as specified by their self-management program (e.g., doubling the inhaled steroid dose when PEF < 75% best), because they are unaware of the drop in PEF. In fact, this disregard for worsening asthma has been suggested as an important contributing factor in episodes of fatal and near-fatal asthma (41,42). Respiratory sensitivity is an issue for adults but not for children, who may be too young to report worsening symptoms. In the case of children, worsening asthma can be detected symptomatically by parents, but only if parents are educated about what symptoms to look out for and how to respond to those symptoms. In the case of children, worsening asthma may require a different and a more cautious approach (e.g., requiring doctor consultation) than with adults.

The advantage of regular PEF monitoring is clear for such patients. However, compliance with regular PEF monitoring is poor. Cote and colleagues used electronically monitored PEF meters—patients were unaware of this monitoring—and found 30% never or almost never used their PEF right from the beginning, and 60% were using their PEF meter <25% of the time at 12 months, with fabricated PEF entries written onto diary cards (31). However, PEF monitoring may not be needed for all patients. For some patients, symptoms may be as accurate as PEF in detecting worsening asthma. If regular monitoring of PEF is not needed (other forms of use include occasional use and checking when symptoms occur) then telling patients that PEF measuring is essential may have an adverse impact on other aspects of compliance, because it increases the burden of treatment. Treatment burden (see later) is one reason for failing to comply.

Patients:

- Forget to take it
- Forget which one to take when
- Forget how to take it
- Do not notice deterioration

IV. Reasons for Intentional Noncompliance

A. Reasoned Action and Treatment Burden

Many human actions are based on reason. Some patients weigh up the advantages (better asthma control) and disadvantages (inconvenience and cost) of taking their medicine as recommended and decide to do otherwise. Although from the physician's perspective, the patient may not be acting in a rational way, the patient nevertheless thinks that he or she is rational and has come to the best decision. There are several reasons why patients decide consciously to take more or less medicine than recommended. For some patients who have a busy lifestyle, the advantage of

'now which was the one I have
to take twice a day?
Hm..., well the blue one
looks nicer so perhaps it's that one.

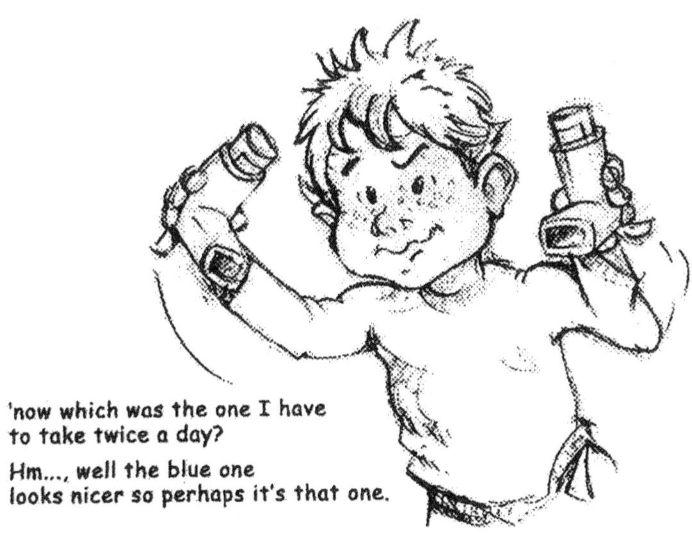

Figure 2

taking their inhaler regularly (i.e., lack of asthma problems) is not considered sufficiently great to justify the time involved. In one study, 17% of patients said that the inconvenience or embarrassment of taking their asthma medicine was a minor bother, 9% said it was a major bother (43). Some patients overuse their inhaler by taking the dose recommended only for exacerbations on the supposition that that dose must be safe if recommended by the doctor and so why bother to allow exacerbation. In both cases, patients weigh up the advantages and disadvantages of acting according to the recommendation of the physician. Clinicians should raise the issue of cost and benefits directly when discussing options for asthma management. Patient compliance will be optimized when patient preference can be incorporated into the choice of therapy.

For others it is the financial cost of the medicine. Indeed many patients undermedicate specifically as a cost cutting measure. It should be noted that the factors determining cost-benefit analysis may differ between asthmatic adults and parents of children with asthma. Parents may be more prepared to spend money on their children than themselves, though in some health care systems the cost of medicines for the child is free.

Where cost is a factor in noncompliance, the patient may attempt to ration medication by adopting a constant reduced dose. The physician can help the patient in some cases by change of prescription to a more cost-effective (for the patient) regimen—though this may not be possible within the constraints of the health care system. Because patients are often embarrassed to admit to difficulties paying for medications, the first step in addressing this barrier to compliance is sensitivity and open communication (prior to prescribing) that directly assesses if cost constraints are present.

There are circumstances where it is in the patient's financial interest to have symptoms or at least to report symptoms. Patients who realize they can use their asthma to obtain a state benefit (e.g., the Disability Living Allowance in the U.K.) may either overreport symptoms or undermedicate specifically to obtain this benefit. Of course, not all patients use their asthma in this way, but the possibility should be considered if decisions are in the process of being made about state benefit. A reduction in symptoms after the decision is made is a possible indicator of benefit-induced symptom reporting.

B. Health and Illness Beliefs

It is an interesting paradox that some patients will happily take vitamins but be reluctant to take their inhaled steroids. Willingness to take one form of medication (vitamins) but not another (drugs) illustrates the importance of beliefs about treatment. Patients sometimes distinguish between (1) the improvement of health and (2) the treatment of illness as being two essentially different processes. Vitamins, from this perspective, are often thought to improve health, whereas medicines are seen as harming health, even though they treat illness. Patients vary as to the extent to which they are health-focused versus illness-focused (44); however, many believe in the importance of health independent of illness. Consistent with this view, studies show that patients do not mind taking their inhalers for short periods of time when they have exacerbations but do not wish to take their medicine over long periods of time (45,46). In one study (33), 86% of the parents of asthmatic children said that medicine should not be used for long periods, 43% said that the medicine was unnatural and harmful to children, and 31% said children's bodies were too small to cope.

The idea that some medicines disturb the body's "balance" is consistent with Chinese and Ayurvedic medicine (48); therefore the idea that health-promoting actions (e.g., vitamin taking) create balance whereas illness-treating actions (e.g., taking steroids) create imbalance may be more common among those patients sympathetic to complementary or alternative medicine or from cultures where traditional medicine is practiced. Although the distinction between health promotion and disease prevention is consistent with modern definitions of health (49), modern medicine does not accept the idea that the body can be become "unbalanced"—drugs can produce localized side effect but not this generalized imbalance which is believed by patients and features in complementary medicine. Thus, doctors and patients have different views about the dangers of steroids. When doctors say steroids are safe, they mean that they do not have specific side effects. Patients, on the other hand, worry about something else—the long-term effect of steroids creating imbalance in a distributed, health-harming way. Despite being inconsistent with much of modern medicine, patients' concerns are not theoretically implausible. Recent research on networks suggests that a more generalized form of network fault may give rise to the known inflammatory mediators (50). From the perspective of compliance, however, the important message is that doctors and patients interpret the word *safe* in different ways. Telling patients that a drug has few measurable side effects will not reassure those who are concerned about long-term, generalized effects on health.

Patient beliefs about illness and therapy are strongly rooted within cultural norms that may be discordant with the traditional biomedical model of the physician. Pachter has described clinical encounters as "an interaction between two cultures—the 'culture' of medicine and the 'culture' of patients" (51). When there are differences between the patient's explanatory model for the causes and treatments of asthma and that of the physician, the resulting miscommunication can lead to poor compliance with therapy. Some patients may elect to use home remedies as an adjunct to prescribed regimens, or reject prescribed therapies outright, and these practices will not usually be revealed in the standard consultation.

Some patients simply do not like taking medicine of any kind because of the potential negative impact on health. As already noted, some patients under-medicate on their bronchodilator (52). However, some patients particularly dislike steroids, and this particular dislike may stem from misinformation—such as a misunderstanding of the difference between oral and inhaled steroids and the fact that the media reports athlete's steroid taking as a bad thing to do. However, in other cases, dislike of steroids is based on nothing other than a general mistrust of powerful drugs coupled with knowledge that steroids can have side effects.

Dislike of medicine can lead to a variety of noncompliant behaviors, including a constantly reduced dose and symptomatic use of the prophylactic inhaler, both behaviors having the intention of minimizing drug intake.

The effect of symptomatic use of a prophylactic inhaler is not always easy to evaluate. This approach to asthma management is so widespread that informal clinical report indicates that many health professionals who have asthma, including respiratory consultants and respiratory nurses, manage their asthma symptomatically. The asthma guidelines have always allowed for an increase in inhaled steroids and recent guidelines also include information for stepping down. However, in the case of patients who use symptomatic control, the stepping down is much more rapid than would be recommended in the guidelines. The exact consequence of this symptomatic control of asthma with inhaled steroids is not known. To some extent its success depends on the insight the patient has into the disease process. A patient who responds rapidly to a worsening of asthma with a higher dose of inhaled steroid may do better than a patient whose response is slower.

Management of symptomatically controlling patients depends crucially on outcome. A patient who employs symptomatic use of prophylactic medicine but has repeated hospital visits needs different management from one who uses this technique effectively. In the former case, it is a good strategy to explain the clinical disadvantages of, for example, repeated courses of oral steroids in contrast to a higher maintenance level of inhaled steroids.

Health beliefs are difficult to change but respond best to balanced, two-sided arguments rather than single-sided arguments. Sensitivity to the patient's concerns about medicine will have a greater impact on the patient than a simple overall assertion that the medicines are safe. In addition, patients who believe that there is an underlying state of health or balance that is independent of illness may feel that the evidence that steroids are safe is the wrong kind of evidence because it does not relate to what they understand by health. Patients who are antagonistic to medicine may be more responsive to "health promoting" advice, including trigger avoidance, exercise, and diet.

Patients can believe that "powerful" drugs

- Are good at curing illness
- Are harmful for health

The presentation of the drug may affect how powerful it is perceived to be. For example, once-daily treatment may be perceived as less powerful than twice daily therapy. If so, once-daily therapy will be more acceptable for regular use, with twice-daily accepted for exacerbations when a more powerful treatment is needed.

C. Self-Perception and Denial

The label *asthma* is interpreted differently by different people and in different cultures. However, for some, the stigma attached to the label leads to negative self-perceptions (53); in general, people are strongly motivated to avoid negative self-perceptions (54). For some patients, noncompliance reflects the negative self-perception that arises from taking asthma medicine—that is, the perception that the patient is an "ill person" which is a message that the use of inhalers can give. The negative message given by an inhaler is culture-specific, as socially acceptable means of delivering drugs differ between cultures (e.g., suppositories are more acceptable in France). Patients therefore fail to comply with treatment and fail to attend the clinic or school because either of these actions reinforces a negative self-image.

For example, Adams et al. (55) examined self-perceptions in a sample of asthmatic patients who had been prescribed prophylactic medications. Over half

"No . . . . I don't
have asthma . . . .
Just sometimes
have these
asthma attacks."

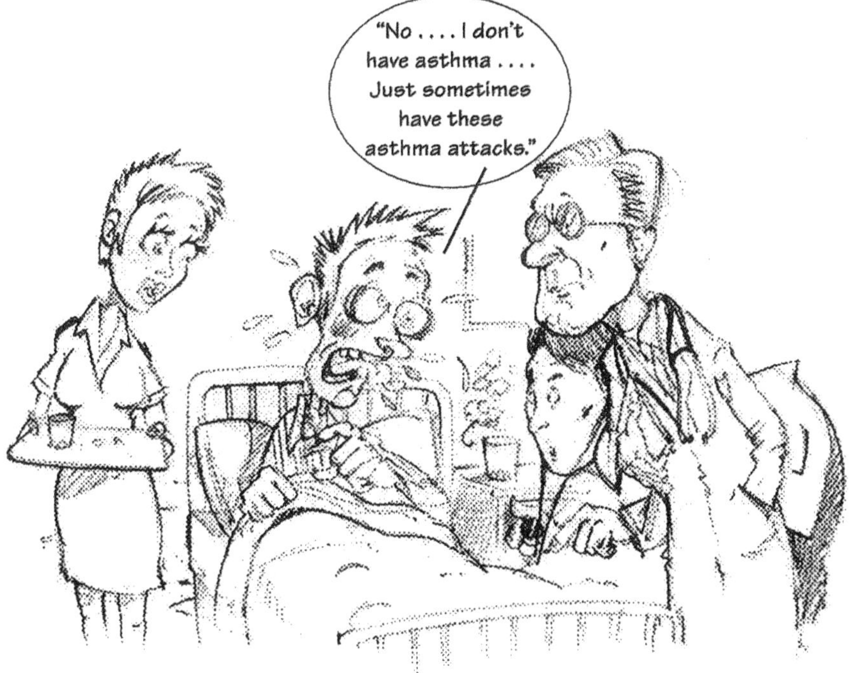

Figure 3

the sample either claimed that that they did not have asthma (despite a clinical diagnosis and prescribed medications) or reported that they had "slight" or "not proper" asthma. Interviewing revealed that these patients frequently used their reliever surreptitiously and that none of these patients were using their prescribed prophylactic asthma medications. All of these individuals refused to accept the stigmatizing (in their view) label of "asthmatic" and instead relabeled their breathing problems as an acute, situation-specific problem or as a "bad chest."

Asthmatics at any age can be sensitive to the effects of asthma self-perception, but greater sensitivity may occur in adolescents whose self-concept may be in flux. Indeed adolescents and young adults are particularly at risk for this reason. It is possible, though by no means certain, that the design of an inhaler will affect health beliefs. For example, if a child's inhaler is visually "fun" to look at, then there may be less of a negative impact on self-perception than with an inhaler that looks as though it had been issued by a hospital pharmacy. Some manufacturers make stickers which can be added to an inhaler to make the inhaler more individualized and user friendly. However, not everyone agrees with the concept of presenting inhalers as a "normal" consumer object due to concern over misuse. However, for patients for whom the thought of asthma creates negative self-perceptions, an approach to treatment which appears less medicalized may help. Less frequent dosing and, when available, effective oral medication may help for this kind of patient.

D. Coping Style

People cope with the ups and downs of life in different ways. It is common to distinguish two broad categories of coping, problem-focused coping and emotion-focused coping (56,57). Problem-focused coping means finding a way of dealing with the problem produced by life stresses (e.g., planning a solution, finding out how others have coped); emotion-focused coping means dealing with the emotion produced by life stresses (e.g., complaining to others, distraction, getting drunk). People vary in the style of coping but some people tend to have a disposition to be problem-focused whereas others have a disposition to be emotion-focused—many people combine both forms of coping.

In a sense, asthma schools and asthma clinics are designed for problem-focused copers. They are designed for people who want to find out about asthma and do something about it. Problem-focused copers generally manage their asthma well. They are the sort of patients who will find out what they can about asthma, and follow self-management plans carefully. These may be the kinds of patients who has found out about asthma on the Internet and come to the clinic armed with a list of the "best" inhalers. However, asthma clinics are, from a psychological perspective, not designed for patients who are emotion-focused. They are not designed for people for whom the experience of going to an asthma clinic or school is in itself emotionally distressing. Such patients cope with their asthma by ignoring their asthma, by finding some form of distraction from their asthma, and by doing anything but deal with the problem directly. Emotion-focused copers represent a difficult management problem because such patients, by their very nature, are not predisposed toward effective management. Like those for whom asthma leads to negative self-perceptions, emotion copers avoid managing asthma as a way of avoiding the emotion caused by recognition of asthma. Although emotion-focused coping leads to short-term emotional gains, it is less effective in the long term, as the stressful event is not addressed and the asthma is not managed.

Emotion-focused copers represent a major problem for asthma management. They tend to deny that they have asthma (e.g., "I don't have asthma, I just sometimes have asthma attacks") and appear to accept what the clinician recommends but do something else. An authoritarian approach with such patients is unlikely to be successful. Instead, the clinician should try to develop a positive and understanding relationship with the patient, where the patient may be cajoled into a different course of action. Sometimes a more conservative management plan may be advisable, in which the patient is advised to seek medical assistance at an earlier stage than normal.

E. Checking/Drug Holidays

Some patients decide to stop taking asthma medicines on specific occasions. For example, a patient may decide that medicine should not be needed when going on holiday. This attitude lets the patient off the burden of taking medicine, just as it lets people off other lifestyle burdens, such as work. Some patients check to see whether they have been "cured" of asthma and so periodically stop taking their medicine to see if they are better. In effect, these patients step down their treatment more rapidly than recommended in the guidelines, but do not, of course, tell the physician about their experimentation. Such patients clearly pose a risk for themselves, but only at irregular intervals. Failing to take an inhaler on holiday is particularly troublesome because, in a new environment, the patient may be exposed to new allergens for which medical care is uncertain. Ceasing medication in order to check whether the patient still has asthma is dangerous only if the patient fails to monitor the worsening of asthma, but patient optimism may lead to a failure in monitoring.

Management of checking/drug holidays is best achieved through a positive relationship between the clinician and patient. If the patient thinks that experimentation or changes of action will receive an authoritarian response if discussed, then the patient is less likely to initiate discussion. The clinician needs to remember that patients will always do odd things if they want to, but advice from the clinician can make those odd things less dangerous if the advice is perceived by the patient as being positive and constructive.

V. Issues in Pediatric Compliance

Despite parents' good intentions, children's adherence with asthma therapy has generally been found to be as problematic as adult adherence with therapy (16,17,58,59). While the consequences of periodic nonadherence with therapy among children with mild asthma may be insignificant, for some children drug holidays or chronic underuse of preventer medications can result in serious asthma flares (17), unnecessary emergency room visits (59,60), and increased risk of fatal or near-fatal asthma attacks (61,62). Just as in adult adherence with asthma therapy, factors which have been associated with increased risk of pediatric nonadherence include knowledge and beliefs about asthma and asthma therapy (63,64), regimen complexity (16), as well as social and cultural resources and barriers (65,66). Unique to pediatric adherence, however, is the contributing role family conflict and poor family communication have been have found to play in children's nonadherence with therapy, particularly among adolescents (67–69).

Pediatric adherence with asthma therapy is necessarily an evolving and developmentally dynamic behavior. As children grow, responsibility for medication administration generally shifts from total parent management for a young child, to shared medication management for the school-age child, to finally, complete self-management for the older adolescent. Factors such as parent beliefs and family functioning will influence the parent's willingness and ability to follow prescribed therapy. Parents' opinions about the value and role of asthma medications for their children do not necessarily match those of the treating physician. For example, parental concerns about children becoming "addicted" to asthma medications or a belief that asthma medicines will loose effectiveness if used too often, may lead parents to use as little medication as possible (64). For many parents, daily use of medication is troubling, particularly when a child is not symptomatic. In some families home remedies or over-the-counter drugs (teas, coffee, cough medicines, decongestants, etc.) for asthma may be common and viewed as "safer" than conventional prescribed asthma medications (62,64).

The age at which a child becomes responsible for self-administration of asthma medications is highly variable and may be based more on family circumstances than on a carefully supervised transition of responsibility as the child matures (70). In some families a child may be expected to manage his or her own medication administration quite young, less because the child has demonstrated sufficient responsibility, and more because the parent believes the child is "old enough to do it" or because family circumstances (e.g., working parents) dictate the need. Medication management responsibility may be shared among a diverse and changing cast, including the child, parents, day care providers, school health aides, grandparents, and siblings. In chaotic, troubled families, primary responsibility for medication monitoring may be confused. Because of the potential for highly variable and often shifting family responsibility for a child's medication use, it is therefore necessary for health care providers to review with both the parent and the child medication use habits in order to develop an adherence profile.

Research in asthma and other chronic pediatric diseases has underscored the particular vulnerability of the adolescent to medication adherence problems (67–69). Normal adolescent independence behaviors, including rule-testing, acting out, and rejection of parental authority can significantly interfere with responsible asthma management. Some adolescents may deny disease severity and undertreat or ignore asthma symptoms (68,69). While all adolescents may be at increased risk of nonadherence with therapy, clinicians should be aware that marked family conflict or a denial of disease severity in an adolescent with severe asthma are red flags for a higher risk of a dangerous asthma event (67).

Tips for managing adolescents

- Sometimes adolescents will admit to noncompliance only in the absence of their parents.
- It is important to "decriminalize" noncompliance. Discussion should focus on what the adolescent can manage, not what should or should not be done.

VI. Diagnosing Noncompliance

A. Clinical Outcome

Not all noncompliance leads to poor outcome, and it therefore seems most time effective for the physician to concentrate on that compliance which has poor outcome. When a patient presents with symptomatic, uncontrolled asthma a nonjudgmental, careful review of compliance should be undertaken. Poor outcome will include reduced quality of life, as well as increased medical care (hospital attendance, nebulisations, unscheduled visits etc.). Whereas increased medical attendance is normally obtained from objective data, quality of life requires report from the patient. Some patients experience quality of life deficits but fail to report them to the doctor because they believe those deficits are worth suffering if a reduced level of inhaler is taken. An automatic record of unscheduled care provides the clinician with a useful picture about the patient's asthma control, as well as occasional specific questions (e.g., "How many times are you awakened at night due to asthma?" rather than "Are you often awakened at night due to asthma?"). However, poor outcome serves merely as an alert for the possibility of noncompliance, and further investigation is needed.

A review of compliance should begin with asking the patient to describe in detail the patient's understanding of the prescribed therapy. If possible, have the patient bring in all unused medication and demonstrate how each medication is used. This approach often uncovers patient confusion about which inhaler to use on a daily basis or a misunderstanding of the dosing schedule. Discussing patterns of use and "drug holidays" can be illustrative for both the patient and clinician in uncovering the relationship between noncompliance and asthma exacerbations.

B. Asking Questions and Listening

A good relationship between the physician/health professional and the patient is an essential first step for understanding asthma management from the patient's perspective. While physicians may endorse the importance of assessing patient compliance with therapy, all too often patients are never directly asked about their compliance with prescribed treatments. The ability of a physician to effectively gather compliance information from patients, and identify patient nonadherence has been shown to be highly variable and dependent on interviewing skill and style (71,72). Further, physician's self-assessments of their own communication skills are not related to observer ratings of their communication skills (73,74).

Physician interviewing skills and the qualities of the patient-provider interaction are important in both measuring and facilitating adherence behaviors. Use of an information-intensive and nonjudgmental style of interviewing has been suggested as a strategy for improving the accuracy of patient self-reported adherence. Steele et al. (72) examined audiotaped interactions between patients and providers and concluded that a nonaccusatory, open-ended, information-intensive approach can be a sensitive and productive tool for the diagnosis of a patient's compliance status.

Thoughtful, nonjudgmental interviewing presents an opportunity to the clinician to explore and understand the nature of the patient's compliance difficulties. Several questions can be asked which provide additional insight into the patient's preferred mode of self-management. For example, patients' use of analgesics, whether they often take painkillers for headaches or whether they prefer not to take painkillers, is a useful indicator of patients' attitudes towards medicines in general. Similarly, questions about the patient's attitudes to vitamins indicates the patient's preparedness to engage in health promoting behaviour in contrast to illness preventing behaviour. Questions which elicit information about coping strategies (for example, whether the patient normally responds to stress in an emotion-focused way or a problem-focused way), can also be useful in anticipating how the patient copes with asthma.

However, the most important (and often scarcest) resource for forming a relationship with a patient is having the time to listen. Patients will often want to give the clinician information, information which may not be clinically relevant. Listening to what a patient wants to say conveys to the patient that the clinician really cares about the patient as a person. Patients respond to small nonverbal cues that can have a substantial impact on the relationship and hence the trust of the patient for the clinician. An example of this is the hospital consultant who feels the patient's pulse after looking at the patient's notes. The message to the patient is "I know the nurses have taken your pulse, but you are such an important patient that I want to check for myself." Giving that message can motivate compliance.

C. Bronchodilator/Prophylactic Ratio

As discussed above, pharmacy data can provide insight into a patient's pattern of medication use and reveal compliance problems. Because many patients' noncompliance takes the form of underuse of anti-inflammatory therapy and overuse of bronchodilators, a bronchodilator/prophylactic ratio which is inconsistent with the guidelines may indicate poor asthma control, and possibly poor compliance. Some clinics have an electronic automatic alert facility that alerts the clinician when this ratio becomes too imbalanced, and the ratio is also an important aspect of asthma audit. However, there are a number of reasons why the bronchodilator/prophylactic ratio should be treated with caution.

First, the bronchodilator/prophylactic ratio will not detect the patient who intentionally undermedicates both on bronchodilators and prophylactics. As described in the previous section some patients do not like to take any kind of medicine. Second, the bronchodilator/prophylactic ratio does not guarantee that the patient has actually taken the medicine for which scripts have been written. It is not unusual for patients to find their treatment expensive and take only the bronchodilator, as it is the treatment which seems to work most effectively. Third, even when the cashing of scripts is checked so that the clinician knows that patient has actually purchased or received the inhaler, there is no guarantee that the patient is actually taking it. There are occasional reports of relatives bringing in a carrier bag full of inhalers that belonged to someone who has recently died. Inhalers can be collected at the back of a cupboard. Fourth, and finally, in some health care systems the cost of medicines differs between family members. For example, in the U.K., medicine is dispensed at no cost for children but not for adults. Under such circumstances "inhaler sharing" sometimes occurs, and the clinician cannot really tell from the clinical records who is using which inhaler within a family.

Despite these disadvantages, the bronchodilator/prophylactic ratio can be useful as a system of alerting the clinician to possible compliance problems. The rule is that if the bronchodilator/prophylactic ratio is poor, then there is probably a problem. However, if the bronchodilator/prophylactic ratio is good, one cannot guarantee that there is no problem.

D. Electronic Monitors

Patients can be asked to keep diary records of PEF and inhaler use. However, such records may be constructed retrospectively by the patient just prior to going to the clinic. As the technology improves and then cost decreases, electronic inhaler and PEF monitoring devices will become more commonly available to assess compliance in the clinical setting.

These electronic monitoring devices should be used with care in clinical practice, because insensitive use can adversely affect the relationship between clinician and patient. Failing to inform the patient about the electronic monitor may lead to distrust as patients perceive the clinician is trying to catch them out. Even where the patient is told about the monitor in advance, the clinician should be careful not to give the impression that the patient is perceived as lying. However, such devices can be used effectively if presented to the patient as a shared tool to be used by the patient and clinician to find out about how the patient is managing. Clinicians do differ in their opinion on the circumstances in which electronic monitoring is useful.

When using an electronic monitor to detect noncompliance, the clinician should introduce the topic from a problem-focused perspective. After discussing whether the patient has any idea why poor outcome is being achieved, the clinician can outline the options, which include measuring exactly how the medicines are being used. Statements such as "People find it very easy to forget to take these inhalers, so we usually check to see how much forgetting occurs" may present the monitoring in a normalized and non-emotionally threatening manner. The important point to remember is that patient must not feel that he or she is being singled out as a suspected incompetent person.

E. Diagnosing Type of Noncompliance: Summary

The diagnosis of type of noncompliance when it is expected requires skill and experience. In setting the scene for a positive therapeutic relationship with a patient, a useful first question is "In what way would you like me to help you with asthma?" Such a question emphasizes the cooperative, helping role of the physician in which patients are encouraged to talk about their aims so that the management plan is *concordant* with the patient, rather than reflecting only the objectives of the clinician. The philosophy of concordance requires a different approach to managing the patient to the philosophy of the passive compliant patient.

Once effective and open communication has been established with patients, the clinician should check for unintentional noncompliance by reviewing the patient's understanding of the regimen. For example, a check should be made of inhaler technique and then some questioning about "how you manage to remember to take the inhaler twice a day." In the case of intentional noncompliance, information about the cost of medicine to the patient and health beliefs may throw some light on the situation. Particularly in the case of intentional noncompliance it is important not to appear judgmental. For example, patients may feel uncomfortable saying that they are reluctant to take the recommended medicine because they cannot afford it. If patients feel that the clinician is on their side rather than a judge then they are likely to be more honest.

VII. Targeting Device/Oral Therapy According to Patient Profile and Individualizing Advice

Patients differ in terms of their psychology just as they differ in terms of their physiology. Two patients whose asthma is identical from a physiological perspective may nevertheless need to be treated quite differently due to psychological differences. Management needs to be individualized according to the needs and abilities of patients. A patient with poor cognitive development who wants to be "told what to do" will respond better to a simpler management plan than an educated patient who wants to take control of his or her asthma management. The extent to which the patient rather than the clinician is responsible for changes in treatment (e.g., stepping up and stepping down) should also be individualised according to the patient's capacities and preferences. Some patients want to take control of their treatment, and will do so whatever the doctor advises. Such patients will read a considerable amount of literature on the subject and will often demand particular types of therapy from the doctor. Other patients, who have a lower need for control and are more emotionally focused will want much less involvement in their asthma management. They will need more support and a simpler management plan.

Equally, not all patients should receive the same inhaler. Different inhalers have different implications for unintentional noncompliance and they may also have implications for intentional noncompliance. Selecting the optimum inhaler is as important as selecting the optimum drug, and giving the optimum instructions in the optimum manner. The importance of individualizing treatment will become more apparent as new treatments for asthma are developed which increase the range of options open to the clinician.

VIII. Summary and Further Research

This chapter has shown that there are different types of noncompliance, which occur for different reasons, and with different outcomes. Rather than managing noncompliance in a particular, fixed way, the type of noncompliance requires diagnosis before appropriate management can be initiated. Although we know a good deal about the nature and reasons for noncompliance, we know surprisingly little about optimal strategies for dealing with it in its various forms. For example, although nurse-led asthma education has been found to be helpful (75), we do not know exactly which aspects of this kind of intervention is most helpful and for which kinds of patients. Although we know that many patients would prefer once-daily therapy (76) to twice daily therapy, we do not know how changing to once-daily therapy affects compliance.

Future research on noncompliance needs to move away from a theoretical model where classification implies similarity. Although all asthmatic patients have the same disease, asthma, they are all psychologically different and these differences underlie differences in response to different kinds of management. There *is* no one single good method of managing noncompliance. The skilled physician uses a range of methods, appropriately selected for different patients, and research should build on this intuitive skill—which undoubtedly exists in all areas of good practice. Further research into asthma requires us to think of patients as people, people with free choice who have their own agendas on their own beliefs about their bodies. In conclusion, further research requires (1) a classification of different types and reasons for noncompliance and (2) an investigation into how different types of intervention affect those different types of people.

References

1. Hayes-Bautista DE. Modifying the treatment: patient compliance, patient control and medical care. Soc Sci Med 1976; 10:233–238.
2. Barofsky I. Compliance, adherence and the therapeutic alliance: steps in the development of self-care. Soc Sci Med 1978; 12:369–
3. Marinker M. Compliance is not all. Br Med J 1998; 316:150–151.
4. Weintraub M. Intelligent non-compliance with special emphasis on the elderly. Contemp Pharm Pract 1981; 4:8–11.
5. Dugdale A. Non-compliance or rational decision. Lancet 1993;342:1426–1427.
6. Rand CS, Wise RA. Adherence with asthma therapy in the management of asthma. In: Szefler SJ, Leung DYM, eds. Severe Asthma: Pathogenesis and Clinical Management. New York: Marcel Dekker, 1996:435–464.
7. Fryday M. Noncompliance rights. Nurs Stand 1997; 12:37–39.
8. Holm, S. What is wrong with compliance? J Med Ethics 1993; 19:108–110.
9. Coy JA. Autonomy-based informed consent: ethical implications for patient noncompliance. Phys Ther 1989; 69:826–833.
10. Lowe M, Kerridge IH, Mitchell KR. These sorts of people don't do very well: race and allocation of health care resources. J Med Ethics 1995; 21:356–360.
11. Johnsen AR. Ethical issues in compliance. In: Haynes RB, Taylor DW, Sackett DL,

eds. Compliance in Health Care. Baltimore: John Hopkins University Press, 1979:113–120.

12. Thompson J. Compliance. In R Fitzpatrick, J Hinton, S Newman, G Sambler J Thompson. The Experience of Illness. London: Tavistock, 1984: 109–131.
13. Kleiger JH, Dirks JF. Medication compliance in chronic asthmatic patients. J Asthma Res 1979; 16:93–96.
14. vanEs SM, LeCoq EM, Brouwer AI, Mesters I, Nagelkerke AF, Colland VT. Adherence-related behavior in adolescents with asthma: results from focus group interviews. J Asthma 1998; 35:637–646.
15. Osman LM. How do patients' views about medication affect their self-management plans in asthma? Patient Educ Counsel 1997; 32:S43–S49.
16. Coutts JAP, Gibson NA, Paton JY. Measuring compliance with inhaled medication in asthma. Arch Dis Child 1992; 67:332–333.
17. Milgrom H, Bender B, Ackerson L, Bowry P, Smith B, Rand C. Noncompliance and treatment failure in children with asthma. J Allergy Clin Immunol 1996; 98:1051–1057.
18. Rand CS, Wise RA, Nides M, Simmons MS, Bleecker ER, Kusek JW, Li VC, Tashkin DP. Metered-dose inhaler adherence in a clinical trial. Am Rev Resp Dis 1992; 146:1559–1564.
19. Yeung M, O'Connor SA, Parry DT, Cochrane GM. Compliance with prescribed drug-therapy in asthma. Respir Med 1994; 88:31–35.
20. Hyland ME, Kenyon CAP, Allen R, Howarth P. Diary keeping in asthma: comparison of written and electronic methods. Br Med J 1993; 306:487–489
21. Kelloway JS, Wyatt RA, Adlis SA. Comparison of patients' compliance with prescribed oral and inhaled asthma medications. Arch Intern Med 1994; *154:1349–1352.*
22. Steiner JF, Fihn SD, Blair B, Inut TS. Appropriate reductions in compliance among well-controlled hypertensive patients. J Clin Epidemiol 1991; 44:1361–1371.
23. Chmelik F, Doughty A. Objective measurements of compliance in asthma treatment. Ann Allergy 1994; 73:527–532.
24. Mawhinney H, Spector SL, Kinsman RA, Siegel SC, Rachelefsky GS, Katz RM, Rohr AS. Compliance in clinical trials of two nonbronchodilator, antiasthma medications. Ann Allergy 1991; 66:294–298.
25. Spector SL, Kinsman R, Mawhinney H, Siegel SC, Rachelefsky GS, Katz RM, Rohr AS. Compliance of patients with asthma with an experimental aerolized medication: Implications for controlled clinical trials. J Allergy Clin Immunol 1986; 77:65–70.
26. Bosley CM, Parry DT, Cochrane GM. Patient compliance with inhaled medication—does combining beta-agonists with corticosteroids improve compliance? Eur Respir J 1994; 7:504–509.
27. Apter AJ, Reisine ST, Affleck G, Barrows E, ZuWallack RL. Adherence with twice-daily dosing of inhaled steroids—socioeconomic and health-belief differences. Am J Respir Crit Care Med 1998; 157:1810–1817.
28. Sears M. Fatal asthma: a perspective. Immunol Allergy Proc 1988; 9:259–259.
29. Spitzer WO, Suissa S, Ernst P, Horwitz RI, Habbick B, Cockcroft D, Boivin J, McNutt M, Buist AS, Rebuck AS. The use of B-agonists and the risk of death and near death from asthma. N Engl J Med 1992; 326:501–506.

30. British Thoracic Society. Guidelines for the management of asthma in adults: 1. Chronic persistent asthma. Br Med J 1990; 301:651–653.
31. Cote J, Cartier A, Malo JL, Rouleau M, Boulet LP. Compliance with peak expiratory flow monitoring in home management of asthma. Chest 1998; 113:968–972.
32. Roter D, Hall J, Katz N. Patient-physician communication: a descriptive summary of the literature. Patient Educ Counsel 1988; 12:99–119.
33. Donelly JE, Donelly WJ, Thong YH. Parental perceptions and attitudes towards asthma and its treatment: a controlled study. Soc Sci Med 1987; 24:431–437.
34. DeBlaquiere P, Christensen DB, Carter WB, Martin TR. Use and misuse of metered-dose inhaler. Am Rev Respir Dis 1989; 140:910–916.
35. Hanania NA, Wittman R, Kesten S, Chapman KR. Medical personnel's knowledge of and ability to use inhaling devices: metered dose inhalers, spacing chambers, and breath-activated dry powder inhalers. Am Rev Respir Dis 1993; 147:SSA983.
36. Kelling JS, Strohl KP, Smith RL, Altose MD. Physician knowledge in use of canister nebulizers. Chest 1983; 83:612–614.
37. Mas JC, Resnick DJ, Firschein DE, Feldman BR, Davis WJ. Misuse of metered dose inhalers by house staff members. Am J Dis Child 1992; 146:783–785.
38. Chapman KR, Hanania NA, Kesten S. Medical personnel's knowledge of the ability to use inhaling devices. Chest 1995; 107:290.
39. Dompeling E, van Grunsven PM, van Schayck CP, Folgering H, Molema J, van Weel C. Treatment with inhaled steroids in asthma and chronic bronchitis: long term compliance and inhaler technique. Fam Pract 1992; 9:161–166.
40. Kendrick AH, Higgs CMB, Whitfield MJ, Laszlo G. Accuracy of perception of severity of asthma: patients treated in general practice. Br Med J 1993; 307:422–424.
41. Strunk RC. Identification of the fatality-prone subject with asthma. J Allergy Clin Immunol 1989; 83:477–485.
42. Zach, MS, Karner U. Sudden death in asthma. Arch Dis Child 1989; 64: 1446–1451.
43. Hyland ME, Ley A, Fisher DW, Woodward V. Measurement of psychological distress in asthma and asthma management programmes. Br J Clin Psychol 1995; 34:601–611.
44. van Zuuren FJ, Dooper R. Coping styule and self-reported health promotion and disease detection behaviour. Br J Health Psychol 1999; 4:810.
45. Osman LM, Russell IT, Friend JA, Legge JS, Douglas JG. Predicting patient attitudes to asthma medication. Thorax 1993; 48:827–830.
46. Osman LM. How do patients' view about medication affect their self-management in asthma? Patient Educ Counsel 1997, 32:S43–S49.
47. Kaptchuk TJR. Chinese Medicine. London: Rider, 1983.
48. Gerson S. Ayurveda. Rockport, MA: Element Books, 1993.
49. World Health Organization. The constitution of the World Health Organization. *WHO* Chronicle 1947; 1:29.
50. Hyland ME. A connectionist theory of asthma. Clin Exp Allergy 1999; 29:1467–1473.
51. Pachter LM. Culture and clinical care: folk illness beliefs and behaviors and their implications for health care delivery. JAMA 1994; 271:690–694.

52. Kinsman RA, Dirks JF, Dahlem NW. Noncompliance to prescribed as needed (PRN) medication use in asthma: usage patterns and patient characteristics. J Psychosom Res 1980; 24:97–107.
53. Sibbald B, White P, Pharoah C, Freeling P, Anderson HR. Relationship between psychosocial factors and asthma morbidity. Fam Pract 1988; 5:12–17.
54. Higgins Tory E. Self-discrepancy: a theory relating self and affect. Psychol Rev 1987; 94:319–340.
55. Adams S, Pill R, Jones A. Medication, chronic illness and identity: the perspective of people with asthma. Soc Sci Med 1997; 45:189–201.
56. Carver CS, Scheier MF, Weintraub JK. Assessing coping strategies: a theoretically based approach. J Personality Soc Psychol 1989; 56:267–283.
57. Lazarus RS Folkman S. Stress, Appraisal, and Coping. New York: Springer, 1984.
58. Gibson NA, Ferguson AE, Aitchison, TC, Paton JY. Compliance with inhaled asthma medication in preschool children. Thorax 1995; 50:1274–1279.
59. Wood PR, Casey R, Kolski GB, McCormick MC. Compliance with oral theophylline therapy in asthmatic children. Ann Allergy 1985; 54:400–404.
60. Sublett JL, Pollard SJ, Kadlec GJ, Karibo JM. Non-compliance in asthmatic children: a study of theophylline levels in pediatric emergency room population. Ann Allergy 1979; 43:95–97.
61. Birkhead G, Attaway NJ, Strunk RC, Towsend MC, Teutsch S. Investigation of a cluster of deaths of adolescents from asthma: evidence implicating inadequate treatment and poor patient adherence with medications. J Allergy Clin Immunol 1989; 84:484–491.
62. Fraser PM, Speizer FE, Waters SDM, Pole R, Mann MM. Circumstances preceding death from asthma in young people in 1968–69. Br Med J 1971; 65:71–84.
63. Donnelly JE, Donnelly W J, Thong YH. Inadequate parental understanding of asthma medications. Ann Allergy 1989; 62:337–341.
64. Rand CS, Butz AM, Huss K, Eggleston P, Thompson L, Malveaux F. Adherence with therapy and access to care: the relationship to excess asthma morbidity among African-American children. Pediatr Asthma Allergy Immunol 1994; 8:179–184.
65. Pachter LM, Weller SC. Acculturation and compliance with medical therapy. J Dev Behav Pediatr 1993; 14:163–168.
66. Butz AM, Malveaux FJ, Eggleston P, Thompson L, Schneider S, Weeks K, Huss K, Murigande C, Rand CS. Use of community health workers with inner-city children who have asthma. Clin Pediatr 1994; 33:135–141.
67. Christiaanse ME, Lavigne JV, Lerner CV. Psychosocial aspects of compliance in children and adolescents with asthma. J Dev Behav Pediatr 1989; 10:75–80.
68. Jay S, Litt IF, Durant RH. Compliance with therapeutic regimens. J Adolesc Health Care 1984; 5:124–136.
69. Varni JW, Wallander JL. Adherence to health-related regimens in pediatric chronic disorders. Clin Psychol Rev 1984; 4:585–596.
70. Winkelstein M, Huss K, Butz A, Eggleston P, Vargas PA, Rand C. Factors associated with medication self-administration in children with asthma. Clin Pediatr 2000. In press.
71. Roter DL, Hall JA. Physician's interviewing styles and medical information obtained from patients. J Gen Intern Med 1987; 2:325–329.

72. Steele DJ, Jackson TC, Gutmann MC Have you been taking your pill? The adherence-monitoring sequence in the medical interview. J Fam Pract 1990; 30:294–299.
73. Francis V, Korsch BM, Morris MJ. Gaps in doctor-patient communications. N Engl J Med 1969; 280:535–540.
74. Mushlin AI, Appel FA. Diagnosing potential non-compliance: physician's ability in a behavioral dimension of medical care. Arch Intern Med 1977; 137:318–321.
75. Madge P, McColl J, Paton J. Impact of a nurse-led home management training programme in children admitted to hospital with acute asthma: a randomised controlled study. Thorax 1997; 52:223–228.
76. Venables TL, Addlestone MB, Smithers AJ, Blagden MD, Weston D, Gooding T, Carr EP, Follows RMA. A comparison of the efficacy and patient acceptability of once daily budesonide via Turbohaler and twice daily fluticasone propionate via a disc-inhaler at an equal dose of 400 mcg in adult asthmatics. Br J Clin Res 1996; 7:15–32.

INDEX

A

B

C

D

G

H

I

J

M

N

O

P

Q

R

S

T

U

V

W

X

Y

Z

SUBJECT INDEX

A

B

C

D

E

F

G

H

N

O

P

R

S

T

U

V

Y

Milton Keynes UK
Ingram Content Group UK Ltd.
UKHW020006071024
449327UK00031B/2680